Behavioral Endocrinology

Behavioral Endocrinology

Second Edition

edited by Jill B. Becker, S. Marc Breedlove, David Crews, and Margaret M. McCarthy

A Bradford Book
The MIT Press
Cambridge, Massachusetts
London, England

This book was set in Melior and Helvetica on 3B2 by Asco Typesetters, Hong Kong and was printed and bound in the United States of America.

Library of Congress Cataloging-in-Publication Data

Behavioral endocrinology / edited by Jill B. Becker ... [et al.]. — 2nd ed.
   p. ; cm.
 "A Bradford book."
 Includes bibliographical references and index.
 ISBN 0-262-02511-6 (hc : alk. paper)
 1. Psychoneuroendocrinology. I. Becker, Jill B.
 [DNLM: 1. Behavior—drug effects. 2. Hormones—metabolism. 3. Psychophysiology.
WK 102 B419 2002]
QP356.45 .B444 2002
152—dc21   2001056208

Contents in Brief

Contents in Detail

Preface to the Second Edition

Welcome to the second edition of *Behavioral Endocrinology*. It's hard to believe that it has been ten years since we edited the first edition. A lot has happened. Human and mouse genomes have been cloned and there is great excitement about molecular approaches to the study of brain and behavior. We share this enthusiasm for molecular approaches, and yet remain convinced that the study of the ultimate causes of behavior are among the most important and fascinating questions a scientist can investigate. On the other hand, we believe that in the field of behavioral endocrinology the application of knowledge about the relations between gene function and behavior will yield important results in the next few years. With that in mind, Margaret M. McCarthy, an expert in the application of molecular techniques to the study of behavior, has joined us as a co-editor for this new edition.

But we are getting ahead of ourselves. As students, you are probably wondering what behavioral endocrinology is all about. So let's begin at the beginning. All of us understand the importance of behavior—it is the fabric of society. Endocrinology is the study of hormones, the chemical messengers that travel through the bloodstream to transmit information from one part of the body to another. The brain is often either a source or a target of these messengers, and because behaviors originate from brain activity, hormones often have a powerful effect on behavior. During the past sixty years or so, the field of behavioral endocrinology has arisen to study how hormones alter behavior and also how behavior affects hormone release.

Why should anyone take a course in behavioral endocrinology? Many people in our society already believe that hormones can affect our moods and behavior. It is widely accepted that some athletes taking anabolic steroids can become dangerously aggressive, that some women experience intense mood shifts during parts of their menstrual cycle, and that men and women are biologically destined to differ in mathematical and other intellectual abilities. There are also strongly held but quite divergent opinions about whether people are "born with" a homosexual orientation, whether hormones force men to be promiscuous, and whether the mental abilities of women are affected by their menstrual cycle, as well as about the extent to which males and females differ and are similar.

Although many of our social policies and attitudes are built upon these opinions, remarkably little solid information is available to evaluate most of them. However, we do have some information, some hints about what is going on, and scientific research reveals important issues and complications in all these questions, which we can use to temper our judgments and decisions. We are not suggesting that instruction in behavioral endocrinology should be required of all students, just that the questions addressed in such a course are relevant to all our lives.

Psychologists and neuroscientists have long been interested in how thoughts, memories, and behavior patterns are physically represented in the nervous system. These are very challenging questions that will not be fully answered for a long time. The only practical approach to the study of these questions is to compare individuals who display a particular behavior to individuals who do not display that behavior. If the nervous system of one group has a different structure or physiological response than the nervous system of the other group, then that difference may be responsible for the differences in the behavior.

Hormones are excellent candidates as causes of such differences: If animals treated with a hormone act differently from animals not treated with that hormone, then we can examine where the hormone goes in an animal's body and what the hormone does there, keeping a special lookout for effects on the nervous system. If we track down the answers to these two questions with enough ingenuity and care, we will eventually discover the changes in the structure or function of the nervous system that caused the change in behavior. As we will see, scientists have made considerable progress in answering these questions for simple behaviors in animals. By building upon this knowledge, we should one day understand the factors affecting more complicated human behaviors.

Biologists have long recognized that hormones can have profound influences on the physiology of animals. But sometimes overlooked are the effects these same hormones can have on behavior and the effects of the behavioral experience of the animals on hormone release. Also, because males and females produce different hormones, it is important for biologists to be aware of how these different hormones may affect their anatomical and/or physiological measures. Furthermore, many stressful experiences, including some found in the laboratory, can cause the release of hormones that will affect most physiological processes. Even nonstressful experiences, such as exposure to an animal of the opposite sex, can affect hormone release. Finally, because hormones are released in particular patterns across the day, a drug or manipulation that has one effect on an animal in the morning may have no effect (or an opposite effect) in the late afternoon. Only by learning how hormones affect behavior and how behavior affects hormones can biologists remain alert for such complications.

Because we believe these issues are important and interesting, we have tried to create a textbook on behavioral endocrinology for undergraduates who have had little previous exposure to physiology. Our aim is to reach students who have taken an introductory survey course in biology or in physiological psychology. This book will allow those students to learn in some detail what hormones are, how they affect cells, and how such effects can alter the behavior of animals. We assume that the reader will need a bit of a refresher course and have therefore written an introductory chapter that covers this basic material. That means that the first chapter is longer than is traditional for textbooks these days. However, much of that chapter will be familiar to all students, although most students will find some material that is new to them. Furthermore, nearly all the topics in chapter 1 will resurface later and will be dealt with in more detail in subsequent chapters.

For the second edition, we have added a second introductory chapter to review some of the techniques used in molecular biology that have become standard tools of the trade. We think that these two chapters will help you with the rest of the book, especially when you read some of the primary research articles that discuss the use of these methods.

As teachers, we used the first edition to teach undergraduate and graduate level courses, and also used it as a reference source. In the second edition, to make the information more accessible to scientists using this book as a reference source we have adopted the scientific style of reference citation within the text, and references appear at the end of each chapter (instead of being compiled at the end of the entire book). We hope this is not too disruptive to students.

Every textbook reflects the strengths and interests of its authors, and in the present case, three such themes are apparent. First of all, we felt it was important to address the question of whether hormones also alter the behavior of that most fascinating and troublesome animal species, humans. Because the data for humans are, in almost all respects, less conclusive and more conflicting than that for animal research, we believe it is important to review it with an open yet critical mind. Some students will be uncomfortable with the ambiguity inherent in such a careful discussion, but we believe that in reviewing the human data, it is important that our conclusions be thorough and cautious. More research is needed to determine how many hormones affect behavior in humans. However, only by accurately and objectively representing what is currently known can we hope to ask the important questions in future research.

Second, we wanted to produce a text that considered more than just rats, mice, and humans, despite the fact that the vast majority of studies focus on these three species. As Frank Beach, one of the founders of behavioral endocrinology, has stated, an appreciation of the variety of ways different species solve life's problems (mate selection, copulation, and food gathering, among others) has importance for understanding both the general and the special ways in which hormones and behavior are interrelated. Thus, we will discuss the effects of hormones on the behavior of frogs, snakes, lizards, birds, fish, and insects. Because rats are far and away the most studied species, we still talk about them a great deal, but we hope to stir interest in other organisms as well.

Finally, we decided to present a broad continuum of levels of analysis, from the molecular to the evolutionary. We will discuss in some detail the ways genes work, the structure of cells, the interactions of endocrine organs, the behavior of individuals, the structure of social hierarchies, and the evolution of mating systems. There are very few other fields of study in which one could even attempt such integration.

For some of us, this diversity of approach is another attraction of behavioral endocrinology as a field of study. Because of the diversity of expertise this approach represents, however, we have asked experts in each field of research to write chapters for this book. We hope readers find that each author's enthusiasm for his or her research comes through and gives you a feeling for the excitement of research in behavioral endocrinology. So get started, think hard, have fun, and let us know what you think about this text and this field.

Contributors

Michael J. Baum
Department of Biology
Boston University
Boston, Massachusetts

Jill B. Becker
Department of Psychology
University of Michigan
Ann Arbor, Michigan

S. Marc Breedlove
Program in Neuroscience
Michigan State University
Berkeley, California

Eliot A. Brenowitz
Department of Psychology
University of Washington
Seattle, Washington

C. Sue Carter
Department of Psychiatry
University of Illinois at Chicago
Chicago, Illinois

Christopher L. Coe
Department of Psychology
University of Wisconsin
Madison, Wisconsin

David Crews
Departments of Zoology and Psychology
University of Texas at Austin
Austin, Texas

Michael R. Gorman
Department of Psychology
University of California, San Diego
San Diego, California

Elizabeth Hampson
Department of Psychology
University of Western Ontario
London, Ontario, Canada

Thomas R. Insel   Department of Psychiatry
Emory University School of Medicine
Atlanta, Georgia

Darcy B. Kelley   Department of Biological Sciences
Columbia University
New York, New York

Lance J. Kriegsfeld   Department of Psychology
Columbia University
New York, New York

Theresa M. Lee   Department of Psychology
University of Michigan
Ann Arbor, Michigan

Margaret M. McCarthy   Department of Physiology
University of Maryland School of Medicine
College Park, Maryland

Robert M. Sapolsky   Department of Biological Sciences
Stanford University
Stanford, California

Rae Silver   Department of Psychology
Barnard College and
Department of Anatomy and Cell Biology
Columbia University College of Physicians and Surgeons
New York, New York

James W. Truman   Department of Zoology
University of Washington
Seattle, Washington

Christina L. Williams   Department of Psychological and Brain Sciences
Duke University
Durham, North Carolina

Larry J. Young   Department of Psychiatry
Emory University School of Medicine
Atlanta, Georgia

I   Introduction

1 Introduction to Behavioral Endocrinology

Jill B. Becker and S. Marc Breedlove

In this first chapter we review the basic principles of how hormones and the nervous system work. That means that this information will be packed rather densely. But students should have been exposed to most of the information before, and virtually all of these topics will be dealt with in specific examples in later chapters. This chapter is intended to be used as a reminder and a reference source for the basic concepts needed to appreciate the information given in the chapters that follow.

Some of the questions you should focus on while reading this chapter include: What are hormones, what are the different kinds of hormones, and how do they change biological processes? How does the brain control hormones, and how do hormones affect the brain? How do we measure behavior and hormones?

The Study of Behavioral Endocrinology

Behavioral endocrinology is the study of how hormones influence an animal's behavior. A. A. Berthold is credited with conducting the first formal experiments in behavioral endocrinology in 1849. We have learned a great deal since Berthold's time, but the basic logic and experimental design used for demonstrating a causal relationship between hormones and behavior is the same now as it was then.

Berthold removed the testes of a rooster and observed the animal's behavior. He found that the rooster no longer crowed or engaged in sexual or aggressive behavior. When Berthold reimplanted one testis in the body cavity, the castrated rooster once again began crowing and also exhibited normal sexual behavior and aggression. The reimplanted testis did not reestablish nerve connections, so Berthold concluded that some chemical, produced by the testes and released into the general circulatory system, influenced the rooster's behavior.

We now know that the effect produced by the grafted testis can be mimicked by administering the hormone **testosterone** to a castrated rooster. Testosterone is the main hormone synthesized and released by the testes of male vertebrates. A causal relationship between the presence of a certain hormone (testosterone) in the circulatory system and behavior (crowing, sexual behavior, aggressive behavior) is established by conducting experiments to show that when the hormone is present, certain behaviors are more likely to occur.

The same kinds of experiments are conducted in behavioral endocrinology today. In order to show that a particular hormone influences a particular behavior, the scientist must demonstrate that the frequency of the behavior changes when the endocrine gland producing the hormone is removed. Then the scientist must show that the frequency of the behavior can be returned to normal by providing the animal with the missing hormone.

Berthold's experiment also shows that the study of behavioral endocrinology is the study of two related systems. First, we must learn about the endocrine system, represented by the testes in this case. Of course, neither the testes nor the testosterone these glands released into the bloodstream completely determined the rooster's behavior. Other factors such as the time of day and the presence of a hen or a rival rooster also made a difference. But the testosterone released from the testes reached the brain. There the hormone acted on nerve cells (neurons) in various brain regions and changed the likelihood that those behaviors would appear under the appropriate circumstances. Therefore, to understand how the hormone influenced behavior, we must study a second system, the nervous system.

Inherent in our discussion of how hormones can influence an animal's behavior is the idea that if hormones produce a change in an animal's behavior, there has been some sort of change in the animal, probably in its brain. We can try to find out which parts of the brain have been changed, how they have been changed, and how those modifications have caused an alteration in behavior. Conversely, if hormones cause alterations in the brain, there should be a corresponding change in the behavior or the physiology of the animal that we may be clever enough to detect.

Behavioral Methods: Field versus Laboratory Studies
Experiments in behavioral endocrinology obviously require the assessment and measurement of behavior. Most people assume that this is the easy part: Sit and watch. However, there are many ways to measure behavior, including ways that may not be valuable. To discuss the issues involved in methodology, we must first consider two very different types of research—laboratory and field. Surely the best way to understand behavioral endocrinology is to observe the creatures of interest in their normal habitat: deer in the woods, mice in the fields, and monkeys in the jungle. But research in the field is a great challenge. Conditions are not very comfortable for humans. Many important variables are beyond inspection or control. Unexpected turns of events are common. Therefore, it is difficult to observe the exact same phenomena twice. Consequently, two researchers trying to study the same things may observe and report very different field results. The difficult task of field researchers is to achieve consistent, repeatable results. Only then can they feel confident that they understand the phenomena.

The consistency field researchers strive for is, in fact, the great advantage of laboratory research because the investigator in the laboratory can control many variables and keep them constant. Temperature, humidity, food and water availability, and even, in some cases, the genetic make-up of the subjects, can all be controlled. If laboratory rats of strain X are kept in conditions

Y and given hormone Z, then they should display the same behaviors each time, and to a great extent they do. As will become obvious at various places in this book, however, there are plenty of individual differences even in a laboratory setting. But as more and more conditions are standardized to achieve consistency in laboratory results, you run a risk that what you are learning is applicable only to the laboratory.

This demonstrates an important strength of field research—validity. If you do learn something in the laboratory and can repeat this observation in the field, you know it is valid for the world-as-it-is. Ideally, laboratory workers read the field reports to help them judge which phenomena may be relevant outside the laboratory and therefore valid. In turn, if field researchers suspect, for example, that hormones are affecting a particular behavior, they may try to test that notion under the more controlled conditions of the laboratory.

To obtain results in the laboratory that approximate conditions in the field, the scientist must approach the experimental question from the perspective of the animal. If your subject is a rat, you need to "think like a rat." In other words, you should design your behavioral tests to take advantage of the normal behavior of the animal in the wild. I. Q. Whishaw et al. described in exacting detail the methods that can be used to analyze the behavior of a laboratory rat. Some of these ideas are summarized in table 1.1.

This approach can be applied to the study of other species in the laboratory. The exact details of the behavioral tests will vary with the species, but the methods used to observe, analyze, and challenge the neurological functions of an animal can be generalized to any species. These authors argue that with the careful observation and description of an animal's appearance and behavior, "meaningful generalizations about the organization of the nervous system [can] later be made" (Whishaw, Kolb, and Sutherland 1983). This is also true for the behavioral endocrinologist who wants to make meaningful generalizations about the influence of hormones on the nervous system.

Experimental Design

The challenge of obtaining meaningful behavioral results in the laboratory can also be addressed by careful construction of the experimental procedures. There are a number of important things to consider when designing an experiment. For example, let's say that you have decided to investigate the effect of estrogen on sexual behavior in female rats. What groups will you compare? In order to control circulating estrogens in your animals, you may want to begin with animals that have had their own source of estrogen (the ovaries) removed (i.e., **ovariectomized** animals).

One way to test the effect of estrogen on sexual behavior in these ovariectomized rats would be to test all the animals first without estrogen. Then you could give the animals estrogen and repeat the behavioral test (this is known as a sequential design, repeated measures, or a within-animal comparison). One thing you need to be aware of, however, is that sometimes experimental procedures themselves can change an animal's behavior. For example,

Table 1.1 Behavioral Assessment of Neurological Function in Animals: Summary of Features of Behavior and Appearance That Can Be Examined

MEASURE	SPECIFIC FEATURE
Appearance	Body weight, core body temperature, eyes, feces, condition, genitals, muscle tone, pupils, responsiveness, saliva, teeth, toenails, vocalizations
Sensory and sensorimotor behavior	Response to auditory, olfactory, somatosensory, taste, vestibular, and visual stimuli presented both in home cage and open field
Posture and immobility	Behavior when spontaneously immobile; posture and muscle tone when immobile; tonic immobility or animal hypnosis; environmental influences on immobility
Movement	General activity, movement initiation, turning, climbing, walking, swimming, righting responses, limb movements, mouth and tongue movements
Species-typical behaviors	All species-typical behaviors including grooming, food hoarding, foraging, taste aversion, sleep, maternal behavior, sexual behavior, play, nest building, and burying
Learning	Classical conditioning, instrumental conditioning, and learning sets, especially including measures of spatial learning, avoidance learning, and conditioned taste aversion

From Whishaw et al. 1983.

perhaps the experience of the first test would affect performance in the second test regardless of hormone treatment. So it is important to run a control group that is tested a second time without receiving the hormone.

Another way to conduct the experiment is to use a simultaneous design (between-animal comparison). With this experimental design, each ovariectomized rat would be tested only once. One group would receive the hormone treatment—say, estrogen dissolved in peanut oil—while the control group would receive injections of the peanut oil vehicle without the estrogen. The behavior of the two groups of animals during the test would then be compared to see if the hormone has affected the behavior.

The advantage of the sequential design is that usually fewer animals are needed. The behavior of each animal during the two tests can be compared, and this tends to reduce variability in the data. On the other hand, if your procedures are causing changes in the animals' behavior for reasons other than the hormone treatment, a simultaneous design may be the best way to test your hypothesis. There are more complex experimental designs, but they are essentially variations and combinations of these two basic protocols.

Behavioral Observations

Next, you must decide how you will define and quantify the behavior. You must also choose your testing environment and procedures. Most behavioral

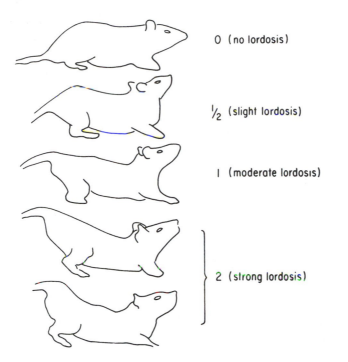

0 (no lordosis)

½ (slight lordosis)

1 (moderate lordosis)

2 (strong lordosis)

Figure 1.1 Lordosis in the female rat. These drawing were traced from single frames of films of rat mating encounters. Note the arching of the back with the elevation of the head and rump. (From Brink et al., 1978.)

experiments involve procedures that require an observer to make decisions about the animals' behavior. For example, before she is mounted by a male, a female rat exhibits a number of behaviors that have been termed "proceptive" behaviors: She will hop and dart and display ear wiggling in response to a male. You must decide if you are going to record these behaviors; if so, you must define them so that they are always scored in the same way. When a male rat mounts a receptive female rat, she will arch her back (head and rump are elevated) and deflect her tail to one side. This is a reflexive behavior known as **lordosis** which permits the male to achieve intromission (i.e., place his penis in her vagina). You must also decide how to quantify this behavior. You could count the number of times the rat displays lordosis in proportion to the number of mounts, measure the amount of time the rat is in lordosis, judge the completeness of the lordosis (figure 1.1), or make-up some combination of these. For each behavior you must come up with a written definition that you and the other observers agree on.

Because behavioral observation often requires making subtle judgments, it is also important that the observer be unaware of the specific treatment that an animal has received (this is known as being "blind" to the experimental conditions). This is usually achieved by coding the animals or treatments to hide their identity from the observer in order to prevent the observer's expectations from coloring his or her judgment. It is also a good idea to have more than one observer score the behavior to test the reliability of the data across observers. In other words, do both observers score the behavior in the same way? This knowledge is important for several reasons. First, you want to be sure that the data have internal consistency, i.e., that all animals were scored in the same way. Second, you want to be sure that your definitions are precise enough to allow two observers using these definitions to obtain the same results. If so, then other investigators will be able to repeat your methods and replicate your results.

Other Considerations

Other things that need to be considered include when to make your behavioral observations and what dose or treatment regimen to use for the hormone administration. When in doubt, it is best to be guided by endogenous, physiological concentrations of the hormone (if they are known) and by what is already known about the temporal relations between the endogenous hormone fluctuations and the behavior under consideration.

When considering the dose, some investigators might be tempted to begin with high doses of a hormone just to be sure that they see an effect. Results from high doses, however, can be very misleading. A bell-shaped curve showing the relationship between a hormone and a behavior is frequently found in behavioral endocrinology. This means that within a physiological range of doses, the higher the dose, the more effective the hormone at producing a change in a behavior. On the other hand, higher doses of the hormone might have no effect or even an opposite effect on the behavior.

Alternatively, when a behavior is altered *only* by a large dose, it is possible that the extremely high dose has made the animal sick or disoriented and thereby has had a crude effect on behavior that is unrelated to the normal actions of the hormone. This latter concern is especially important when a large dose of a drug or hormone *decreases* a behavior, because the animal may display the behavior only when it is feeling comfortable and relaxed. Similarly, you must always be concerned when a treatment alters behavior in the same way that general stress might alter it; perhaps the treatment distressed the animal and thereby changed the behavior, which reflects nothing about the normal influence of that hormone on that behavior.

There are many ways to administer hormones. Steroid hormones are not very soluble in water, so they are usually dissolved in oil and injected just under the skin (subcutaneously). Another way to administer hormones is to pack solid hormone into a piece of silicone rubber (the brand name is Silastic) tubing and seal the ends. This Silastic implant is placed under the animal's skin. The hormone will slowly diffuse out of the tubing. By varying the thickness and length of the tubing, the amount of hormone to be delivered and the duration of hormone delivery can be adjusted. This method has the advantage that a hormone can be delivered for long periods of time without the repeated stress of frequent injections. The disadvantages are that you do not always know how much hormone you are delivering, and, as we will learn, endogenous hormones are not released in such a constant fashion.

It may be desirable in some experiments to deliver hormone directly to specific areas of the brain in order to localize the brain area mediating a particular behavior. In order to do this, a small cannula (a hollow piece of stainless steel tubing) is tamped full of hormone at one end. The end of the cannula containing the hormone is then introduced into an animal's brain in a specific location. If the behavior is changed by this local application of hormone, you need to make sure that the effect is specific to the hormone and that it acted in that particular area of the brain. Maybe the cannula damaged the brain, causing the observed effect, or perhaps the hormone diffused to another area of the brain a few millimeters away. Therefore, to be sure of your result, you need to find out if cannulae containing control hormones (i.e., biologically inactive versions of the same hormone) and cannulae containing the active hormone placed in other brain regions produce the same effect.

Thus, the study of hormones and behavior in the laboratory requires a design that will accurately measure and evaluate the effect of experimental manipulation on the behavior. In order to produce results that can be generalized to animals outside the laboratory, it is a good idea to use behavioral tests that reflect naturally occurring behaviors and hormone treatments that closely approximate endogenous hormone secretions.

Relating Behavior to Brain: Highlights of Chapters to Follow

Using procedures such as these and others, scientists have investigated how hormones affect behavior, and that is the topic of this book. Investigators have studied the way hormones affect neuronal function as well as how the brain is organized. For example, we know that specific areas of the brain are responsible for sexual behavior and that the areas of the brain important for sexual behavior are different for males and females. In chapter 3 you will learn how the hormones produced by the fetus are responsible for the sexual differentiation of the brain. In fact, some hormones determine whether certain neurons live or die (chapters 3 and 11). You will learn how this exciting field of research has demonstrated that sex differences in both reproductive behavior and brain morphology are determined by the hormonal milieu in which neurons develop.

In the second section of the book, the consequences of hormonal influences on brain development for sexual behavior, courtship, and parental behavior will be explored in greater detail. In chapter 4 you will learn about the intricate hormonal cycle that coordinates the simultaneous production of eggs with the onset of sexually receptive behavior in many female mammals. You will also learn that more than one strategy has evolved to maximize the possibility that fertilization of the egg will take place. In chapter 5 you will learn, among other things, how scientists have been able to determine that different areas of the brain are important for sexual arousal and sexual motivation in males. Then, in chapter 6, you will be asked to consider how the data from nonhuman animals relates to what we know about hormonal influences on sexual behavior in humans.

In chapter 7 you will learn more about the diversity of hormone-behavior relations that have evolved in various species. You will see that even though the hormone-behavior relations may appear to be very different, the same neuroendocrine systems are involved in controlling reproductive behaviors. In some species getting together in order to reproduce is more challenging than for others. These species have evolved elaborate courtship behaviors. Frogs, birds, and fish have evolved different mechanisms to convey to members of their own species information about their reproductive status and fitness. Hormonal influences on sensory receptors, muscle development, and the electrical activity and morphology of neurons in the brain all play a role in ensuring that males and females of a species find and select their mates. But there is a rich diversity among species in where and when hormones produce their effects. Part II concludes with a discussion in chapter 9 of how the hormones of pregnancy also facilitate the initiation of parental behavior. Since the main goal of reproduction is to produce viable young, parental behavior is an additional way that hormones act in the brain to ensure survival of a species.

In Part III you will examine the interactions among hormones and regulatory functions. For example, you will learn in chapter 10 that the immune system is quite sensitive to neuroendocrine signals. Conversely, chronic stress has a profound impact on the secretion of hormones by the adrenal gland, and in chapter 11 you will learn that these hormones can have dire consequences for an animal, affecting energy availability, growth, reproduction, and the immune system. Then, in chapter 12, you will learn how endogenous biological rhythms coordinate the many endocrine systems, serving as one of the major organizing forces for hormone-behavior relations.

In Part IV you will learn that hormones can act on specific areas of the brain to affect sensorimotor and cognitive function. Basic studies, described in chapters 13 and 14, have investigated some of the possible underlying neural processes involved in these functions for nonhuman animals, and correlative experiments, discussed in chapter 15, have suggested that hormones have similar effects on cognitive function in humans.

In the final part of the book, you will learn how intimately hormone-behavior relations are related. Even though hormones have profound effects on brain and behavior, the environment in which an animal lives and the behavior it engages in impact its hormones. All in all, it is a delicate and fascinating arrangement wherein our hormones and our day-to-day experiences interact—hormones influencing behavior and behavior influencing hormones. For example, in chapter 16 you will learn that hormones can affect eating and drinking and that these behaviors affect the secretion of many hormones. Chapter 17 describes the research on invertebrate systems that has demonstrated the ways in which various behaviors triggered by different hormones interact to ensure successful metamorphosis. We will see many examples of the ways in which secreted hormones alter behavior, but conversely, exposure to stimuli and even the execution of behavior itself can affect hormonal secretions in turn. Chapter 18 describes many of the various ways in which behavior and experience can affect hormones. Input from each of our senses affects our neuroendocrine systems and serve to coordinate neuroendocrinology and behavior.

Each chapter in this book describes what is known about how hormones affect behavior and the underlying neural mechanisms mediating these hormone-behavior relations. This means that in addition to understanding how behavior is studied, we must also have a basic understanding of both the nervous system and the endocrine system. In every chapter, whenever possible, we have included some of the latest information from modern molecular biology. In chapter 2 we will spend some time telling you about those methods. But first, let's review the basics.

Basic Concepts in Cell Biology

Experiments similar to those performed by Berthold are still conducted today to establish hormone-behavior relations. Of course, today's behavioral endocrinologist can investigate the underlying neural mechanisms mediating hormone-behavior relations, the subcellular events that occur in response to hormones, and even the molecular biology of those subcellular responses. Therefore, today's student of behavioral endocrinology must become familiar with the basic mechanisms of neural and cellular function to understand hormone-brain interactions.

Before we discuss how and where hormones act in the brain to influence various components of an animal's behavior, we will first review some basic facts and principles of biology, endocrinology, and biopsychology. As mentioned earlier, these ideas will be important for an understanding of the topics to be discussed later in the book. This discussion is not intended to be a comprehensive review or "everything you ever wanted to know" about the brain and endocrine systems. Instead, it is a brief review of some basic ideas, which can be referred to when reading the rest of the book if questions arise. For more details and further explanations of the subject material, additional readings are suggested at the end of this chapter.

The Biology of Eucaryotic Cells

All complex biological organisms are made up of individual eucaryotic cells that contain a spherical-shaped nucleus, in which the genetic material for the organism is stored, and a surrounding cytoplasm, which contains many subcellular organelles that perform diverse functions. While the number of cells in an organism and the complexity of relations between cells varies considerably across species, most of the cellular processes that eucaryotic cells carry out are found in all species. In particular, the ways in which genes store or encode the information needed to produce an organism is a fascinating story that seems to change little across species from worms and flies to people. The modern behavioral endocrinologist takes advantage of the principles and methods of the genetic code and its regulation when asking questions about hormones and behavior. Because many chapters in this book discuss the effects of hormones that produce their effects by activating specific genes, a brief overview of how the instructions contained in the genome are carried out will help you understand how hormones produce their effects.

THE GENETIC CODE

The genetic information for each cell is stored in fiberlike structures called chromosomes. The chromosomes are actually long, twisted molecules of **deoxyribonucleic acid** (or **DNA**) that remain in the cell's nucleus. DNA is composed of four different molecules called **nucleotides** (because they were originally isolated from cell nuclei). The nucleotides form a long chain with a sugar (deoxyribose), linking them together. Two of these DNA chains wind around each other in the famous double helix. DNA codes for the sequence of amino acids that go into individual proteins. Some of these proteins are packaged by the cell for export; others are enzymes that allow the cell to make other molecules or perform certain functions. Amazing as it may seem, all genetic instructions come down to which particular proteins are to be made in different cells at different times.

A particular piece of DNA that contains the instructions for making a protein is known as a gene. In order for DNA to produce a protein, the gene must first be **transcribed** (figure 1.2). During this process of transcription, a single strand of DNA serves as a template for the assembly of a string of nucleotides forming **ribonucleic acid (RNA)**. Each of the four different DNA nucleotides have a tendency to pair with only one particular RNA nucleotide. There are, therefore, four different RNA nucleotides, each complementary to a DNA nucleotide. The newly transcribed string of RNA nucleotides forms a molecule known variously as the "message," the "transcript," or the messenger RNA (**mRNA**).

Since each DNA nucleotide is transcribed as a specific RNA nucleotide, the code for an amino acid sequence is now contained within the series of RNA nucleotides. The mRNA leaves the nucleus for the cytoplasm, where protein synthesis occurs when the genetic instructions encoded in the mRNA transcript are **translated** into a chain of amino acids. A series of three nucleotides constitutes the name (also referred to as the **codon**, or code) for which of the 20 or so different amino acids will be added to the chain. A long series of such triplets codes for a long series of amino acids, and that is what constitutes a protein. This flow of information from the gene to a protein is the foundation upon which modern molecular biology is built (figure 1.2).

SUBCELLULAR ORGANELLES

Outside the nucleus but within the cytoplasm of the cell are a number of subcellular organelles that serve different specific functions. For example, **mitochondria** provide energy to the cell. **Ribosomes** (themselves made up of special ribosomal RNA) are the site of protein synthesis, i.e., translation. The **endoplasmic reticulum** (literally, a network of membranes) and **Golgi appa-**

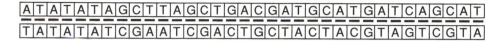

1. DOUBLE STRANDED DNA

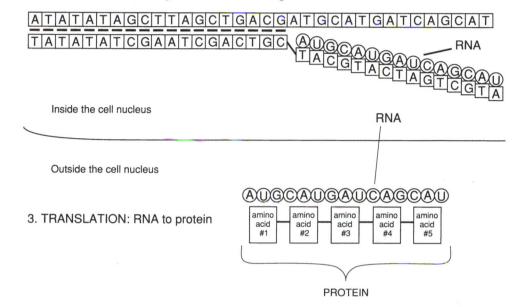

2. TRANSCRIPTION: single strand DNA to single strand RNA

Inside the cell nucleus

Outside the cell nucleus

3. TRANSLATION: RNA to protein

PROTEIN

Figure 1.2 The four nucleotides that make up each DNA molecule (adenine, thymine, guanine, and cytosine) are represented schematically in this figure by boxes with the letters A, T, G, and C, respectively. The four nucleotides in RNA (adenine, uracil, guanine, and cytosine) are represented by circles with the four letters A, U, G, and C.
1. In forming the double-stranded DNA molecule, each nucleotide is always paired with only one of the other base pairs: C with G, T with A. Normally the two strands are tightly twisted around each other in a "double helix."
2. In order for transcription to occur, the two strands of the DNA molecule must first unwind. The single strands of DNA can then serve as templates for synthesis of single strands of RNA. Each of the four DNA nucleotides always codes for only one of the four RNA nucleotides (C for G, G for C, T for A, and A for U). The newly synthesized RNA can then leave the nucleus.
3. Translation of the sequence of amino acids to make up a protein occurs outside the nucleus. Each series of three RNA nucleotides is the code for one particular amino acid to be added to the chain. A short series of amino acids is called a peptide; a long series of amino acids is a protein.

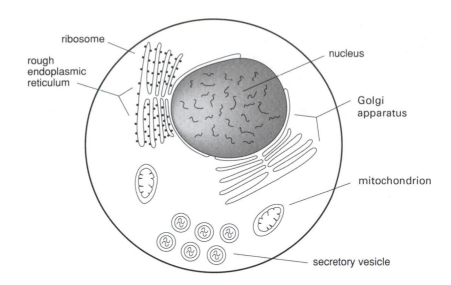

Figure 1.3 Schematic drawing of some of the subcellular organelles found in eucaryotic cells. The genetic material (large strands of DNA coiled into chromosomes) is sequestered within the nucleus of the cell (depicted as fibers within the nucleus). Protein synthesis occurs on the ribosomes in the rough endoplasmic reticulum. Additional processing takes place in the Golgi apparatus where proteins that were synthesized for export are sequestered in secretory vesicles. Mitochondria provide energy for cellular metabolism.

ratus assist with protein synthesis and transport within the cell. Proteins that are destined for secretion from the cell or insertion into the cell's own membrane are synthesized on ribosomes found within the endoplasmic reticulum. Together, the ribosomes and endoplasmic reticulum are referred to as the **rough endoplasmic reticulum** because in electron micrographs the ribosomes appear as bumps on the membranes of the endoplasmic reticulum. This is illustrated schematically in figure 1.3.

THE SECRETORY PROCESS

All cells in an organism engage in protein synthesis. However, some cells use proteins or other chemicals produced by enzymes (which are themselves proteins) for communication between cells. We will be interested in three different types of these intercellular chemical messengers: (1) **hormones**, produced by endocrine cells and released into the circulatory system, (2) **neurotransmitters**, produced by neurons and released at the synapse, and (3) **neurohormones**, produced by specialized neurons known as neurosecretory cells. The three types of chemical messengers differ in where they are produced, where they are released, and the distance the chemical has to travel to produce an effect. These methods of communication differ, therefore, in the speed of the message and the type of information they convey. Nevertheless, cells using these different methods produce, package, and secrete their different chemical messengers in much the same way. With this idea in mind,

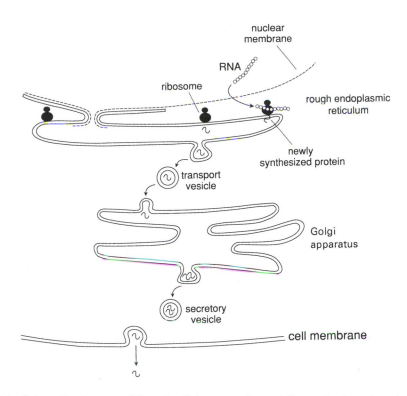

Figure 1.4 Schematic close-up of the subcellular organelles and the synthesis and packaging of protein into secretory vesicles for release by exocytosis. mRNA leaves the nucleus and protein synthesis occurs on the ribosomes in the rough endoplasmic reticulum. Newly synthesized proteins undergo additional processing in the rough endoplasmic reticulum and are then transported to the smooth endoplasmic reticulum where they are packaged into secretory vesicles for release by exocytosis. The movement of the protein from where it is synthesized, to where it is packaged, and then released by exocytosis is indicated by the arrows.

we shall examine the mechanisms involved in a generic model of the secretory process in all cells.

The general model for the secretory process is based on the now-classic work of George Palade. Investigating the synthesis and secretion of proteins by the pancreas, Palade followed the fate of the radioactively labeled amino acids as they were incorporated into newly synthesized proteins. He determined that amino acids were first incorporated into proteins as they were produced by the ribosomes of the rough endoplasmic reticulum (Palade and Farquar 1981). The radioactive protein was later found packaged into transport **vesicles** (sphere-shaped sacks). Still later, these radioactivity-filled vesicles were found in the Golgi complex.

In the Golgi complex, the protein was packaged into **secretory vesicles** and was released from the pancreas by a process known as **exocytosis** (figure 1.4). Exocytosis is the fusion of a secretory vesicle with the extracellular membrane and the subsequent discharge of the vesicle contents outside the cell. Exocytosis is an active process that requires both energy and the presence of

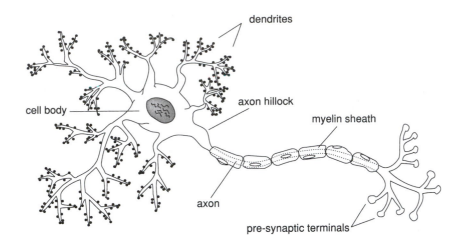

Figure 1.5 In neurons, as in other eucaryotic cells, the nucleus is sequestered in the cell body or soma. Dendrites project in treelike formation from the soma and receive information from other neurons. A single axon projects from the cell body. When the membrane potential at the axon hillock reaches a certain threshold, an action potential is generated and transmitted down the axon to the presynaptic terminal where the neurotransmitter is released by exocytosis, to transmit information to other neurons.

free calcium ions. Endocrine cells, neurons, and neuroendocrine cells all use exocytosis to release secretory products.

In the synthesis of some hormones and neurotransmitters, the secretory product and its packaging into vesicles differ from this model. In fact, steroid hormones are probably not packaged into vesicles at all. But in all other cases, the Golgi apparatus (or an analogous structure) is involved in the formation of the secretory vesicles, the secretory product is packaged into secretory vesicles, and release occurs by exocytosis.

These are the general processes mediating protein synthesis and secretion. In order to understand the ideas discussed in the following chapters, you need to be familiar with these basic relations between DNA, RNA, and proteins. (A more detailed look at these processes is the topic of chapter 2.) Now we are ready to consider the details of the nervous and endocrine systems.

Basic Concepts in Neurobiology

The adult human brain contains from 30 to 100 billion neurons, whereas in the tobacco hornworm moth (*Manduca sexta*) it is estimated that there are 30 to 100 thousand neurons. But in both moths and humans neurons behave very much alike—they share characteristics that allow them to receive, process, and transmit information.

Parts of the Neuron

Most neurons have three structural components: the **cell body**, the **dendrites**, and the **axon** (figure 1.5). Neurons have an outer membrane made of a double layer of fatlike molecules (lipids) with proteins that float within the lipid membrane. As in almost all other cells, the neuronal cell body (or soma) has a nucleus as well as the various subcellular organelles typical of eucaryotic cells.

Extending from the cell body are two different types of projections, axons and dendrites (figure 1.5). Dendrites are usually widely branching fibers that receive information from other neurons. Axons are single fibers that extend from the cell body and transmit information to other neurons. The site where the axon leaves the cell body appears to be slightly swollen and is therefore called the **axon hillock**. The axon usually branches many times at its terminal end, so that multiple contacts can be made with many different target neurons. At the end of each axon branch is a swelling known as the **presynaptic terminal**. The site where the presynaptic terminal contacts another neuron is known as a **synapse**.

The Membrane Potential and Action Potentials

Neurons can receive and transmit information because, unlike most other types of cells, their membranes are electrically excitable. Because there are more negatively charged ions inside neurons than outside, the cells have a **polarization** or electrical charge across the membrane, called the **resting potential**. All cells have a resting potential that they actively defend, but it is a change in the membrane potential that is the result and cause of the transmission of information between neurons.

If an electrical stimulus is applied to the neuronal membrane to make the potential across the membrane *less* negative (i.e., the inside becomes less negative than the outside), then we say that the membrane has become **depolarized**. If an electrical stimulus makes the potential across the membrane *more* negative (i.e., the inside becomes even more negative than the outside), then the membrane is said to be **hyperpolarized**. Such changes in membrane polarization can be caused by an experimenter using electrical stimulation, but in the normally functioning nervous system, changes in membrane polarization are brought about by different means, as we shall soon see.

However the membrane polarization is altered, and whether the alteration is a depolarization or a hyperpolarization, the membrane will **passively conduct** this change in potential along the membrane away from the site that was stimulated. This type of conduction is called **decremental conduction** because the change in membrane potential is smaller and farther from the site of stimulation. The analogy frequently used is that a wave created by dropping a pebble into a pool of calm water becomes smaller as the distance from the site of impact increases. The change in membrane potential created is also referred to as a **graded potential**. This is because the size of the change in membrane potential is proportional to the size of the stimulus. As our analogy illustrates, if you drop a large rock into the pool of calm water, you will produce bigger waves than you would with a pebble.

The events that normally produce changes in neuronal membrane potential occur at the synapse. A **presynaptic** neuron releases its **neurotransmitter**, and this produces changes in the membrane potential of the **postsynaptic** neuron. The postsynaptic response in the next neuron is passively conducted by decremental conduction. The response is also a graded potential, so it is proportional to the amount of neurotransmitter released at a synapse. Throughout the dendrites and cell body, any stimulation of the neuron results in a graded potential and decremental conduction of that potential away from the many sites of stimulation. Because it is literally covered with synapses, each neuron receives input from thousands of other neurons. The neuronintegrates the many depolarizations and hyperpolarizations received by the dendrites and cell body. But it is at the axon hillock that the *net* polarization determines whether this neuron has become sufficiently depolarized to pass on the information to other neurons.

If the net depolarization of the membrane potential at the axon hillock reaches a certain threshold, the axon becomes depolarized, an **action potential** is generated, and the neuron is said to "fire." This action potential is an all-or-none phenomenon: Once an action potential has been generated in the axon hillock, it cannot be stopped, and the strength of the signal does not diminish as it travels down the axon at some 10 to 100 miles per hour (mph). If, as is usually the case, the axon branches, the action potential travels down each branch, and available neurotransmitter is released at each synapse. Action potentials are relatively easy to measure by a variety of electrophysiological techniques.

Synaptic Transmission

The process of communication between two neurons relies on the release of a chemical messenger, the **neurotransmitter**. When the action potential arrives at the presynaptic terminal, the terminal releases a neurotransmitter. The released neurotransmitter crosses the synapse and is detected by postsynaptic receptors. Release of a neurotransmitter and its reception by the postsynaptic neuron is a process known as **synaptic transmission**. This term reflects two important aspects of this process—*synaptic*, because it occurs only at a synapse, and *transmission*, because information is communicated or transmitted between two cells. Synaptic transmission relies on (1) the availability of the neurotransmitter, (2) the release of the neurotransmitter by exocytosis, (3) the binding of the postsynaptic receptor by the neurotransmitter, (4) the response of the postsynaptic cell, and (5) the subsequent removal or deactivation of the neurotransmitter.

AVAILABILITY OF NEUROTRANSMITTER: SYNTHESIS AND PACKAGING INTO VESICLES

Most neurotransmitters are small molecules, about the size of a single amino acid, but neurotransmitters can also be larger proteins or peptides. Some of the substances that are currently thought to be neurotransmitters are listed in

Table 1.2 Partial List of Putative Neurotransmitters and Releasing Factors

Monoamines	*Peptides*
Acetylcholine	Dynorphin
Catecholamines	Enkaphalin
Dopamine (DA)	Substance P
Norepinephrine (NE)	Neurotensin
Epinephrine (EPI)	Bombesin
Indoleamines	Somatostatin
Serotonin (5-hydroxytryptamine or 5-HT)	β-Endorphin
istamine	Neuropeptide Y
	Cholecystokinin (CCK)
Amino acids	Oxytocin
Glutamate	Vasopressin
Gamma-aminobutyric acid (GABA)	Angiotensin II
Glycine	Vasoactive intestinal polypeptide (VIP)
Aspartate	Corticotropin releasing hormone (CRH)
	Growth hormone releasing factor (GRF)
Purines	Thyrotropin releasing hormone (TRH)
Adenosine	Gonadotropin releasing hormone (GnRH)

table 1.2. The synthesis of a neurotransmitter varies according to the size of the molecule. Protein and peptide neurotransmitters are synthesized as described above, in the cell body, and then packaged into secretory vesicles (which in neurons are called **synaptic vesicles**). Once the proteins or peptides have been manufactured and packaged into vesicles in the cell body, they are transported down the axon to the presynaptic terminal for release. If the neurotransmitter is a small molecule, then synthesis does not occur only in the cell body. The enzymes for neurotransmitter synthesis are assembled in the cell body and transported to the presynaptic terminal. The neurotransmitter is then synthesized and packaged into synaptic vesicles in the presynaptic terminal, close to where it will be needed.

EXOCYTOSIS

When a neuron fires, the arrival of the action potential at the presynaptic terminal causes calcium influx into the terminal. The availability of free calcium results in the release of the neurotransmitter from the presynaptic terminal by exocytosis. The neurotransmitter diffuses across the synaptic cleft, where it contacts postsynaptic receptors—large protein molecules or multiprotein complexes that recognize and bind to the neurotransmitter (figure 1.6).

RECEPTOR BINDING

When the neurotransmitter contacts the postsynaptic receptor, the two molecules are thought to fit together in such a way that for a short time they are bound to each other. Because a particular neurotransmitter will fit into only some receptors, such **receptor binding** is usually conceptualized as a "lock and key" association between the two molecules. But the binding is

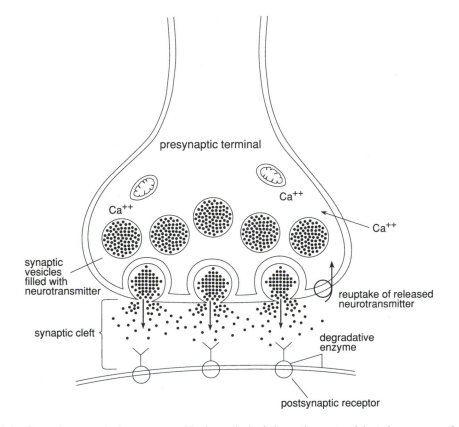

presynaptic terminal

Ca^{++}

Ca^{++}

Ca^{++}

synaptic
vesicles
filled with
neurotransmitter

reuptake of released
neurotransmitter

synaptic cleft

degradative
enzyme

postsynaptic receptor

Figure 1.6 Synaptic transmission occurs with the arrival of the action potential at the presynaptic terminal. This causes an increase in calcium (Ca^{++}) influx and results in movement of the synaptic vesicles filled with neurotransmitter to the presynaptic terminal membrane where the membranes fuse and neurotransmitter is released by exocytosis. The neurotransmitter diffuses across the synaptic cleft to bind to the postsynaptic receptors where a graded potential is generated in the postsynaptic cell. (The synaptic vesicles are depicted with only one membrane, but their membranes are also lipid bilayers as depicted for the extracellular membrane.)

like Velcro—when two complementary strips come in contact, they stick together, but they can also be pulled apart with no change in the shape or usefulness of either. Thus, when the two are attached, they are bound to each other, but this is not a permanent attachment. Similarly, a neurotransmitter has an affinity for its receptor, so it sticks to the receptor for a brief time and then is easily released.

The binding of the neurotransmitter at the postsynaptic receptor induces changes in the electrical potential of the postsynaptic neuronal membrane. The change in membrane potential is proportional to the amount of neurotransmitter released. A neurotransmitter can produce either inhibition (by hyperpolarization) or excitation (by depolarization) of the membrane of the postsynaptic cell. The particular neurotransmitter and the particular postsynaptic receptor determine the direction of the response. If the postsynaptic response is hyperpolarization, the chance of depolarization occurring at the axon hillock is ultimately reduced, and therefore the cell is inhibited from firing. Conversely, if the postsynaptic response is depolarization, the cell is excited. In either case, the information from this synapse is summated with all the other information arriving at this postsynaptic neuron, and when the **threshold** is reached at the axon hillock, this neuron will fire.

DEACTIVATION OF THE NEUROTRANSMITTER
A neurotransmitter is available only briefly to bind to the postsynaptic receptors and then it is rapidly deactivated. Deactivation occurs through either degradative enzymes present in the synaptic cleft or removal of the neurotransmitter by reuptake into the presynaptic terminal. Nevertheless, a brief exposure of the receptor to the neurotransmitter is quite effective at producing a postsynaptic response.

Some Simple Pharmacology

To investigate how specific neural systems interact with the endocrine system, it is often helpful to be able to manipulate neuronal activity. Because pharmacological manipulations are frequently used, it is a good idea to become familiar with the general principles and terminology used to describe the ways in which drugs can influence neuronal activity.

Drugs that act on the brain to influence an animal's behavior usually do so by altering neurotransmitter activity, and there are a number of different ways that drugs can produce their effects. Many drugs act on specific neurotransmitter systems and therefore alter activity in specific populations of neurons. For example, **neurotransmitter synthesis** can be prevented or decreased by drugs that affect the *synthetic enzyme for a neurotransmitter*. When neurotransmitter synthesis is blocked, the amount of neurotransmitter available for release is decreased, so there is decreased neurotransmitter activity. Alternatively, **storage** in synaptic vesicles can be prevented with drugs that make *synaptic vesicle membranes leaky*. This results in depletion of neurotransmitter stores and also decreases neurotransmitter activity.

Other drugs block or stimulate the **release** of specific neurotransmitters. Still other drugs act by **blocking receptors**, so that the real neurotransmitter cannot bind to the receptors. Drugs that *prevent a neurotransmitter from binding* to its receptor are called receptor **antagonists**. For example, drugs used to treat patients with schizophrenia such as haloperidol, chlorpromazine, and clozapine (i.e., neuroleptics or antipsychotic drugs), are antagonists at receptors in the brain for the neurotransmitter dopamine. Other drugs act by binding to a receptor and *mimicking the normal neurotransmitter*. Such drugs are called receptor **agonists**. An example of a receptor agonist is Valium, a benzodiazepine that mimics the effect of the endogenous neurotransmitter gamma-aminobutyric acid (GABA) to decrease anxiety. Other drugs interfere with the **deactivation** of a neurotransmitter after it has been released, thereby prolonging the action of a neurotransmitter. This can be done by blocking reuptake (as cocaine does for catecholamines) or inhibiting

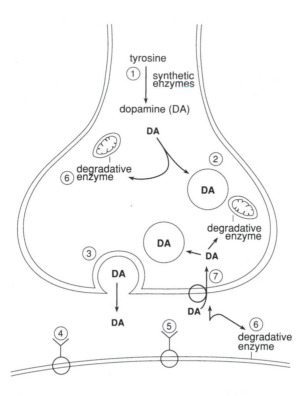

Figure 1.7 Possible sites of drug action in a dopamine (DA) neuron. These same sites can be affected by drugs in neurons that use other neurotransmitters. Drugs can also influence the endocrine system by acting at analogous sites: 1. synthesis; 2. storage; 3. release; 4. receptor-agonist; 5. receptor-antagonist; 6. degradative enzymes; 7. reuptake. (Adapted from Cooper, Bloom, and Roth 1996.)

degradative enzymes. Finally, drugs that **prevent an action potential** from occurring can *block neuronal activity* throughout the brain and the peripheral nervous system. Drugs such as tetrodotoxin (pufferfish poison) and others that block neural activity are usually lethal. The various ways in which drugs can affect neuronal activity are illustrated schematically in figure 1.7 for a neuron that uses dopamine (DA) as its neurotransmitter.

Basic Concepts in Neuroendocrinology

In vertebrates, the central nervous system develops from a long hollow tube of cells called the neural tube. As the brain develops, the neural tube forms three outpouchings. The adult brain is divided into subdivisions based on these embryological formations of forebrain, midbrain, and hindbrain (table 1.3). In mammals, the cerebral hemispheres of the forebrain comprise the largest portion of the brain. These include the cerebral cortex, the basal ganglia, and the limbic system. The cortex can be subdivided into four lobes: frontal, parietal, occipital, and temporal (figure 1.8). However, behavioral endocrinologists, are most interested in a relatively small region at the base of the forebrain, a part of the diencephalon called the hypothalamus. As we

Table 1.3   Major Subdivisions of the Vertebrate Brain

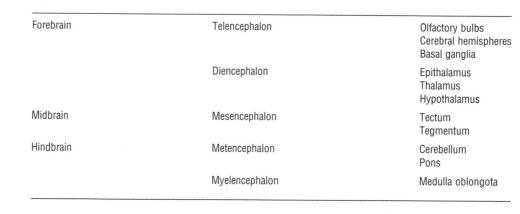

Forebrain	Telencephalon	Olfactory bulbs Cerebral hemispheres Basal ganglia
	Diencephalon	Epithalamus Thalamus Hypothalamus
Midbrain	Mesencephalon	Tectum Tegmentum
Hindbrain	Metencephalon	Cerebellum Pons
	Myelencephalon	Medulla oblongota

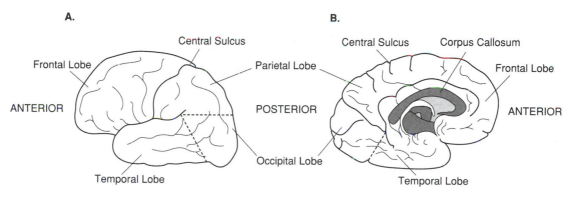

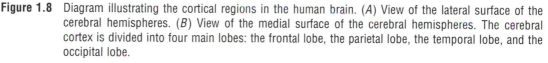

Figure 1.8   Diagram illustrating the cortical regions in the human brain. (*A*) View of the lateral surface of the cerebral hemispheres. (*B*) View of the medial surface of the cerebral hemispheres. The cerebral cortex is divided into four main lobes: the frontal lobe, the parietal lobe, the temporal lobe, and the occipital lobe.

will see, the hypothalamus warrants this attention because it exerts a profound influence on the secretion of nearly every known hormone (figure 1.9)

Hypothalamic-Pituitary Relations in Vertebrates

By definition, hormones are substances produced by a gland and carried by the circulatory system to a distant target organ to cause an effect. The brain is a target organ for many of these hormones and in turn the brain regulates hormone secretion. Although the relations between the brain and the endocrine system in vertebrates are conceptually simple, as with most biological systems the details can be quite complex.

In vertebrates, the hypothalamus is the neural control center for all endocrine systems. Although it is relatively small, it contains a number of specialized nuclei (i.e., functional groups of neurons) (figure 1.10). These nuclei are involved in the regulation and integration of endocrine and physiological functions and behaviors. For example, the suprachiasmatic nucleus (named

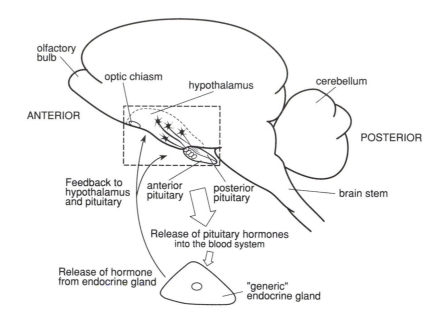

Figure 1.9 The hypothalamic-pituitary-endocrine gland feedback system. A "generic" case. In this figure, the brain is viewed from the side. There are two different classes of neurosecretory cells in the hypothalamus, as illustrated schematically in this figure. The first class of hypothalamic neurosecretory cells send their axons to the median emminence (see figure 1.10). There the cells deliver releasing factors onto blood vessels in the hypophysial portal system. The releasing factors travel to the anterior pituitary to stimulate or inhibit the release of anterior pituitary hormones. The second class send their axons down the pituitary stalk and terminate near blood vessels in the posterior pituitary. When these neurons fire, they release neurohormones (either oxytocin or vasopressin) directly into the circulatory system. Hormones from the anterior pituitary or neurohormones from the posterior pituitary reach their target glands and induce hormone release. Hormones released from the endocrine gland feed back to both the hypothalamus and pituitary. Stippled box indicates region of close-up in figure 1.10.

after its location above the optic chiasm) is involved in the maintenance and coordination of biological rhythms, and the medial preoptic area and ventromedial hypothalamus are involved in sexual behavior (among other functions). In the chapters that follow, you will learn much more about the various hypothalamic nuclei and their many functions.

Specialized types of neurons that allow the brain to influence the secretions of the endocrine system have evolved in the hypothalamus. These neurons, which communicate directly with endocrine systems, are called **neurosecretory cells** because they release their products not into a synapse but into blood vessels that carry the neurotransmitter to other organs to produce its effect. Such neurotransmitters can be thought of, therefore, as **neurohormones**.

The hypothalamus is directly above a very important endocrine gland, the **pituitary**. The pituitary gland (sometimes called the **hypophysis**) is sandwiched between the roof of the mouth and the hypothalamus. Cradled in a small nook in the cranium, the pituitary is actually attached to the hypothalamus by a slender stalk. As we will see, the hypothalamus receives information about external conditions from other brain regions and, using this information, controls secretions from the pituitary. However, the hypothalamic neurosecretory cells exert their control over the pituitary in two quite different ways.

As illustrated schematically in figure 1.9, neurosecretory cells in the hypothalamus are associated with the both the anterior and posterior lobes of the pituitary gland (there is also a slim intermediate zone in the pituitary, but it will not concern us). One type of neurosecretory cell releases its neurohormones onto specialized blood vessels that supply the *anterior* pituitary to stimulate the release of hormones. These neurohormones are also called **releasing factors** because they stimulate or inhibit the release of hormones by cells in the anterior pituitary gland. The other type of hypothalamic neurosecretory cell sends axons into the *posterior* pituitary to release its neurohormones directly into the general circulatory system.

HYPOTHALAMIC CONTROL OF THE ANTERIOR PITUITARY

It was widely accepted for some time that the hypothalamus produced releasing factors that acted on the anterior pituitary to stimulate or inhibit pituitary hormone secretion. However, isolation of a releasing factor did not occur until the early 1970s. The convention now is to call a substance a "releasing factor" until it has been chemically isolated and characterized. Once its chemical structure is known, it is called a **releasing hormone**. We will use the term **releasing factor** as a generic term to refer to both.

Releasing factors are secreted into a specialized system of blood vessels that runs between the base of the hypothalamus and the anterior pituitary lobe (or **adenohypophysis**) rather than the posterior pituitary lobe (or **neurohypophysis**). The hypothalamic-pituitary portal system is actually a profuse tangle of small blood vessels (i.e., capillaries) that use blood flow to deliver the hypothalamic-releasing factors to the pituitary. There are many different types of cells in the anterior pituitary: Some release growth hormone (GH) and are called somatotrophs; other cells (lactotrophs) release prolactin (Prl), and so on (table 1.4). Each of these specialized pituitary cells is controlled by specialized hypothalamic releasing factors. The pituitary cells respond to the releasing factors by either increasing or decreasing their production and release of pituitary hormones (see figure 1.10).

The pituitary hormones are released into the bloodstream and subsequently act on peripheral endocrine glands to stimulate or inhibit *their* function and hormone release. The hormones produced by the various endocrine target glands then feed back to both the hypothalamus and the pituitary. In this way, the hormonal production of the endocrine glands can be continuously monitored and regulated by the brain (see figures 1.9 and 1.10).

For example, the hypothalamus manufactures and releases corticotropic-releasing hormone (CRH) into the portal blood system. CRH reaches the

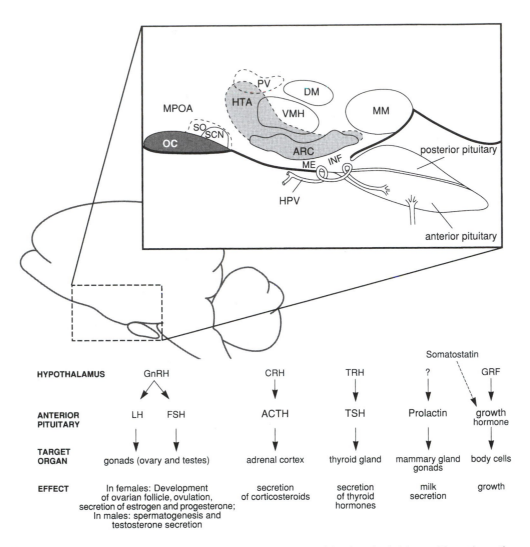

Figure 1.10 A close-up of the hypothalamus and pituitary region indicated by the stippled box, with a schematic representation of the relations between hypothalamic-releasing factors, pituitary hormones, and their target glands. A solid arrow indicates a stimulatory effect; a dashed arrow indicates an inhibitory effect. The releasing factors are released by neurons in the hypothalamus and diffuse through the hypophysial portal blood vessels (HPV) to the anterior pituitary.

1. Gonadotropin-releasing hormone (GnRH) stimulates the pituitary to release luteinizing hormone (LH) and follicle stimulating hormone (FSH). LH and FSH in turn stimulate their primary target organs, the gonads, to promote spermatogenesis in the testes or the development of eggs in the ovary.

2. Corticotropic hormone (CRH) stimulates the pituriary to release adrenocorticotropic hormone (ACTH), which acts primarily on the adrenal cortex to induce the release of corticosteroids.

3. Thyrotropic hormone (TRH) stimulates the release of thyroid stimulating hormone (TSH) from the pituitary, which acts primarily on the thyroid gland to stimulate the release of thyroid hormones.

4. Scientists are still uncertain about the hypothalamic-releasing factor that induces prolactin release. At high concentrations, dopamine will inhibit prolactin release. Prolactin has a wide range of actions in the body and the brain. Prolactin gets its name from its effect on the mammary gland to promote milk secretion. Prolactin also acts in conjunction with LH to promote gonadal function.

pituitary and stimulates corticotrophs there to release adrenocorticotropic hormone (ACTH) into the general circulation. ACTH travels to the adrenal glands (just above the kidneys) which in turn release various corticosteroid hormones (such as cortisol) into the bloodstream. This pattern of control holds for all the anterior pituitary hormones: Neurosecretory cells in the hypothalamus release their releasing factors into the portal system. The releasing factors act on specific pituitary cells to stimulate or inhibit the release of their particular hormone. The anterior pituitary hormone travels through the general circulation to affect the hormonal secretions of the target organ(s).

We can use this same example to illustrate another basic feature of hypothalamic-pituitary interactions: negative feedback. The adrenal steroids, released in response to pituitary ACTH (itself released in response to hypothalamic CRH), travel through the bloodstream to reach the entire body, including the brain and the pituitary. At these two sites, the adrenal hormones act to stem the flow of CRH from the hypothalamus and inhibit the responsiveness of pituitary adrenotrophs. Both actions result in decreased ACTH release. Lowered ACTH levels then result in a decrease in any additional release of adrenal hormones. The negative feedback loop of information means that the release of adrenal cortex hormones is (normally) self-limiting. The adrenal cortex hormones turn off the stimulus that caused them to be secreted in the first place. In turn, as the blood concentration of adrenal cortex hormones falls, CRH and ACTH levels are released from inhibition, and adrenal cortex hormone levels rise again. Thus, the negative feedback aspect of this loop helps to maintain relatively constant levels of adrenal hormones. If they get too high, CRH and ACTH levels are inhibited. If blood concentrations of adrenal cortex hormones fall too low, CRH and ACTH levels rise to bring them up again.

This negative feedback effect is a general phenomenon characteristic of the regulation of the hypothalamus and the anterior pituitary. To cite another example, the hypothalamus also makes and releases thyrotropin-releasing hormone (TRH). TRH stimulates the pituitary to release thyroid-stimulating hormone (TSH). TSH stimulates the thyroid gland to release thyroxine and other thyroid hormones. These thyroid hormones then have a negative feedback effect, reducing hypothalamic release of TRH and pituitary release of TSH. When thyroid hormone levels fall below a certain level, TRH and TSH are released again to restore them.

Figure 1.10 (continued)

5. Somatostatin inhibits, and growth hormone relasing factor (GRF) stimulates, the release of growth hormone (GH) from the anterior pituitary. GH stimulates growth of cells; this includes bone growth as well as growth of other cells in the body. ARC, arcuate nucleus; DM, dorsomedial nucleus; HPV, hypophysial portal vessels; HTA, hypophysiotrophic area; INF, infundibular stalk; ME, median emminence; MM, mammilary nucleus; MPOA, medial preoptic area; OC, optic chiasm; PV, paraventricular nucleus; SCN, suprachiasmatic nucleus; SO, supraoptic nucleus; VMH, ventromedial hypothalamic nucleus. (Adapted from Shepard 1988.)

Table 1.4 Vertebrate Endocrine Glands and Some of the Hormones They Are Known to Secrete

ENDOCRINE GLAND	HORMONES SECRETED
Anterior pituitary	Growth hormone (GH) Prolactin (Prl) Melanaphore stimulating hormone (MSH) Adrenal corticotrophic hormone (ACTH) Luteinizing hormone (LH) Follicle stimulating hormone (FSH) Thyroid stimulating hormone (TSH)
Posterior pituitary	Arginine vasopressin (AVP), also known as antidiuretic hormone (ADH) Oxytocin
Thyroid gland	Thyrotoxin Calcitonin

Adrenal cortex	Glucocorticoids
	   Corticosterone
	   Cortisol
	Mineralicorticoids
	   Aldosterone

Adrenal medulla	Epinephrine Norepinephrine Enkephalins Endorphins
Kidney	Renin
Liver	Preangiotensin
Pancreas	Insulin Glucagon
Stomach and intestines	Gastrin Secretin Cholecystokinin (CCK) Vasoactive intestinal peptide (VIP) Bombesin Somatostatin Leptin Orexin
Pineal	Melatonin

Gonads: ovary	Estrogens
	   Estradiol (E2)
	   Estriol
	   Estrone
	Progesterone

Gonads: testes	Androgens
	   Testosterone (T)
	   Dihydrotestosterone (DHT)
	   Androstendione

While the negative feedback loop tends to keep hormone concentrations in blood relatively constant, there are also conditions under which the feedback system results in regular cycles of varying hormone concentrations. This occurs during the reproductive cycle in females (chapter 4), during pregnancy (chapter 9), and with endogenous rhythms (chapter 12). For example, during the female reproductive cycle, estrogen exerts both negative and positive feedback effects on the hypothalamus. During initial development of an egg (or oocyte), a small amount of estrogen is produced and released by the ovary (see figure 4.1). This inhibits hypothalamic release of gonadotropins-releasing hormone (GnRH) and pituitary release of luteinizing hormone (LH) as a negative feedback effect. Then, as the oocyte becomes mature, there is a rapid increase in estrogen release from the ovary. Instead of inhibiting GnRH and LH release, however, this rapid increase in estrogen has the opposite effect. It *stimulates* a pulse of GnRH release from the hypothalamus. This GnRH pulse induces a pulse of LH release from the pituitary, which is crucial for the final maturation and release of the mature egg (see chapters 3 and 4).

HYPOTHALAMIC NEUROSECRETORY CELLS AND THE POSTERIOR PITUITARY

Oxytocin and vasopressin are hormones made by neurosecretory cells in the hypothalamus. Oxytocin and vasopressin are both neurohormones and neurotransmitters. Some of these cells send their axons down to the median eminence and into the posterior pituitary. When these neurons fire, oxytocin or vasopressin is released from the posterior pituitary directly into the bloodstream. You can think of oxytocin and vasopressin as hypothalamic neurohormones that affect target organs directly, without using pituitary cells or their hormones as intermediaries. However, not all neurons that make oxytocin or vasopressin project to the posterior pituitary. Some of the hypothalamic cells that make these hormones project to the brain and spinal cord, synaptically releasing their products upon neurons.

Oxytocin released into the bloodstream triggers milk ejection during nursing and uterine contractions for childbirth. In fact, hospitals often administer a synthetic version of oxytocin, called pitocin, to induce or speed delivery. Vasopressin is vital for fluid conservation. Additional functions of oxytocin and vasopressin will be discussed in chapters 4, 9, and 16. Oxytocin and vasopressin are "sister" hormones—their chemical structures are very similar. This structural similarity probably reflects a common evolutionary origin. Amphibians, for example, have only one such hormone, called vasotocin, which has actions reminiscent of both oxytocin and vasopressin.

Most vertebrates produce vasopressin and oxytocin or vasotocin, but there are species variations in the molecular structure of the actual hormones produced and in the functions of these hormones. Table 1.4 lists some of the endocrine glands and the hormones that they produce in most vertebrate animals (mammals, reptiles, amphibians, fishes, and birds). The relations among the hypothalamic-releasing factors, the anterior pituitary hormones, and their target endocrine glands are illustrated schematically in figure 1.10. Each releasing factor stimulates the release of a specific hormone (or, in the case of GnRH, the release of two hormones). These hormones are released by the pituitary into the bloodstream and are then carried to their target organs, where they produce their specific effects, usually stimulating the target organs to release hormones of their own.

Mechanisms of Hormone Action

OVERVIEW: STEROIDS VERSUS PEPTIDE HORMONES
Hormones fall into two general classes based on their molecular structures. The first class comprises steroid hormones produced by the gonads and the adrenal cortex and the steroidlike hormones produced by the thyroid gland. The steroid hormones are all synthesized from the common precursor cholesterol (see figure 3.2). The thyroid hormones have a steroidlike three-dimensional structure that influences their chemical properties, making them behave like steroids. Because these hormones share many common properties they are usually discussed together. The second class of hormones comprises the glycoprotein hormones (LH and follicle-stimulating hormone [FSH]) and protein or peptide hormones. As we hinted earlier, these different hormones are synthesized and packaged for secretion in different ways.

The protein and peptide hormones are chains of amino acids and are processed like most proteins (see p. 15). The glycoprotein hormones undergo additional processing in the Golgi apparatus, where a sugar group (glycogen is the basic building block in sugars, hence the "glyco" prefix) is added to the protein prior to packaging into vesicles. Steroid hormones, on the other hand, are synthesized from precursors in the smooth endoplasmic reticulum, processed further in the mitochondria, and then returned to the smooth endoplasmic reticulum for final processing. The thyroid hormones are synthesized from amino acids that form a complex steroidlike structure. It is currently believed that, unlike protein hormones, steroid and steroidlike hormones are not stored in vesicles. It is thought that they simply diffuse out of cells after synthesis. Release of these hormones is, therefore, governed primarily by the rate at which they are synthesized.

The molecular structure of a hormone is also important because of the way it can act upon other cells. Protein, peptide, and glycoprotein hormones do not readily pass through cell membranes, so they usually act upon receptors found in the outer membrane of responsive cells. Only cells containing the appropriate receptor can respond to a particular hormone. Like a neurotransmitter and its receptor, the hormone and the receptor have complementary shapes that result in the binding of the hormone to the receptor. Protein, glycoprotein, and peptide hormones bind to specific receptor molecules that span the cell membrane, which triggers intracellular chemical reactions that can have a wide range of effects, as we will see.

In contrast, because steroid hormones are lipid soluble, they are thought to pass through the extracellular membrane. Inside the cell, steroid hormones bind to specific receptor proteins, and this steroid-receptor complex then binds to DNA. The binding of the hormone to DNA results in an increase or decrease in the synthesis of specific proteins, which can begin a wide range of effects.

PROTEIN HORMONES

Among the vertebrates, protein hormones include the hypothalamic-releasing factors as well as the pituitary hormones (see table 1.4). The posterior pituitary hormones oxytocin and vasopressin are both peptides composed of only nine amino acids. Insulin, another vital protein hormone, consists of about 100 amino acids and is released from the pancreas. Like other proteins, the molecular structure of these hormones is coded for by genes in DNA.

The binding of a protein hormone to its receptor sets into motion a chain of chemical events inside a cell. One of the first events is the activation of a second messenger system that results in a cascading series of reactions within the cell. The exact second messenger varies among the protein hormones, but all are thought to employ second messenger systems to induce a response in target cells. The initial response of the target cell is much like that of a neuron responding to a neurotransmitter, i.e., a change in membrane potential. The particular chain of subsequent events depends upon the type of receptor that was activated and the state of intracellular events that existed before the hormone arrived. Figure 1.11 is a diagram of the rather complicated cascade of chemical reactions triggered by the arrival of a glucagon molecule at a target cell.

The regulation of receptors for protein hormones is thought to be mediated by negative feedback mechanisms similar to those operating at neurotransmitter receptors. In general, the number and activity of these receptors are inversely regulated by the amount of hormone or neurotransmitter available. When neurotransmitter release or protein-hormone release is high, a "down-regulation" of receptors occurs, so that even more hormone is needed to induce a biological response. In contrast, when hormone release is low, the receptors' response can become supersensitive to stimulation by protein hormones, i.e., less hormone is required to produce the same biological response. This negative feedback system serves to maintain a relatively constant biological response even when the endocrine system is damaged or altered. For each hormone and receptor, however, there are also other factors that are important in the regulation of receptor activity, including the regulation of receptors by steroid hormones.

One example of the operation of the negative feedback mechanism carried to an extreme occurs in people with adult onset diabetes (also known as type II, or insulin-independent diabetes mellitus). This form of diabetes, as suggested by its name, develops late in life and is usually associated with

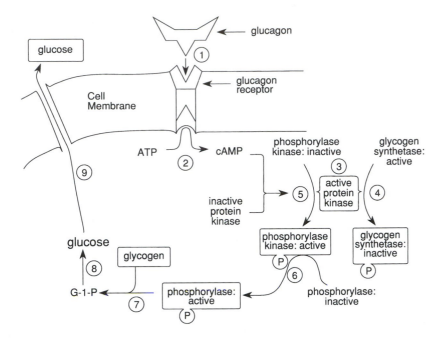

Figure 1.11 Cascade of events triggered by the arrival of a glucagon molecule at a target cell. Glucagon binds to its cell membrane receptor (1). This stimulates the activity of an effector enzyme that promotes the formation of cyclic adenosine monophosphate (cAMP) from adenosine triphosphate (ATP) inside the cell (2). cAMP, known as the second messenger, activates one of a class of enzymes known as protein kinases (3). This particular protein kinase catalyzes the phosphorylation (i.e., the addition of phosphate groups (P)) to other specific enzymes (4), (5), and (6), which in turn catalyze the metabolism of glycogen to glucose-1-phosphate (G-1-P) (7) and then the generation of glucose (8) which is released from the cell (9). (Adapted from Norman and Litwack 1997.)

obesity. Unlike type I diabetes (in which individuals do not produce enough insulin), in type II diabetes insulin secretion is elevated and peripheral insulin receptors are reduced in number and insensitive to insulin. It is as though the elevated insulin secretion has desensitized the insulin receptors. Alternatively, it may be that the decreased receptor response has resulted in an increased insulin secretion. Frequently, after weight loss, these individuals regain normal insulin secretion and sensitivity (Norman and Litwack 1987). Why some individuals develop this abnormality in the negative feedback response to insulin is not known.

STEROID HORMONES

In vertebrates, steroid hormones are often referred to by the organ of their origin. For example, the hormones produced by the ovaries and testes (or gonads) are referred to as the gonadal steroids. The principal products of the testes are the androgens, testosterone and dihydrotestosterone. The ovaries primarily make two types of steroid hormones, estrogens and progestins. Examples of estrogens include estradiol, estriol, and estrone. Progesterone is the principal progestin, so named because it promotes gestation or pregnancy. It should be noted, however, that testosterone is a precursor to estrogen and the ovaries also make testosterone. Conversely, estrogen is a metabolite of testosterone, so the testes also produce some estrogen.

The hormones secreted by the cortex of the adrenal gland are known as the adrenal steroids or corticosteroids. The corticosteroids include two classes of steroid hormones. These are the glucocorticoids and the mineralocorticoids. The glucocorticoids, in general, increase circulating glucose. Cortisol and corticosterone are examples of glucocorticoids. Cortisone is a synthetic version of cortisol that is used medicinally. Androgens (testosterone, dehydro-epiandrosterone, and so on) are also produced by the adrenal cortex; they are released in response to ACTH, like the mineralocorticoids that regulate water balance (e.g., aldosterone). In fact, over 50 adrenal steroid hormones can be released in response to ACTH from the pituitary. As we will learn in chapter 11, scientists suspect that there are other hormones determining which steroids the adrenals will produce.

One word of caution may be needed here. Although the principal secretion of the testes in most male vertebrates is testosterone, the testes also secrete small amounts of estrogens, as noted earlier. Similarly, ovaries and adrenals also produce androgens. Thus, the idea that androgens are ''male'' hormones while estrogens are ''female'' hormones is overly simplistic; both sexes make both classes of hormone, albeit in quite different proportions (see chapter 3). The proportions and specific androgens or estrogens that are produced also vary with the species. For example, the stallion has exceptionally high concentrations of estradiol.

The third organ to release steroidlike hormones is the thyroid gland. As noted before, the thyroid hormones look and behave very much like steroids in that they are lipid soluble and not released by exocytosis. The principal thyroid hormones are triiodothyronine, abbreviated as T3, and thyroxine (also known as tetra-iodothyronine, abbreviated as T4).

Steroid hormones (and thyroid hormones) act quite differently from protein hormones. They are lipophilic and therefore readily cross the lipid cell membrane. Target cells are those that contain protein receptor molecules that recognize and bind to a particular steroid. Once the steroid binds to its receptor, the steroid-receptor complex binds to DNA and thereby manages to either increase or decrease the transcription of specific genes (probably by triggering the winding or unwinding of DNA coils), changing the production of a wide variety of proteins. Thus, steroid hormones can **regulate gene transcription** (or expression) and can therefore expert powerful influences upon the development and differentiation of cells.

Another difference between steroids and protein hormones occurs in the regulation of their receptors. Steroid hormone receptors are sometimes regulated by a positive feedback system. In other words, in the absence of testosterone, for example, the number of testosterone receptors decreases.

Therefore, it is sometimes necessary to treat an animal repeatedly with a steroid hormone to induce sufficient numbers of receptors to get a biological response. The number of receptors that can be induced by this mechanism is finite, however, so that if excess hormone is present for a prolonged period of time, eventually no receptors will be available to bind the hormone.

Selective gene activation or regulation is an important concept. Even though all the cells in an animal contain the same genetic material (about 100,000 genes in a human), the genes used, or **expressed**, by individual cells vary. Genes that are expressed in a cell are those genes that are transcribed to produce proteins. Most cells will express the genes that contain the information needed to produce the synthetic and housekeeping organelles, so some genes are expressed in most cells. Then there are some genes that are expressed only in a particular cell type. For example, it has been estimated that liver cells express about 30,000 genes and various neurons express about 50,000 genes, and that about 20,000 of these genes are common to both liver cells and neurons. It is also important for a cell to be able to adapt to the changing needs of an organism. So the expression of genes is regulated by information obtained from within the cell and by information from external sources. One way that the expression of genes can be regulated is through hormonal input. You will learn more about hormone receptors and how they work in chapter 2.

Endocrine Methods

BIOASSAYS

In the old days, the only way to measure the concentration of a hormone in blood or in an organ was to reconstruct in the laboratory some physiological system that normally responds to the hormone. For example, what if you wanted to measure the testosterone concentration in a sample of blood plasma from a bull? You could castrate adult male rats, thereby depriving them of their own gonadal steroid hormones; you would then notice that the prostate glands surrounding the urethra become smaller afterward and that injections of testosterone make them bigger again. The weight of these glands can serve as a biological assay, or **bioassay**, of androgen concentrations. If you now inject the rat with a solution containing hormones extracted from the plasma of a steer (i.e., a castrated bull), kill the rat, and then weigh its prostate, you would see little or no growth, whereas if you injected the rat with a solution of hormones extracted from the plasma of a bull, you should see considerable growth of the rat's prostate. Such bioassays are effective but not very convenient or sensitive. Furthermore, minor differences in the way the rats are treated or the glands are dissected can dramatically affect the bioassay results. This makes it sometimes difficult to compare the results of bioassays from different investigators because not all laboratories measure a substance in the same way.

RADIOIMMUNOASSAYS

These days the most common method for measuring hormone concentrations in blood is the **radioimmunoassay**, or RIA. The RIA was invented by Rosalyn Yalow and Seymour Berson, for which they won the Nobel prize. To measure the testosterone concentrations in bull plasma with an RIA, you need three things: (1) testosterone (T) of known purity that was either expressly manufactured (known as "synthetic hormone" because it was synthesized by humans in either a chemistry laboratory or by the enslavement of bacteria) or was "purified" from some animal product (testes perhaps) by the use of biochemical methods; (2) testosterone that has been radioactively labeled (T*). By detecting the radioactive particles given off by the radioactive isotopes, it is possible to quantify the total radioactivity and therefore the total number of so-called "hot" T* molecules. Nonradioactive T molecules may be referred to as "cold" T; and (3) an **antibody** that recognizes and attaches itself to testosterone. Antibodies are large, complex proteins made by an organism to attach to invaders and mark them for destruction (see chapter 10). We can inject a rabbit with the substance of interest and later withdraw some of the rabbit's plasma to harvest the antibodies it made to the substance of interest—in this case, testosterone.

With these three reagents (which can be purchased commercially for most hormones), it is possible to assay the concentrations of testosterone in the sample of bull plasma. We refer to the bull's own testosterone as endogenous testosterone because it was made inside the bull in contrast to exogenous testosterone, which was introduced in either the bull or the plasma sample by researchers. If we were to add the antibodies that recognize testosterone to the sample, they would bind the testosterone more or less irreversibly. Unfortunately, there are no simple ways to count the antibodies. On the other hand, if we added the antibodies to our exogenously supplied "hot" T*, then separated the leftover free T* from the T* bound by antibodies, we could use Geiger counter–like machines to detect the antibody-T* complexes by measuring the radioactive T*.

So what would happen if we added a known amount of hot T* to our plasma sample and then added the antibodies? After waiting awhile for the antibodies to bind to both T and T*, we would separate out the leftover, unbound T*. If there were no endogenous testosterone in the sample, we would get just as many antibody-T* complexes (measured by the amount of radioactivity) as we'd get if we added antibody and T* to water instead of plasma. But if there were some endogenous testosterone in the plasma sample, some of the antibodies would stick to that testosterone (which of course would not be "hot"), and therefore fewer antibody-T* complexes would be made. In fact, if more endogenous testosterone is present, more hot molecules will be displaced and therefore fewer antibody-T* complexes will be detected when we measure the radioactivity. We can find out how much hot T* will be displaced by a given amount of testosterone by measuring out different amounts of "cold" T of known purity (say 50, 100, 250, and 500 micrograms [μg] worth) and seeing exactly how much T* is displaced by each. From this information we could generate a standard curve that would allow us to determine exactly how much testosterone exists in each of our biological samples.

Summary

Behavioral endocrinology joins together the fields of neuroscience, endocrinology, and psychology to ask important and exciting questions about how changes in the endocrine system influence the brain and behavior. In this chapter we have reviewed some of the basic concepts important to the study of the nervous and endocrine systems. Some of the most important concepts are summarized below.

1. The methods used to measure and evaluate behavior must be just as precise and exacting as the methods used to quantify hormones. In many ways, the behavioral component of experiments is much more difficult than the biochemical methods used to quantify the behavior because it frequently depends on visual observation. Thus, a great deal of time is needed to conduct precise and accurate measures of behavior.

2. You will study three different types of intercellular messengers: neurotransmitters, neurohormones, and hormones. Most of these intercellular messengers are packaged into secretory vesicles for release by exocytosis. Differences among these messengers lie in where they are produced, where they are released, and the distance that must be traveled to produce an effect. Neurotransmitters are produced by neurons in the brain, released at the synaptic terminal, and diffuse across the synaptic cleft to produce a response at the postsynaptic membrane. Neurohormones are produced by neurons in the brain, released from synaptic terminals into the bloodstream, and produce their effects at target organs. Hormones are produced by endocrine cells, released into the bloodstream, and produce their effect at distant target organs.

3. Communication between neurons occurs through the release by exocytosis of chemical messengers known as neurotransmitters. The neurotransmitter is released at the synapse and binds to a postsynaptic receptor. This process is known as synaptic transmission. The binding of the neurotransmitter to the receptor results in a change in the membrane polarization of the postsynaptic cell. This influences whether or not the postsynaptic cell will fire an action potential. Drugs that produce changes in neuronal activity usually do so by influencing one or more components of synaptic transmission.

4. Neurohormones known as releasing factors are released by neurosecretory cells in the hypothalamus. These releasing factors travel through a specialized system of blood vessels to reach the anterior pituitary which controls the release of pituitary hormones. The pituitary hormones enter the bloodstream to regulate the release of hormones from the peripheral endocrine glands.

Negative and positive feedback from the endocrine glands to the brain and pituitary results in coordination of the neuroendocrine systems.

5. Hormones are classified according to their molecular structures as either steroid or protein hormones. Both kinds of hormones produce their effects on target tissues by binding to specific receptors. The process induced by the binding of a hormone to a receptor depends on whether the hormone is a protein or a steroid. Protein hormones induce their effects by binding to membrane-associated receptors and inducing intracellular changes by activation of a second messenger system. Steroid hormones bind to intracellular receptors, and the steroid-receptor complex alters gene expression.

6. Genetic information is coded by the DNA found in the nuclei of eucaryotic cells. Particular lengths of DNA known as genes are transcribed into a string of specific RNA nucleotides that leave the nucleus. In the cytoplasm of the cell, RNA is translated into a specific sequence of amino acids. A short sequence of amino acids is called a peptide; a long sequence is called a protein. The genetic code is important for our understanding of information in later chapters for two reasons. First, steroid hormones produce their effects by altering gene expression, and this can be shown to be related to the behavioral effects of steroid hormones. Second, releasing factors, neurotransmitters, and some hormones are proteins or are synthesized from proteins. One way to measure changes in production of these molecules is to quantify the production of the mRNA that codes for these proteins.

Study Questions

1. You are observing your favorite species in the wild, the gastric brooding frog, and you would like to be sure that your observations of the animal's mating behavior will be reproducible. What steps would you take to obtain reliable, reproducible data? How would you determine if hormones are involved in this behavior?

2. What are the differences among oxytocin, LH, and estrogen? Include a discussion of the chemical structure, how the hormone is released, where it is released from, and the receptors on which the hormones act.

3. What are the differences between positive feedback and negative feedback in the control of hormone secretion? Give examples of each.

4. How do psychoactive drugs produce their effects in the brain? Be specific.

5. What is selective gene expression? How would you determine if a hormone was altering gene expression?

Sources of Additional Information

Textbooks

Cooper, J. R., Bloom, F. E., and Roth, R. H. (1996) *The Biochemical Basis of Neuropharmacology*, 7th edition. New York: Oxford University Press.
Norman, A. W., and Litwack, G. (1997) *Hormones*, 2nd edition. San Diego: Academic Press.

Rosenzweig, Mark R., Breedlove, S. M., and Leiman, A. L. (2002) *Biological Psychology: An Introduction to Behavioral, Cognitive, and Clinical Neuroscience*, 3rd edition. Sunderland, Mass.: Sinauer.

Review Articles

On the secretory process in eucaryotic cells: Palade, G. E. and Farquar, M. G. (1981) Cell biology. In L. H. Smith and S. O. Thie (Eds.), *Pathophysiology: The Biological Principles of Disease*. Philadelphia: W. B. Saunders, pp. 1–56.

On behavioral techniques in the laboratory: Whishaw, I. Q., Kolb, B., and Sutherland, R. J. (1983) The analysis of behavior in the laboratory rat. In T. E. Robinson, (Ed.), *Behavioral Approaches to Brain Research*. New York: Oxford University Press, pp. 141–202.

Reference Cited

Brink, E., Modianos, D. and Pfaff, D. W. (1979) Ablations of epaxial deep back muscles. Effects on lordosis behavior in the female rat. *Brain Behav. Evol.* 17: 67–88.

2 Molecular Approaches to Behavioral Neuroendocrinology

Margaret M. McCarthy and David Crews

There has been an explosion of information about the way changes in gene expression impact brain and behavior. Since hormones produce many of their effects on the body and on behavior by altering gene expression in their target cells, the modern behavioral endocrinologist must become familiar with the techniques of molecular biology.

How do you know if a hormone has turned on a gene in its target cells? What do you do if you want to clone a gene? What is a transgenic animal? This chapter was designed to help you become more familiar with new techniques and the exciting questions that can now be answered with them.

Introduction

Now that you have reviewed some of the basic concepts of behavioral neuro-endocrinology, you are prepared to review some of the more sophisticated approaches that are becoming increasingly important in the field. Of particular note is the increased emphasis on understanding the molecular or genetic basis for hormonal modulation of behavior. Nowadays behavioral neuro-endocrinologists can choose from a wide range of techniques and can customize a particular method or combine several approaches to suit their needs.

By and large, hormones exert their effects by influencing the expression of particular genes. As we saw in chapter 1, this is accomplished via different pathways for peptide versus steroid hormones. In the case of steroid hormones, this is generally achieved by a direct interaction with the DNA, whereas peptide hormones usually bind to membrane receptors and activate a signal transduction cascade that may ultimately activate gene expression. As a result of their different sites and mechanisms of action, steroids and peptides can generally be distinguished by their effects being relatively slow (hours to days) versus extremely fast (milliseconds to minutes), respectively. Changes in gene expression alter the protein composition of a cell, thereby altering its function and perhaps changing its influence on other cells as well. We will begin with a more detailed review of the receptors. This will be followed by a discussion of some of the techniques used to measure and characterize messenger RNA (mRNA), DNA, and proteins. Then we will look at some of the new techniques for altering gene expression that are being used by behavioral neuroendocrinologists.

Mechanisms of Hormone Receptor Action

Peptide Hormone Receptors

As you saw in chapter 1, peptide hormone receptors are found on the surface of cells. In order for them to influence the expression of genes, the signal must be transduced to the nucleus. This is referred to as the **signal transduction pathway** (Albers et al. 1994). The peptide or protein hormone binds to its receptor and this results in changes in intracellular molecules and, in some cells, the production of **second messengers**. A number of second messengers are produced (depending on the cell and the receptor), including cAMP and the inositol phospholipids, better known as IP3. Recent evidence suggests that calcium ions also function as important second messengers.

METABOTROPIC RECEPTORS

Probably the most broadly distributed type of receptor are the **G-protein coupled receptors**, sometimes called **metabotropic receptors**. These are large proteins with a structure that spans the extracellular membrane 7 times (referred to as 7-transmembrane domains) with a piece of the protein that extends into the extracellular space and binds to its ligand. Intracellularly, these receptors are associated with the G-proteins. Binding of the receptor to the ligand extracellularly activates the G-protein complex inside the neuron and, as a consequence, enzymes are activated that result in the production of second-messenger molecules such as cAMP and IP3. These types of receptors are utilized by many peptide hormones such as oxytocin, gonadotropin releasing hormone (**GnRH**), **corticotropic releasing hormone** (**CRH**), and the glycoprotein hormones luteininzing hormone (LH) and follicle stimulating hormone (FSH).

LIGAND-GATED ION CHANNELS

A second type of extracellular receptor are the **ligand-gated ion channels**. This type of receptor tends to be the exclusive domain of acetylcholine and the amino acid transmitters GABA, glutamate, and glycine. Interestingly, progesterone and some progesterone metabolites are known to bind to a subunit of the GABA-A receptor, which enhances the receptor response to GABA. So here we have a receptor that looks like it should respond to peptide hormones but responds to steroid hormones.

RECEPTOR KINASES

Finally, the **receptor kinases** are receptors that function as enzymes and phosphorylate other proteins to regulate their activity. Growth factors such as nerve-growth factor (NGF) or brain-derived neurotrophic factor (BDNF) use receptors of this type.

Thus, the majority of peptide hormones we are concerned with act through G-protein-coupled receptors. Different hormones will activate receptors that selectively increase either cAMP or IP3. For instance, GnRH increases IP3, and ultimately the level of free calcium in a cell, whereas the factors it releases from the pituitary, LH and FSH, both bind to G-protein coupled receptors that increase cAMP. Ultimately, the increased calcium released by IP3 and cAMP can influence gene expression by activating a protein called CREB (cAMP-response-element-binding protein) which finds a site on the DNA and binds to it. This is analogous to the hormone-response elements we discuss below for steroid receptors. A brief summary of these different signal transduction pathways is schematically illustrated in figure 2.1.

Steroid Hormone Receptors

ACTIVATION OF SELECTIVE GENE EXPRESSION

Because of their ability to interact directly with the DNA, steroid hormone receptors are referred to as **transcription factors**; in other words, they either increase or decrease the transcription of particular genes. As we learned in chapter 1, the first step in steroid-hormone action involves the steroid passing through a cell's exterior plasma membrane. Inside the cell, the steroid molecule encounters unoccupied (or unactivated) receptors. These receptors are present as individual proteins (monomers) that are part of a complex of multiple chaperone proteins. These chaperone proteins (that include inhibitory heat shock proteins) serve to lock the receptor in a high affinity state for ligand binding. After the steroid ligand binds to its receptor, the inhibitory heat shock proteins dissociate and the receptor is activated. Activated receptors bound to their ligand dimerize (two receptor-ligand units bind together) and then interact with the DNA.

Before interacting with the DNA, the steroid receptors may bind to other proteins, forming part of a **transcriptional complex**. This complex consists of multiple proteins, many of which are enzymes that will unwind the DNA and help transcribe it into mRNA. Some of these additional proteins are referred to as **co-activators** and **co-repressors**. Their presence in the transcriptional complex can be essential for steroid responsiveness. For instance, the first of these co-activators to be discovered is called steroid receptor co-activator 1 (SRC-1). If levels of this co-activator are reduced, animals do not show normal development of secondary sex characteristics or expression of sexual behavior (Auger et al. 2000; Xu et al. 2000).

One important function of steroid hormone receptors in this transcriptional complex is to confer specificity. It would not be very useful to have the complex randomly settling down on the DNA and turning on genes. Instead, the steroid hormone receptor will only interact with a specific sequence of nucleotides that must be present in the upstream or **promoter** region of a gene. The promoter is just as it sounds, a part of the gene that promotes its expression by specific factors as a result of its specific nucleotide sequence (keep in mind that not all portions of a gene are transcribed into mRNA). For steroid receptors, this sequence is referred to as a **hormone response element or HRE**.

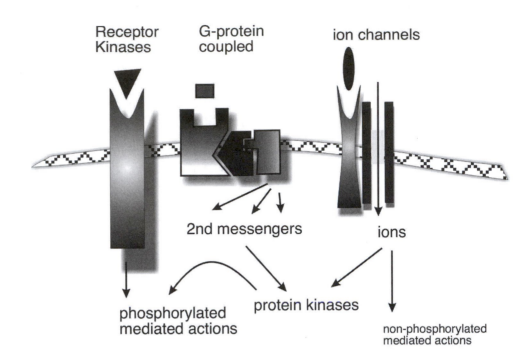

Figure 2.1 Signal transduction following membrane receptor binding. There are three general types of membrane receptors: (1) the kinase receptors, (2) G-protein-coupled receptors, and (3) ligand-gated ion channels. Kinase receptors bind growth factors, thereby activating their intrinsic enzymatic activity to phosphorylate various substrates, inducing a cascade of cellular changes. The G-protein-coupled receptors may bind peptides, neurotransmitters, or prostaglandins. They can be coupled to the production of cAMP or to the phosphotidylinositol pathway that can release internal calcium from the endoplasmic reticuluum. The ligand-gated channels are ionophores, which are permeable to various ions (Cl^-, K^+, and Ca^{++}) and which bind neurotransmitters, in particular, the amino acids GABA and glutamate.

There is a different HRE for the estrogen receptor than for the progesterone receptor and so on. The sequence is about 6 to 15 nucleotides long and is usually a palindrome (something that is the same when read forward or backward, like the name HANNAH). For instance, the HRE for the estrogen receptor is $\frac{\text{AGGTCANNNTGACCT}}{\text{TCCAGTNNNACTGGA}}$ where the N refers to any nucleotide. The DNA binding site on the estrogen receptor will specifically recognize and bind to this sequence on the DNA and either activate or suppress the associated gene. The estrogen receptor also contains a binding site for its ligand, estrogen, and several other domains that are highly conserved across species (Rollerova and Urbancikova 2000).

The androgen, progesterone, estrogen, and glucocorticoid receptors, along with thyroid receptors and an even larger group of proteins termed orphan receptors (meaning that their ligands and/or function are as yet undetermined), are members of a nuclear receptor superfamily. Almost all members of this family act as transcription factors that exert broad influences on gene expression. For some receptors, such as the androgen receptor, both testosterone (T) and dihydrotestosterone (DHT) operate through a single receptor, but their effect on gene expression can be quite distinct. For example, as will be discussed in more detail in chapter 3, T is required for the development and differentiation of the internal accessory sexual organs, including the transformation of the Wolffian ducts into the epididymis, vas deferens, and seminal vesicles. On the other hand, DHT is required for the development of the penis, scrotum, and prostate.

To further complicate things, steroid hormone receptors exist in multiple forms. For example, in most avian and mammalian species, the progesterone receptor is expressed as two major DNA-binding forms, PR-A and PR-B. Another example is estrogen receptor alpha (α), beta (β), and now gamma (γ) (Hawkins et al. 2000). It seems likely that additional forms of steroid receptors will continue to be discovered in the near future. Having multiple forms of a receptor is another mechanism by which the cell can selectively regulate its response to a steroid.

NONTRADITIONAL STEROID EFFECTS

When a steroid binds to its receptor and induces gene transcription, this is referred to as a genomic action and has long been considered the classic or traditional form of steroid action. This distinction is important because for all the steroid hormones, actions have been reported that occur very rapidly in cells devoid of the classical intracellular receptors (see chapters 4 and 13); these rapid effects are referred to as "nontraditional" steroid effects. In the past they were referred to as "nongenomic" steroid actions, but it is now clear that this terminology should be avoided because it can easily be confused with rapid effects that result in genomic activation or with transgenerational effects such as the influence of maternal behavior, handling, intrauterine position, temperature, and so on.

Exactly how the rapid effects of steroid hormones are exerted in the cell is still under investigation. Many reports have implicated a metabotropic receptor in the rapid effects of estrogen in the striatum (for example, Mermelstein et al. 1996; chapter 13). Recently, however, it was found that the traditional nuclear receptor can incorporate into a cell's lipid bilayer, with the steroid-binding pocket of the receptor actually extruding through the membrane (Razandi et al. 1999) and possibly picking up passing molecules of steroid. This was a surprising finding and may help explain many anomalies regarding the rapid versus traditional effects of steroids. It also highlights the fact that steroid effects cannot be easily pigeonholed into one type or another.

LIGAND-INDEPENDENT ACTIVATION

Another surprising discovery was that the traditional nuclear steroid receptor also moonlights as a signal transduction protein and interacts with various signaling pathways in the cytoplasm of a cell. Estrogen receptors, for example, can associate with specific cytoplasmic proteins to activate kinases, enzymes that phosphorylate and thereby activate other proteins. This will set in motion a signaling cascade that eventually ends in the nucleus with the induction of gene transcription (Singh et al. 2000). The spark that ignites this pathway may or may not be a steroid hormone molecule. In another example, dopamine binding to the D_1 dopamine receptor can result in activation of the progesterone receptor in certain cells (see chapter 4 for more details). This results in what is known as ligand-independent activation of steroid receptors. Such discoveries of novel and unexpected ways in which steroid receptors can be activated and interact with other cellular proteins has upended the traditional view and greatly expanded our concept of steroid hormone action. As a result, the terms nongenomic and genomic actions of gonadal steroids have gone the way of the dial phone and become obsolete.

Techniques for Measuring Gene Expression

What do we mean when we say "gene expression"? How does a gene express itself? A diamond nose ring and purple hair dye? No, much more mundanely, unfortunately. As we discussed in chapter 1, gene expression refers to an increase (or decrease) in the transcription rate of a gene to produce more (or less) mRNA, which may (or may not) ultimately result in more (or less) protein. To measure gene expression, we usually resort to measuring the product: mRNA or the protein produced. We have several technical approaches to doing this. *Molecular Cloning* by Sambrook, Fritsch, and Maniatis (1989) has done for the laboratory what the *Joy of Cooking* did for the home kitchen.

A number of the techniques currently in use to measure gene expression will be described below (so don't worry about what the names mean for the moment). First, it is important to clarify what question you are asking and which technique will best answer it. For instance, if you need to know whether a gene expressed ubiquitously and in abundance is changing within a tissue, then you will want to take advantage of the quantitative aspects of

Northern Blots. Alternatively, if the gene is widely distributed but rare, you will probably want to exploit the sensitivity of RNase protection assay or quantitative PCR. Often, however, a particular gene may be modulated only in a subset of cells, such as those that express androgen receptors; then you may want to retain the cellular resolution afforded by in situ hybridization. Lastly, it may be that your gene of interest has not even been cloned yet, in which case you must begin by fishing your gene out of the pool and sequencing it.

All of this may sound rather daunting, but in fact the development of techniques for research in molecular genetics has been transformed into a growth industry with simplified kits and reagents that allow virtually any laboratory, no matter how small, to study gene expression. The two most important criteria are attention to detail and excellent laboratory procedure. For example, in all RNA-based work, the investigator must be aware that the enzyme RNase will instantly chew up RNA, so it is important that all glassware and other items be free of this enzyme. Unfortunately, one of the major sources of this enzyme is the oil on your hands, making the use of latex or rubber gloves a must.

Measuring mRNA

Measuring the mRNA level for a particular gene requires having a probe specific to that gene. This allows us to distinguish our needle (i.e., gene) in the haystack (the hundreds of thousands of other mRNAs). The probes come in a variety of types, distinguished mostly by their length and whether they are made of RNA or DNA. If you are lucky, the sequence for your gene of interest is already known and you simply design a probe complementary to the mRNA sequence. What does complementary sequence mean? Remember that DNA is double-stranded, but only one strand of DNA codes for mRNA to synthesize the protein your gene codes for. That strand of DNA is complementary to its mRNA and will bind or hybridize with its mRNA under the right conditions. So you can order a short synthetic stretch of DNA complementary to your mRNA, known as an **oligonucleotide**, from any number of companies.

Sometimes, however, either your gene has not been cloned and sequenced because you are breaking new ground by studying the gastric-brooding frog, or you desire a probe of a different sort which requires you to make it yourself. The most common approach is to use primers selective for a portion of a particular gene to extract a chunk of that gene from the RNA with the use of polymerase chain reaction (PCR). We will discuss these steps in more detail below.

NORTHERN BLOTS

The most direct way to determine how much of a species of mRNA, DNA, or protein you have is to do electrophoresis to isolate and characterize your molecule of interest. If you are doing an analysis of mRNA on your tissue, you would do what is called a **Northern blot**. This odd-sounding procedure is named in response to another technique we will discuss below, the Southern blot, which gets its name from its inventor, E. M. Southern (Southern 1975). Rather than measuring the mRNA as it exists in the cell, the Northern blot technique requires breaking open the cell, extracting the mRNA with chemicals, and then separating it by size using electrophoresis. Electrophoresis refers to passing an electric current through a gel or matrix, which results in molecules separating along a gradient by size. After this step is achieved, the gradient of mRNAs is transferred to a membrane and then this membrane is probed using a radioactively labeled antisense probe for the mRNA (an antisense probe is the complementary sequence of RNA which will bind or hybridize only to the mRNA that mirrors its sequence.) After various washings to eliminate nonspecific hybridizations, the membrane is apposed to X-ray film, and if all has gone well, a band will appear on the film at the location that corresponds to the original place that the mRNA was separated in the gradient on the gel by electrophoresis.

To determine the molecular weight of your particular band, you will use a molecular weight marker that appears as a ladder on the gel and consists of different-sized bands of RNA. If the size of the band corresponds to the known size of your mRNA, then you are in business. The darkness of the band is directly proportional to the amount of mRNA that was in the original sample. For example, say you have the idea that estradiol will stimulate transcription of the gene coding for oxytocin in a particular part of the brain (we will discuss how to isolate parts of the brain in a moment). To test this hypothesis, you will use female rats whose ovaries have been removed. You create two groups, one in which you inject a small amount of estradiol and the other in which you inject the same volume of vehicle, but lacking the hormone (sometimes called the vehicle control). If the hypothesis is supported, you will find a much darker band in the mRNA prepared from the estradiol-treated females than from the vehicle-control females.

In such studies, it is important to have a way of determining that your measure of gene expression is specific. For this you will use a "housekeeping gene," a gene found ubiquitously in all cells and presumably not regulated by estradiol. Actin is a commonly used housekeeping gene that can be probed on the same membrane as the control. An advantage of Northern blot hybridization, as well as of in situ hybridization, is that you can often use the probe from another species if that particular sequence has not been cloned in your species. But unlike in situ hybridization, substantially more tissue is required with Northern blots. This can be a potential drawback when dealing with rare species (like our frog) or endangered species.

It is important to keep in mind that you can never be sure that what you are measuring is newly synthesized mRNA, since changes in mRNA stability or half-life could also result in changes in mRNA levels between conditions. In fact, estrogen has been found to increase the stability of vitellogenin (an egg yolk protein) and, in some cases, GnRH, independent of any effects on transcription. So this caveat must always be borne in mind when using quantitative assays for mRNA levels. Nonetheless, these tools are very powerful and are an important part of the technical arsenal of any neuroendocrinologist.

REVERSE TRANSCRIPTASE POLYMERASE CHAIN REACTION (RT-PCR)

The development of the **reverse transcriptase polymerase chain reaction** (RT-PCR) resulted in a Nobel prize for Kary Mullis in 1993 and depended in large part upon the Nobel prize–winning discovery of an enzyme that would transcribe RNA into DNA awarded to David Baltimore and Howard Temin in 1975. The name of the technique actually describes it quite effectively. We begin by extracting the mRNA from cells, in exactly the same manner as we would do for a Northern blot. The difference in this case is that we add an enzyme called reverse transcriptase, which will transcribe RNA into DNA. In other words, it is the *reverse* of the normal process (DNA to RNA). Once that is accomplished, you have what is known as cDNA or copyDNA. This can then undergo the polymerase chain reaction (Erlich 1991).

The word "polymerase" refers to the enzyme DNA polymerase, an essential enzyme used to copy DNA during cell replication or mitosis. In this case, however, the DNA polymerase is of a special form in that it can tolerate very high temperatures, close to boiling. These special polymerases were discovered in bacteria living in the deep ocean next to vents that release steaming hot water warmed by the earth's core, and in the bubbly cauldrons familiar to any visitor to Yellowstone National Park. The enzymes are called *Vent* polymerase or *Taq* (from *Thermus aquaticus*) polymerase, depending on where they were discovered. The function of these enzymes is to recognize the end of a short stretch of double-stranded DNA formed by the primer and the cDNA and then elongate it so that the entire length of that piece of DNA becomes double stranded. The initial stretch of double-stranded DNA is generated by you, the investigator, by adding the primers discussed below along with free nucleotides and the DNA polymerase.

The key step is that you design the primers so that they are specific only to your cDNA of interest. In other words, with hundreds of thousands of mRNAs present in a cell, this method lets you pick out and amplify just one. These primers are oriented so that their growing ends are directed toward each other. If two such primers flank the target DNA sequence, over a million-fold amplification of a single starting target sequence can be achieved. This is because the amplification comes about as part of a chain reaction, or exponential process. This is achieved by successively heating and cooling the sample so that the double strands of DNA will fall apart (when heated) and then the primers will reanneal (when cooled) and be extended again by the DNA polymerase. Since there is an excess of single-stranded DNA available, each cycle will increase the number of copies, so it is like a chain reaction (figure 2.2). After the reaction is completed, usually allowing for 30 to 35 cycles of amplification, melting, reannealing and amplification, the resulting DNA must be separated by gel electrophoresis and visualized to assure that a band of the appropriate molecular weight has been achieved. In this case, the band is visualized

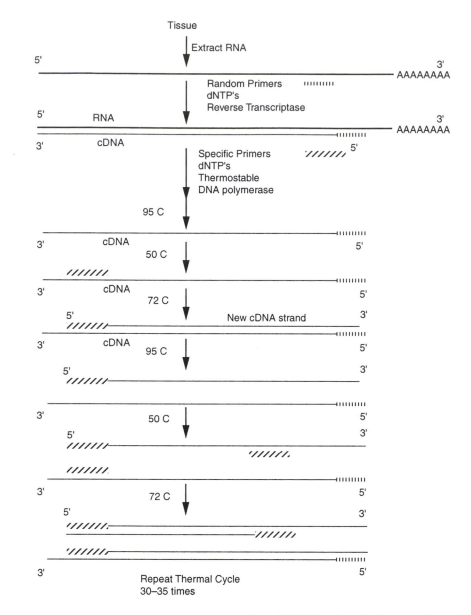

Figure 2.2 Reverse transcriptase polymerase chain reaction: RT-PCR begins with the extraction of RNA from a tissue known to contain an mRNA of interest. This is then converted into DNA using the enzyme reverse transcriptase. The addition of specific primers would then allow for the amplification of only the original mRNA of interest so that it could be selectively amplified from all the others. Repeated cycles of heating and cooling allow for annealing of the primers, primer extension (amplification of the cDNA), and denaturation (separation of the DNA strands so that they can be amplified again). The result is an exponential increase in the rate of synthesis of a particular stretch of cDNA. As indicated in the text, a nested primer strategy will increase the likelihood of obtaining the correct mRNA.

directly in the gel used for electrophoresis by soaking it in ethidium bromide, a chemical that naturally intercalates into double-stranded DNA and fluoresces when exposed to ultraviolet light.

The RT-PCR technique has many uses and, as you can imagine, is extremely sensitive. With this method you are able to detect a single copy of mRNA. Under very carefully controlled conditions, the amount of PCR product produced can be related to the amount of mRNA originally found in the sample and can therefore give a quantitative estimate.

IN SITU HYBRIDIZATION

A frequently asked question in behavioral neuroendocrinology is how do steroids or other stimuli influence the expression, or mRNA levels, of a particular gene. There are a variety of techniques available for quantifying mRNA. We now have the ability to measure the mRNA in an individual cell maintained in its natural place in the brain. *In situ* means "being in place." This is accomplished by first cutting the brain area of interest into very thin slices, usually while the brain is kept frozen. The sections are placed on slides and then a solution that contains a probe for a particular mRNA is pooled on top of the section. This solution optimizes conditions so that the probe can hybridize with the mRNA. Hybridization takes place in airtight plastic containers such as Tupperware lined with moistened paper towels to keep the incubation chamber humid. The container is then placed in an oven and the reaction allowed to proceed overnight at temperatures of 37 to 50 °C. The reason the probe can hybridize to a specific mRNA is that it is a piece of either synthetic DNA or RNA that consists of a nucleotide sequence that is complementary to a portion of the mRNA of interest. In other words, the probe is an antisense sequence to the sense sequence of the mRNA.

A commonly used control is a synthetic sense sequence that is now identical to, not complementary to, the mRNA and therefore will not hybridize. Instead, when the tissue undergoes a series of washes, this sense probe will be washed away. Of course, hybridization kinetics are not perfect and some of the antisense and sense probes will stick to the tissue. As much as possible of this nonspecific hybridization is removed by the washing procedure, which increases by a property known as stringency. By lowering the salt concentration and raising the temperature, i.e., increasing the stringency, it is made increasingly difficult for the nonspecific hybridization to be maintained. When completed, the overwhelming majority of the remaining probe should only be hybridized to the mRNA of interest.

All that is required now is to visualize the remaining probe. In most cases, the probe has been radiolabeled with an isotope attached to one or more of the nucleotides. The probe can then be detected in one of two ways. One way is to appose the slides to X-ray film in the dark for a period of time. This will give an **autoradiogram**, or a film image of the entire section (figure 2.3). Areas where there is a lot of probe will appear dark on the film and areas where

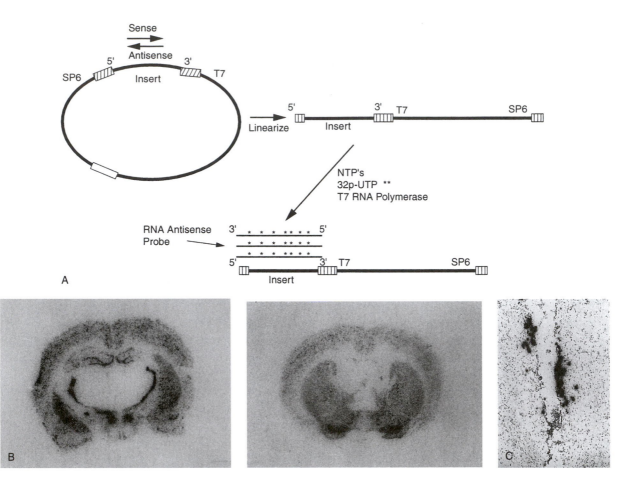

Figure 2.3   In panel (*A*) you see a schematic representation of how a riboprobe used for in situ hybridization detection of an mRNA is generated from a plasmid insert. The circular plasmid is linearized using a restriction enzyme that cuts only one place. Then enzymes specific to the SP6 or T7 promoters will transcribe the insert in either the antisense or sense direction. Radioactive UTP is used in the reaction and incorporated into the probe, which can now be detected by autoradiography or on photographic emulsion. The images in panel (*B*) are autoradiograms made on film by a radioactive probe for the enzyme glutamic acid decarboxylase (GAD), which synthesizes GABA. These are coronal sections, one through the mediobasal hypothalamus and the hippocampus and the other through the preoptic area. Darker areas indicate regions of high mRNA expression, and light areas indicate that little to no mRNA is present. Note how there is a heterogenous distribution of the mRNA for this enzyme throughout the brain. The image in panel (*C*) is a high magnification of cells lining the third ventricle in the turkey brain, which are expressing GnRH. The dark grains are in the emulsion that coats the slide and are generated by the radioactivity released from the probe used to detect the GnRH mRNA in the brain section.

there is little probe will appear light. However, this makes resolution of individual cells impossible.

A second way to detect the probe, which will yield resolution of individual cells, is to dip the slides in photographic emulsion, which is essentially liquid film. This process must be done in the dark. The emulsion is allowed to dry on the slides, which are then stored in light-protected boxes for a period of days to weeks after which the emulsion is "developed" just like a photograph. Only in this case, the photograph consists of small black dots or silver grains that form as the radioactive particles being released by the probe on the tissue pass through the emulsion. The cells themselves are visualized by counterstaining the tissue with a Nissl stain such as cresyl violet. Cells that contain a high level of probe will have lots of silver grains over their surface whereas cells that do not have probe should have few to no grains over their surface. In fact, the number of grains per cell can actually be counted and this can be used as an index of how much mRNA there was in that particular neuron. A comparison can then be made between brain sections from two different conditions, such as male versus female, estrus versus proestrus, and young versus old.

As with all techniques, in situ hybridization histochemistry has its drawbacks. One is that it is considered "semiquantitative," meaning that it is often difficult to obtain highly reliable quantitative data because there are numerous sources of variation in the protocol. A second drawback is that the technique uses radioactivity to interact with the photographic emulsion, which is of concern to many scientists. Methods for conducting in situ hybridization without radioactivity have been developed and are likely to become more common as their resolution is improved. Radioactive in situ hybridization is also a procedure that can take weeks to months to complete (Eberwine et al. 1994). Since you are afraid that the gastric-brooding frog is on the verge of extinction, time is of the essence and it would be advisable to seek a faster technique for quantifying your estrogen receptor mRNA.

RNASE PROTECTION ASSAY

The RNase protection assay is a quantitative method used to measure RNA levels in homogenized tissues or cells which is relatively quick compared to in situ hybridization. The procedure is sometimes called solution hybridization because the hybridization reaction occurs in a solution in the tubes containing samples or standards. This is in contrast to the application of probe to tissues as in in situ hybridization, or hybridization of probe to RNA that has been immobilized on a filter, as in the case of Northern Blot.

In the RNase protection assay, an RNA probe is allowed to hybridize with RNA in extractions of dissected tissues or cell cultures. Additionally, a standard curve is produced using increasing amounts of known sense, or reference, RNA. The antisense riboprobe is allowed to hybridize with RNA in these standards. This standard curve is later used as a basis of comparison for quantification of the absolute amount of RNA in the unknown samples. You may have noticed that this is similar to the technique employed in radio-immunoassay (see chapter 1) in which known amounts of hormones are used to produce a standard curve. One advantage of the RNase protection assay is that it allows absolute as opposed to relative amounts of the RNA to be quantified.

The methodology of the RNase protection assay is as follows: First, a plasmid containing the cDNA sequence of interest is linearized. Often the cDNA insert is cloned into a plasmid containing two RNA promoter sites, one at the 5' end and one at the 3' end, which can be used to make both sense and antisense RNAs. For the antisense RNA, a radiolabelled ribonucleotide (e.g., alpha^{32}P UTP) is used in the transcription of the probe. This radioactivity is later used for quantitation of how much the probe hybridizes with the sample or standards for analysis (McCarthy 1998). Once the probe is made, it is added in excess to the standard curve dilution tubes as well as to the homogenized and extracted RNA samples containing unknown amounts of the specific RNA, such as oxytocin receptor in the rat or estrogen receptor in the whiptail lizard.

The samples hybridize overnight and then a buffer containing a mixture of two RNases is added to the reaction. These RNases are enzymes that specifically digest single-stranded RNA. Thus, any double-stranded hybrids formed by the binding of the probe to the sample or standard are spared from the digestion. However, excess unbound probe and any unbound RNA not complementary to the probe (which is the majority of the RNA in the unknown sample tubes) will be digested by this RNase mixture. It is this step that gives the procedure the name RNase protection assay, or RPA; that is, the double-stranded hybrids are protected from RNase digestion.

After RNase digestion, samples are processed to purify and concentrate the RNA hybrids. The molecules are then separated by molecular size using electrophoresis and the gels exposed to X-ray film to produce an autoradiogram. The amount of radioactivity in the standard curve increases linearly with amount of RNA in the standard, and a regression analysis is performed to relate the amount of radioactivity to the absolute amounts of RNA in the standard curve. This regression analysis is used to calculate how much RNA is in each unknown sample, since the amount of radioactivity in each sample can be quantified, and the amount of RNA extrapolated from the regression curve can be calculated from the standard curve.

Ribonuclease protection assays are quite sensitive and allow detection of RNA amounts as low as picogram (10^{-12}) quantities. Another advantage is that many different RNA transcripts (up to 12 at last count) can be measured in the same sample. This is accomplished using riboprobes of differing molecular sizes. Each probe will hybridize specifically to its complement, thereby enabling multiple RNAs to be quantified without interfering with the hybridization of other probes. During electrophoresis, multiple hybridized RNA bands can be resolved on the gel as long as the probes are different lengths.

Therefore, if we wanted to and we planned correctly, we could simultaneously measure the receptors for estradiol, progesterone, and oxytocin in the same sample of rat brain.

But the brain is a highly heterogeneous structure and not all neurons in an estrogen-concentrating area will have receptors for estradiol, progesterone, and oxytocin; that is, a particular gene might be regulated by estradiol in only a few select cells. Pooling together large chunks of tissue could dilute or wash out any specific effects of the estradiol on individual neurons. This lack of anatomical specificity can be overcome in part, however, if specific brain areas are examined. The most common method is to place thick (~ 300 μM) frozen sections of the brain on microscope slides (making sure they are RNase-free). Then, using a dissection microscope and hollow tubing, usually a spinal tap needle (also RNase-free), you can remove or "punch" those areas of the brain of particular interest (Palkovits 1988). You might think of this as the cookie-cutter method. These punches, which may be a circumscribed brain nucleus like the VMH, can then be assayed. Still, even these procedures do not replace the cellular level of specificity afforded by in situ hybridization.

QUANTITATIVE PCR

We have already discussed the technique of PCR at some length as a tool in cloning. However, given its sensitivity and selectivity, this technique also lends itself to quantification. The procedure is essentially the same as the RNase protection assay with two notable changes. One is that great care is taken to use the exact same amount of starting mRNA for each reaction that is being compared in a particular experiment. The second is that an internal control is included in the reaction. This control can be one of two types. It can be a standard template with its own primers that you include in the reaction and use to compare across reactions. This will control for differences in the rate of the reaction or slight differences in the amount of enzyme, template, nucleotides, and so on that were added to the reaction tube.

Given that PCR involves exponential amplification of mRNA, it is not hard to imagine that small variances in any of these parameters can have big effects on the amount of final PCR product. This approach allows for relative comparison between samples. The second type of control involves creating a competitive template that your primers will compete for. The competitive template is identical to your PCR product of interest but has been mutated so that a large piece is missing. This allows you to distinguish the endogenous PCR product and the template when separated by electrophoresis. This approach has the additional advantage of allowing for the construction of a standard curve (similar in principle to that described for the RNase protection assay) so that the absolute amount of the endogenous mRNA can be calculated. Again, the lack of cellular resolution that comes from homogenizing chunks of tissue can be lessened if micropunches are taken of the target and control brain areas.

Isolating and Cloning a Gene

SOUTHERN BLOTS

A **Southern blot** is essentially the same as a Northern blot with the exception that instead of extracting mRNA from the cell, the genomic DNA is extracted. In general, for behavioral neuroendocrinologists, this technique is used to confirm that a particular gene or allelic variant of a gene is or is not present in one or two copies in a particular animal. The genotyping of transgenic animals uses this technique to determine if an animal is a homozygote, heterozygote, or wild-type.

In fact, unless you limit your studies to a species where the entire genome has been cloned and mapped, at some time in your illustrious career you are likely to need to clone a gene. Let's say you want to know whether an estrogen-receptor gene's expression is controlled by day length, diet, or behavioral interactions. To your dismay, the gene has not yet been cloned in the gastric-brooding frog. This will require you to get out your toolbox of molecular biology tricks, roll up your sleeves, and subclone it yourself.

TISSUE CHOICE AND RNA ISOLATION

In order to isolate your gene, you start with cells that make the product of your gene. First, you choose a tissue that contains abundant levels of the target RNA transcript needed, and then you can use the mRNA to pull out the DNA you are looking for. Let's use a steroid hormone receptor as an example. Since the mRNA of steroid hormone receptors is rare in the brain, you'll want to use another tissue that is rich in the hormone receptor you are interested in—the uterus, for instance, which contains abundant estrogen receptor mRNA that can be enriched further with an injection of exogenous estradiol into the animal. You harvest the tissue and immediately freeze it in liquid nitrogen until enough has been accumulated. Usually several grams are collected, but methods have been developed recently that enable you to suck up the contents of a single cell and apply some of the techniques described below. In most instances, a total RNA preparation is then performed from which the mRNA is isolated, usually comprising only 1 to 2% of the total RNA. This isolation is done by selecting the mRNA from the total RNA using reagents that bind the mRNA at the poly-A tail. Quantification of pure mRNA is then confirmed using an ultraviolet spectrophotometer. With this material in hand you are now ready to do some molecular genetic analyses.

PRIMER DESIGN

Your next step in the cloning process is an intellectual one, the designing of the primers to be used for the PCR which you are going to use again, this time to pull out the DNA you are interested in isolating. If you pick the right primers, your job will be easier. As before, primers are short stretches of synthetic DNA, usually 18 to 22 bases long, that are complementary to a portion of our gene of interest. Remember that all DNA is double stranded, but only one of the strands codes for our gene; the other strand is said to be *complementary*. So, one of our complementary primers is "upstream" on the gene (toward the 5' end) and the other is "downstream" (toward the 3' end). When we do PCR with these two primers, we get a product that is the complementary sequence from the first primer through the end of the second primer. The distance by which they are separated will dictate the size of our PCR product. For instance, if the primers are separated by ~300 base pairs, the PCR reaction will produce a product that is ~300 base pairs long.

The nucleic acid sequence for steroid receptors was first elaborated for conventional animal species such as the mouse, rat, guinea pig, monkey and human. In many instances this work has been extended to domesticated species such as the chicken, dog, pig, cow, and horse, and in some instances, wild species of bird, fish, amphibian and reptile. With this diverse group of species, we find there is substantial overlap at the amino acid level in the DNA-binding and ligand-binding domains; this is called serial homology and usually is expressed as the percentage of amino acid residues identical to the sequence of the mouse, rat, or human (figure 2.4).

Conservation at the amino acid level doesn't necessarily guarantee conservation at the nucleotide level due to the **degeneracy** of the genetic code (some amino acids are coded by as many as six different codons). Even with this caveat, however, the amino acid–sequence information can be used to create degenerate oligonucleotide primers, which usually consist of 10 to 20 nucleotides. These primers will amplify the "sense" or "+" strand and are used in conjunction with an "antisense" or "−" primer, which is the reverse complement of the receptor sequence. When working with steroid receptors, these primer sequences are usually located in the Hormone- or ligand-Binding Domain (HBD) because it is a highly conserved region.

In cloning and sequencing by RT-PCR, sometimes it is advisable to use a "nested primer" approach. The advantage of this strategy becomes apparent when cloning a member of a family of genes, such as steroid hormone receptors. A characteristic of these families is that they share a number of conserved regions or domains that are very similar (e.g., portions of the HBD and the hinge region, the intervening domain between the HBD and the DNA binding domain). In the nested approach there are two rounds of 25 cycles of PCR amplification. The primers in the first round of PCR amplification may amplify not only the desired gene, but also related members of the gene family. This leads to multiple products and more extensive screening to identify the desired target. Using a second pair of primers that lie between, or are internal to, the original pair of primers during the second round of PCR frequently leads to the selective amplification of the desired target.

So, for the case of the gastric-brooding frog, you would design nested PCR primers based on the sequence from the most closely related species you could find. Next, you would isolate some RNA from a collection of steroid hormone–concentrating tissues such as gonads, oviducts, vas deferens, and liver, conduct the PCR under highly permissive conditions, and *voila*! You've got it.

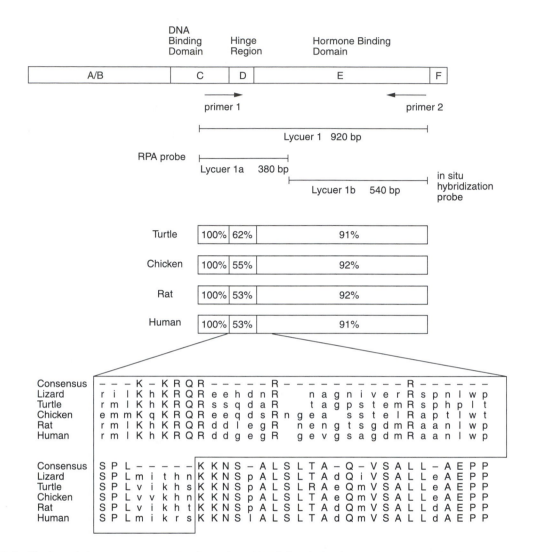

Figure 2.4 Cloning of the estrogen receptor from the whiptail lizard. At the top is a schematic diagram of functional domains of the estrogen receptor cDNA. Below that is a depiction of the clones and subclones generated to characterize the estrogen receptor of the whiptail lizard, *Cnemidophorus uniparens*. The 920 bp PCR clone of the whiptail lizard estrogen receptor spans from the DNA-binding domain to the end of the hormone-binding domain. Subclones of the fragment can be used as probes for RNase protection assay and in situ hybridization, as indicated. The remainder of the figure is a comparison of the deduced amino acid sequence of the whiptail lizard estrogen receptor to published sequences of estrogen receptor of the turtle, chicken, rat, and human. The sequences shown are comparisons of the relatively nonconserved hinge region (boxed) and a portion of the hormone-binding domain. Percentages indicate the degree of serial homology among the different vertebrate species listed. Dashes indicate nonconserved amino acid in the consensus sequence; space indicates an amino acid deletion. (From Young et al. 1994.)

LIGATION OF THE PCR PRODUCT INTO THE PLASMID VECTOR

The next step is to clone the DNA that has just been isolated. To do this, the PCR product must be ligated or joined to a vector for subsequent transformation into a bacterial host. A **plasmid** is a special form of chromosome found in bacteria which is circular and exists outside the nucleus. This unusual feature gives the unique advantage of letting us make lots of plasmid by growing up large numbers of bacteria. The PCR product is inserted into a vector (or plasmid) using enzymes that cut open the circular DNA and then insert the PCR product, creating a recombinant hybrid molecule (figure 2.5). Once transformed into bacteria, these hybrids replicate in the same manner as the original plasmid would. Therefore, as the bacteria multiply, so do the recombinant plasmids within them. The ultimate outcome is the production of large amounts of the clone from the bacterial hosts. Different types of plasmids have been engineered by molecular biologists and can be chosen to fit with your particular experimental needs. You need only thumb through the catalog and go shopping for the right size, style, and color

TRANSFORMATION OF LIGATED VECTOR INTO E. COLI

Once the PCR product has been ligated into the vector, it is introduced into a bacterial host. This process, called **transformation** or transfection, involves the uptake of the exogenous hybrid DNA by the bacteria through its plasma membrane. Bacterial cells that are treated to perform this task are referred to as competent cells. The transformed cells are grown in media and then plated on ampicillin-containing agar plates. Ampicillin, you might recall, is an antibiotic. Since the transformed cells have a gene that confers resistance to ampicillin, only bacteria that have been successfully transformed with the insert will grow. The next thing is to make sure that your cells are producing the gene that you have isolated.

A colorometric assay is often used to provide a second level of selection. For example, a vector may contain a portion of the *lac*Z gene, which normally codes for the enzyme beta-galactosidase. When your cells are grown under the right conditions, white colonies are produced when a recombinant vector containing the *lac*Z gene has been transformed into the host. While the appearance of white cells tentatively indicates that the vector possesses an insert of some sort, it does not guarantee that the PCR insert contained the desired target product (i.e., both the *lac*Z gene and your PCR product). Thus, a number of white colonies must be selected for further analysis by restriction mapping and DNA sequencing to establish the clone that has the desired target gene. Each colony is then digested with restriction endonuclease enzymes that recognize short DNA sequences and catalyze the cleavage of double stranded DNA (dsDNA) at specific sites at or near the recognition sequence. A specific pattern of digestion products is predicted from a known sequence. If the pattern generated experimentally matches that predicted, then you have subcloned what you think you have. A second replica of the original colonies

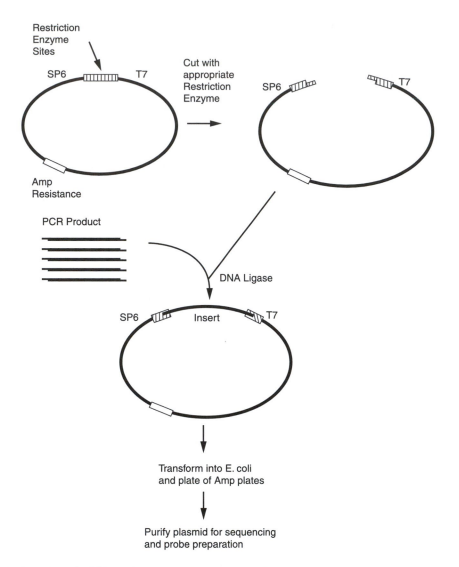

Figure 2.5 Insertion of a PCR product into a plasmid vector. Plasmids are naturally occurring circular pieces of DNA found in bacteria. They contain DNA sequences which can be cut by specific enzymes, called restriction enzymes. The plasmid DNA can be cut at a single site, opening up the circle, and under the appropriate conditions, a piece of DNA that has been generated by PCR can be inserted into this spot and the circle closed again with an enzyme called DNA ligase. The plasmid is then reinserted into its bacterial host and grown in large numbers. This will allow for the subsequent use of the plasmid to generate probes for in situ hybridization, RNase protection assay, and Northern blots.

that does not undergo restriction endonuclease digestion is kept and can be used for additional purposes.

SEQUENCING THE PRESUMPTIVE CLONES

The presumptive clones are sequenced today using kits. For example, a kit may employ the dideoxy-DNA sequencing method from a single-stranded DNA template. In this procedure, the plasmid template is denatured to separate the dsDNA. Oligonucleotide primers added to the reaction tube are allowed to anneal to its target sequence on the clones. A sequencing buffer solution containing a mixture of deoxynucleotides to serve as the reaction substrate is also added to the reaction tube. One of these deoxynucleotides is radioactively labeled with Sulfur-35 to facilitate detection and visualization of the reaction products on an autoradiographic film. The sequencing reaction is initiated by adding the sequencing enzyme to the reaction tube.

The sequencing reaction contents are given a quick spin in a microcentrifuge, which allows the dideoxynucleotides to participate in the sequencing reaction. The sequencing reaction generates a variety of nucleic acid fragments of varying lengths with a fixed 5′ end and variable 3′ ends that depend on when the dideoxynucleotide is incorporated into the nucleic acid. These fragments are then separated on a denaturing polyacrylamide gel, which can resolve single nucleotide bases. Lastly, voltage is applied to the sequencing gel apparatus to separate the nucleic acid fragments. The DNA sequence is then read directly from the autoradiographic film, starting at the bottom of the film and working to the top. This corresponds to the 5′ to 3′ direction, which is the convention for reporting nucleic acid sequences.

If all has gone well, you will be able to read the sequence of your subclone and compare it to the published sequences for large numbers of genes, which are available on the Internet at a site called the Genbank. Using very simple commands, you can compare your sequence to all those already existing and see if there is any match that would indicate significant serial homology. As you can see in figure 2.4, the estrogen receptor cloned from the whiptail lizard is highly homologous to the estrogen receptor of other vertebrates.

Although it is important to understand the basic principles used for nucleotide sequencing, it is unlikely that you will find yourself in the position of ever actually using this technique. The advent of automated sequencers that can efficiently sequence large numbers of nucleotides at a reasonable cost is rapidly making manual sequencing seem as quaint as a black and white television. It is now much more common to send your DNA sample to a sequencing facility which will then e-mail you results that you can quickly check against the databases available at Genbank. All too often you may find you have actually cloned a contaminant from a neighboring lab bench instead of the estrogen receptor of the gastric-brooding frog; however, with greater attention to working on clean surfaces with pure reagents, you will succeed. Once you do clone the desired gene and a probe has been successfully manufactured, you can move on to the process of using it to ask questions about how gene expression changes under various experimental conditions. Several different approaches can be taken at this point, each with its own advantages and disadvantages.

cDNA ARRAYS

We noted previously that the RNase protection assay is sometimes referred to as "solution hybridization" because the assay is carried out in liquid. A variant of this assay involves attaching a template for a particular gene to a substrate, such as a nylon filter, and then allowing your probe to hybridize to this immobilized substrate. This is referred to as "slot blot" hybridization since probes are sometimes administered through a slot in an apparatus.

Recently biotech companies have carried this approach to another level by manufacturing arrays of multiple genes immobilized on a suitable substrate such as glass (DNA sticks to glass). These arrays may contain hundreds of identified genes. The investigator prepares a unique set of probes from each experimental condition, only in this case, rather than being a probe for a single gene of interest, all of the mRNAs represented in a sample are labeled and available to hybridize to the immobilized cDNA array. In this way, if several genes exhibit altered expression, in a particular experimental condition, either down or up, they can be detected simultaneously. The most advanced form of this technology, called "DNA chip technology," involves tens of thousands of genes immobilized on a glass microchip smaller than a postage stamp. These displays look like New York City on a clear night viewed from an airplane. This exciting new technology is likely to change the way we investigate gene expression in the near future.

Techniques for Measuring Proteins

In addition to knowing the levels of gene expression, it is often of equal if not greater importance to assess the level of protein for a particular receptor or gene product. In fact, levels of mRNA do not necessarily translate into equivalent levels of protein. Differences in the rate of translation, stability, and half-life of the mRNA can all contribute to variance between levels of mRNA and protein. Since the protein is one step closer to the physiological outcome, it is often more important to quantify protein levels. Unfortunately, our techniques for measuring proteins are more restricted than those for measuring gene expression.

WESTERN BLOTS

The **Western blot** is analogous to the Northern and Southern blot techniques. The advent of the Western blot heralded a whole new direction in this type of analysis in that it involves the measurement of the actual protein rather than the mRNA or DNA. Most of the steps are essentially the same as for the Northern or Southern blots, except that the cellular content extracted is protein instead of nucleic acids and the probe consists of an antibody to the protein rather than a synthetic antisense RNA or DNA.

The procedure requires the generation of an antibody to a particular protein, which is accomplished by injecting a pure form of the protein into another species, which will recognize it as foreign (i.e., an antigen) and make antibodies to it. A commonly used species for antibody production is the rabbit, which will be injected with rat or human estrogen receptor or whatever other protein is of interest, such as oxytocin receptor. This would be referred to as a rabbit-anti-rat antibody and is the **primary antibody**. Fortunately, this primary antibody can often be used in a variety of other species but that has to be determined on an experimental basis. An antibody made for estrogen receptor in the whiptail lizard might very well work in the gastric-brooding frog, but it just as well might not.

The primary antibody is labeled with a substrate for an enzyme that when reacted will release light and can therefore be detected by X-ray film in the same manner as radioactivity. Again a molecular weight ladder of proteins of various sizes must be used to confirm that your band appears at the appropriate place, and more problematically, that there is only one band. The latter criterion is particularly important since antibodies are notorious for their ability to crossreact with more than one protein. Nonetheless, this can be an extremely powerful approach. For instance, although you may see a 50-fold increase in the mRNA levels of the progesterone receptor following estradiol treatment, this does not mean there has been a commensurate change in the receptor protein levels. By using a Western blot you can confirm or deny that there is a similar level of change between mRNA and protein.

IMMUNOCYTOCHEMISTRY
We have just discussed the use of Western blot to measure protein in chunks of whole tissue. This is an antibody-based procedure and, if you are lucky, the same antibody used in a Western blot can also be used for immunocytochemistry. As its name implies, immunocytochemistry is an antibody-based procedure; however, it involves maintaining the integrity of the cell so that proteins can be visualized in their appropriate intracellular location. It also allows for an assessment of cellular heterogeneity within the brain where one neuron may express a particular protein, such as the estrogen receptor, but the neuron immediately next door may not.

Immunocytochemistry requires two antibodies. First, the primary antibody, which is generated to the protein you want to visualize. Then it is necessary to have a secondary antibody, which is made in another species. The secondary antibody serves the purpose of recognizing all antibodies made by the first species. So, for instance, a goat will be immunized against a rabbit, and this is referred to as goat-anti-rabbit and is the **secondary antibody**. The secondary antibody is conjugated to some sort of signal marker, such as a biotin-strepavidin, or more commonly, to an enzyme such as alkaline phosphatase, which due to its catalytic nature will amplify the signal. In the case of alkaline phosphatase, the substrate is diaminobenzadine (DAB) which when reacted makes a brown reaction product that allows us to visualize the antibody.

Sometimes secondary antibodies are conjugated to fluorescent markers and can be visualized directly using a fluorescence microscope.

In either case, it is the secondary antibody we actually see, not the primary, but we can see it only if we have conjugated some signal marker to the secondary. The careful reader might now ask, but why use the secondary antibody at all? Why not just visualize the primary antibody? There are two reasons. One is that conjugating a signal molecule to the primary antibody could easily compromise its ability to bind to the target antigen, such as the estrogen receptor. The second is that the chemical procedure of labeling the antibody is wasteful, because up to half the antibody can be lost in the procedure. Antibodies generated against an entire species, such as goat-anti-rabbit, can be obtained by the proverbial bucket load, whereas a highly selective antibody to estrogen receptor in the gastric-brooding frog might only be generated by the thimbleful. So we take advantage of the ease of generating secondary antibodies to help us in visualizing our precious primary antibody.

The good news is that many primary and secondary antibodies are commercially available and kits containing all the ingredients you need for immunocytochemistry make these procedures fairly straightforward these days. If all goes well, only those cells containing our protein of interest will bind the primary antibody, and therefore the secondary as well, and we will be able to see which cells selectively have the protein. However, it is difficult to make quantitative statements about proteins visualized in this manner and we usually have to resort to an "all or none" or "high versus low" statement. Sometimes under very carefully controlled conditions, comparisons can be made between treatments so that one animal can be said to have relatively more protein/cell than another does. The development of new quantitative ("stereological") techniques has enabled a more reliable quantitative analysis of amounts of protein visualized by immunocytochemistry.

CIRCUIT MAPPING WITH THE USE OF IMMEDIATE EARLY GENES
One avenue in which immunocytochemistry has proven to be of great benefit is in the detection of what are known as **immediate early genes**. This refers to a family of genes that are some of the first turned on in response to a stimulus. These genes are often not detected until the cell is stimulated; in other words they are "inducible." The most famous and frequently used of these is *fos*, and its protein product Fos. Also of frequent interest are the gene *jun* and its protein product Jun. Just like steroid receptors, Fos and Jun are transcription factors, and they can interact (dimerize) with each other and, in the case of Jun, with themselves. Fos/Jun and Jun/Jun dimers then interact with the DNA at a particular place on a gene called an AP-1 site, where AP stands for "activator protein". Steroid receptors, such as the estrogen receptor and the glucocorticoid receptor, can also interact with Fos/Jun complexes and thereby indirectly influence transcription at AP-1 sites.

Because they are transcription factors, Fos and Jun are nuclear proteins and they are readily visualized by immunocytochemistry. In the nervous system, when a neuron is activated or "depolarized" it will frequently express the *fos* gene as a consequence. The usual time course is an increase in Fos protein by 30 minutes, with levels diminishing within 2 to 4 hrs (there is a rapid negative feedback loop between Fos protein and *fos* gene expression). This attribute has proven of great benefit to behavioral neuroendocrinologists since it can be used to essentially map which neurons are activated in response to the expression of a particular behavior or exposure to a particular stimulus. For instance, when female rats display the sexually receptive posture of lordosis, neurons in the ventromedial hypothalamus and preoptic area express high levels of Fos (Flanagan-Cato and McEwen 1995; Auger et al. 1996; Pfaus et al. 1996). Similarly, male rats exposed to the odors of a sexually receptive female exhibit high levels of Fos in the amygdala (Coolen et al. 1997).

A further advantage of Fos immunocytochemistry as a marker for neuronal activation is that in many cases it can be combined with assays for a cytoplasmic protein, allowing the investigator to establish the neurochemical identity of a particular cell. For instance, you may wish to know whether oxytocin neurons are particularly activated following mating behavior. The picture in figure 2.6 demonstrates the activation of GnRH neurons occurring at the time of the LH-surge in a female rat (Hoffman et al. 1990). Many examples of the use of Fos as a marker will be apparent throughout the text.

IN VITRO RECEPTOR AUTORADIOGRAPHY

There is one other way to visualize proteins in the brain that can be very useful and is quantitative, but it is restricted to the detection of receptors. Most commonly, this technique is used for peptide receptors, such as those for neurotransmitters. The approach is quite simple. Very thin slices of the brain mounted on glass slides and maintained at a cold temperature are incubated in a buffer containing the ligand of interest and binding is allowed to occur. The ligand is tagged with a radioisotope such as tritium (^{3}H) or iodine 125 (^{125}I). After a series of washes to remove the unbound ligand, the slides containing the tissue sections are apposed to isotope-sensitive film, which is placed in the dark and allowed to expose for a number of days to weeks (short for iodine, long for tritium). When the film is developed, there is an image of where in the brain the ligand is bound to the receptor. For example, the GABA-A receptor is distributed widely throughout the brain, whereas the oxytocin receptor is found more selectively in the amygdala and ventromedial hypothalamus of the female rat (figure 2.7). If a set of standards with which to generate a standard curve is included in the assay, absolute amounts of the protein can be quantified using a technique called densitometry, which simply refers to measuring the density of signal of a particular area on the film. One drawback of this technique with peptide receptors is that cellular resolution is lost because the image of the brain slice obtained is not of sufficient resolution to allow the detection of individual cells.

Steroid receptors can also be visualized by receptor autoradiography but with some challenging twists. The incubation and washing procedures

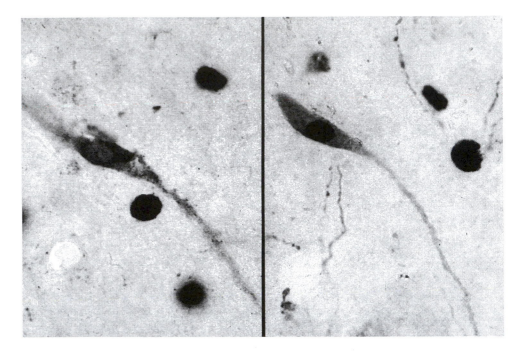

Figure 2.6 Combined immunocytochemistry for Fos and GnRH. The immediate early gene Fos is a nuclear protein and appears as a dark black circle. It is detected by a conventional immunocytochemical technique but enhanced with nickel sulfate to appear black. The lighter-stained material in the cell cytoplasm is the neuropeptide GnRH, also detected by conventional immunocytochemistry and having a grayish caste. These are cells from the preoptic area. The panel on left is from a brain just before the LH-surge, and you can see there is no Fos protein in the nucleus. The panel on the right is from a brain at the time of the LH-surge, when GnRH neurons are activated, as evidenced by the Fos signal in this neuron. Note that other cell types are also activated, as indicated by the presence of a dark nucleus, but the neurochemical identity of those cells remains unknown. (Courtesy of G. E. Hoffman.)

routinely used as a part of this technique will uncouple the steroid ligand from its receptor and all resolution will be lost. Therefore, the steroid ligand must be injected into the animal and allowed to bind in vivo. Remember that the ligand is radioactive, which makes it expensive (mostly because of the costs of disposal, not synthesis), so when using mammals such as rats or monkeys, it is usually given to the animal via an indwelling catheter into the jugular vein; with relatively small animals weighing 20 grams or less, the radioactive hormone can be injected in the peritoneal cavity. After an hour or so, the animal is killed and the brain removed and sliced very thin (10–20 μM thick), a process called "sectioning", which is also used for in situ hybridization and immunocytochemistry. However, in this case, the sections must be placed onto slides that are already coated with emulsion, the liquid film we referred to above in the section on in situ hybridization. It is important not to expose the emulsion to light, which would defeat the whole purpose. Thus, the brains must be sliced and placed on the emulsion-coated slides in the dark.

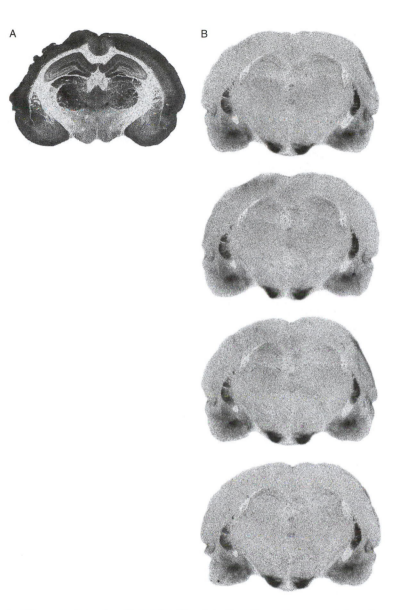

Figure 2.7 In vitro receptor autoradiography. The detection of membrane receptors for neurotransmitters in the brain can be accomplished with the use of a radioactive ligand. Brain slices placed on glass slides are incubated in a buffer containing the ligand and the excess removed by washing. The slides are then exposed to X-ray film for a period of time and an image of where the ligand has bound is obtained. Panel (*A*), on the left, shows the distribution of the GABA-A receptor, which is broadly distributed throughout the brain, and panel (*B*), on the right, is for the oxytocin receptor, which exhibits a relatively restricted distribution, being mostly expressed in the ventromedial nucleus of the hypothalamus.

Fortunately, a dim red light will not excessively expose the emulsion so the investigator has some assistance, avoiding an epidemic of fingerless behavioral neuroendocrinologists. After a period of exposure in the dark (sometimes for months), the slides are developed the same way as for in situ hybridization, and those cells which contain steroid receptors will have a dense collection of silver grains over their surface. This technique was used to generate the first atlas of estrogen-concentrating cells in the brain (Pfaff and Keiner 1973), which remains a valuable resource to this day.

Techniques for Altering Gene Expression

The origin of changes in behavior, physiology, and morphology in many cases stems from changes in gene expression. Understanding the underlying genetic mechanisms has put us in the position where we can alter the patterns of gene expression. Here we describe some of the most commonly used methods.

So far we have been talking exclusively about the ability to measure differences in mRNA or gene expression under varying conditions. Throughout this book, points will be made about the important contribution of expression of a particular gene to the manifestation of a hormonally influenced behavior. Traditionally, these types of inferences could only be made by comparing genetically distinct strains of animals or by correlating changes in gene expression with changes in behavioral states. The last decade or so has presented an array of new tools to the behavioral neuroendocrinologist, which allow the investigator to selectively manipulate the genome or gene expression of individual animals. Some manipulations result in permanent alterations in the genome of an animal, whereas others involve only temporary and restricted changes.

Transgenics

What is a **transgenic animal**? In Webster's New Collegiate Dictionary, one of the many definitions attributed to the word "trans" is "beyond, across, so as to change." In that light, the term transgenic could not be more apt since it refers to an animal that has received a gene from beyond itself or across species, which changes its phenotype. Transgenic sheep, cows, goats, chickens and fish have all been generated. But by far the most popular and most successful has been the transgenic mouse. The making of a transgenic animal requires equal parts of molecular biology, reproductive endocrinology, and animal husbandry.

The process of making a transgenic animal is relatively straightforward. Step number one is the creation of the desired DNA "construct," or, more simply, gene. This gene may be a mutated form of a naturally occurring gene that will be over-expressed, and thereby swamp the effect of the normal gene (often called a "dominant negative"), or it may be a normal allelic variant of a gene. Alternatively, it might be a gene that codes for cytotoxic molecules or even a bacterial gene used as a marker for other cellular processes. What genes can be used to generate transgenics is limited only by the imagination of the investigator (Fukamizu 1993). However, in order for the **transgene** to be expressed, it must contain all the necessary accoutrements that accompany the coding sequence of any gene. These include the promoter region, which may or may not be tissue specific, the 5' and 3' untranslated regions, and the polyadenylation site that codes for the poly-A tail necessary for stability of the mRNA. Creating this DNA construct may sound like an overwhelming task best left to the molecular jocks, but in fact with the increasingly available technology, it is essentially a cut-and-paste operation accessible to all life scientists.

The second major step is the preparation of the mouse. This actually requires two female mice, one to be the donor of the fertilized eggs into which the transgene, or DNA construct, will be injected, and one to serve as the incubator for the injected eggs. The first female is induced to superovulate (produce more than the usual number of eggs) by treatment with the gonadotropins FSH and LH, allowed to mate normally with a fertile male, and then her fertilized eggs are harvested before the first cleavage. This results in the demise of the original female, so another female must be tricked into thinking she is pregnant (a physiological state called pseudopregnancy) to receive the transgenic embryos.

The third critical step is the difficult business of injecting the transgene into the fertilized eggs. The site of injection is the male pronucleus formed after the sperm fuses with the egg. Usually about 100 to 300 copies of the transgene are microinjected using a microscope at 200× magnification and a micromanipulator. As you might imagine, this is not a trivial process and is usually performed by highly trained experts skilled in this particular technique.

The last step is taken by nature. During the normal processes of recombination and meiosis, the transgene is randomly inserted into the genome of the embryo. The number of copies of the gene inserted may vary from 1 to 200, although when multiple copies are inserted it is usually in a head-to-tail orientation at the same site. Since the integration of the transgene occurs before the first cell division, all the cells, including the germ line, will be heterozygous for the transgene. The ultimate level of expression of the transgene can vary greatly between animals and depends on such factors as the number of copies, the site of integration, and the intrinsic efficiency of the transgene promoter.

Only a small percentage of the injected embryos will ever become live mouse pups and actually express the transgene. Those select few that do reach this status are termed "founders." The next step is to mate founders with wild-type mice to generate some heterozygote offspring. These, as well as the founders, can be identified by extracting DNA from a small piece of the mouse's tail and probing for the presence of the transgene by PCR or Southern blot. Once the F1 heterozygotes have been identified, they are mated to each other to generate homozygotes and the arduous process of assessing the phenotype can begin. The protocol for generating a transgenic mouse is illustrated in figure 2.8.

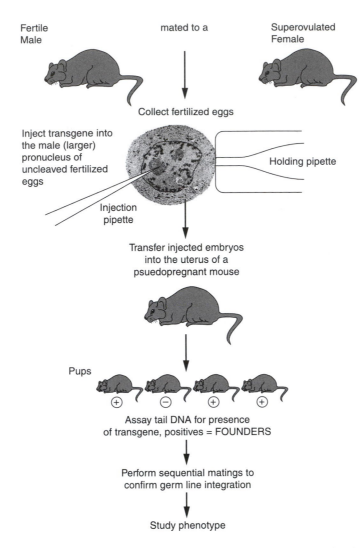

Fertile Male · mated to a · Superovulated Female

Collect fertilized eggs

Inject transgene into the male (larger) pronucleus of uncleaved fertilized eggs

Holding pipette

Injection pipette

Transfer injected embryos into the uterus of a psuedopregnant mouse

Pups

⊕   ⊖   ⊕   ⊕

Assay tail DNA for presence of transgene, positives = FOUNDERS

Perform sequential matings to confirm germ line integration

Study phenotype

Figure 2.8 Generation of a transgenic mouse. A female mouse is superovulated to maximize the harvesting of fertilized embryos following mating to a fertile male. These eggs are then directly injected with multiple copies of the transgene and then inserted in the uterus of a pseudopregnant female. Once the pups are delivered, they must be genotyped to test for the presence of the transgene by extracting DNA from a small piece of the tail. The transgene is detected by PCR or Southern blot. If positive, the animals are grown to adulthood, mated to wild-type mice, and heterozygous offspring obtained. These heterozygotes can then be bred together to generate homozygotes and the phenotype characterized. (Adapted from Shuldiner 1996.)

Knockouts

What is a **knockout mouse**? Basically, a knockout mouse is a specific type of transgenic mouse in which a naturally occurring gene is disrupted, rather than allowing a pre-constructed gene to be inserted randomly into the genome (Galli-Tallidoros et al. 1995). The terms "gene disruption," "gene targeting," and "targeted gene replacement" all refer to the process by which a specific gene is manipulated via homologous recombination. This refers to a naturally occurring process in which identical sequences (homologs) will align and be recombined. The experimenter constructs a gene in which portions are homologous to the targeted gene but other portions are severely mutated or missing. When this construct lines up with the naturally occurring gene on the chromosome, in a small number of cases it will be substituted for that gene.

Unlike the generation of transgenic animals, knockouts do not begin with a fertilized egg but start with embryonic stem cells (ES cells). Stem cells are the precursors to the germ cells of the mature gonad. The DNA construct that will be used for homologous recombination is referred to as the "targeting vector." In addition to containing the mutated or disrupted gene, the targeting vector includes markers that will allow for the selection of the ES cells that have incorporated the gene into the correct site and thereby disrupted the naturally occurring gene of choice. This selection procedure is usually based on resistance to antibiotics. So, for instance, the disrupted gene might contain what is called a "neomycin-resistance cassette," with neomycin being a commonly used antibiotic. When the stem cells are treated with the neomycin, only those that contain the cassette, and hence the transgene, will survive. This is not because stem cells are bacteria, but rather because most antibiotics act by blocking gene transcription or protein translation and the cells will quickly die without these cellular processes.

After this selection procedure, the ES cells that meet criteria are inserted into a developing mouse embryo at the blastocyst stage (this is when the embryo has formed a fluid-filled ball with a knot of cells at one end that eventually will become the developing fetus). This recipient embryo is of a different strain than the mouse strain that the ES cells came from. It is important to be able to distinguish the strains, so strains having different coat colors are used; if working with fish, the investigator will use strains with different pigmentation patterns. The embryos are implanted into a host female and, when they grow to the point of developing hair, the mice that have the ES cells incorporated can be detected by their coat color. The chimeric (multicolored) males are mated to wild-type females to generate heterozygotes, as before, which in turn are mated. Mendelian genetics insures that one in four offspring will carry the disrupted gene in both alleles of the gene, i.e., a homozygous knockout.

The nomenclature for these animals is often an acronym for the gene, such as ER for estrogen receptor, followed by the traditional genomic nomenclature for dominant versus negative genes, only in this case they refer to wild type versus knockout. So ER−/− is a homozygous knockout, ER−/+ is a heterozygote, and ER+/+ is a wild-type littermate. If heterozygotes having different null mutations are mated, it is possible to obtain "double knockouts," or offspring that will carry disruptions in both genes. To continue with the estrogen receptor example, recently mice have been generated with both the estrogen receptor α and the estrogen receptor β knocked out (Ogawa et al. 2000).

To date, the technology for generating knockout vertebrate animals has been limited to mice and zebra fish and in invertebrates to fruitflies and worms; and this situation may remain for some time. However, major progress is being made in overcoming one of the frequent criticisms of this technology, namely, that the organism lacks the gene throughout its lifespan. For example, an ER α−/− mouse develops and grows up without a functional estrogen receptor α. Thus, estrogen-dependent changes in behavior may be due to the pleiotropic consequences of missing that gene rather than due to the gene's function during adulthood. Recently the development of tissue-specific and temporally constrained knockouts has enabled the researcher to control where and when a particular gene can be turned on or off. These preparations are sometimes called "conditional knockouts" or "tissue-specific knockouts" and, while difficult to produce at this time, will no doubt be a valuable and frequently used tool in the very near future.

ANTISENSE OLIGONUCLEOTIDES

Elegant in its simplicity, **antisense technology** exploits the fact that single-stranded mRNA will hybridize with a complementary sequence of synthetic DNA. You can use antisense sequences of DNA with in situ hybridization to visualize where mRNA has been made, or you can use antisense sequences to look at the functional consequences of preventing gene expression. The formation of a duplex between the antisense sequence and mRNA in the animal will disrupt the ability of the mRNA to be translated into protein. Because the formation of the duplex is dependent on the sequence specificity of the genetic code, it is theoretically possible that one and only one gene product will be disrupted (figure 2.9). The requirements for the investigator are relatively few. If the sequence of the targeted mRNA is known, then a short piece (15 to 20 bps) of synthetic DNA can be ordered from any number of companies or university facilities. So after subcloning and sequencing the estrogen receptor from the gastric-brooding frog, you can order up your antisense. This antisense **oligonucleotide** (a generic term for a short synthetic stretch of DNA) is injected directly into the brain and a behavioral endpoint is monitored.

There are a number of advantages to antisense technology in behavioral neuroendocrinology (McCarthy 1998; Stein and Krieg 1998; McCarthy et al. 2000). For instance, a gene product can be selectively reduced in only one brain region and only for a short period of time. However, the gene product can only be reduced, not knocked out, and sometimes it can only be reduced

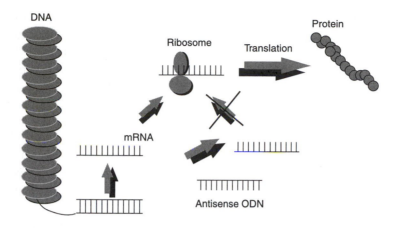

Figure 2.9 Antisense technology. A short (15–22 mer) piece of synthetic DNA that is complementary to mRNA is known as an antisense oligonucleotide and can be used to selectively disrupt gene expression. The antisense oligo is administered directly into the brain where it gains access to cells. There it will hybridize with its complementary mRNA, and only that mRNA, and will prevent it from being translated into protein. This process may involve a variety of mechanisms, including the prevention of proper splicing of the mRNA, blocking of the ribosomal complex that is needed to transcribe the mRNA and inducing the degradation of the mRNA by selective enzymes. (Drawing by A. P. Auger.)

by 20 to 30%. In addition, the investigator must conduct numerous controls to demonstrate a lack of general toxicity before a conclusion can be reached regarding the role of a particular gene product in a behavioral response. These would include making sure that general locomotion has not been impaired and that animals continue to eat well and lack any signs of overt illness, which have been witnessed following some antisense treatments (Spanagel et al. 1998). Nonetheless, because the primary action of steroid hormone receptors is inducing gene expression, this technique has been very informative in the field of behavioral neuroendocrinology.

VIRAL VECTORS

In some circumstances it would be useful if an antisense construct could be continuously expressed, rather than administered intermittently as is most commonly done. This has been achieved by actually infecting neurons with viruses that then express at high levels an antisense that is mRNA (rather than DNA). The most commonly used viruses are the adenovirus and the herpes simplex virus, both of which have been inactivated so that they cannot replicate and wreak the havoc that viruses so often do. The generation of additional virus is accomplished by growing them in special cell lines that possess the replication proteins that the virus is missing. The use of these viruses is similar to that of the plasmids we discussed earlier in that they are vectors and we can insert our gene construct of choice. This can be an antisense construct or some other variant of a naturally occurring gene; it could even be an unmodified gene that we simply want to try and express in a different part of the brain (Kaplitt et al. 1993; Akli et al. 1993). The virus carrying our gene construct is then injected into the brain where it is taken up by neurons in a process called transfection, just like transforming bacteria with plasmid. Not all cells will take up the virus so we make sure that it also expresses a marker protein that we can detect, such as green fluorescent protein or beta-galactasidase. This approach is just beginning to be used by behavioral neuroendocrinologists.

Summary

In this chapter we have reviewed some of the basic principles of hormone action and the techniques commonly used for measuring gene expression in behavioral neuroendocrinology. We have also discussed recently developed techniques that allow for the control of gene expression, either by knocking out or overexpressing specific genes, or by temporarily dampening translation of mRNA into protein. These points can be summarized as follows:

1. Peptide hormones bind to receptors on the cell membrane. There are three basic types of these receptors: kinases, G-protein coupled, and ligand-gated ion channels. Different receptor types are linked to specific signal transduction pathways, but there is overlap and crosstalk between these pathways.
2. Steroid hormones combine with nuclear receptors and together they are integral components of a transcription complex that induces gene expression.
3. Steroids and their receptors can interact with proteins in the membrane and in the cytoplasm and modulate gene expression indirectly.
4. In order to study the expression of a gene it is necessary to know its nucleotide sequence. This may require subcloning the gene and sequencing it yourself.
5. Once the nucleotide sequence is known, levels of mRNA can be measured by in situ hybridization, Northern blot, RNase protection assay, or quantitative PCR. Each approach has distinct advantages and disadvantages.
6. Specific proteins can be measured by Western blot, immunocytochemistry, or in the case of receptors, autoradiography. Again, each approach has distinct advantages and disadvantages.
7. Transgenic mice are animals in which a novel gene has been inserted and is expressed in addition to, or instead of, a naturally occurring gene.
8. Antisense technology is a tool for temporarily dampening the translation into protein of a particular mRNA.

Study Questions

1. What is the difference between the mode of action of steroid and peptide hormones?
2. What techniques are available for studying gene expression and why would you choose a particular approach?
3. What techniques are available for measuring protein levels and why would you choose a particular approach?

4. How are transgenic animals generated and what advantages do they offer to a behavioral neuroendocrinologist?

References

Albers, B., Bray, D., Lews, J., Raff, M., Roberts, K., and Watson, J. D. (1994) Cell signaling. In *Molecular Biology of the Cell*. New York: Garland Publishing, pp. 721–785.

Akli, S., Caillaud, C., Vigne, E., Stratford-Perricaudet, L. D., Poenaru, L., Perricaudet, M., Kahn, A., and Peschanoki, M. R. (1993) Transfer of a foreign gene into the brain using adenovirus vectors. *Nature Genet.* 3: 224–228.

Auger, A. P., Moffatt, C. A., and Blaustein, J. D. (1996) Reproductively-relevant stimuli induce fos-immunoreactivity within progestin receptor-containing neurons in localized regions of female rat forebrain. *J. Neuroendocrinol.* 8: 831–838.

Auger, A. P., Tetel, M. J., and McCarthy, M. M. (2000) Steroid receptor coactivator-1 (SRC-1) mediates the development of sex-specific brain morphology and behavior. *Proc. Natl. Acad. Sci. USA* 97: 7551–7555.

Coolen, L. M., Peters, H. J. P. W., and Veening, J. G. (1997) Distribution of fos immunoreactivity following mating versus anogenital investigation in the male rat brain. *Neuroscience* 77: 1151–1161.

Eberwine, J. H., Valentino, K. L., and Barchas, J. D. (1994) *In Situ Hybridization in Neurobiology. Advances in Methodology*. New York: Oxford University Press.

Erlich, H. A. (1991) *PCR Technology. Priniciples and Applications for DNA Amplification*. New York: W. H. Freeman.

Flanagan-Cato, L. M., and McEwen, B. S. (1995) Pattern of fos and jun expression in the female rat forebrain after sexual behavior. *Brain Res.* 673: 53–60.

Fukamizu, A. (1993) Transgenic animals in endocrinological investigation. *J. Endocrinol. Invest.* 16: 461–473.

Galli-Talidadoros, L. A., Sedgwick, J. D., Wood, S. A., and Korner, H. (1995) Gene knock-out technology: A methodological overview for the interested novice. *J. Immuno. Meth.* 181: 1–15.

Hawkins, M. B., Thornton, J. W., Crews, D., et al. (2000) Identification of a third distinct estrogen receptor and reclassification of estrogen receptors in vertebrates. *Proc. Natl. Acad. Sci. USA* 97: 10751–10756.

Hoffman, G. E., Lee, W. S., Attardi, B., Yann, V., and Fitzsimmons, M. D. (1990) LHRH neurons express c-fos after steroid activation. *Endocrinology* 126: 1736–1741.

Kaplitt, M. G., Rabkin, S. D., and Pfaff, D. W. (1993) Molecular alterations in nerve cells: Direct manipulation and physiological mediation. *Curr. Topics Neuroendocrinol.* 11: 169–191.

McCarthy, M. M. (1998) *Modulating Gene Expression by Antisense Oligonucleotides to Understand Neural Functioning*. Boston: Kluwer.

McCarthy, M. M., Auger, A. P., Mong, J. A., Sickel, M. J., and Davis, A. M. (2000) Antisense oligodeoxy-nucleotides as a tool in developmental neuroendocrinology. *Methods* 22: 239–248.

Mermelstein, P. G., Becker, J. B., and Surmeier, D. J. (1996) Estradiol reduces calcium currents in rat neostriatal neurons through a membrane receptor. *J. Neurosci.* 16: 595–604.

Ogawa, S., Chester, A. E., Hewitt, S. C., Walker, V. R., Gustafsson, J. A., Smithies, O., Korach, K. S., and Pfaff, D. W. (2000) Abolition of male sexual behaviors in mice lacking estrogen receptors α and β (αβERKO). *Proc. Natl. Acad. Sci. USA* 97: 14737–14741.

Palkovits, M., and Brownstein, M. J. (1988) *Maps and Guide to Microdissection of the Rat Brain*. New York: Elsevier.

Pfaff, D. W., and Keiner, M. (1973) Atlas of estradiol-concentrating cells in the central nervous system of the female rat. *J. Comp. Neurol.* 151: 121–158.

Pfaus, J. G., Marcangione, C., Smith, W. J., Manitt, C., and Abillamaa, H. (1996) Differential induction of Fos in the female rat brain following different amounts of vaginocervical stimulation: Modulation by steroid hormones. *Brain Res.* 741: 314–330.

Razandi, M., Pedram, A., Greene, G. L., Levin, E. R. (1999) Cell membrane and nuclear estrogen receptors (ERs) originate from a single transcript: Studies of ERalpha and ERbeta expressed in Chinese hamster ovary cells. *Mol Endocrinol.* 13: 307–319.

Rollerova, E., and Urbancikova, M. (2000) Intracellular estrogen receptors, their characterization and function. *Endocrin. Reg.* 34: 203–218.

Sambrook, J., Fritsch, E. F., and Maniatis, T. (1989) *Molecular Cloning. A Laboratory Manual,* 2nd edition. Cold Spring Harbor Laboratory Press.

Sanger F., Nicklen S., and Coulson, A. R. (1977) DNA sequencing with chain-terminating inhibitors. *Proc. Natl. Acad. Sci. USA* 74: 5463–5467.

Shuldiner, A. R. (1996) Molecular medicine. Transgenic animals. *N. Engl. J. Med.* 334: 653–654.

Singh, M., Setalo, G., Guan, X., Grail, D. E., and Toran-Allerand, C. D. (2000) Estrogen-induced activation of the mitogen-activated protein kinase cascade in the cerebral cortex of estrogen receptor-α knock-out mice. *J. Neurosci.* 20: 1694–1700.

Southern, E. M. (1975) Detection of specific sequences among DNA fragments separated by gel electrophoresis. *J. Mol. Biol.* 98: 503–17.

Spanagel, R., Schobitz, B., and Engelmann, M. (1998) Non-specific effects of centrally administered oligonucleotides. In M. M. McCarthy (Ed.), *Modulating Gene Expression by Antisense Oligonucleotides to Understand Neural Functioning,* Kluwer Academic, pp. 27–41.

Stein, C. A., and Krieg, A. M. (1998) *Applied Antisense Oligonucleotide Technology.* New York: Wiley-Liss.

Xu, J., Liao, L., Ning, G., Yoshida-Komiya, H., Deng, C., and O'Malley, B. W. (2000) The steroid receptor coactivator SRC-3 (p/CIP/RAC3/AIB1/ACTR/TRAM-1) is required for normal growth, puberty, female reproductive function, and mammary gland development. *Proc. Natl. Acad. Sci. USA* 97: 6379–6384.

Young, L. Y., Lopreato, G. F., Horan, K., and Crews, D. (1994) Cloning and in situ hybridization analysis of estrogen receptor, progesterone receptor, and androgen receptor expression in the brain of whiptail lizards (*Cnemidophorus uniparens* and *C. inornatus*). *J. Comp. Neurol.* 347: 288–300.

3 Sexual Differentiation of the Brain and Behavior

S. Marc Breedlove and Elizabeth Hampson

The final introductory chapter is made necessary by a quite fundamental fact of life on this planet: sex. Almost all of the more complex animals on earth are either male or female, and this difference has remarkably wide-ranging consequences for both physiology and behavior. The processes that lead to external and internal differences between the sexes are fairly well understood, and, as you will see, hormones play a pivotal role in these differences. We even know something about how the brains of males and females came to be different, but deciding how those differences affect behavior remains a challenge.

How do males and females develop differently, what controls those differences, and when do they arise? What biological factors influence sex differences in behavior, and are such factors at work in humans? How might environmental and biological influences interact during the development of sex differences?

Introduction

Every toddler quickly learns that humans come in two basic anatomical packages. Thereafter, the tendency to classify animals, people, and inanimate objects (e.g., boats, cars, and so on) and their behavior as either feminine or masculine becomes, for most of us, deeply ingrained and virtually reflexive. We're used to thinking that the ultimate criterion for gender is based upon external genitalia: is there a penis or a vagina? But many other parts of the body, including the brain, are also different in males and females and, as we shall see, it is possible for an individual to be masculine in some body regions and feminine in others.

We will explore what is known about how males and females develop different bodies, brains, and behaviors—a process known as "sexual differentiation." The principles for the development of sex differences in the body have already proven to be very much the same for humans as for other mammals. However, when we consider sex differences in behavior and the structure of the nervous system, it has been more difficult to decide whether the processes at work in other animals apply to humans. Our strategy will be to gain a firm understanding of sexual differentiation in animal models and then see which mechanisms apply to humans. Chapter 7 will discuss the ways in which sexual differentiation in some nonmammalian vertebrates (frogs, electric fish, and songbirds) is similar to, and the ways in which it is different from, mammals.

Sexual Reproduction

Almost all vertebrates reproduce sexually. However, you should keep in mind that mammals are the minority and that for most animal species on this planet (i.e., invertebrates), there is only one sex. Some animals can reproduce by **parthenogenesis** (literally "virgin birth"). These parthenogenetic females give rise to daughters that are genetically identical to the mother. You will learn more about a parthenogenetic vertebrate in chapter 7. Many invertebrate species (e.g., slugs, worms, and jellyfish) are **monoecious** (all individuals are alike) and **hermaphrodites** (each individual has both male and female reproductive organs and can reproduce as either or both). Note that, unless the hermaphrodite self-fertilizes, it is still reproducing sexually.

On the other hand, almost all vertebrates and many invertebrate species are **dioecious** (there are two distinct sexes). Another term with a similar meaning is "gonochorism"—the specialization of **gonads** (i.e., ovaries or testes) in the two sexes to produce different **gametes** (i.e., eggs or sperm) for reproduction. Sexual reproduction, by combining chromosomes from different individuals, clearly helps to bring together in a single individual many advantageous mutations which arose in many separate individuals (Bodmer 1970). However, evolutionary theorists have yet to reach a consensus on why almost all vertebrates reproduce sexually.

Sex Determination

You probably already know that sex chromosomes normally determine whether we develop as boys or girls. The mother's egg always contains one X chromosome, and if it is fertilized by a sperm carrying another X chromosome, the baby will be a female, but if the father contributes a Y chromosome, the baby will be a male. These rules of **sex determination** hold for mammals, and will be discussed below.

First, however, you should be aware that the mechanisms of sex determination vary dramatically across other vertebrates. In birds, the female has two different sex chromosomes (known as W and Z), while the male has two Z chromosomes. Consequently, it is the mother's contribution that determines the sex of the offspring, depending upon which sex chromosome was carried by the egg before fertilization. Some reptiles have sex chromosomes, but in other reptile and amphibian species, it is the temperature at which the eggs are incubated that determines the sex (Bull and Vogt 1979).

Among the invertebrates, many species have no sex determination at all since, as mentioned above, each individual has both sets of reproductive organs. Other invertebrates have two distinct sexes and, like mammals, use sex-determining chromosomes—for example, the well-studied fruit fly, *Drosophila melanogaster*. Finally, some invertebrate species have some individuals that are hermaphroditic, while other individuals are one sex or the other.

Sexual Differentiation in Mammals

The process during development through which an individual becomes either male or female is known as sexual differentiation. How does the presence of the Y chromosome cause male development and the absence of a Y chromosome result in female development? The chain of events during sexual differentiation is well understood in placental mammals such as ourselves, and was largely worked out by Alfred Jost in the 1950s and 1960s (Jost 1979). A simplified summary is that genetic sex determines gonadal sex, and gonadal sex determines phenotypic sex. Recall that an individual's **phenotype** is the sum total of all the physical characteristics she or he possesses. Clearly our phenotype changes with time, and we call those changes across time "development" or "ontogeny" or "aging." In contrast, our **genotype**, that is, the sum total of all genetic information contained in our DNA, is fixed at fertilization. Except for rare mistakes in duplication in cells which continue to divide throughout life, our genotype does not change. So what do we mean by saying genetic sex determines gonadal sex which determines phenotypic sex?

Genetic Sex Determines Gonadal Sex

The Y chromosome does not seem to do very much (as many people have guessed). Early in development, both XX and XY individuals have gonads that do not yet resemble either testes or ovaries, and are therefore called "**indifferent gonads**" (figure 3.1A). The one crucial task performed by at least one gene on the Y chromosome is the transformation of this originally indifferent gonad into a testis. This gene on the Y chromosome is called the **sex-determining region of the Y** (*Sry*). If the cells of the indifferent gonad contain a Y chromosome with the *Sry* gene, they begin to develop as a testis. In the absence of a *Sry* gene, the gonad will develop as an ovary. Thus, genetic sex (whether the individual is XX or XY) determines gonadal sex (whether there will be ovaries or testes). Thereafter, the rest of sexual differentiation will be driven not by the sex chromosomes directly, but by the hormones secreted by the gonads.

Gonadal Hormones Determine Phenotypic Sex

If the indifferent gonad develops as an ovary, it appears to secrete very little hormone prenatally, and the fetus develops into a female. But if the gonad develops into a testis, several hormones will be secreted, and these hormones instruct the rest of the body to develop in a masculine fashion. Thus genetic sex, via the presence or absence of *Sry*, determines gonadal sex, which, via hormonal secretions, determines phenotypic sex. In other words, differences between males and females arise indirectly, as a function of the hormones secreted by the gonads, not under the direct influence of sex chromosomes.

ANTI-MÜLLERIAN HORMONE

Two testicular hormones drive masculine development: the steroid hormone testosterone and the peptide hormone known as anti-müllerian hormone (AMH), also known as müllerian-regression hormone or müllerian-inhibiting substance. At first, both XX and XY individuals have two sets of ducts connecting the indifferent gonad to the exterior: the müllerian ducts and the wolffian ducts (figure 3.1A). AMH is secreted only by testes and, true to its name,

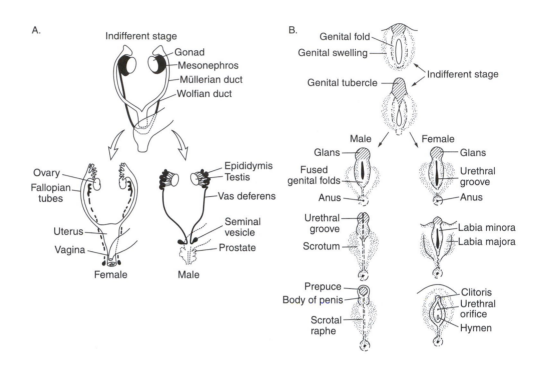

Figure 3.1 Fetal development of male and female reproductive tracts. (*A*) Early in development (*top*), internal organs are "indifferent" because they appear identical in the two sexes. Two duct systems, the müllerian and the wolffian, connect the indifferent gonads to the body wall. In females (*lower left*), the müllerian ducts grow and differentiate to form the fallopian tubes, the uterus, and the inner portion of the vagina. In males (*lower right*), it is the wolffian ducts that develop, forming the epididymis, vas deferens, and seminal vesicle; the prostate arises from nearby tissues. (*B*) External genitalia also begin as indifferent (*top*). In males (*left*), the genital tubercle grows to form a penis, and genital folds fuse, forming the scrotum and enclosing the urethral groove to form the urethra. In females (*right*), the genital tubercle develops into the clitoris, and genital folds form the labia and outer vagina. Hormones drive this sexual differentiation of the urogenital system. (From Wilson et al. 1980.)

causes the müllerian ducts to regress. Ovaries do not secrete AMH and consequently the **müllerian ducts** in females develop into the fallopian tubes, uterus, cervix, and inner vagina. In adult females, these structures form the pathway through which the ripened egg will be fertilized, the embryo will be nurtured, and the fetus brought to the outside world.

TESTOSTERONE

The second testicular secretion directing sexual differentiation is the steroid hormone **testosterone (T)**. T has masculinizing effects on many parts of the developing body including, as we will see later, the brain. One effect of T is the acceleration of development in the wolffian ducts—a process known as virilization. In the absence of T, the wolffian ducts will remain only as tiny remnants. But with T stimulation, the **wolffian ducts** form the epididymis, vas deferens, and seminal vesicles in males. In the adult male, these structures lead from the testis to the penis and deliver sperm for reproduction.

T also directs the masculine development of the genital skin into the penis and scrotum (the pouch of skin that holds the testes). In the absence of T, these genital regions will form a clitoris, the outer vagina, and the labia surrounding the vagina (figure 3.1B). An enzyme called **5-α-reductase**, which is present in the genital skin and converts T to **dihydrotestosterone (DHT)** (figure 3.2), amplifies the masculinizing influence of T on the external genitalia. DHT binds the androgen receptors more effectively than T does, and thus the reductase enzyme serves to locally amplify the effects of androgen. We know that the virilization of the wolffian ducts does not require this amplification because little or no reductase is found there during that period.

Anomalies in Sexual Differentiation

Occasionally individuals are born with an abnormal complement of sex chromosomes. **Turner's syndrome** results when only a single sex chromosome is present (denoted as XO). Such individuals develop abnormal but recognizable ovaries and, in the absence of testicular secretions, a feminine body. Unfortunately, they also usually suffer from reduced IQ and other defects that result from the poorly understood consequences of having only one X. No individuals have been found without any X—that is, there are no known cases of YO, which indicates that such a condition is lethal during early development. In XXY (**Klinefelter's syndrome**) or XYY individuals, the gonads develop as testes and result in a masculine phenotype, again with reduced IQ and sterility. These chromosomal abnormalities underscore the simple rule that when a Y chromosome is present, the indifferent gonads will develop as testes.

On the one hand, sexual differentiation appears rather simple since testicular secretions drive masculinization. However, in order to produce the male phenotype, *Sry*, two hormones (AMH and testosterone), many enzymes (including 5-α-reductase and the enzymes needed for steroid manufacture), and several receptors (those for androgen and those for AMH) must all be expressed by the individual's genes. Thus, there are many steps where a missing or defective gene can cause things to go awry. Because such mistakes are not lethal, each has been found in humans (table 3.1).

TESTICULAR FEMINIZATION MUTATION
One interesting anomaly in sexual differentiation is the **testicular feminization mutation (TFM)**, usually referred to in humans as **androgen insensitivity syndrome (AIS)**. These individuals have a defective structural gene for the androgen receptor and therefore they fail to respond to androgen. The gene for the androgen receptor is on the X chromosome. Some females carry the TFM mutation on one X chromosome, and have a normal androgen receptor gene on the other X chromosome. Half of the eggs produced by such a carrier will receive the X with the TFM gene. If an X-bearing sperm fertilizes such an egg, another female carrier will result. But when a Y-carrying sperm fertilizes an egg with the TFM gene, anomalies arise. The resulting offspring will develop testes (due to normal *Sry* activity from the Y), and the testes will

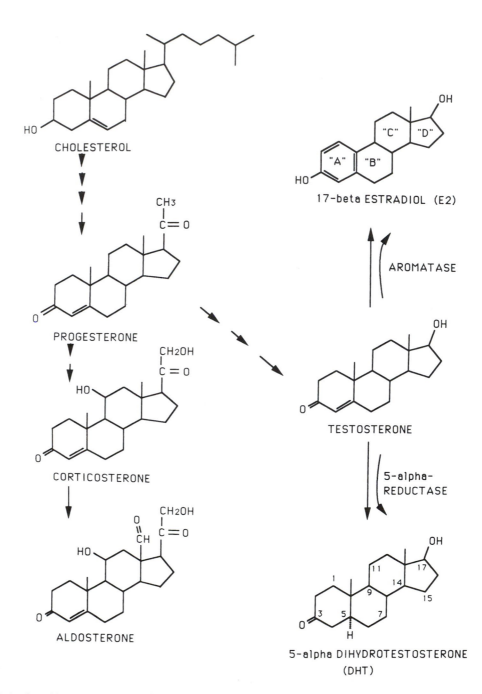

CHOLESTEROL

17-beta ESTRADIOL (E2)

PROGESTERONE

CORTICOSTERONE

ALDOSTERONE

AROMATASE

TESTOSTERONE

5-alpha-
REDUCTASE

5-alpha DIHYDROTESTOSTERONE
(DHT)

Figure 3.2 Steroids are synthesized from cholesterol that is either eaten or manufactured from simpler compounds. Cholesterol (*top left*) consists of four connected rings of carbon atoms. In chemical convention, each line represents a bond between carbon atoms and double lines represent double bonds, but most of the Cs are omitted for clarity. Cholesterol can be converted to progesterone via four chemical reactions (represented by four arrows), each catalyzed by a specific enzyme. Progesterone in turn can be converted to the glucocorticoid called corticosterone, which in turn can be converted to the mineralocorticoid aldosterone (*bottom left*). Alternatively, a series of enzymes can

Table 3.1   Possible Genetic Defects Resulting in Abnormal Sexual Phenotype

Predict for each of the cases below the sexual phenotype of the following structures: gonads, müllerian duct features, wolffian duct features, and external genitalia. Later, after we have discussed sex differences in neural structure, you may want to deduce whether they would appear feminine or masculine in these instances. We provide an answer for the first two cases.

1. An XY individual in which both testes fail to develop (or are removed).

Here you would predict that there would be no gonads and, in the absence of anti-Müllerian hormone, the müllerian duct structures would develop in a feminine fashion and, due to the absence of androgen, wolffian ducts and external genital features would be phenotypically female.

2. An XY individual in which one testis fails to develop (or is removed).

The single testis should produce enough androgen to masculinize, at least partially, the external genitalia and wolffian duct structures. It turns out that anti-Müllerian hormone (AMH) must act locally, because when this experiment is performed, the müllerian duct structures partially develop on the side where the testis is removed.

3. An XX individual in which both ovaries fail to develop.

4. An XY individual in which androgen receptors are absent (i.e., TFM).

5. An XY individual in which the enzyme 5-α-reductase is absent.

6. An XO individual (Turner's syndrome).

7. An XY individual in which AMH is defective or absent.

8. An XY individual in which AMH receptors are defective or absent.

9. An XY individual with an additional X chromosome (47 XXY; Klinefelter's syndrome).

10. An XY individual with an additional Y chromosome (47XYY).

secrete AMH, which will cause the müllerian ducts to regress. Furthermore, the testes will also secrete T but, because the individual lacks functional androgen receptors, the genital epithelium fails to respond to the androgen and therefore develops in a feminine fashion, that is, with a clitoris, labia, and a shallow vagina. Thus, individuals will be born looking like normal females, and in humans they may not be detected until puberty, when the absence of menstruation brings the attention of a doctor.

Androgen-insensitive humans look, act, and think of themselves as females, despite their XY genotype, testes, and infertility. TFM defects have also been found in mice, rats, cats, and goats (Stanley et al. 1973). One aspect of sexual differentiation unique to humans that is illustrated by androgen insensitiv-

Figure 3.2   (continued)

transform progesterone to testosterone (T) (*middle right*). The various carbon atoms of steroids are numbered by convention (*lower right*). The enzyme 5-α-reductase acts to reduce the number 5 carbon atom by adding a hydrogen atom to it. This hydrogen is added in the "alpha" position, meaning that it projects slightly below the plane of the figure (indicated by a broken line). A hydrogen atom is also added to the number 4 carbon (not shown), and hence the result is known as dihydro-testosterone (DHT). 5-alpha DHT is an important androgen. If the hydrogen is added to the number 5 carbon in the beta direction (catalyzed by 5-β-reductase), the resulting 5-beta DHT has no biological activity. An enzyme called aromatase, because it aromatizes the "A" ring of carbon atoms, converts T to 17-beta estradiol (E2) (*upper right*). The hydroxy group (OH) attached to the number 17 carbon atom is in the "beta" position, meaning that it projects slightly above the plane of the figure. 17-alpha estradiol has no biological activity. The conversion of T to either estrogen or DHT is a one-way process, i.e., neither E2 nor DHT are converted back to T.

ity is the development of breasts. The extent of breast development seems to depend on the ratio of estrogens to androgens—the higher the ratio the greater the development. These steroids have their greatest effect upon breast development during puberty, exerting only subtle effects thereafter. Human TFM individuals typically develop phenotypically female breasts, because their testes and adrenals secrete small amounts of estrogen. This does not amount to much estrogen, but due to inadequate androgen receptors, the *functional* ratio of estrogens to androgens is high. There are also instances of incomplete androgen insensitivity that result in an intermediate sexual phenotype that may be obvious at birth.

CONGENITAL ADRENAL HYPERPLASIA

Sexual differentiation of genetic females can also be perturbed by early exposure to androgen. The most common such syndrome is **congenital adrenal hyperplasia (CAH)**, so-called because the individuals are born with enlarged adrenal glands. These individuals lack one of several enzymes needed to produce cortisol from the adrenal cortex. Because there is little cortisol to provide negative feedback, the hypothalamus releases more corticotropic releasing hormone (CRH). This causes the pituitary to release more adreno-corticotrophic hormone (ACTH). Consequently, the adrenal gland grows larger (hence the term "hyperplasia," an excessive number of cells) and releases more steroid hormone in response to ACTH. However, some of the precursors that would normally be converted to cortisol are instead made into androgen as a spill-over product. Since the adrenal cortex is unable to make cortisol to bring CRH and ACTH levels back down, this high androgen secretion will continue unless the individual is treated. When this prenatal condition occurs in females, their bodies are exposed to androgen and are therefore partially masculinized—that is, the phallus is intermediate in size between a clitoris and a penis, while the folds of skin appear intermediate between labia and scrotum. We call such a configuration, which is intermediate between normal male and female phenotype, an **intersex phenotype**.

Administering exogenous cortisol will reduce ACTH release and thereby halt any further androgen production, but will not undo the fetal masculinization of the periphery. Such individuals are usually identified at birth and recent treatment has been to surgically reduce the phallus to resemble a more normal clitoris. Such individuals are sometimes referred to as hermaphrodites. This term is not quite correct because they do not possess testes and, unlike true hermaphrodites, cannot reproduce as males. Thus, CAH cases are more properly called "pseudo-hermaphrodites." Not so long ago, they were often untreated and they and their families experienced a good deal of confusion about their actual gender. Today there are adult CAH women who were surgically altered as babies, and many of these adults advocate avoiding surgery until the children are adults and can make their own decisions about whether to have surgery.

OTHER SYNDROMES

Some XY individuals lack either AMH or the receptors to respond to AMH. Such individuals look like men, but abdominal surgery (for unrelated reasons) reveals a moderately developed uterus and remnants of fallopian tubes!

Especially intriguing human examples of abnormal sexual differentiation are those cases where inadequate 5-α-reductase (which is required to convert testosterone to DHT in the external genitalia) is produced by an XY fetus. A child with such **reductase deficiency** is born with intersex genitalia—labia-like folds of skin (with testes inside) and an enlarged clitoris. This partial masculinization is presumed to be the result of testicular testosterone acting without the amplification provided by reductase in the external genitalia (Imperato-McGinley et al. 1974). The individuals are usually raised as females, but at puberty the rise in testicular androgen secretions causes the phallus and scrotum to grow and the body to develop in a male fashion, that is, with narrow hips, a malelike chest, a muscular build and, eventually, a slight beard growth. This genetically transmitted condition is fairly common in one area of the Dominican Republic where such individuals are known as *guevedoces* or "eggs (slang for testes) at 12." Once the testes descend at about age twelve, these individuals start wearing male clothes, assume male tasks, and have girlfriends. We will come back to this syndrome later in the chapter.

In summary, for placental mammals, sex chromosomes guide the development of the gonads, and then gonadal secretions coordinate the sexual differentiation of the body. Both males and females have the capacity to respond to the masculinizing influence of testicular secretions, and both male and female bodies can develop in a feminine fashion in the absence of those hormones.

Ovulatory Competence in Rodents

Testicular steroids also masculinize the ability to ovulate. The first demonstration that early steroids could permanently masculinize the nervous system took place in 1933, but was not originally recognized as such. It was known that the pituitary was crucial for **ovulation** (i.e., the production and expulsion of a mature egg), because when the pituitary was removed, ovulation ceased. Furthermore, when bits of ovary were implanted in the chamber of the eye (a hospitable environment because it is so highly vascularized) of female rats, the ovarian fragments would still ovulate. This finding demonstrated that hormones alone could control ovulation, even when the nerves innervating the ovary were cut. We will discuss ovulatory cycles further in chapter 4. But when Carol Pfeiffer (1936) implanted bits of ovary in the eyes of male rats, the fragments did not ovulate. Pfeiffer very reasonably concluded that the male rats' pituitary could not support ovulation.

Pfeiffer then went on to show that testicular secretions in the first few days of life determined whether a rat would later, as an adult, be competent to induce ovulation. When male rats were castrated shortly after birth, they would support ovulation (in surgically implanted ovaries, of course) as adults. When newborn female rats were given subcutaneous grafts of testicular tissue, they could not support ovulation as adults in either their own or surgically provided ovaries. (Later experimenters showed that a single injection of testosterone during the first week of life had the same effect as a testicular graft: the rat became permanently incompetent to support ovulation.) Pfeiffer concluded that exposure to androgen early in life somehow masculinized the pituitary and that ovulatory incompetence was an indication of the masculinization that took place.

OVULATORY COMPETENCE IS CONTROLLED BY THE BRAIN

In the meantime, Geoffrey Harris was championing the idea that while the pituitary was the "master gland" for regulating hormone secretion, it was in turn being controlled by the brain. The idea that the brain plays a role in triggering ovulation was supported by the existence of **induced-ovulators** (such as rabbits and cats; see chapter 4). In these animals, ovulation is triggered by the stimulation of copulation itself. Rabbits could be induced to ovulate by gently stimulating the vagina and cervix with a blunt glass rod. These findings indicated that the nervous system must be somehow involved in the control of ovulation. Since there were no nerve fibers from the brain to the anterior pituitary, Harris proposed that the sensory stimulation of copulation eventually reached a part of the brain called the **hypothalamus** and that the hypothalamus in turn released some chemical factor to stimulate the pituitary. Harris and others had previously noted that the hypothalamus was close enough to the pituitary to allow such chemical control. In fact, electrical stimulation of the hypothalamus could itself induce ovulation. Harris's vision of hypothalamic domination of the pituitary was amply confirmed (Harris 1964) (see chapter 1).

Did Pfeiffer's hormone manipulations of rats masculinize the pituitary or the hypothalamus? Harris proved that the pituitary of male rats could, in fact, support ovulation. He removed the pituitary of the female rat and, in a very demanding surgery, implanted the male rat's pituitary in its place. If he succeeded in getting the blood supply (that is, the hypothalamic-pituitary portal system) to the pituitary, the rat could support ovulation (Harris and Jacobson 1952). This result proved that the male's pituitary was competent to support ovulation.

Pfeiffer's experiments therefore needed to be reinterpreted. By elimination, one would conclude that the brain, probably the hypothalamus, had been permanently altered, made incompetent for ovulation, by early androgen exposure. This idea would eventually be proved correct. Specifically, for ovulation to take place, the female rat's hypothalamus must release a surge of GnRH in response to estrogen stimulation. This transient **positive feedback** effect of estrogen on GnRH differs from the more usual case when steroids inhibit further GnRH release (the negative feedback described in chapter 1). The pulse of GnRH causes the pituitary to release a pulse of LH, which causes the ovary to expel the egg. We now know that the hypothalamus of male rats does not show the positive feedback effect and therefore does not release the pulse of LH needed for ovulation.

Interestingly, primates differ from rodents in this regard. Males can show a positive feedback response to estrogen. In fact, male monkeys receiving an ovarian implant can support ovulation (Norman and Spies 1986). No one knows why primates differ from rodents in this way. But in rodents, the same testicular signals that instruct the body to develop a male phenotype also masculinize (or, more properly, defeminize (Whalen 1982)) the brain to prevent ovulatory capacity.

Reproductive Behavior

Testicular steroids early in life masculinize behavior and the absence of androgens results in the feminization of sexual behavior. This has been studied extensively in rodents, where for copulation to take place the female must arch her back to elevate the rump and head and, in species that have a tail, move the tail to one side (see figure 1.1). This posture, called **lordosis**, can serve as a measure of the female's receptivity to mating.

ACTIVATIONAL EFFECTS OF GONADAL HORMONES ON THE BRAIN

As you will learn in more detail in chapter 4, normally female rodents exhibit the lordosis reflex in response to mounting from a male only during a particular part of the ovulatory cycle. When the ovaries are removed, the animal becomes behaviorally unreceptive (i.e., she fails to exhibit lordosis). You can cause a female rat to become receptive again by giving her injections of estrogen for 1 to 2 days, and then a single injection of progesterone. This regimen simulates the sequence of steroids normally produced during the ovulatory cycle. Approximately 6 hours after the progesterone injection, the female becomes receptive—that is, for a few hours she will display the lordosis posture in response to the mounting of a male. We say that the estrogen and progesterone **activate**, or have an **activational influence** on, the lordosis behavior.

When the same hormonal regimen that activates behavioral receptivity in ovariectomized females is given to a castrated male, the male shows almost no lordosis in response to another male's mounting. (Normal male rats will readily mount and thrust their pelvis against the backside of just about any other rat they bump into, especially if that rat is smaller. If the mounted rat is a male and, as in the case just mentioned, fails to show a lordosis response, the first male will eventually stop mounting him.) The fact that males are not induced to show lordosis after being given the same hormones that activate lordosis in females indicates that male and female rats must be different. Because the CNS mediates behavior, it seems likely that the nervous system holds the difference. In other words, the male and female nervous systems are not alike in their behavioral responsiveness to hormone.

ORGANIZATIONAL EFFECTS OF GONADAL HORMONES ON THE BRAIN
Charles Phoenix, Robert Goy, Arnold Gerall, and William Young (1959) asked
whether the same factor that masculinized the bodies and ovulatory competence of rodents also masculinized their ability to show a lordosis response
to adult steroids. They found that female guinea pigs that had been exposed
to testosterone prenatally showed little or no lordosis behavior when given
estrogen and progesterone in adulthood. This result inspired the **organizational hypothesis**, namely, that early androgens permanently alter the developing brain, causing it to function in a masculine manner in adulthood. In
other words, sexual differentiation of the nervous system, and consequently
behavior, is guided by the same steroid cues that drive sexual differentiation
of the body. These organizational effects of steroids, permanently altering the
developing nervous system, were often contrasted with the activational effects
of steroids, transiently influencing the adult brain.

Testicular steroids normally exert a masculinizing influence on the body
early in development, during the first trimester of pregnancy in humans.
After that time, androgens come to be increasingly less effective, so that by
adulthood, steroids can exert only modest effects on these structures. Little is
understood about why the body stops responding to steroids, but restricted
sensitive periods such as this are common in development. The organizational hypothesis proposed that the nervous system, too, was sensitive to the
masculinizing influence of steroids for only a brief period in development.
In rats, for example, injections of testosterone on the day of birth or up to the
tenth day of life can render a female anovulatory and unlikely to display lordosis. However, by the twelfth day of life, even large doses of steroids have
little effect on these measures.

The organizational hypothesis had an immediate and profound effect upon
the field of behavioral endocrinology. Many researchers tried to see whether
other sex differences in adult behavior were determined by early androgen
exposure. In each case, the prediction was clear—exposure of young animals
to androgen should make their behavior more masculine in adulthood, while
the absence of early androgen should result in more feminine (and less masculine) adult behavior. Furthermore, particular behaviors could be affected
by steroid treatment only during a sensitive period, which varied from species to species and for different behaviors. Although there were some interesting exceptions (Arnold and Breedlove 1985), these predictions were often
borne out for many other behaviors (e.g., taste preferences, aggression, rough
and tumble play, and masculine copulatory behavior).

The organizational hypothesis presented a nice clear picture: the same
hormonal signals that guided the sexual differentiation of the genitalia also
guided the sexual differentiation of the brain. So individuals with penises
will not bother with the neural circuitry to support ovulation or display lordosis behavior, while those individuals with vaginas will develop lordosis
"circuits" and therefore show the sex-appropriate behavior. In the case of
both the genitalia and the nervous system, androgen secretions from the fetal

testes drive masculine development. If you expose a newborn female rat to androgen, it may be too late to cause a penis to develop, but she will grow up unable to support ovulation and unlikely to display lordosis. If you deprive a newborn male rodent of his testes, he will still have a penis in adulthood (because the testes did their prenatal work), but he will act like a female: given the right hormones in adulthood, he will show lordosis behavior.

Aromatization of Testosterone to Estrogen

Paradoxically, early estrogen treatment can also masculinize the CNS. Not only will a single injection of T permanently masculinize the behavior of a newborn female, but so will a single injection of estrogen! Such early estrogen treatment has little or no effect on genitalia, but drastically masculinizes ovulatory competence and lordosis behavior (Feder and Whalen 1965; Booth 1977). In fact, microgram for microgram, **estradiol** (**E2**) was more effective than T for masculinizing ovulation and lordosis behavior. These findings at first challenged the organizational hypothesis. Why should an ovarian steroid cause masculinization? Why don't estrogens from the newborn female's ovaries (or prenatal estrogen from the mother's ovaries) masculinize them normally? The organizational hypothesis was rescued from these vexing questions by a very helpful offspring: the **aromatization hypothesis**.

The chemical structure of T and E2 are very similar. In fact, T can be converted to E2 by a single chemical reaction, the substitution of an hydroxy-group for a double-bonded oxygen and simultaneous losses of a hydrogen atom and a methyl group. These substitutions make the A ring resemble benzene, a process that chemists refer to as "aromatization" (see figure 3.2). Originally this term referred to the fact that benzenelike compounds were literally aromatic (fragrant). The aromatization of T to E2 is greatly facilitated by the enzyme **aromatase**. Importantly, the reverse reaction, converting estrogens back to T, is energetically very expensive, very rare, and functionally insignificant. These biochemical facts of life mean that tissues containing aromatase can convert T to E2 and thereby make use of estrogen receptors.

It was soon demonstrated, in adult (Naftolin and MacLusky 1984) and newborn (Reddy et al. 1974) rats, that the hypothalamus contained aromatase. Furthermore, when rats were injected with radiolabeled T, a small but significant amount of radiolabeled estrogen appeared in the brain (McEwen and Krey 1984), and some of that estrogen was bound to estrogen receptors. Thus, systemic T could wind up stimulating estrogen receptors in the hypothalamus. The aromatization hypothesis proposed that it was, in fact, the aromatized, estrogenic metabolites of testosterone that masculinized the developing rodent brain by acting upon estrogen receptors rather than androgen receptors. That was why injections of E2 to newborn females could permanently render them anovulatory and less likely to display lordosis. If it seems paradoxical to you that a "feminine" hormone like estrogen could be responsible for masculinization, remember that both sexes normally secrete the same steroids, albeit in different proportions. Also remember that T is a normal

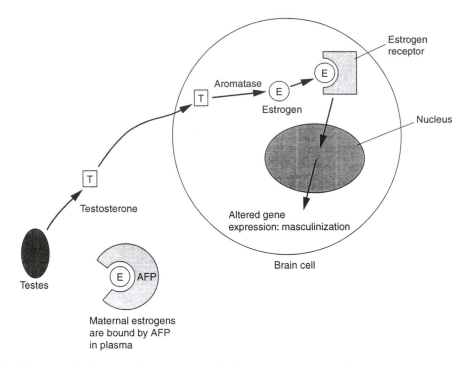

Figure 3.3 The aromatization hypothesis is that testicular androgens such as T can sometimes be aromatized in the brain by the enzyme aromatase to form estrogens, such as estradiol. The estradiol can then bind to and activate estrogen receptors (rather than androgen receptors) to trigger a chain of events. There is excellent evidence that the perinatal rodent brain is masculinized through such an aromatization of androgens to estrogens. T, testosterone; E, estrogen; AFP, alpha-feto-protein. (From McEwen and Krey 1984.)

precursor for the synthesis of estrogen. It seems that natural selection shows no concern for our labels of what is feminine or masculine.

The Role of Alpha-Feto-Protein

There was a problem with this theory of course—how do females normally escape masculinization? While the ovaries of fetuses and newborns secrete very little steroid, all fetuses are exposed to rather high levels of estrogens produced by the mother's ovaries during pregnancy. (Steroids readily pass through the placental barrier.) What prevents these maternal estrogens from masculinizing female offspring? A protein called **alpha-feto-protein (AFP)** was found in the plasma of perinatal rodents. AFP binds estrogen but not testosterone. AFP works in rat fetuses of both sexes to bind maternal (or fetal) estrogen and limit its entry to the developing brain (figure 3.3). The male fetuses circumvent this barrier by secreting T, which bypasses AFP. The T enters brain cells, where it is locally aromatized to estrogen beyond the reach of AFP, and triggers (via estrogen receptors) some cascade of events that prevents the normal expression of ovulation and lordosis. Injections of exogenous estrogens swamp the AFP molecules, allowing some estrogen to reach the brain. Interestingly, while a clear homologue of rodent AFP is found in primates, it does not bind estrogen. As we will see, this and other findings cast doubt on the role of aromatization in the masculinization of the human CNS.

In several situations hormonal crosstalk between mother and fetus or between fetuses can affect sexual differentiation. For example, farmers have known for centuries that a female calf born with a male twin may be sterile as an adult. The likelihood that such cows, known as *freemartins*, will be sterile correlates with the amount of overlap between the twins' placentas (Lillie 1916). In rats there is a similar but subtler effect on the receptivity of females developing near males in utero (Clemens et al. 1978; Meisel and Ward 1981). For both cows and rats, fetal testicular hormones appear to be able to cross from one fetus to the other and thereby influence sexual differentiation. In humans, women who had a twin brother display slightly masculinized features of their hearing (McFadden 1993), which may be a result of fetal exposure to androgen. Male fetuses of pregnant rats exposed to stress have slightly lower than normal levels of fetal androgen and adult masculine copulatory behavior (Ward and Reed 1985), due to maternally secreted opiates damping fetal GnRH release and therefore T secretion.

Finally, from the discussion above you might think that the sexual differentiation of the brain and sexual behavior are passive on the part of the female. But some research suggests that the presence of a small amount of estrogen (from the mother prenatally and/or the developing ovary postnatally) may be necessary for the full expression of feminine sexual behavior and other sex-related behaviors in female rats and mice (Toran-Allerand 1981; Dohler et al. 1984). Thus, AFP may serve to regulate or prolong, not completely prevent, estrogen's access to the female brain.

Detailed Mechanisms of Sexual Differentiation

Sex differences in neural structure were discovered in the 1970s. Up until then, almost all researchers agreed that early steroid exposure could indeed permanently alter the structure of the brain and thereby permanently alter behavior. However, this belief rested on indirect evidence. Just as particle physicists spoke of atoms, electrons, and so on without ever actually seeing them, behavioral endocrinologists spoke of androgenic organization of the neural structure without actually seeing any changes in the brain. They inferred the organization of the brain by the changes in behavior. Since the nervous system controls behavior (barring the existence of spirits or demons), sex differences in behavior imply that there are sex differences in neural structure. While there were those who worried that sex differences outside the nervous system, most obviously in the structure of the genitalia, might be responsible for differences in behavior (Beach 1971), later studies would amply vindicate the notion that male and female brains are built differently.

Sexual Dimorphism in the Hypothalamus

Darwin coined the term **sexual dimorphism** to refer to the tendency in many species for the two sexes to have very different body shapes or sizes. For example lions, peacocks, and gorillas exhibit moderate to great sexual dimorphism, but seagulls, hyenas, and many snakes and fish show little to none.

PREOPTIC AREA (POA)

One of the first reports of sexual dimorphism in neural structure to generate a great deal of interest was from Raisman and Field (1973), who examined the **preoptic area** (**POA**) of the hypothalamus in rats. Using electron microscopy, they carefully classified and counted synapses in this area, and found that females had more of a particular synapse type than males did. Furthermore, in complete accord with the organizational hypothesis, early androgen manipulations could reverse the sex difference seen in adulthood. Because earlier work had shown that lesions or stimulations of the POA could alter reproductive behavior and ovulation and because synapses were known to play a crucial role in neural function, this finding generated a great deal of enthusiasm and admiration (especially because the work involved was very tedious and time-consuming). This was also the exact sort of sexual dimorphism researchers were prepared for—subtle and requiring great technological skills to detect.

MACROSCOPIC SEXUAL DIMORPHISMS IN THE BRAIN

In 1976 the assumption that neural sexual dimorphisms would be subtle was blown apart. Nottebohm and Arnold (1976) reported that the brain nuclei of songbirds displayed sex differences that were so large one could detect them without a microscope. Each of these nuclei (remember that a cluster of neurons found within the CNS is known as a nucleus and is different from an individual cell's spherical repository of chromosomes, also known as a nucleus) had been shown by lesion and electrical stimulation experiments to be involved in birdsong production. Nottebohm and Arnold, studying canaries and zebra finches, where males do almost all the singing, found **vocal control regions** in the brain that were 5 to 6 times larger in males than in females (figure 3.4).

Soon after, a deluge of sex dimorphisms in neural structure were reported, some subtle, some large, involving the number or shape of synapses, the length of dendrites, the number of neurons, the amount of neurotransmitter, and so on (for reviews, see Arnold and Gorski 1984; Cooke et al. 1999; DeVries et al. 1984). Some brain regions are larger in males; others are larger in females (Simerly 1998). By now the list of articles describing sex differences in neural structure is too long to be reviewed comprehensively. Instead, we will concentrate on a few of the well-studied systems in this chapter and the ontogeny of several other interesting systems will be discussed in chapter 8.

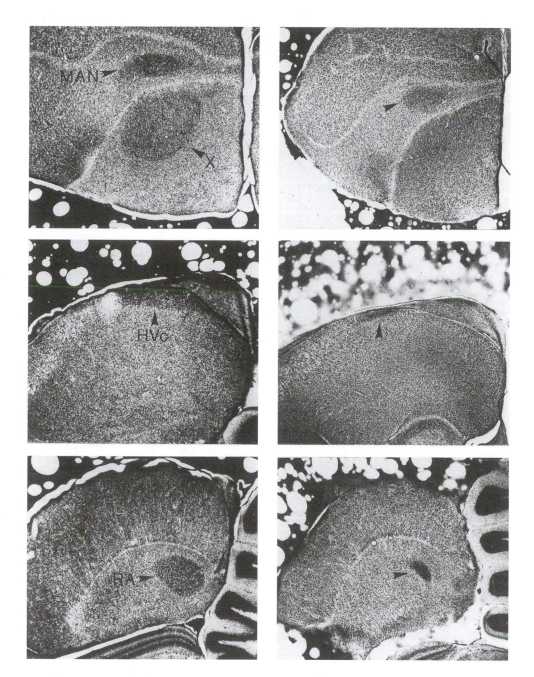

Figure 3.4 Sexually dimorphic neural regions of the songbird brain. In these frontal sections of Nissl-stained material you can compare the sizes of nuclei MAN and Area X (*top*) between males (*left*) and females (*right*). Middle panels depict nucleus HVC, bottom panels depict nucleus RA. All of these nuclei are involved in song learning or production, which is primarily performed by males in both canaries and zebra finches. The volume of these nuclei is greater in males than in females because of the early actions of steroids (see also chapter 8). For a schematic representation of the connections between these nuclei, see figure 8.9. (Courtesy of Arthur Arnold.)

SEXUALLY DIMORPHIC NUCLEUS OF THE POA (SDN-POA)

We have already mentioned the preoptic area (POA)—lesions of the POA stop male copulatory behavior in a striking variety of species (Hart and Leedy 1985). Thus, Roger Gorski and his colleagues carefully examined the POA and found within this region a nucleus that was 5 to 6 times larger in males than in females, a difference so prominent that one could distinguish brain slices from the two sexes with the naked eye (figure 3.5). They named this region the **sexually dimorphic nucleus of the POA** (**SDN-POA**) (Gorski et al. 1978). The sex dimorphism of the SDN-POA obeyed beautifully the rules of the organizational hypothesis: castration of males on the day of birth caused their SDN-POAs to be smaller (i.e., less masculine) in adulthood, while androgen treatment of newborn females caused their SDN-POAs to be larger in adulthood. In fact, if females were exposed to androgens both before and just after birth, their SDN-POAs were as big as those of normal males. In other words, early androgen exposure determined the size of the SDN-POA in adulthood. The greater the early androgen exposure, the larger the SDN-POA (figure 3.5). Furthermore, manipulations of androgens in adulthood had no effect on the volume of the SDN-POA. There was great excitement, therefore, that the SDN-POA might provide an anatomical signature of the androgen's masculine organizing influence upon the rat nervous system (Gorski 1984).

How do early androgens orchestrate the masculine development of the SDN-POA? First of all, one can look at the ontogeny of the SDN-POA: when does it first become detectable and when does the sex difference in size first arise? Jacobson and Gorski found that the SDN portion of the POA was visible as early as the twentieth day of gestation, but the volume did not differ between the sexes until the day of birth (the twenty-third day of gestation), and became most prominent on the tenth day of life (Jacobson et al. 1980). Of course, just because the sex difference in SDN-POA volume is not visible before birth does not mean that androgen is not driving processes before birth that will cause the later dimorphism. In fact, there is a sex difference in the production of neurons in the SDN before birth.

When a cell duplicates its DNA (in order to provide a full set to each daughter cell), it must use thymidine and other nucleotides to synthesize a new set of chromosomes (see box 3.1). Jacobson and Gorski (1981) injected pregnant rats with radiolabeled thymidine. If the fetuses are killed a few hours later, all the radioactivity is found along the rim of the brain's ventricles, in the *ventricular zone*, indicating that the dividing cells are found there. Several days after injecting the thymidine, some neurons have radioactivity in their nuclei, indicating that a cellular "ancestor" of that neuron was about to divide on that day the thymidine was injected. In the parlance of the trade, people talk about the "birth date" of cells, that is, the day of the final division that produced that cell and its sister cell. Thus, the thymidine is used to determine the time of **neurogenesis**, the generation of a cell that soon becomes a neuron. It turns out that all the neurons of the SDN-POA are born by the eighteenth day of gestation. What's more, on the seventeenth day of gestation,

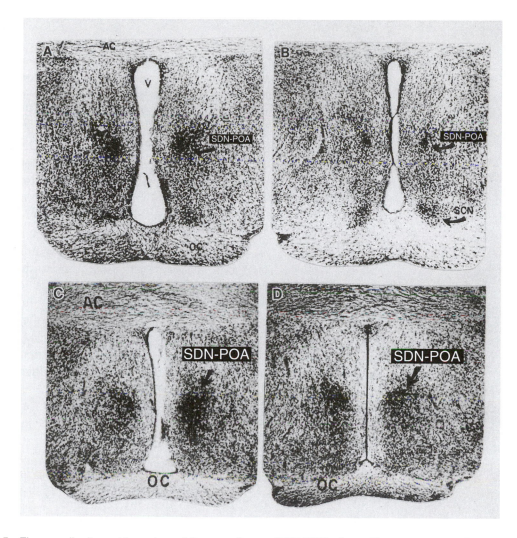

Figure 3.5 The sexually dimorphic nucleus of the preoptic area (SDN-POA) of rats. This region is 3 to 5 times larger in male (*A*) than in female rats (*B*). The masculine development of the SDN-POA depends upon the perinatal effects of estrogens, normally obtained as aromatized metabolites of testosterone. Thus, perinatally androgen-treated females (*C*), or females perinatally treated with estrogen (*D*) have an enlarged SDN-POA in adulthood. AC, anterior commissure; OC, optic chiasm; SCN, suprachiasmatic nucleus; V, ventricle. (Courtesy of Roger Gorski.)

Box 3.1 Thymidine Autoradiography to Detect the Time of Neurogenesis

Even we multicellular organisms begin as a single cell. The zygote duplicates the DNA and divides, leaving both daughter cells with a complete genetic blueprint. Cycles of mitosis continue to form an embryo, a fetus, a juvenile and an adult. Even in adulthood, some cells, like blood cells and glia, continue to divide. But the cells that give rise to neurons generally stop dividing early in life, shortly after birth in humans. The time of that final division that gave rise to a neuron is the "birth date" of that cell. The timetable of the divisions that give rise to different neuronal populations is relatively fixed—motoneurons are born well before birth, interneurons later, and glia continue to be born in the adult CNS. Outer cortical neurons are born later than neurons of the inner cortex, and so on. The birth date of particular cells can be determined by labeling the DNA that is copied before division. If we inject a radiolabelled precursor to DNA called thymidine, it will be used to provide the thymine (see figure 1.2) in new DNA being produced at that time. Once the animal grows up, we can examine cells to see whether they have radioactivity in their nuclei. If so, then one of their "ancestors" was preparing to divide back when we injected the thymidine. If injections of thymidine before day 14.5 of development result in labeled motoneurons in adulthood, but injections after 14.5 days never label them, we can conclude that those cells are all born by 14.5 days. In rats, neurons of the POA are generally born between 14 and 16 days post-conception. However, neurons in the SDN portion of the POA are born a little later, 16 to 18 days of gestation. This later birthdate coincides with a time during which males have elevated systemic levels of androgen. Furthermore, male rats appear to be producing more neurons during this later period than females are, so it may be that androgen augments neurogenesis in the SDN-POA, and thereby makes the nucleus larger. In chapter 8 we will learn about systems in which animals continue to give rise to new neurons in adulthood.

more SDN-POA neurons are being born in males than in females (Jacobson and Gorski 1981). It is important to note that a consequence of this early sex difference in neurogenesis will not manifest itself as a sex difference in the volume of the SDN-POA for another 5 to 6 days.

There is also evidence that more cells die in the SDN-POA of female rats than of male rats around the seventh day of life (Davis et al. 1996; McCarthy et al. 1997). So the sex difference in prenatal androgen exposure seems to promote an immediate sex difference in neurogenesis (favoring males) and a later sex difference in cell death (favoring females), leading to a larger SDN-POA in males.

The next obvious questions about the SDN-POA are these: When during development can steroids exert their effects, and which steroids are effective? We mentioned briefly above that testosterone could affect the volume of the SDN-POA only when administered perinatally. More specifically, it was found that either prenatal or neonatal injections of testosterone could masculinize the SDN-POA of females. However, the prenatal injections were more effective than the postnatal, and androgen had to be given during both periods to completely sex-reverse SDN-POA volume (i.e., make it as big as in normal males). As far as which hormone does the work, perinatal estrogen is more effective than testosterone at masculinizing SDN-POA volume, and the other major active metabolite of testosterone, DHT, has no measurable effect upon the SDN-POA. It appears then that in normal males testicular testosterone is aromatized to estrogen (possibly within the developing SDN-POA itself), and that estrogen is actually guiding the masculine development of the nucleus. This inference is supported by the examination of TFM rats. While these XY individuals produce testes and testosterone, they lack the androgen receptors to respond, and therefore develop a feminine exterior phenotype. However, the TFM animals possess estrogen receptors (Attardi et al. 1976) and aromatase (Rosenfeld et al. 1977) and, in accord with the aromatization hypothesis of brain sexual differentiation and in contrast to their feminine bodies, TFM animals have a large, masculine SDN-POA. Thus, androgen receptors per se do not appear to cause the masculinization of the SDN-POA of rats. Rather, by acting upon estrogen receptors, it is the aromatized metabolites of testosterone that direct the masculine development of this nucleus. The SDN-POA not only follows the rules of the organizational hypothesis, but of the aromatization hypothesis as well. Another demonstration of the importance of estrogen receptors is the finding that infusions of antisense oligonucleotides (see chapter 2) to the estrogen receptor leads to a smaller SDN-POA (McCarthy 1994).

The excitement about the SDN-POA was slightly diminished for a time when Gorski's group reported no deficit in masculine sexual behavior caused by lesions of the SDN-POA (Arendash and Gorski 1983), even though similar-sized lesions of dorsal POA outside the SDN region significantly decreased the likelihood of ejaculation. However, another group found that lesions of the SDN portion of the POA decreased male sexual behavior in rats who were sexually naive (De Jonge et al. 1989). Specifically, lesioned animals were less likely to reach ejaculation and took longer to mount, achieve intromission, and ejaculate than normal males. The deficit caused by the lesion was relatively subtle, disappearing with additional sexual experience.

Sexually Dimorphic Spinal Nucleus of the Bulbocavernosus

One way to overcome the problem of understanding the functional significance of a sex difference in the nervous system is to deliberately choose a system so simple that its function is relatively obvious. Such a simple sexual dimorphism is found in the spinal cord. The muscles which attach to the penis (figure 3.6) are quite likely to play a role in sexual behavior, and so too are the spinal motoneurons which innervate and control those muscles. Thus, the striated muscles **bulbocavernosus (BC)**, **levator ani (LA)**, and ischiocavernosus (IC), all of which attach to the base of the penis, became an object of the study of neural sexual differentiation. The BC and IC are present in human males (the BC is under voluntary control and is used to eject the last drops of urine) and in females (except in this case they attach to the base of the clitoris—the BC, under voluntary control in women, constricts the opening of the vagina). The BC and IC are smaller in women than in men, but in rats the sexual dimorphism of these muscles is much more drastic. Adult female rats lack them altogether.

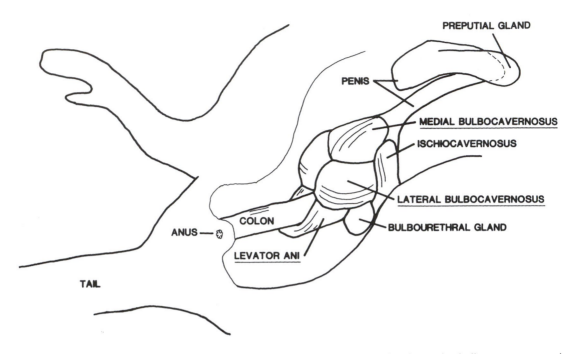

Figure 3.6 Schematic drawing of the perineal region of a male rat. The striated muscles bulbocavernosus and levator ani are innervated by the spinal nucleus of the bulbocavernosus (SNB). The levator ani, which attaches to the base of the penis and wraps around the colon, is sometimes called the dorsal bulbocavernosus. The bulbocavernosus looks similar in males of many species, including humans, but the levator ani may be restricted to rodents. (From Breedlove 1984.)

Given the sexual dimorphism in the muscles of the perineum (the pelvic floor region that includes the genitalia), it is not surprising that the spinal motoneurons controlling these muscles would also display a dimorphism. These motoneurons innervating the BC and LA are found in a distinctive position and collectively are called the **spinal nucleus of the bulbocavernosus (SNB)**. There are more SNB cells in male rats than in females, and they are larger in males (figure 3.7). The motoneurons innervating the external anal sphincter are also located in the SNB region, and it is these cells which occupy that nucleus in female rats.

Female rats begin life with BC, LA, and IC muscles attached to the base of the clitoris (Cihak et al. 1970), and SNB motoneurons have made functional synapses with the muscles (Rand and Breedlove 1987). Despite all this effort, the SNB cells and perineal muscles die in the first weeks of life in female rats. The naturally occurring death of cells, which is quite common during development, is known as *apoptosis*. The apoptosis of the SNB system is averted in males by the intervention of androgen, and you can permanently save the SNB system in females with a single injection of androgen early in life (Breedlove and Arnold 1983a,b). Aromatized metabolites of testosterone do not seem to affect the survival of SNB cells or their targets (Breedlove et al. 1982). For example, TFM rats (which possess normal levels of testosterone,

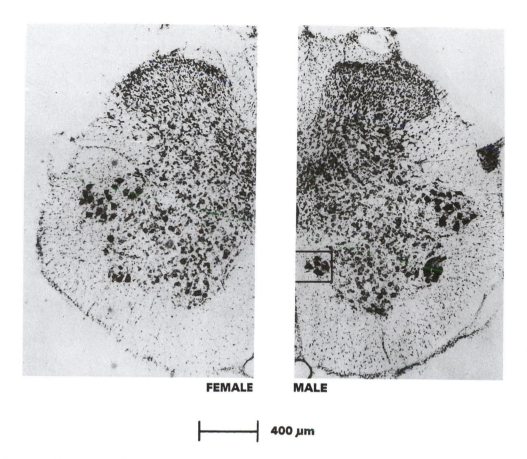

FEMALE   MALE

├──────┤ 400 μm

Figure 3.7 Photomicrographs of cross-sections of the lumbar spinal cord of adult female (*left*) and male rats (dorsal is up). The spinal nucleus of the bulbocavernosus (SNB) is a readily recognized, discrete nucleus of motoneurons in males (*box*). Most of these motoneurons innervate either the bulboca-vernosus or levator ani, but some innervate the external anal sphincter, and it is these scattered motoneurons that occupy this area in female rats. The human homologue of the SNB occupies a more ventral position and is known as Onuf's nucleus. (Adapted from Breedlove and Arnold 1981.)

aromatase, and estrogen receptors) develop a completely feminine SNB system, apparently because they lack the androgen receptors to prevent the death of these cells. Once the SNB cells and their target muscles have died, androgen cannot resurrect them. Thus, the basis of the sensitive period for steroids to organize the SNB system is determined by how far the degeneration has proceeded. If the organizational actions of steroids in other systems involve the prevention of cell death, a similar mechanism may be behind other sensitive periods (Konishi and Akutagawa 1985).

How does early androgen prevent the death of BC/LA muscles and their SNB motoneurons? It appears that androgen directly prevents the degeneration of the muscles and that the survival of the SNB motoneurons is a secondary response to the sparing of their muscle targets. Several lines of evidence support this idea. First, androgen can maintain the muscles in newborn females even after the motoneurons have been removed (Fishman and Breedlove 1988a). Second, androgen receptor blockers interfere with testosterone's effects better when they are injected directly into the muscle rather than into general circulation (Fishman and Breedlove 1988b). Furthermore, while the BC muscles of newborn rats can bind androgen (Fishman and Breedlove 1992), neither SNB cells nor other spinal motoneurons can accumulate steroid until after the sensitive period for sparing the system (Jordan et al. 1989). Finally, SNB motoneurons producing a defective androgen receptor are just as likely to be spared by early androgen as those motoneurons using a functional androgen receptor (Freeman et al. 1996). Thus, androgens affect the target of SNB neurons and thereby spare them from cell death, leading to the sexual differentiation of the spinal cord. Forger has gathered evidence that androgen causes the BC muscles to produce a **neurotrophic factor**, a protein that keeps neurons alive. There are many different neurotrophic factors, but the one that seems to keep SNB motoneurons alive is one related to, but different from, ciliary neurotrophic factor (Forger et al. 1997).

Many features vary between the sexes. Notice that this diversity of sex differences makes it very difficult to refer to someone as being simply "male" or "female," because it is possible for an individual to be masculine in some body or brain regions and feminine in others. With our more informed view of sexual differentiation, we need to specify which characteristic we are interested in before deciding whether it is masculine or feminine. We can also use the more refined terms, feminization and masculinization. When a normally masculine characteristic develops, we can describe that process as "masculinization" and a treatment that prevents that structure from forming is called demasculinizing. Similarly, the development of a feminine characteristic is "feminization," while the prevention of the appearance of a female characteristic is defeminization. Normally, of course, males are both masculinized (in terms of genital structure, copulatory behavior, SDN-POA, SNB, and so on) and defeminized (in terms of müllerian duct structures, ovulatory competence, lordosis responsiveness, and so on). Females are normally both feminized and demasculinized. In most discussions, one refers to any move in the female direction as feminization and any move in the male direction as masculinization.

Sexual Differentiation of the Human Nervous System

There is no doubt that men and women look and act differently. The sex differences in behavior are more prominent in some cultures than in others, but never quite absent (Ford and Beach 1951). What is controversial is the question of *how* boys and girls grow up to be so different—is it the result of inborn biological differences or the result of their different experiences while growing up? This question is a subset of the ongoing nature-versus-nurture debate—to what extent is our behavior affected by our genome (nature) or our experience (nurture)? This is a complex and sometimes emotional debate that is of interest to almost everyone. Several different disciplines, including behavioral genetics (Plomin et al. 1990), animal behavior (Alcock 2001), and developmental neurobiology (Purves and Lichtman 1985) address this question, each with a slightly different approach.

Nature versus Nurture

In the field of behavioral endocrinology, the nature-nurture debate is so confined that it may one day be resolved. Because so much is known about sexual differentiation of the body, the question of sexual differentiation of the brain and behavior can be boiled down to this—if there is a biological influence on the sexual differentiation of human behavior, then steroid hormones mediate that influence. So we can ask, do differences in early steroids alter the human nervous system and/or behavior? It is a great intellectual advantage to be able to pare down a question to such a readily comprehensible form that can be tested. Nonetheless, the complexity of behavior and the nervous system, coupled with the difficulties and limitations of working with human subjects, has so far given us only a partial answer.

Remember that the principles by which testicular secretions direct masculine development of the body are much the same in all mammals, including humans. Do the sex differences in prenatal steroid exposure also cause sex differences in the development of the human nervous system and therefore sex differences in behavior? To address that question, we can first ask whether there is sexual dimorphism in the human nervous system.

Overall Brain Size Relative to Body Weight

Nineteenth century researchers noted that men have heavier brains than women, and some of these (male) workers viewed this finding as the natural result of the intellectual superiority of men (for reviews, see Gould 1981; Swaab and Hofman 1984). Of course, men have larger bodies than women and if you measure brain weight relative to body weight or height, the sex difference disappears or favors women. There is a tendency to dismiss the obvious sex difference in brain weight because of the sex difference in body size, but it is worthwhile to examine this tendency. How does brain size come to mirror body size? There are three general ways it could come about: (1) The nervous system might monitor body size and adapt itself to follow suit, (2) The nervous system might instruct the body how much to grow, or (3) Some other signal(s) (e.g., growth and/or thyroid hormone) might independently control body and brain growth. Which of these three mechanisms cause men to have heavier brains than women? We don't know. Whichever mechanism is at work, it seems likely that the sex difference in body/brain size is the result of biological influences, specifically hormones. This idea is supported by the fact that a small (2–3%) but reliable sex difference in human brain weight (heavier in males), corrected for height, arises by 2 years of age (Pakkenberg and Voigt 1964; Swaab and Hofman 1984), presumably (but not necessarily) before parents' treatment of infants could have much effect.

Table 3.2 Anatomical Studies Showing Sex Differences in the Human Brain

Crichton-Browne (1880)	Weight differences between left and right hemispheres less marked in females than in males
Rabl (1958), Morel (1948), Davie and Baldwin (1967)	Agenesis of massa intermedia more frequent in males than in females
Wada et al. (1975)	Planum temporale larger on right more often in females than in males (but usually larger on left in both sexes)
Wada (1976)	Cuneate area of occipital lobe larger on right in females, larger on left in males
Gur et al. (1982)	Higher rates of cerebral blood flow in females
deLacoste-Utamsing and Horvath (1985)	At 13 weeks gestational age, entire right cortex more developed in males and left prefrontal cortex in females
Baxter et al. (1987)	Higher cerebral glucose metabolic rates in females
Swaab and Fliers (1985), Allen et al. (1989)	Nuclei of the POA hypothalamic area larger in males than in females
Witelson (1989)	Isthmus of the corpus callosum proportionately larger in females than in males; genu larger in males
Allen and Gorski (1991)	Anterior commissure at the midsagittal plane larger in females
Allen and Gorski (1990), Zhou et al. (1995)	Regions of the bed nucleus of the stria terminalis larger in males than in females
Schlaepfer et al. (1995), Witelson et al. (1995)	Volume of gray matter and neuronal cell densities larger in females than in males in language-related cortex

Our knowledge of sex differences in the human brain has expanded dramatically. Many sex differences have been identified (table 3.2). Differences might be present in measures as diverse as neuronal packing density, the size of particular nuclei or fiber tracts, the localization of functions in the cortex of men and women, among others. We also know from other species that similar appearing macroscopic brain structures can be built from sexually dimorphic neurotransmitter systems. Scientists are coming to recognize that sexual differentiation also encompasses metabolic differences between the brains of men and women. Even though women's brains tend to be smaller, they have a higher glucose utilization rate and blood flow per unit of tissue. As a student, therefore, you must be careful not to fall into the "my brain's bigger than your brain" trap. Functional capacity is an emergent property of the brain and depends on many factors besides overall size.

SDN-POA

The two prominent sex differences in the rat CNS that we discussed above, the SDN-POA and the SNB, have both been examined in human tissues. The first group to describe a sexual dimorphism in the human POA named the nucleus the SDN-POA, and found it larger in men than in women (Swaab and Fliers 1985). This human nucleus has a somewhat different shape than the rat

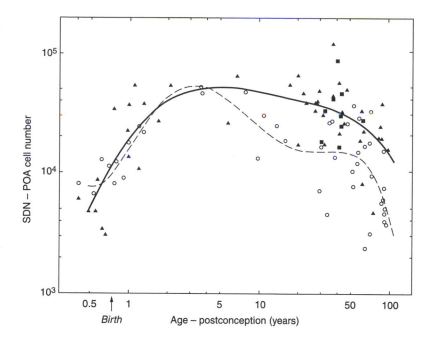

Figure 3.8   The change with age in the number of neurons seen in the human SDN-POA (INAH-1). Because this sex difference in the human POA arises sometime between the ages of 6 and 10 years, we do not know whether a sex difference in exposure to fetal androgens or a sex difference in social experience is responsible. (Adapted from Swaab et al. 1992.)

SDN-POA, and the degree of sexual dimorphism is much less pronounced than in rats. Is this human nucleus in the POA really the equivalent of the rat SDN-POA, or is the human nucleus really a different nucleus that just happens to be dimorphic? This difficult question may never be fully answered. Even if the human POA nucleus turns out to be unrelated to the rat SDN-POA (i.e., the result of evolutionary convergence), it seems unlikely than anyone would have noticed the sexual dimorphism in humans without the impetus provided by the animal research.

Interestingly, the sex difference in the number of neurons in the human SDN-POA does not occur until about 10 years of age (figure 3.8) (Swaab et al. 1992). The rat SDN-POA shows a delayed response to androgen, as prenatal androgens cause a sexual dimorphism to arise a week later. Perhaps prenatal androgens program for a later increase in the SDN-POA of human males. On the other hand, it is possible that the sex difference in experience (people treat little girls differently from little boys) in the first years of life causes this brain nucleus to develop differently in the two sexes. Thus, we don't know whether fetal hormones or early socialization is responsible for this sexual dimorphism.

When Laura Allen and Roger Gorski examined the human POA, they described four related nuclei and named them the "interstitial nuclei of the anterior hypothalamus" (INAH), numbering them 1 through 4 (Allen and Gorski

1991, 1992). INAH-1 is the region Swaab and Fliers named the SDN-POA. Gorski's group did not see a sexual dimorphism in INAH-1, but that could be due to a smaller sample size. However, they did see a sexual dimorphism in INAH-2 and INAH-3. Both nuclei were slightly larger in men than in women. So there is sexual dimorphism in the human POA, but we don't know whether fetal androgens are responsible for these sex differences. As we'll see later, INAH-3 was later examined in gay and straight men.

Sexually Dimorphic Spinal Nucleus of the Bulbocavernosus

The SNB is more easily defined for humans—it is the group of motoneurons that innervate the BC and IC muscles, which are present in both men and women and look very much the same in male rats and humans. The nucleus of motoneurons innervating these perineal muscles is called **Onuf's nucleus** (Onuf 1899). Onuf's nucleus looks much the same in humans, monkeys, cats, and dogs, but is found in a slightly different location in the spinal cord than the rat SNB. Since women have smaller BC and IC muscles than men do, one might expect a sex difference in the number of Onuf's nucleus motoneurons, and men do, in fact, have more cells there (Forger and Breedlove 1986). Also, as one might expect, the sex difference is subtler in humans than in rats, where females lose the BC altogether after birth. Furthermore, dogs also have a sex difference in the number of Onuf's motoneurons (again favoring males), and prenatal androgen treatment of females leaves them with a masculine number of cells in Onuf's nucleus. Thus, it seems likely that the sexual dimorphism in human Onuf's nucleus is in fact biologically determined by sex differences in prenatal steroid secretion, just like its rat homologue, the SNB.

Lateralization of Brain Structures and Functions

Another area of research into human sexual dimorphisms revolves around the issue of cerebral asymmetry or lateralization. As you may know, some higher cognitive functions seem to be primarily controlled in one cerebral hemisphere or the other. For example, speech seems to be controlled by the left cerebral hemisphere in most of us (including most left-handed people). This conclusion was first reached in the 19th century by neurologists examining the postmortem brains of stroke and accident victims whose injuries made them aphasic (i.e., unable to speak and/or understand speech). Spatial reasoning, on the other hand, is usually carried out by the right hemisphere. The extent to which a function is carried out by one hemisphere rather than another is referred to as **lateralization** (Springer and Deutsch 1997).

There have been several reports of a sex difference in the degree of lateralization of cognitive functions (McGlone 1980); in general, women seem to display less lateralization of cortical function than men do. Other sex differences in the arrangement of functions within the cortex might also exist, and these will be discussed thoroughly in chapter 15. When such sex differences are seen, they are often subtle, and there have been many studies which failed to find a difference at all (Feingold 1988). A complication in studying such differences is that cortical functions are not directly measurable—there isn't an anatomical marker that we can search for in the cortex that identifies which regions control which functions. Direct anatomical studies have, however, been successful in identifying other types of sex differences that may be linked to lateralization or to the ability of the two hemispheres to communicate with each other.

PLANUM TEMPORALE

An exciting finding of the 1970s was that of Wada and his colleagues, who reported that the **planum temporale**, a flat region of the human temporal lobe thought to be involved in speech, was usually larger on the left than on the right (Wada et al. 1975). This anatomical asymmetry fitted well with what was known about the functional lateralization of speech. What's more, the scientists reported that the asymmetry of the planum temporale, while present in both sexes, was more prominent in men. That is, while most women had a larger planum temporale on the left, the right side was occasionally equal to or larger than the left, and women were more likely than men to show this unusual pattern. If the planum temporale is involved in language, these structural sex differences may contribute to a sex difference in patient outcome following stroke: women are more likely than men to retain language after a stroke in the left hemisphere (Inglis and Lawson 1981).

What made the report from Wada and his colleagues exciting was the possibility that the sex difference in structural asymmetry might be a reflection of sex differences in functional asymmetry. There were several reports that indicated that various functions were more evenly distributed on the left and right brain halves of women than of men. For example, most of us can pick words out of noise better with our right ear (and hence the left side of our brain) than with our left ear. But, in general, women show less discrepancy in the performance of the two ears than men do. It makes sense that the left side of the brain, which performs most language processing, would have a larger planum temporale. Furthermore, if women are less lateralized in auditory processing than men are, the more symmetrical planum of women may be partly responsible. Similarly, men are more likely to detect written words briefly flashed to their right visual field than to their left visual field. While women also perform better with right visual field presentation, they are more likely than men to do about as well on either side (see chapter 15). Again, the explanation for this is hypothesized to be the more symmetrical distribution of language functions in the female brain.

Planum asymmetry develops before birth. It was already visible by the 29th week of gestation in Wada's study, the youngest brains they examined. Another observation in the fetus comes from work by de Lacoste and associates who examined fetal brains from the famous Yakovlev brain collection. They found that by 13 weeks gestational age, the entire right cortex in males was more visibly developed than the left, while in females, the development of the two hemispheres was more nearly equal or favored the left hemisphere, particularly in frontal cortex (de Lacoste et al. 1991; de Lacoste-Utamsing and Horvath 1985). It is around this time that testicular androgens reach peak concentrations in the male fetus. In adult humans, there is little evidence for any persisting difference in hemispheric growth patterns, although as far back as 1880 Crichton-Browne noted in postmortem brain tissue that the two hemispheres are more nearly equal in weight in females than in males. In males, it is the right hemisphere that is heavier.

CORPUS CALLOSUM

The major pathway that transmits information from one half of the brain to the other is the **corpus callosum** (CC). The CC consists of the axons from millions of neurons that carry information from one hemisphere to the other. It was reported that the caudal end of the CC, the splenium, was more bulbous in females than in males (DeLacoste-Utamsing and Holloway 1982). But there have been several problems with the interpretation of the finding of sexual dimorphism in human CC. First, there may not be a sex difference in the number of axons because there is no sex difference in the overall cross-sectional area of the CC, only in the shape of the caudal end. Perhaps that means that women invest a greater proportion of their CC axons in one task than another, but no one has found a way to demonstrate that.

A second problem has been the failures of other researchers to replicate the original finding (e.g., Witelson 1985). To see the sex difference in shape, you must adhere very strictly to a remarkably complicated series of steps to define the splenium. If you deviate from these steps in measuring the splenium, you find no sex difference. The very particular steps you must go through to see a sex difference illustrates how subtle the difference is, and how difficult it is to understand just what the difference really means.

If you accept that there is a sexual dimorphism in the CC, it is possible that sex differences in the cognitive or social experiences of young children are responsible for the sex difference in CC. There is a report that the sex difference in the CC is present in fetal human material (DeLacoste et al. 1986), which would suggest that prenatal factors such as hormones are responsible for the dimorphism in CC. Unfortunately this report, too, is contested (Bell and Variend 1985). A recent review of 43 studies of the corpus callosum (Driesen and Raz 1995) concluded that in absolute size the splenium is, if anything, larger in men, but that the corpus callosum area is larger in women as a proportion of their total brain size. We are left with the impression that there may be a sexual dimorphism in human CC, but it is subtle.

Results for another callosal subregion, the isthmus, have been more consistent. This region is defined as the posterior segment of the corpus callosum just anterior to the splenium. Several studies, beginning with Witelson (1989), report that the midsagittal area of the isthmus is larger in women than in men, at least in right-handers. Whether any sexual dimorphism in the CC is the cause or the result of sex differences in the lateralization of cognitive function, or completely unrelated to lateralization, is also unclear.

OTHER PATHWAYS BETWEEN HEMISPHERES

The CC is not the only large connection between the two hemispheres that is said to be sexually dimorphic. Of the five major fiber pathways that interconnect the two cerebral hemispheres—the CC, the anterior commissure (AC), posterior commissure, massa intermedia (MI), and the hippocampal commissure—sex differences have been reported in at least 3. Besides the CC, the MI and the AC have been studied. Several studies have found that the massa intermedia, a band of neural tissue that connects the two halves of the thalamus across the third ventricle, is more frequently absent in men than in women. In people who do have an MI, its cross-sectional area is typically larger in women (Allen and Gorski 1991). Lansdell and Davie (1972) noted that males without the MI tended to have higher scores on nonverbal items on a test of general ability than do males with the MI present.

Finally, Allen and Gorski (1991) calculated the midsagittal area of the AC in 100 human brains ranging in age from 4 to 84 years. Although the male brains were larger, as expected, the AC was about 12% larger in area in females than in males. It is not known whether the commissural differences that have been reported so far represent a greater number of fibers traversing the cerebral commissures in women or simply a greater diameter of fibers.

Sexual Orientation

Many people would like to know whether the biological influences upon the developing nervous systems of animals are also at work in humans. Specifically, some have wondered whether early prenatal steroid exposure influences sexual orientation. Do heterosexual men and homosexual women prefer female sexual partners because androgen organized their developing brains in a "masculine" fashion? Or conversely, is the sexual orientation of homosexual men and heterosexual women (i.e., a preference for male partners) the result of low prenatal androgen levels? It's easy to pose these questions conversationally, but exceedingly difficult to answer them scientifically. It is impossible to monitor prenatal steroid levels without incurring substantial risk to the fetus. Also, it would be unethical to manipulate the prenatal steroid environment of humans to try to alter sexual orientation. Thus, the only way to answer this question is to make use of correlational data, and that data, as you might have guessed, gives equivocal answers at best.

First of all, there have been many studies which failed to find any difference between heterosexual and homosexual men (or women) in terms of adult plasma androgen or estrogen levels (Meyer-Bahlburg 1984). Of course, animal models might suggest that any androgenic effect on sexual orientation should occur early in life, perhaps even prenatally. However, there is no technically feasible way to monitor fetal steroid levels in a large number of individuals. There have been reports that homosexual and heterosexual men differ in their response to injections of estrogen (Dorner 1976; Gladue et al. 1984). Specifically, it is reported that homosexual men show a pattern of LH release in response to an injection of estrogen that falls in between heterosexual men and heterosexual women—that is, they show more of a "positive feedback" response. The rat models of sexual differentiation would suggest that this positive feedback response is feminine. The reasoning continues that a prenatal androgen shortage might result in only a partial masculinization of brain circuits concerned with sexual orientation and ovulatory competence.

However, you may remember that primates are not very sexually dimorphic in terms of ovulatory capacity, so it is not clear that this is indeed an exclusively feminine trait in humans. Furthermore, there have been several failures to replicate these observations (Hendricks et al. 1989). Finally, rather than prenatal androgen altering both sexual orientation and gonadotropin regulation, it is always possible that something about the homosexual experience causes the subtle changes in gonadotropin regulation. In that case, development of adult sexuality might be unrelated to prenatal steroids. Similarly, although homosexual men have a more feminine pattern of cognitive lateralization, this could be interpreted in two ways—perhaps a difference in brain organization led to development of a homosexual orientation, or development of a homosexual orientation may have led to a difference in brain organization.

In 1991, Simon LeVay confirmed the earlier report that INAH-3 was larger in men than in women and expanded his observations to find that INAH-3 was smaller in gay men than in heterosexual men (LeVay 1991). Almost all the gay men whose brains were examined had died of AIDS, so you might be concerned that the disease caused INAH-3 to shrink. But LeVay also had a sample of brains from heterosexual men who had died of AIDS, and these men had a large, masculine INAH-3 (figure 3.9). However, because the nucleus was examined only in adulthood, we do not know whether the structure of INAH-

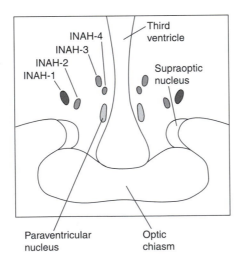

Figure 3.9 The interstitial nuclei of the anterior hypothalamus (INAH) of humans are numbered 1 through 4. Two different labs have reported that INAH-3 has a greater volume in men than in women. Simon LeVay also reported that INAH-3 was smaller in gay men than in heterosexual men.

3 affected the development of sexual orientation, or whether the development of sexual orientation affected the structure of INAH-3. It is even possible that adult experience affected the structure of INAH-3 (Breedlove 1997; Cooke et al. 1999). Homosexual men have also been reported to resemble heterosexual women in having a larger anterior commissure than heterosexual men (Allen and Gorski 1992). So far, however, we have no direct evidence that in humans either INAH-3 or the anterior commissure is susceptible to the organizational effects of steroids.

Besides looking at homosexual men, we can also look to the clinical anomalies we discussed earlier in the chapter for information about the possible role of hormones in the development of sexual orientation. People with AIS typically are sexually attracted to men (Meyer-Bahlburg 1984). But this could be due to learning, not hormones, because these individuals have a characteristic female appearance and are raised as women. What AIS individuals do tell us is that, unlike the case of rodents, estrogenic metabolites of testosterone cannot play a major role in the sexual differentiation of the human hypothalamus. If they did, then we would expect AIS women to behave in a masculine fashion, just as TFM rats have a masculine SDN-POA despite their feminine exterior.

What about females with congenital adrenal hyperplasia (CAH) who are exposed to high levels of androgen before birth? Since they are raised as girls, this condition more clearly teases apart the influences of early hormones and upbringing. There does seem to be some increase in bisexuality or homosexuality in women who have CAH (Ehrhardt et al. 1968; Money et al. 1984; Zucker et al. 1996), although this is not always expressed in overt behavior. This would seem to favor a predisposing influence of early androgen exposure. But the presence of genital anomalies or surgical correction that isn't always optimal for sexual functioning makes this issue very complex (Mulaikal et al. 1987). A smaller increase in the incidence of bisexuality or homosexuality has also been reported in women who were exposed prenatally to diethylstilbestrol (DES) (Ehrhardt et al. 1985; Meyer-Bahlburg et al. 1995). This is a synthetic estrogen that was widely used at one time to try to prevent miscarriages. It does not result in genital virilization but does have masculinizing or defeminizing effects in the developing CNS in other species. It is hard to know whether the DES data are meaningful or whether there could be some alternate interpretation. The large majority of DES-exposed women (>75%) are still exclusively heterosexual. And as you know, it is still far from clear whether estrogen is at all important in sexual differentiation of the primate brain. Two putative markers of early androgen exposure, the pattern of finger lengths (Williams et al. 2000) and otoacoustic emissions (McFadden and Pasanen 1998), have been found to be slightly more masculine in lesbians than in heterosexual women. This is consistent with the idea that elevations in early androgen exposure increase the likelihood of lesbianism in women, but neither measure indicates that gay men were exposed to less androgen than were straight men.

Thus, there is no irrefutable evidence that prenatal hormones affect sexual orientation in humans. The subjective experience of the majority of homosexuals and heterosexuals is that, from their very earliest remembrance, the object of their sexual interest has been unchanged. Of course, while this experience is consistent with a prenatal determination, it proves nothing. Our earliest memories of language may be of English, but of course that is because of experiences which predate our memories, not because we were "born English." Interestingly, sexual orientation seems to be more malleable in women than in men. On the other hand, there is very strong evidence of a heritable component to human sexual orientation in both sexes. About half the variance in sexual orientation in our culture can be attributed to variance in the genome. More specifically, there is good, but not undisputed, evidence that a gene on the X chromosome can affect the likelihood that a male will become gay (Hamer et al. 1993). All of this evidence comes under close public scrutiny because of the legal and ethical debate about equal rights for homosexuals.

Gender Identity

We conclude with a brief mention of gender identity. Gender identity is defined as a person's primary identification with one or the other sex, in other words, whether we view ourselves as male or female. While this is closely allied with sexual orientation, it is not the same thing. A gay man, for example, might have a male gender identity but an alternative sexual orientation. Does prenatal exposure to sex steroids influence our fundamental sense of ourselves as male or female?

In a review of the literature, Ehrhardt and Meyer-Bahlburg (1981) concluded that the prenatal hormone environment exerts little influence on gender identity. This conclusion was based mainly on case histories showing that gender identity appears to depend largely on the sex of rearing, even when this is in contrast to some of the biological markers of sex (Money and Ehrhardt 1972). For example, children born with ambiguous genitals were reported to develop a gender identity that agrees with their assigned sex, provided steps were taken early in life to correct the physical ambiguity and there was no ambiguity in the parental upbringing. Proponents of this view argue that the sex of rearing is the major factor in determining gender identity, which is thought to be established irrevocably by about 3 to 4 years of age.

Recent evidence has drawn the strict social learning view into question. You may recall our earlier description of the **guevedoces**. Imperato-McGinley (Imperato-McGinley et al. 1974; Imperato-McGinley et al. 1979) described a group of males in the Dominican Republic, called "guevedoces" by the locals, who had 5α-reductase deficiency. Although genetically male, these individuals were raised as girls because they were born with female-appearing external genitals due to the enzyme deficiency. At puberty, they suddenly became virilized as T levels rose to adult concentrations. They experienced penile growth, the descent of the testes into the scrotum, and the deepening of the voice. Despite being raised as girls, 17 of 18 males made a relatively effortless change in gender identity at puberty in response to the physical changes. This would not be expected from the strict social learning perspective. It has been suggested that these cases prove that early testosterone masculinizes the brain in terms of gender identity and that social influences contribute relatively little. Imperato-McGinley's work is controversial because in our culture other reports of sudden virilization at puberty have suggested that a change in gender identity requires a very long and difficult period of readjustment (Ehrhardt and Meyer-Bahlburg 1981). It is hard to rule out the possibility that the villagers treat these children differently from normal girls. Certainly the existence of a nickname for the condition means they are aware of the possibility. Furthermore, there are considerable advantages to be gained from being a male in Dominican society. Thus, an alternative explanation is that early hormones have no influence on gender identity, that humans are quite malleable and, if confronted with an altered body and residing in a society that permits it, can change sexual identities at puberty. The truth probably lies somewhere in between.

Recently another piece of evidence has come to light that reinforces the view that biology may be important in the formation of gender identity after all (Diamond and Sigmundson 1997). It is the case of a young boy who lost his penis in a circumcision accident while still an infant. After great debate, a decision was made to raise "John" as a girl ("Joan"). Accordingly, his testes were removed to prevent further virilization and his parents ensured he was given a female upbringing. Initially, "Joan" was described as developing into a normally functioning girl, and the case was widely cited as evidence of the primacy of the social environment. A recent long-term follow-up, however, revealed a very different picture: despite a supposedly female upbringing, John felt from a very early age that he was not really a girl. Even though he had no knowledge of his early accident, John felt so utterly unnatural as a female that by puberty he'd decided to seek formal sex re-assignment. He has been living happily as a male ever since.

Although this evidence would seem to implicate hormonal factors, you must keep in mind that not all the evidence supports this interpretation. In particular, most females with CAH retain a female gender identity despite prolonged exposure to high levels of androgens in utero.

Summary

1. During sexual differentiation, the presence of a Y chromosome transforms the indifferent gonad into a testis. The absence of the Y chromosome results in the gonad becoming an ovary. Thereafter, the sexual differentiation of the male relies on the fetal testis production of AMH and testosterone. This means that both primary sex characteristics (penis, scrotum, etc.) and secondary sex characteristics (facial and axillary hair, muscle, etc.) are depen-

dent upon hormonal secretions for phenotypic expression. The absence of testicular secretions results in development of feminine primary and secondary sex characteristics.

2. The brain is also organized by the presence or absence of testicular secretions during perinatal development. In rodents, testosterone masculinizes the brain to prevent ovulatory capacity and establish male-typical sexual behavior. Estrogen is equally capable of masculinizing the brain. In the male this is thought to reflect the conversion of testosterone to estrogen (aromatization) within the brain. Female rodents are protected from their own and their mother's estrogen by the presence of alpha-feto-protein in the blood. This protein binds to estrogen and limits its entry into the brain. However, a small amount of estrogen gains access to the brain in females and this may be important for the expression of feminine sexual behavior in the adult.

3. Primates may be very different from rodents in the mechanism(s) mediating sexual differentiation of the hypothalamus. Two points are important to note. First, it does not seem likely that the aromatization of testosterone to estrogen is important for sexual differentiation of the hypothalamus in primates. Second, male primates, unlike male rodents, retain the capability of supporting ovulation.

4. The number of brain regions that have been found to be sexually dimorphic in rodents is substantial and the number will undoubtedly continue to increase as more brain regions are investigated. Processes mediating the expression of sex-related differences vary with the brain region. Gonadal steroid hormones can exert effects both directly on neurons as well as by having a trophic effect on the target muscles of motoneurons. In both cases, it seems that there are gonadal hormone effects on both neuron survival and the morphology of the surviving neurons.

5. While there has been considerable effort expended throughout the years to document sexual dimorphisms in the brains of humans, the origin of these sex differences remains uncertain. Evidence in support of sex-related differences in the hypothalamus and spinal cord is the most compelling. Other sex-related differences tend to be subtler. There is no conclusive evidence that hormones establish neural sexual dimorphism, sexual behavior, or sexual preference in humans.

Study Questions

1. You are a famous behavioral endocrinologist studying the behavior of a new species in which the males and females exhibit very different behaviors as adults. What experiments could you do to determine whether the sex differences in behavior are due to organizational rather than activational effects of gonadal hormones? How do you determine when the sensitive period is? If you only had access to adult animals (so you couldn't do developmental hormone manipulations), how could you determine whether sex differences in behavior are organizational rather than activational effects of gonadal hormones?

2. Describe the ways in which hormones can act on neurons to influence sexual differentiation of the brain.
3. Discuss the roles of estrogen, testosterone, and dihydrotestone in sexual differentiation of the POA versus SNB.
4. What evidence is there that the brains of humans are sexually dimorphic? Discuss.

References

Alcock, J. (1989) *Animal Behavior. An Evolutionary Approach.* Sunderland, Mass.: Sinauer.

Allen, L. S., and Gorski, R. A. (1991) Sexual dimorphism of the anterior commissure and massa intermedia of the human brain. *J. Comp. Neurol.* 312: 97–104.

Allen, L. S., and Gorski, R. A. (1992) Sexual orientation and the size of the anterior commissure in the human brain. *Proc. Natl. Acad. Sci. USA* 89: 7199–7202.

Arendash, G. W., and Gorski, R. A. (1983) Effects of discrete lesions of the sexually dimorphic nucleus of the preoptic area or other medial preoptic regions on the sexual behavior of male rats. *Brain Res. Bull.* 10: 147–154.

Arnold, A. P., and Breedlove, S. M. (1985) Organizational and activational effects of sex steroid hormones on vertebrate behavior: A re-analysis. *Horm. Behav.* 19: 469–498.

Arnold, A. P., and Gorski, R. A. (1984) Gonadal steroid induction of structural sex differences in the central nervous system. *Annu. Rev. Neurosci.* 7: 413–442.

Attardi, B., Geller, L. N., and Ohno, S. (1976) Androgen and estrogen receptors in brain cytosol from male, female, and testicular feminized (tfm/y) mice. *Endocrinology* 98: 864–874.

Beach, F. A. (1971) Hormonal factors controlling the differentiation, development and display of copulatory behavior in the ramstergig and related species. In Tobach, E., Aronson, L. R., and Shaw, E. (Eds.), *Biopsychology of Development.* New York: Academic Press, pp. 249–296.

Bell, A. D., and Variend, S. (1985) Failure to demonstrate sexual dimorphism of the corpus callosum in childhood. *J. Anat.* 143: 143–147.

Bodmer, W. F. (1970) The evolutionary significance of recombination in prokaryotes. *Symp. Soc. Gen. Microbiol.* 20: 279–294.

Booth, J. E. (1977) Sexual behavior of neonatally castrated rats injected during infancy with oestrogen and dihydrotestosterone. *J. Endocrinol.* 72: 135–142.

Breedlove, S. M., and Arnold, A. P. (1983a) Hormonal control of a developing neuromuscular system: I. Complete demasculinization of the spinal nucleus of the bulbocavernosus in male rats using the anti-androgen flutamide. *J. Neurosci.* 3: 417–423.

Breedlove, S. M., and Arnold, A. P. (1983b) Hormonal control of a developing neuromuscular system: II. Sensitive periods for the androgen induced masculinization of the rat spinal nucleus of the bulbocavernosus. *J. Neurosci.* 3: 424–432.

Breedlove, S. M., Jacobson, C. D., Gorski, R. A., and Arnold, A. P. (1982) Masculinization of the female rat spinal cord following a single neonatal injection of testosterone propionate but not estradiol benzoate. *Brain Res.* 237: 173–181.

Breedlove, S. M. (1997) Sex on the brain. *Nature* 389: 801.

Bull, J. J., and Vogt, R. C. (1979) Temperature dependent sex determination in turtles. *Science* 206: 1186–1188.

Cihak, R., Gutmann, E., and Hanzlikova, V. (1970) Involution and hormone-induced persistence of the muscle sphincter (levator) ani in female rats. *J. Anat.* 106: 93–110.

Clemens, L. G., Gladue, B. A., and Coniglio, L. P. (1978) Prenatal endogenous androgenic influences on masculine sexual behavior and genital morphology in male and female rats. *Horm. Behav.* 10: 40–53.

Cooke, B. M., Tabibnia, G., and Breedlove, S. M. (1999) Activational effects of adult androgen on the sexually dimorphic medial amygdala. *Proc. Natl. Acad. Sci. USA* 96: 7538–7540.

Davis, E. C., Popper, P., and Gorski, R. A. (1996) The role of apoptosis in sexual differentiation of the rat sexually dimorphic nucleus of the preoptic area. *Brain Res.* 734: 10–18.

De Jonge, F. H., Louwerse, A. L., Ooms, M. P., Evers, P., Endert, E., and Van de Poll, N. E. (1989) Lesions of the SDN-POA inhibit sexual behavior of male wistar rats. *Brain Res. Bull.* 23: 483–492.

deLacoste, M.-C., Holloway, R. L., and Woodward, D. J. (1986) Sex differences in the fetal human corpus callosum. *Hum. Neurobiol.* 5: 93–96.

deLacoste, M.-C., and Horvath, D. S. (1985) Sex differences in the development of morphological asymmetries in human fetuses. *Am. J. Phys. Anthropol.* 66: 163.

deLacoste, M.-C., Horvath, D. S., and Woodward, D. J. (1991) Possible sex differences in the developing human fetal brain. *J. Clin. Exp. Neuropsychol.* 13: 831–846.

deLacoste-Utamsing, C., and Holloway, R. L. (1982) Sexual dimorphism in the human corpus callosum. *Science* 216: 1431–1432.

DeVries, G. J., DeBruin, G. J., Uylings, H. M. B., and Corner, M. A. (1984) *Progress in Brain Research: Sex Differences in the Brain.* Amsterdam: Elsevier.

Diamond, M., and Sigmundson, H. K. (1997) Sex reassignment at birth: Long-term review and clinical implications. *Arch. Pediatr. Adolesc. Med.* 151: 298–304.

Dohler, K. D., Coquelin, A., Davis, F., Hines, M., Shryne, J. E., and Gorski, R. A. (1984) Pre- and postnatal influence of TP and DES on differentiation of the SDN-POA in male and female rats. *Brain Res.* 302: 291–295.

Dorner, G. (1976) *Hormones and Brain Differentiation.* Amsterdam: Elsevier.

Driesen, N. R., and Raz, N. (1995) The influence of sex, age, and handedness on corpus callosum morphology: A meta-analysis. *Psychobiology* 23: 240–247.

Ehrhardt, A. A., Evers, K., and Money, J. (1968) Influence of androgen on some aspects of sexually dimorphic behavior in women with the late-treated adrenogenital syndrome. *Johns Hopkins Med. J.* 123: 115–122.

Ehrhardt, A. A., and Meyer-Bahlburg, H. F. L. (1981) Effects of prenatal sex hormones on gender-related behavior. *Science* 211: 1312–1318.

Ehrhardt, A. A., Meyer-Bahlburg, H. F. L., Rosen, L. R., Feldman, J. F., Veridiano, N. P., Zimmerman, I., and McEwen, B. S. (1985) Sexual orientation after prenatal exposure to exogenous estrogen. *Arch. Sex. Behav.* 14: 57–75.

Feder, H. H., and Whalen, R. E. (1965) Feminine behavior in neonatally castrated and estrogen-treated male rats. *Science* 147: 306–307.

Feingold, A. (1984) Cognitive gender differences are disappearing. *Am. Psychol.* 43: 95–103.

Fishman, R. B., and Breedlove, S. M. (1988) Neonatal androgen maintains sexually dimorphic perineal muscles in the absence of innervation. *Muscle Nerve* 11: 553–560.

Fishman, R. B., and Breedlove, S. M. (1988) Sexual dimorphism in the developing nervous system. In Meisami, E. and Timiras, P. (Eds.), *Handbook of Human Growth and Developmental Biology.* Boca Raton: CRC Press.

Fishman, R. B., and Breedlove, S. M. (1992) Local perineal implants of anti-androgen block masculinization of the spinal nucleus of the bulbocavernosus. *Devel. Brain Res.* 70: 283–286.

Ford, C. S., and Beach, F. A. (1951) *Patterns of Sexual Behavior.* New York: Harper.

Forger, N. G., and Breedlove, S. M. (1986) Sexual dimorphism in human and canine spinal cord: role of early androgen. *Proc. Natl. Acad. Sci. USA* 83: 7527–7531.

Forger, N. G., Howell, M. L., Bengston, L., MacKenzie, L., DeChiara, T. M., and Yancopoulos, G. D. (1997) Sexual dimorphism in the spinal cord is absent in mice lacking the ciliary neurotrophic factor receptor. *J. Neurosci.* 17: 9605–9612.

Freeman, L. M., Watson, N. V., and Breedlove, S. M. (1996) Androgen spares androgen-insensitive motoneurons from apoptosis in the spinal nucleus of the bulbocavernosus in rats. *Horm. Behav.* 30: 424–433.

Gladue, B. A., Green, R., and Hellman, R. E. (1984) Neuroendocrine response to estrogen and sexual orientation. *Science* 225: 1496–1498.

Gorski, R. A. (1984) Critical role for the medial preoptic area in the sexual differentiation of the brain. *Prog. Brain Res.* 61: 129.

Gorski, R. A., Gordon, J. H., Shryne, J. E., and Southam, A. M. (1978) Evidence for a morphological sex difference within the medial preoptic area of the rat brain. *Brain Res.* 148: 333–346.

Gould, S. J. (1981) *The Mismeasure of Man.* New York: Norton.

Hamer, D. D., Hu, S., Magnuson, V. L., Hu, N., and Pattatucci, A. M. L. (1993) A linkage between DNA markers on the X chromosome and male sexual orientation. *Science* 261: 321–327.

Harris, G. W. (1964) Sex hormones, brain development and brain function. *Endocrinology* 75: 627–648.

Harris, G. W., and Jacobson, D. (1952) Functional grafts of the anterior pituitary gland. *Proc. Roy. Soc. B* 139: 263.

Hart, B. L., and Leedy, M. G. (1985) Neurological bases of sexual behavior. A comparative analysis. In N. T. Adler, D. Pfaff, and R. W. Goy (Eds.), *Reproduction*. Vol. 7 in Handbooks of Behavioral Neurobiology. New York: Plenum.

Hendricks, S. E., Graber, B., and Rodriguez-Sierra, J. F. (1989) Neuroendocrine responses to exogenous estrogen: No differences between heterosexual and homosexual men. *Psychoneuroendocrinology* 14: 177–185.

Hines, M. (1982) Prenatal gonadal hormones and sex differences in human behavior. *Psychol. Bull.* 92: 56–80.

Imperato-McGinley, J. I., Guerrero, L., Gautier, T., and Peterson, R. E. (1974) Steroid 5-α-reductase deficiency in Man: An inherited form of male pseudohermaphroditism. *Science* 186: 1213–1215.

Imperato-McGinley, J. I., Peterson, R. E., Gautier, T., and Sturla, E. (1979) Androgens and the evolution of male-gender identity among male pseudohermaphrodites with 5α-reductase deficiency. *N. Engl. J. Med.* 300: 1233–1237.

Inglis, J., and Lawson, J. S. (1981) Sex differences in the effects of unilateral brain damage on intelligence. *Science* 212: 603.

Jacobson, C. D. (1980) The characterization, ontogeny and influence of androgen on the sexually dimorphic nucleus of the preoptic area. Ph.D. dissertation. University of California, Los Angeles.

Jacobson, C. D., and Gorski, R. A. (1981) Neurogenesis of the sexually dimorphic nucleus of the preoptic area in the rat. *J. Comp. Neurol.* 196: 519–529.

Jordan, C. L., Letinsky, M. S., and Arnold, A. P. (1989) The role of gonadal hormones in neuromuscular synapse elimination in rats. I. androgen delays the loss of multiple innervation in the levator ani muscle. *J. Neurosci.* 9: 229–238.

Jost, A. (1979) Basic sexual trends in the development of vertebrates. In *Sex, Hormones and Behavior*. Ciba Foundation Symposium 62. North Holland: Elsevier.

Konishi, M., and Akutagawa, E. (1985) Neuronal growth, atrophy and death in a sexually dimorphic song nucleus in the zebra finch brain. *Nature* 315: 145–147.

Lansdell, H., and Davie, J. C. (1972) Massa intermedia: Possible relation to intelligence. *Neuropsychologia* 10: 207–210.

LeVay, S. (1991) A difference in hypothalamic structure between heterosexual and homosexual men. *Science* 253: 1034–1037.

Lillie, F. R. (1916) The theory of the freemartin. *Science* 43: 611–613.

McCarthy, M. M. (1994) Molecular aspects of sexual differentiation of the rodent brain. *Psychoneuroendocrinology* 19: 415–427.

McCarthy, M. M., Besmer, H. R., Jacobs, S. C., Keidan, G. M., and Gibbs, R. B. (1997) Influence of maternal grooming, sex and age on Fos immunoreactivity in the preoptic area of neonatal rats: Implications for sexual differentiation. *Devel. Neurosci.* 19: 488–496.

McEwen, B. S., and Krey, L. C. (1984) Properties of estrogen sensitive neurons: Aromatization, progestin receptor induction and neuroendocrine effects. In F. Celotti et al. (Eds.), *Metabolism of Hormonal Steroids in the Neuroendocrine Structures*. New York: Raven Press.

McFadden, D. (1993) A masculinizing effect on the auditory systems of human females having male cotwins. *Proc. Natl. Acad. Sci. USA* 90: 11900–11904.

McFadden, D., and Pasanen, E. G. (1988) Comparison of the auditory systems of heterosexuals and homosexuals: Click-evoked otoacoustic emissions. *Proc. Natl. Acad. Sci. USA* 95: 2709–2713.

McGlone, J. (1980) Sex differences in human brain asymmetry: A critical survey. *Behav. Brain Sci.* 3: 215–263.

Meisel, R. L., and Ward, I. L. (1981) Fetal female rats are masculinized by male littermates located caudally in the uterus. *Science* 213: 239–242.

Meyer-Bahlburg, H. F. L. (1984) Psychoendocrine research on sexual orientation. Current status and future options. *Prog. Brain Res.* 61: 375–398.

Meyer-Bahlburg, H. F. L., Ehrhardt, A. A., Rosen, L. R., Gruen, R. S., Veridiano, N. P., Vann, F. H., and Neuwalder, H. F. (1995) Prenatal estrogens and the development of homosexual orientation. *Devel. Psychol.* 31: 12–21.

Money, J., and Ehrhardt, A. A. (1972) *Man and Woman, Boy and Girl*. Baltimore: Johns Hopkins Press.

Money, J., Schwartz, M., and Lewis, V. G. (1984) Adult erotosexual status and fetal hormonal masculinization and demasculinization: 46,XX congenital virilizing adrenal hyperplasia and 46/XY androgen insensitivity syndrome compared. *Psychoneuroendocrinology* 9: 405–414.

Mulaikal, R. M., Migeon, C. J., and Rock, J. A. (1987) Fertility rates in female patients with congenital adrenal hyperplasia due to 21-hydroxylase deficiency. *N. Engl. J. Med.* 316: 178–182.

Naftolin, F., and MacLusky, N. (1984) Aromatization hypothesis revisited. In M. Serio et al. (Eds.), *Differentiation: Basic and Clinical Aspects.* New York: Raven Press.

Norman, R. L., and Spies, H. G. (1986) Cyclic ovarian function in a male macaque: Additional evidence for a lack of sexual differentiation in the physiological mechanisms that regulate the cyclic release of gonadotropins in primates. *Endocrinology* 118: 2608–2610.

Nottebohm, F., and Arnold, A. (1976) Sexual dimorphismn in vocal control areas of the songbird brain. *Science* 194: 211–213.

Onuf, B. (1899) Notes on the arrangement and function of the cell group in the sacral region of the spinal cord. *J. Nervous Ment. Dis.* 26: 498–504.

Pakkenberg, H., and Voigt, J. (1964) Brain weight of the Danes. *Acta Anat.* 56: 297–307.

Pfeiffer, C. A. (1936) Sexual differences of the hypophyses and their determination by the gonads. *Am. J. Anat.* 58: 195–216.

Phoenix, C. H., Goy, R. W., Gerall, A. A., and Young, W. C. (1959) Organization action of prenatally administered testosterone propionate on the tissues mediating mating behavior in the female guinea pig. *Endocrinology* 65: 369–382.

Plomin, R., DeFries, J. C., and McClearn, G. E. (1990) *Behavioral Genetics: A Primer.* New York: Freeman.

Purves, D., and Lichtman, J. W. (1985) Geometrical differences among homologous neurons in mammals. *Science* 228: 298–302.

Raisman, G. and Field, P. M. (1973) Sexual dimorphism in the neuropil of the preoptic area of the rat and its dependence on neonatal androgen. *Brain Res.* 54: 1–20.

Rand, M. N., and Breedlove, S. M. (1987) Ontogeny of functional innervation of bulbocavernosus muscles in male and female rats. *Devel. Brain Res.* 33: 150–152.

Reddy, V. V. R., Naftolin, F., and Ryan, K. J. (1974) Conversion of androstenedione to estrone by neural tissues from fetal and neonatal rat. *Endocrinology* 94: 117–121.

Rosenfeld, J. M., Daley, J. D., Ohno, S., and YoungLai, E. V. (1977) Central aromatization of testosterone in testicular feminized mice. *Experientia* 33: 1392–1393.

Simerly, R. B. (1998) Organization and regulation of sexually dimorphic neuroendocrine pathways. *Behav. Brain Res.* 92: 195–203.

Springer, S. P., and Deutsch, G. (1998) *Left Brain, Right Brain*, 5th edition. New York: Freeman.

Stanley, A. J., Gumbreck, L. G., and Allison, J. E. (1973) Male pseudohermaphroditism in the laboratory rat. *Recent Prog. Horm. Res.* 29: 43–64.

Swaab, D. F., and Fliers, E. (1985) A sexually dimorphic nucleus in the human brain. *Science* 228: 1112–1115.

Swaab, D. F., Gooren, L. J., and Hofman, M. A. (1992) The human hypothalamus in relation to gender and sexual orientation. *Prog. Brain Res.* 93: 205–217.

Swaab, D. F., and Hofman, M. A. (1984) Sexual differentiation of the human brain: A historical perspective. *Prog. Brain Res.* 61: 361.

Toran-Allerand, C. D. (1981) Gonadal steroids and brain development. In vitro veritas? *Trends Neurosci.* 4: 118–121.

Wada, J. A., Clarke, R. A., and Hamm, A. (1975) Cerebral hemisphere asymmetry in humans. Cortical speech zones in 100 adult and 100 infant brains. *Arch. Neurol.* 32: 239.

Ward, I. L., and Reed, J. (1985) Prenatal stress and prepuberal social rearing conditions interact to determine sexual behavior in male rats. *Behav. Neurosci.* 99: 301–309.

Williams, T. J., Pepitone, M. E., Christensen, S. E., Cooke, B. M., Huberman, A. D., Breedlove, N. J., Breedlove, T. J., Jordan, C. L., and Breedlove, S. M. (2000) Finger-length ratios and sexual orientation. *Nature* 404: 455–456.

Witelson, S. F. (1985) The brain connection: the corpus callosum is larger in left-handers. *Science* 229: 665–668.

Witelson, S. F. (1989) Hand and sex differences in the isthmus and genu of the human corpus callosum. *Brain* 112: 799–835.

Zucker, K. J., Bradley, S. J., Oliver, G., Blake, J., Fleming, S., and Hood, J. (1996) Psychosexual development of women with congenital adrenal hyperplasia. *Horm. Behav.* 30: 300–318.

In the next six chapters we will be considering the mysterious and fascinating world of reproductive behaviors. It is in this arena that most people already consider hormones to have a great deal of influence. Indeed, rats are very unlikely to display sexual behavior without the appropriate hormones (either from their internal supplies or administered by an experimenter). This close correlation between hormones and sexual behavior is the reason we devote six chapters (a third of the book) to the behaviors that ensure the survival of a species; few behaviors are so reliably altered by hormone treatment in so many species. In later chapters, we will find that the effects of hormones on some other behaviors are more subtle and more likely to vary from one species to another. This helps us appreciate how reliably and robustly hormones affect reproductive behaviors.

But as you will see, not even rats are hormone-driven automatons. When we give animals hormones, we change the probability that they will show male- or female-like behaviors, but there are still individual differences in response. For example, some male rats refuse to copulate even though they have plenty of the apparently appropriate hormones (i.e., androgens), and some male mice continue to copulate even after castration. Furthermore, even when females are in heat, they can still be rather selective about which males they will allow to mount them if they are given the opportunity to choose.

By the time you read about human sexual behavior in chapter 6, you will be prepared for some ambiguity in the relations between hormones and sexual behavior. Natural selection has also produced species in which hormones have, of necessity, become uncoupled from reproductive behavior, as chapter 7 describes. Hormones also affect many of the courtship behaviors attending copulation, and chapter 8 gives you a glimpse of the remarkable species diversity of such behaviors and the diverse ways in which hormones influence them. Finally, the hormones of pregnancy (which results from the courtship and sexual behavior) ensure infant survival in many species. You may notice that this chapter emphasizes maternal rather than paternal behavior, but that is a reflection of the fact that it is predominantly the mother's behavior that is influenced by hormones. On the other hand, new information presented in chapter 9 suggests that in some species paternal behavior may also have an endocrine component.

These chapters reveal that hormones are not love potions that force animals to copulate but coordinators of reproduction. The same hormones that prepare the production of eggs and sperm and control other physiological processes directly involved in reproduction also prepare the nervous system to display the courtship and copulatory behaviors that are required for reproduction. As hormonal influence upon reproductive organs evolves, so too do the hormonal effects upon the nervous system. The nervous system is a very complex organ that processes a great deal of information at a rapid clip, and hormones are just one source, albeit an important one, of information about reproduction. An animal's previous experiences, level of arousal, and even general health are all integrated by the nervous system and affect the behavior.

4　Neuroendocrinology of Sexual Behavior in the Female

Margaret M. McCarthy and Jill B. Becker

We begin our study of sexual behavior with females. Females display cycles of reproductive function, and behavior is an integral part of that cycle. For example, female rats ovulate about every four days and will, for a period of a few hours during that time, allow males to copulate with them. This receptivity on the part of the female occurs at a particular point in the ovulatory cycle that favors fertilization and pregnancy. The receptive behavior is coordinated by the same gonadal hormones that guide ovulation. The close correlation between female receptivity and gonadal hormones has made it possible to discover a good deal about how hormones affect this and other female sexual behaviors.

What sexual behaviors do females display? Which hormones affect these behaviors? How does hormonal modulation of gene expression affect female sexual behavior? What neural systems mediate female sexual behavior? What neurotransmitters are involved?

Introduction

Sex—whether you are obsessed by it, scared of it, addicted to it, curious about it, or tired of it, one thing is for sure, at some point in your life it will be important. Sex pervades our daily living. It colors our relationship with friends, co-workers, and even strangers. It is used to sell us new cars, the clothes we wear, the TV shows we watch. It determines how we perceive our own bodies and those of others. Relationships are forged and broken by the same pervasive drive to have sex. Why is this drive so powerful that it can lead presidents to risk their office, priests to discard their vows, and ordinary men and women to gamble the security of marriage and family? From an evolutionary standpoint, sexual behavior is a critical component of reproduction. The drive to perpetuate our genes can override all other drives, leading to what at times may seem like irrational behavior. As will be discussed in chapter 11, the short-term need to survive will take precedence over reproductive processes—if you are a zebra being chased down by a hungry lion, you will wait to ovulate at another time. But as soon as safety returns, the forces regulating the processes of seeking a suitable mate, copulating, and ultimately reproducing will come rushing back to the fore.

Reproduction is successful only when the male and female of a species engage in behaviors that result in the two joining in copulation. Reproductive hormones act on the brain to induce the behaviors that bring males and females together (i.e., courtship behaviors) and to induce copulatory behaviors.

How do steroids alter brain functioning to control reproductive behavior? Why do females of most species exhibit sexual receptivity only certain times during their reproductive cycles? Why are humans, some primates, and horses different? What are the variables that determine varying patterns of sexual receptivity across species? Finally, what are the neural substrates as well as the cellular and molecular mechanisms that ultimately determine female sexual behavior? These questions will be the focus of this chapter. The hormonal influences on sexual behavior in the female begins with the process of sexual differentiation of the brain early in life, as discussed in chapter 3. Hormone control of sexual behavior commences at puberty in most species with the onset of reproductive maturity. To completely understand this complex biological process, a researcher needs a working knowledge of steroid action at the molecular, cellular, and organismal level, along with generous doses of neuroanatomy, neuropharmacology, and neuroethology.

Sexual Behavior in the Female

Female sexual behavior evolved to serve a distinct biological function; it allows the fertilization of a female's ova by a male's sperm. Not so obvious is the tight regulation that coordinates the behavioral response of the female, called "receptivity," with the physiological response of ovulation. In the overwhelming majority of species, **female sexual receptivity** is a transient state that occurs only in association with ovulation. Humans, some primates, and horses are a notable exception in this regard. In most species, achieving the coordination between the physiological events of ovulation, preparation of the uterus, and behavioral receptivity is best accomplished by multiorgan responsiveness to the same humoral (blood-borne) signal. Steroid hormones produced by the ovary serve this purpose. Released into the bloodstream, estrogen and progesterone gain access to the brain where they regulate both behavior and the control of the pituitary gland, which ultimately regulates the ovary. While steroids are acting in the brain to induce sexual receptivity, they are also simultaneously preparing the uterus for the possible arrival of a newly fertilized egg. In the event that this does not happen, the ovary ceases steroid production, the uterine lining is reabsorbed or discarded, and behavioral receptivity is terminated.

There are significant species differences in reproductive behaviors, but in spite of this variation it has been possible to compare the behavioral effects of a variety of hormones across species. Most of the available research examining the mechanisms underlying female sexual behavior has been conducted on rodents, such as rats, mice, and hamsters. Most research into the neuro-endocrinology of female sexual behavior has been done on the laboratory rat and we will focus heavily on it as a model species.

The Hormones That Induce Sexual Behavior in the Female Rat

In the rat, as in most vertebrates, estradiol and progesterone are the hormones produced in the largest quantity by the ovaries. The experiments that determined which hormones are necessary for sexual behavior used the standard endocrine manipulations that we discussed in chapter 1. The ovaries were removed from female rats (a surgical procedure called ovariectomy or OVX) to remove the endogenous source of ovarian hormones. When tested for sexual behavior, an OVX female will vigorously resist and protest the attempts by a male rat to mate with her. When an OVX female is treated with estradiol alone, after about 7 to 10 days she will exhibit reproductive behaviors, but the behavior does not look quite normal. Furthermore, the normal estrous cycle of the rat is only 4 to 5 days. So estradiol alone could not be producing sexual behavior during the naturally occurring estrous cycle. If progesterone alone is given, sexual behavior is never induced, even after weeks of progesterone treatment. So progesterone alone is not the answer.

But if estradiol is administered about 48 hours before progesterone, normal-looking reproductive behaviors are induced. What you will learn is that estradiol primes the brain to be sensitive to progesterone by inducing the synthesis of progesterone receptors in the hypothalamus. Progesterone then acts on these receptors to induce sexual behavior. Later in the chapter we will talk more about this priming effect of estradiol and where in the hypothalamus these hormones are acting.

RECEPTIVITY

To study sexual behavior in the rat, a female rat is placed into a cage with a sexually experienced male rat. After some anogenital investigation, the male will usually attempt to mount the female and will stimulate her flanks with his forepaws. A receptive female will stop moving and will exhibit the lordosis posture (see figure 1.1 in chapter 1) in response to this stimulation. A nonreceptive female will either run away, kick at the male, roll on her back, or just generally ignore him. The response of the female to each successful mount by the male is noted by the researcher and the test is usually completed after 10 mounts. The frequency of lordosis responses is then expressed as a quotient — # lordosis / # of mounts × 100—and this is referred to as the **lordosis quotient** (LQ). A female with an LQ in the range of 80 to 100 (meaning she exhibited lordosis in response to 8 out of 10 mounts) is considered highly receptive, whereas a female with an LQ of less than 50 is not considered sexually receptive. The amplitude of the lordosis is also taken as a measure of the level of receptivity. For instance, a female whose back remains arched and shows no elevation of the rump, in other words no lordosis, is scored as having an amplitude of 0. If her back is slightly straightened, the score is 1, if mildly convex, a 2, and if the back is strongly curved and the rump elevated, a 3. These two scores together—the lordosis quotient and the lordosis amplitude—give an accurate picture of the state of sexual receptivity of a female rat.

PROCEPTIVE BEHAVIOR

For many years, female reproductive behavior was studied under these rather artificial conditions. It was assumed that females were passive receptive vessels that exhibited the lordosis reflex in response to stimulation by the male, but that females played no active role in sexual behavior. Recent research has demonstrated that this is not the case. Under seminatural conditions, the female rat will actively control the pace of copulatory behavior by exhibiting proceptive or soliciation behaviors and actively withdrawing from the male. There are three components to a female rat's proceptive behavior: approach, orientation, and runaway, which occur in this sequence. Sniffing and grooming (orienting) follows the approach to the male, as do ear wiggling, hopping, and darting.

Ear wiggling sounds like a nifty party trick but is actually an extremely rapid vibration of the head that makes it appear that the ears are wiggling. Females usually show ear wiggling in response to an approach and contact by a male. If, on the other hand, the male is recalcitrant and not paying proper attention to the female, she will resort to hopping and darting. This behavioral complex consists of a rapid hop with rigid legs combined with fast darting movements away from the male (runaway) and almost always induces the male rat to chase after her. Interestingly, while scientists have thought that these behaviors serve primarily to attract the male to the female, observations in seminatural conditions suggest that in the wild the female may actually use proceptive behaviors to distract the male and delay copulation (McClintock 1984).

The hormones necessary for the induction of proceptive behaviors are estradiol and progesterone. Estradiol alone can induce a low rate of proceptive behavior but both the frequency of proceptive behaviors and the number of females exhibiting proceptive behaviors are greatly increased by progesterone in a dose-dependent manner. In other words, female rats are more likely to exhibit proceptive behaviors with higher doses of progesterone.

PACING BEHAVIOR

In the continuing battle between the sexes, it turns out that the optimal rate of intromissions is different for males and females. This may be because the goal of the male is to achieve an ejaculation and move on, whereas the female wants to maximize the use of that ejaculation for fertilization. By way of controlling the behavior of the male, the female rat will actively engage in proceptive behaviors and in an additional behavior called "pacing behavior." Pacing takes the female away from male contact for several minutes. For the male rat, a rapidly paced series of intromissions (about 30 sec between intromissions) is optimal to induce ejaculation in the fewest number of intromissions. The female rat, on the other hand, requires behavioral activation of a progestational reflex in order to facilitate pregnancy. When intromissions are spaced several minutes apart, this progestational reflex is activated and the chance that insemination will result in pregnancy is significantly enhanced (Adler 1978). We will further discuss this progestational reflex later in the chapter.

In order for a female rat to pace the rate of intromissions there must be a barrier behind which she can escape from the male rat. The importance of this behavior is apparent in the fact that a female rat with no previous sexual experience will almost immediately take advantage of a barrier in the testing apparatus and begin pacing. The rate at which the female withdraws from the presence of the male after a mating bout (the percent of exits) and the time before she returns to the male after a contact (the return latency in min), are used to objectively define the behavior referred to as pacing. A female that is pacing shows higher rates of percent exits and a longer return latency after an ejaculation than after an intromission or mount. These sexually dimorphic mating strategies are optimal for the reproductive success of both males and females. In the wild, mating actually occurs among a group of animals rather than in individual male-female pairs. With rapid intromissions and ejaculation, the mating strategy of the male maximizes the number of females he can inseminate. The pacing behavior of the female increases the probability that pregnancy will occur by activation of a neuroendocrine reflex that promotes implantation due to activation of the corpus luteum (see below) which causes progesterone to be released (Erskine 1989; McClintock 1984).

From this, we see that pacing behavior is dependent on both estradiol and progesterone to induce sexual receptivity. Certain aspects of pacing behavior may be primarily sensitive to estradiol (see chapter 13). On the other hand, the proceptive behaviors that the female rat uses on occasion to delay subsequent male contacts are more dependent on progesterone. Thus, both hormones seem to play important roles in the neural control of pacing behavior.

TERMINATION OF RECEPTIVITY

Once estradiol and progesterone have induced sexual behavior, what causes the behavior to be terminated? Interestingly, if no sexual behavior occurs during the period when the female is receptive to the male, she will stop being receptive 18 to 20 hours later. On the other hand, if the female engages in sexual behavior, receptivity terminates sooner. Furthermore, females who engage in paced mating behavior show termination of sexual receptivity even sooner than those who engage in nonpaced mating (Erskine and Baum 1982).

How does this happen? Investigators have found that progesterone, the same hormone that activates sexual behavior initially, is also responsible for its termination. You will remember that estradiol priming induces the synthesis of progesterone receptors in the brain. Progesterone occupation of these receptors activates sexual behavior, but it also makes the receptors unavailable to further actions of progesterone. If sexual behavior does not occur, the progesterone receptors are occupied by the available progesterone and then deactivated. If mating occurs, additional progesterone is released from the corpus luteum in the ovary (see figure 4.1), and the progesterone binds to its receptors and rapidly deactivates them. With paced mating behavior, the release of progesterone is greater than with nonpaced mating, so pacing results in a more rapid termination of the sexually receptive period. This is what is thought to regulate the onset and offset of sexual receptivity as indicated by a female's lordosis quotient. How other aspects of sexual behavior are terminated in the female have not yet been studied and may be regulated by other mechanisms (Pfaus 1999).

From this we see that the hormones of the estrous cycle have many different and complementary effects on the behavior of the female rat. Estradiol increases a female's attractiveness to a male rat and primes for progesterone receptors. Then progesterone induces sexual receptivity and proceptive behaviors, followed by termination of lordosis behavior.

Female Reproduction Is Cyclic

The hallmark of female reproduction is its cyclicity, which is in turn the result of an intricate hormonal dance between the brain, the pituitary, and the ovary. These cycles may be as short as 4 to 5 days or as long as a year. In humans the cycle lasts about a month. In some species, cycling is replaced by opportunistic fertility. In other words, females only become sexually receptive when in the presence of a male. The rate-limiting step is found in the ovary, which has two major functions, the release of ova (eggs) and the synthesis of steroid hormones. The main functional components of the ovary are the **ovarian follicles**, which house and nurture the eggs. Once the eggs have been released at ovulation, the follicles are converted into **corpora lutea**. Keep in mind that a female is born with all the eggs she will ever have. These remain in a quiescent state until the maturation of the follicle in which a particular egg is stored. The structures of the ovary are illustrated in figure 4.1. The follicle is the site of estradiol production, in particular by the theca and granulosa cells. **Estrogen** gains its name from its ability to induce the behavioral state of **estrus**, or heat, and refers to a collection of steroids which includes the familiar estradiol and the less well-known estriol and estrone.

The corpora lutea is a transient endocrine gland that produces copious quantities of **progesterone** (pro-gestational) in order to prepare the uterus for the implantation of fertilized eggs. In species with a spontaneously functional corpus luteum, if implantation does not occur, the corpus luteum degenerates and new follicles develop. In other species, such as rats, the corpus luteum becomes functional as a consequence of the female engaging in sexual behaviors that activate the progestational reflex. This reflex refers to the fact that neural stimulation caused by mating results in a change in secretions from the anterior pituitary, particularly in prolactin. Prolactin induces the maintenance of the corpus luteum, which in turn secretes progesterone to prepare the uterus for implantation, and this increases the probability that pregnancy will occur.

The Ovarian Cycle

The ovary begins steroid production in response to stimulation by the gonadotropins, LH (leutinizing hormone) and FSH (follicle-stimulating hormone), which are released into the bloodstream from the anterior pituitary. They bind to their respective receptors on the surface of the granulosa and theca

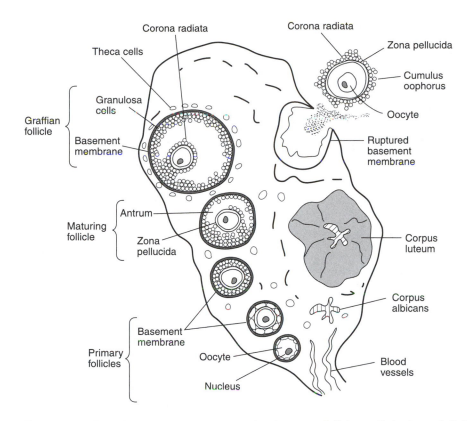

Figure 4.1 The ovary. Individual eggs or oocytes are stored in immature follicles, called primary follicles, until they are recruited to develop during a particular reproductive cycle. In response to stimulation by FSH, the follicle will grow; when it reaches the preantral stage, substantial steroid synthesis by the granulosa cells begins. The development of an antrum is the sign of a maturing follicle. A preovulatory, or Graffian, follicle is poised to ovulate its ova in response to stimulation by LH. The event of ovulation will rupture the basement membrane and allow for increased vascularization of the follicle. An additional action of LH is to stimulate the proliferation of the granulosa cells and the formation of the corpus luteum, a transient endocrine gland that synthesizes large quantities of progesterone. In the event that fertilization does not occur, the corpus luteum will eventually regress, leaving behind a small white scar known as the corpus albicans. (Adapted from Porterfield 1997.)

cells and promote the activity of steroidogenic enzymes. The release of LH and FSH from the pituitary is regulated by a releasing hormone from the brain, referred to as GnRH (gonadotropin-releasing hormone). As steroid synthesis by the ovary increases, levels in the blood rise and eventually gain access to the brain. During the first part of the cycle, estrogens exert a positive feedback effect on the brain to promote increased GnRH release and ultimately the **LH-surge**, which will lead to ovulation. The cellular mechanisms of estrogen-induced positive feedback on LH release are yet to be elucidated, but it is clear that after ovulation estrogens and progesterone exert a negative feedback on the brain, reducing the release of GnRH and ultimately LH and FSH (in males there is only negative feedback, which is why there is no cycle). As the levels of these gonadotropins drop, so does steroid synthesis by the ovary due to the degenerating corpora lutea. The dynamic changes in the structure of the ovary, from the development of follicles to the dramatic event of ovulation and the formation of the corpora luteum, are pivotal events and are used to delineate the various phases of the cycle.

FOLLICULAR PHASE

A new cycle begins with the development of follicles from what is called a preantral stage (the antrum is the opening or space within the follicle where the egg resides) to a fully mature follicle, sometimes called a preovulatory follicle or a graffian follicle. Low levels of FSH from the pituitary mediate follicular development. There is also increased steroidogenesis at this phase due to stimulation by LH. Even in species in which only one fetus is maintained, such as humans, several follicles will develop with each cycle in a process referred to as "recruitment." As the follicular phase progresses, all but one follicle will regress and eventually die or become "atretic." A single dominant follicle will then proceed to ovulation. The selection processes leading to only one mature follicle is poorly understood but may involve differential sensitivity to FSH. This process can be overridden with fertility drugs so that multiple follicles will develop to full maturity and ultimately ovulate, resulting in the risk of multiple births. In humans, the time needed to develop from a preantral follicle to full maturity is about 12 or 14 days, whereas in rodents the time can be as short as 2 or 3 days.

PERIOVULATORY PERIOD

The time just before and after ovulation is a dynamic one, with dramatic changes in circulating hormone levels and a structural reorganization of the follicle. In response to the extremely high levels of estrogens, a surge of LH is released from the pituitary and will precipitate ovulation. Progesterone also rises a few hours prior to ovulation and contributes to this process. The periovulatory period in humans lasts 1 to 2 days, with the surge in LH preceding ovulation by about 24 hours. The recent advent of home kits for predicting ovulation are based on detecting LH in the urine, and because LH levels are sustained at high levels for a full day, the test can be conducted at any time. In rodents, the elevation in LH levels lasts only hours and ovulation is induced much more quickly.

LUTEAL PHASE

Within hours of ovulation, the ruptured follicle will begin to reorganize into the corpora luteum (literally "body yellow"), which is actually a transitory endocrine gland derived from the granulosa cells that are interior to the graffian follicle. During the follicular phase, these cells are essentially starved of a blood supply and therefore make very little steroid. After ovulation, the granulosa cells become vascularized and undergo both hyperplasia (increased number) and hypertrophy (increased size). This process is collectively known as leutinization. The granulosa cells do not possess high levels of the enzymes required to complete steroidogenesis to the point of making androgens and estrogens, and therefore progesterone is the predominant secretory product. The theca interna cells, on the other hand, have high levels of the P450 enzyme, aromatase, which converts testosterone into estradiol.

MENSTRUAL PHASE

In primates, menstruation results from the fall in progesterone and estradiol levels that inevitably follows the degeneration of the corpora luteum. A sloughing off accompanied by some fresh bleeding now reverses the building up of the uterine wall (endometrium) that occurred during the luteal phase. The majority of species do not menstruate but rather reabsorb the endometrial buildup. The adaptive significance of menstruation is still being debated. Two theories that have been advanced but not proven are that menstruation reduces circulating iron (which can generate free radicals) or that it helps flush out harmful pathogens introduced by mating.

The Estrous Cycle

In rodents, all the same phases of the cycle exist (with the exception of the menstrual phase) but they are seldom referred to by those labels. In rats, the cycle is so short we speak of it in terms of days rather than phases, with each day having a distinct name. In general, rats have either a 4- or 5-day cycle. The reason for this short cycle is that the corpora lutea does not fully develop unless the animal engages in sexual behavior that activates the progestational reflex that we discussed above. In rodents, the hormonal events that occur during the estrous cycle are tightly regulated by the light-dark cycle. In hamsters, the regulation is so precise that some investigators joke that you could set your watch by the time of day that female hamsters ovulate. Because most rodents are nocturnal, the hormones are timed so that the onset of sexual receptivity occurs at night when the animal is active. Thus, we will define the days of the cycle as starting when the lights go out in the colony room (or the sun goes down in the wild). You may see others define the days of the cycle as beginning at midnight, but this means essentially breaking the period of sexual receptivity into 2 days, which we believe is artificial and not conducive to defining the behavioral states produced by the antecedent hormonal events.

METESTRUS AND DIESTRUS

It is conventional to consider the first day of the menstrual cycle as the beginning of the follicular phase, so by analogy the first day of the estrus cycle begins when steroid hormones are low. Some researchers consider the first day a transitional one and term it **metestrus** or **diestrus I**, and it is followed by **diestrus II**. There is still some progesterone from the corpora luteum on diestrus I, but in the absence of pregnancy this structure is not maintained, progesterone drops, and after a second day when both estradiol and progesterone are extremely low, the cycle begins again. Just as with the menstrual cycle, the hypothalamus begins secreting GnRH, which triggers the pituitary to release LH and FSH into the bloodstream. These gonadotrophins then induce follicular development in the ovary.

PROESTRUS

Proestrus is analogous to the periovulatory phase of the menstrual cycle. It is the most eventful day of the cycle in rodents, because it is the day of the LH-surge. Rapidly increasing levels of estradiol is the rate-limiting event. Maximum ovarian vein estradiol occurs 18 hours before ovulation and a drastic increase is seen around 6 to 12 hours prior to ovulation. In the peripheral plasma, the levels begin rising 30 hrs prior to ovulation, and peak values occur in the late morning or early afternoon of proestrus (~100 pg/ml). One of the most important functions of increasing estradiol levels is a positive feedback effect to produce the LH surge required for ovulation. This positive feedback is achieved at two levels: One is the regulation of the GnRH neuron and the other is to increase the synthesis and storage of LH by the anterior pituitary. As a result, on the afternoon of proestrus, there is a synchronized bursting of the GnRH neurons, producing a bolus release of LH and FSH from the anterior pituitary into the bloodstream. The pulsatile firing of the GnRH neurons results in a 10-fold increase in GnRH levels in the portal blood supply to the anterior pituitary, and this increase is almost simultaneous with the onset of the LH surge.

A significant increase in progesterone also occurs 4 to 6 hours after the estradiol peak, during the afternoon of proestrus. The serum concentrations of progesterone at the proestrus peak is in the range of 25–50 ng/ml; the baseline is 3–15 ng/ml. Note that this is 1000 times more than estradiol. A substantial portion of this progesterone appears to come from the adrenal gland. Once LH and progesterone are released into the circulation, they rapidly reach their target, the mature Graffian follicle of the ovary, and set into action a series of events that will result in ovulation some 10 to 12 hours later (longer in other species). Although both LH and FSH are released by the pituitary, it is clear that only LH is needed for ovulation. FSH is synthesized by some of the same cells that secrete LH but has not been shown to have a distinct and necessary role in ovulation.

ESTRUS

Estrus (vaginal estrus) is the period of sexual receptivity and occurs on the actual day of ovulation. Sexual receptivity onset occurs shortly after the onset of the dark phase of the light:dark cycle and precedes ovulation by a few hours in most animals. Ovulation, induced by the LH surge on proestrus, occurs 4 to 6 hours after nightfall, and sexual receptivity persists for 12 to 20 hours (depending on whether the female mates or not). Note that behavioral receptivity occurs 36 to 48 hours after the initial increase in estradiol and 4 to 6 hours after progesterone. Baseline serum concentrations of estradiol at vaginal estrus or behavioral estrus are approx. 3–12 pg/ml, but by the time of ovulation, levels have returned to baseline. This is because, as we will discuss later, the effects of estradiol are mediated by the induction of specific genes in neurons in specific areas of the brain, and it takes time for these effects to be seen as a change in the animal's behavior. The hormonal profile of the menstrual cycle, estrus cycle, and reproductive patterns in a few select species are illustrated in figure 4.2.

Species Differences in Female Sexual Behavior

As mentioned above, the hallmark of female reproduction is cyclicity, but cycles are not an absolute and when present can vary widely in character. One criteria that distinguishes reproductive parameters of females is whether they ovulate spontaneously or reflexively. Table 4.1 describes the different categories of female reproductive behavior and gives examples of each.

Spontaneous versus Induced Ovulators

When the release of an ova from the maturing follicle is determined by endogenous stimuli such as hormones, as we have been discussing, this is referred to as spontaneous ovulation. Species that are considered spontaneous ovulators include rats, mice, hamsters, guinea pigs, dogs, sheep, and most primates including humans. Alternatively, in some species the maturation of follicles and sexual receptivity are under hormonal control and considered spontaneous, but ovulation is induced by exogenous stimuli, in particular, the stimulus of mating, which releases the hypothalamic-pituitary hormones required to trigger egg release. Species that exhibit this reproductive pattern include cats, ferrets, and rabbits, and they are considered induced or reflexive ovulators. In other species, both behavioral estrus and ovulation are induced by specific stimuli, as is the case in prairie voles. These animals remain reproductively inactive until stimuli from a male are present. The critical stimuli from the male appear to be chemical signals such as pheromones.

By coincidence, or perhaps design, the two most readily identified species that spontaneously ovulate are predator and prey, cats and rabbits. Rabbits don't have an estrous cycle per se; rather, they have waves of follicular development so that there is always a mature follicle or one shortly on its way. Females will show more or less continuous sexual receptivity throughout the breeding season. For cats, anyone that has heard them mating in the alley at night knows it is a noisy business, with much growling and hissing by the female. This is due to the extensive amount of vaginal-cervical stimulation required to induce ovulation. Sensory stimulation is also an important component of mating in lions, and mating requires that the male bite the back of the female's neck in addition to copulatory stimuli. Hormonally, cats exhibit sexual receptivity in response to estrogen in the absence of progesterone, but will continue to show receptivity after ovulation and the formation of the corpora luteum and the attendant progesterone production.

Being a reflexive ovulator is considered an opportunistic reproductive strategy. In the case of wild cats or other animals with a solitary lifestyle, it assures

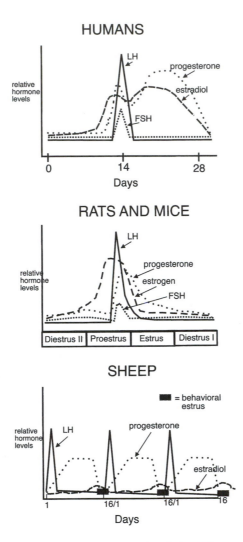

Figure 4.2 Reproductive hormone cycles. Schematic representation of changing hormonal profiles across the cycle in humans, rats and mice, and sheep. Note the basic similarities during the first half of the cycle during which time estradiol is low but slowly rising. The majority of species differences occur after ovulation and is dependent on the duration of the corpus luteum, the major source of progesterone, which can determine the length of the luteal phase of the cycle. In sheep, there is no behavioral estrus after the first cycle because a priming effect of progesterone from the previous cycle is required.

Table 4.1   Reproductive Patterns Used by Females

PATTERN	SPECIES	COMMENTS
Hormonal control of ovarian development, sexual receptivity, and spontaneous ovulation	Rats, mice, guinea pigs, dogs, most primates	Receptivity occurs only around the time of ovulation
Hormonal control of ovarian development, sexual receptivity, and spontaneous ovulation	Humans, horses	Receptivity is independent of ovulation
Hormonal control of ovarian development and sexual receptivity with induced ovulation	Wild and domestic cats, ferrets, rabbits	Mating is required to induce release of the ova
Environmental induction of ovarian development and sexual receptivity	Voles, parakeets	Environmental cue is pheromones in voles, nest box in parakeets
Seasonal breeders	Sheep, syrian hamsters	Hamsters will breed continuously in the laboratory but the males' testes regress when on short days

that the female does not foolishly ovulate her precious egg when the male is busy defending a territory in the next hectare. For rabbits, life is risky all around and having to wait a day or two to ovulate may be too long because there may be no tomorrow. By being ready to ovulate at a moment's notice, rabbits greatly increase the probability of pregnancy and ultimate reproductive success. The clear adaptive advantage of induced ovulation is illustrated by the fact that in many ways there is a continuum between spontaneous and reflexive ovulators. Socially induced estrus and ovulation can be alternative modes of reproduction in animals that are usually characterized as having spontaneous or cyclic ovulation during suboptimal environmental conditions, such as irregular light cycles or limited availability of food or water. Such flexibility in patterns of reproduction is especially characteristic of animals that tend to inhabit highly variable environments.

Seasonal Breeders

Spontaneous ovulators can be further subdivided into those that cycle regularly throughout the year, such as most rodents and humans, and those that time their reproduction to the season, such as sheep. In the Northern Hemisphere, sheep are seasonal breeders with 16-day cycles that start in autumn and cease in spring. The onset of estrus behavior precedes ovulation by 24 to 72 hours and lasts only about one day. The sheep ovary has waves of follicular development like the rabbit, only they are restricted to a single cycle, with each wave producing estradiol but only the last one being of sufficient magnitude to actually result in ovulation. Each wave of follicular development is 4 to 5 days, so in fact the cycle is very similar to rats and hamsters.

However, they are different in that they lack a preovulatory progesterone surge and it appears that it is the withdrawal from postovulatory progesterone that is critical for sexual receptivity. Oddly, this action of progesterone is required for the induction of behavior in the next estrous cycle. Evidence in favor of this is that sheep that have not recently ovulated (i.e., prepubertal or at the beginning of the breeding season), will ovulate but not show sexual receptivity, a so-called "silent estrus" as a result of the lack of a sensitizing action of progesterone from the previous cycle.

As opposed to this strict seasonality, domestic dogs can have an estrous cycle during any season of the year, usually with a 7 or 8 month interval between periods of activity. In this case, proestrus is about 9 days and is marked by vulval swelling and some bleeding, but the female will not accept the male at this time. The beginning of estrus is characterized by the onset of behavioral receptivity and its termination is marked by her refusal to mate— in other words, it is operationally defined. Ovulation occurs during this period of estrus, which has a duration of 9 or 10 days. Preovulatory progesterone is implicated in the onset of receptivity; however, as opposed to most other mammals, sexual receptivity persists for 8 or 9 days after ovulation, during which period estradiol is low but progesterone levels continue to increase as a result of the growth of the corpus luteum.

A major determinant of reproductive parameters is whether the animal is responsive to environmental cues, such as photoperiod or food availability, both of which tend to vary systematically across the year, or social cues like the presence of a suitable mate or a lack of overcrowding. Some species even have very specific requirements for successful breeding that if not available will prevent the female from exhibiting sexual receptivity. Female budgerigars (parakeets), for example, must have an available nest site with an entrance of the correct size and at the correct height before they will mate. These restrictions insure that the nest hole is only big enough for parakeets to get in and out of and is sufficiently high off the ground to deter most predators. Reproduction is both an energetically expensive and risky endeavor, and adaptive selective pressure helps animals living in different environmental conditions to optimize their reproductive success by breeding as frequently as possible within the constraints of that particular environment.

Thus, species such as humans and house mice that essentially breed all year long with little to no seasonality enjoy staggering reproductive success. Pretty much the same can be said for other species that have hitched their reproductive wagons to man's star, including rats, pigeons, house sparrows, starlings, roaches, and many farm animals. When we bring animals into the laboratory to breed under optimal conditions, they can escape naturally imposed environmental constraints. Hamsters, for example, normally hibernate through the winter but will readily breed all year long in the laboratory. Other species, however, cannot overcome the restrictions evolution has placed on them. Cats and dogs do not seem to breed any more frequently when domesticated than when feral, despite the removal by domestication of social constraints that exist in groups of wild animals.

Other Variations in Hormone-Sex Behavior Relations

As mentioned earlier, not all species exhibit female sexual behavior only during the fertile phase of the reproductive cycle. It is well established that women are capable of engaging in sexual behavior at any time during the cycle or after menopause, as can many other female primates. The hormone-behavior relations in women and other primates will be discussed more in chapter 6.

While it is quite rare, there are other nonprimate species where the female will engage in sexual behavior irrespective of the breeding season or ovulatory cycle. The domestic horse is one such animal—the mare will exhibit behavioral estrus and sexual receptivity during anestrus, pregnancy, or after surgical removal of the ovaries (Squires 1993). Why some species have evolved to engage in sex even when not fertile is not known, but as discussed in chapter 6, it is probably due to the constraints and advantages of the social group that a species has evolved within.

Evolutionary Aspects of Female Sexual Behavior

Years of research into the variety and complexity of reproductive patterns have elucidated some general principles. One is that the surest way for an animal to assure its own reproductive success is to inhibit the reproduction of its rivals and to eliminate competition for limited resources such as food, nest sites, and even mates. This inhibition is often accomplished behaviorally via dominance, competition, or even direct interception. The use of chemical communication can also serve this purpose. Studies on house mice have revealed the range and variety of the pheromonal modulation of reproduction. These include the ability of females to inhibit each other's cycles and synchronize their cycles, the male acceleration of female cycles, and the strange male blockade of a recently inseminated female's pregnancy. Ultimately, these chemical modulations of reproductive cycles prove adaptive in that females are prevented from breeding when conditions are too crowded, they are too young, or males are not of optimal fitness. For instance, when female rats or mice are housed together, the "cycles change in length until estrus is synchronized within the social group; as a consequence, females tend to come into heat and ovulate on the same day" (McClintock 1987). When mice are group-housed under conditions that facilitate this synchronization, often several females will deliver on the same day and communally pool their pups into one nest. This allows for group defense, greater heat retention, and more regular feeding bouts, obvious advantages to the rearing of large groups of offspring.

Mediated by the vomeronasal organ, pheromones are an active component in the social structure of a variety of rodents, including rats, voles, lemmings, mice, and hamsters. It is likely we have under estimated their importance in rats due to the emphasis of researchers on inbred laboratory strains rather than wild rats (for obvious and understandable reasons). They also appear to some degree in ungulates such as deer, goats, pigs and cows, marsupials, and various primates, perhaps including humans.

Increasing evidence suggests there is a functional vomeronasal organ in humans, a topic of intense interest to the perfume industry. Regardless of how chemical information is detected, it is clear that humans are responsive to chemical cues from each other. Martha McClintock has demonstrated that in both rats and humans females living together begin to synchronize their reproductive cycles. McClintock's (1971) initial finding was that female coeds living together in a residential women's college showed menstrual cycle synchrony after a period of 4 to 7 months. Apparently it is the amount of time women spend together, not just the sharing of common living quarters, that determines whether two women become synchronized. Over a 4-month period, women who identified themselves as close friends were more likely to develop a synchronous onset of menstruation than those who were just roommates.

McClintock has continued to follow this line of research and has recently published definitive evidence that this phenomenon is mediated by human pheromones (McClintock 1998). Her research demonstrates that odorless compounds (i.e., pheromones) from the armpits of women affect the menstrual cycles of other women. When the compounds are obtained from women during the follicular phase of the cycle, the menstrual cycles of other women are shortened. When the compounds are obtained from women at ovulation, the cycles of other women are lengthened. The reproductive advantage of synchronized ovarian cycles is not known, but it is easy to speculate that females in frequent close contact would also be likely to cooperate in the rearing of offspring born around the same time, as is the case in mice.

A discussion of the variability in patterns of reproductive cycles, copulatory behavior, and how they are regulated could fill volumes and entertain us for some time. However, for our purposes it will prove far more useful to illustrate the mechanistic approach to the study of the neuroendocrinology of reproductive behavior in the female rat. This will serve two purposes: it will allow us to understand the behavior from the bottom up, as opposed to the more traditional top-down approach, and it will illustrate how studies of the reproductive behavior of the female rat have proved not only informative to the understanding of this particular behavior, but have also elucidated many novel principles of brain functioning that have impacted on the field of neuroscience as a whole.

The Neural Circuitry Regulating Lordosis
In rats, lordosis is a behavior that is evoked, meaning it does not occur in the absence of external stimuli. This trait makes it considerably more amenable to study. Pity the poor field researcher who has to sit for hours observing

animals in the hope of seeing some interesting behavior while the student of lordosis need only be sure the subject animal is hormonally primed and that a ready and willing stud male is available, usually not a problem. Lordosis begins with stimulation to the flanks and perineal region. Sensory nerves transmit the information to the spinal cord where it is passed on up through the midbrain and distributed throughout the hypothalamus. Prior treatment with estradiol increases the receptive field of some sensory neurons in the perineal region, but with that exception, hormones appear to play no significant role in the transmittal of information into the brain. Quite the contrary is the case for the neural output that ultimately leads to the behavior. Many researchers are continuing to contribute to the mapping of the lordosis circuitry, but substantial portions of it have been elucidated by the work of Donald Pfaff and his colleagues at the Rockefeller University (Pfaff et al. 1994).

THE VENTROMEDIAL NUCLEUS (VMN)

There is something truly extraordinary about the neural circuitry of lordosis because one major brain site coordinates the entire response, a sort of CPU for lordosis. The VMN of the hypothalamus is a bilateral egg-shaped region that contains a dense collection of estrogen-receptor-containing neurons. The name of this nucleus also refers to its location in the hypothalamus; it is toward the bottom (ventral) and toward the middle (medial). There are further subdivisions within the VMN based on their location. The diagram in figure 4.3 illustrates how the two VMN are like eggs cocked on their sides leaning toward each other. Estrogen-receptor-containing neurons are densely clustered in the ventrolateral portion of the nucleus while relatively few are found in the dorsomedial subdivision. Many neurons in the dorsomedial portion are intrinsic (internal) to the VMN and project to the neurons of the ventrolateral subdivision. The ventrolateral neurons then appear to project out of the VMN towards the midbrain, thereby passing the information downstream toward the spinal cord.

The neurons in the VMN both receive **afferents** from, and send **efferents** to, other estrogen-receptor-containing neurons that are also important modulators of lordosis—the external hard drives, if you will. The importance of the VMN was identified by lesioning it, which abolishes the behavior, and by stimulating it with electricity or chemicals, which induces the behavior. However, lordosis is never reliably induced in the absence of prior treatment with estradiol. Of equal importance is the realization that a critical function of estradiol action in the hypothalamus is to alter the responsiveness to somatosensory input so that previously aversive stimuli from the male now increases the probability that the female will exhibit lordosis. Estradiol acting in the hypothalamus will also alter the behavior of the female in such a way that she spends more time in the vicinity of the male, thereby increasing the likelihood of her receiving the appropriate somatosensory stimulation and subsequent copulation (Pfaff et al. 1994).

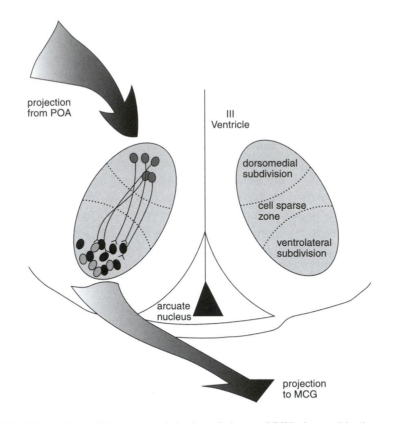

Figure 4.3 The ventromedial nucleus of the hypothalamus (VMN). Located in the mediobasal hypothalamus, the VMN is a key site for estrogen-induction of lordosis responding in female rats. The VMN is subdivided into the dorsomedial and ventrolateral subdivisions with a cell-sparse intermediate zone. The majority of estrogen receptor–containing neurons are in the ventrolateral subdivision (dark circles), and it is these neurons that subsequently project to the midbrain central gray (MCG). Neurons of the dorsomedial subdivision receive afferent inputs from other brain regions, including the POA, and then project locally to neurons of the ventrolateral subdivision.

Further evidence that the VMN is essential for lordosis was demonstrated by implanting estradiol using small stainless steel cannulae (tubes) directly into the VMN of animals in which the ovaries had been removed. This local administration of estradiol was found to be both necessary and sufficient to induce lordosis, demonstrating that hormone action was not essential in other brain regions (Rubin and Barfield 1983). This is not to suggest that the rest of the brain is dispensable, however, and the more we learn about this behavioral response, the more we appreciate the importance of modulating influences from other regions.

In addition, the VMN does not act alone; it must transmit its information down the line, in particular to the spinal cord, where the appropriate back muscles are innervated. With this in mind, we will review the neural circuitry of lordosis from a nose-to-tail perspective. A diagram of the lordosis circuitry is given in figure 4.4.

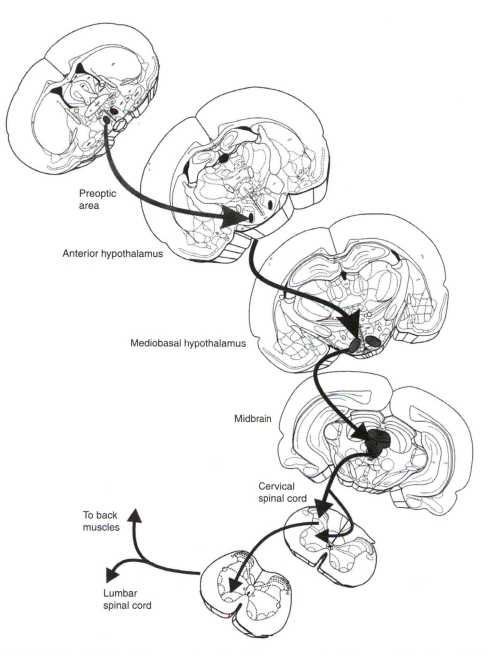

Preoptic area

Anterior hypothalamus

Mediobasal hypothalamus

Midbrain

Cervical spinal cord

To back muscles

Lumbar spinal cord

Figure 4.4 The neural circuitry of lordosis responding. The major components of the neural circuitry controlling lordosis include the preoptic area (POA), ventromedial nucleus of the hypothalamus (VMN), the midbrain central gray (MCG), and the spinal cord. The POA and anterior hypothalamus project directly to the VMN and exert predominantly inhibitory influences over the response, although they also contain facilitating components. The VMN in turn projects directly to the MCG in the midbrain, which in turn projects to the cervical spinal cord, which projects to the lumbar spinal cord and the motor neurons that innervate the back muscles. Many of the neurons along the circuit contain estrogen receptors and thereby constitute the components of a steroid-sensitive neuronal network.

THE PREOPTIC AREA (POA)

Like many brain structures, the preoptic area gets its name from its location. In this case, preoptic refers to being prior to the optic chiasm, the place at the base of the brain where the two optic nerves cross before entering into the brain. While commonly referred to as an "area," the major nucleus in this region is actually called the medial preoptic nucleus but we will refer to it simply as the POA. As will be discussed in chapter 5, the POA is a major brain region regulating male sexual behavior. In the female the POA is generally considered inhibitory to sexual behavior. Lesioning the POA releases the lordosis response from some constraint and stimulating it enhances the response. There is a major projection from the POA directly to the VMN, and this may be the source of the inhibitory influence on lordosis responding. However, as with most things, the reality is not nearly as simple as the initial studies would suggest. Experiments involving anatomically precise pharmacology or electrophysiology indicate that there is also a component of the POA that is facilitatory to lordosis responding. It is not surprising that our initial view of the brain as a series of interconnected boxes that project to and from each other and increase or decrease responses was found to be overly simplistic. This doesn't negate the early principles but rather requires an additional level of complexity. Like learning any foreign language, to learn the language of the brain you must begin with the basics.

THE MIDBRAIN CENTRAL GRAY (MCG)

The MCG is also referred to as the periaqueductal gray or PAG since it is a structure surrounding the 4th ventricle. The gray refers to the appearance of the tissue, which contains very small myelinated fibers that have a grayish caste compared to lighter nearby areas. The MCG is an important way-station on the line but it does more than merely pass along the information; it also integrates and refines the signals coming in from other brain regions. This is a critical function because there are many competing stimuli bombarding the MCG at any particular time. This is a major brain area regulating pain sensitivity (nociception), anxiety, blood pressure, heart rate, and other vegetative functions such as urination (Bandler and Shipley 1994). In order for mating to proceed, many other stimuli must be ignored. Pain and anxiety must be overcome and urination must be suppressed. The MCG serves as a gateway that allows the neural activity relevant to lordosis to pass on down the line but blocks activity related to competing bodily functions. Alternatively, when appropriate, the MCG will block the propagation of impulses specific to lordosis responding in favor of those needed for short-term survival, like running away from a predator or foraging for food. There are estrogen-receptor-containing neurons in the MCG and many of them receive direct input from estrogen receptor-containing-neurons in the VMN (Pfaff et al. 1994). This relationship allows for a steroid sensitive neural circuitry embedded within the main projections from the hypothalamus to the midbrain.

THE SPINAL CORD

Information basically makes two stops in the spinal cord, one at the top (cervical spinal cord) and one near the bottom (lumbar spinal cord). The key component is the activation of motor neurons in the lumbar spinal cord which innervates the back muscles that control the lordosis posture. These are the lateral longissimus and the transverso spinalis. If the spinal cord is cut at about the point where the key motor neurons exit, females cannot exhibit lordosis. There are sparse but significant numbers of estrogen receptors in the spinal cord, and these appear to be located in interneurons which innervate the motor neurons as well as the sensory neurons innervating the flanks and perineal region. The receptive field of these sensory neurons is not particularly altered following estradiol treatment but the threshold for their activation by cutaneous stimuli is substantially lowered. This indicates yet another mechanism by which steroid hormones act to facilitate the expression of this critical behavior (Schwartz-Giblin et al. 1989).

METHODS USED TO MAP THE LORDOSIS CIRCUIT

A fair question to ask at this point is how do we in fact know that these are the major brain areas regulating lordosis? The techniques for mapping out neural circuits continue to increase in sophistication and precision. Early studies are now often considered relatively crude, but they were in fact highly effective at establishing the broad brushstrokes of our increasingly refined picture. An early atlas of the steroid-concentrating neurons of the brain served as a useful guide to the most likely neuroanatomical sites mediating this steroid dependent behavior (Pfaff and Keiner 1973). Clearly the POA and the VMN were major sites of steroid action given the extremely dense levels of estrogen receptors in these regions. Lesioning the POA with chemicals (kainic acid) or electricity, or severing the connections between the POA and the VMN with a Halaz knife, resulted in increased lordosis responding of hormonally primed female rats. The same manipulations performed on the VMN and the connections between the VMN and the MCG had the opposite effect—it eliminated all female sexual behavior. The use of specialized compounds known as tract tracers were then used to establish precise neuroanatomical connections. For instance, a tracer called HRP (horseradish peroxidase) could be injected into the MCG where it is taken up by nerve terminals and transported back to the cell bodies of origin in the VMN. Visualization of the HRP (by standard immunocytochemical techniques) is then combined with either steroid-binding autoradiography or immunocytochemical detection of estrogen receptors. The number of VMN neurons that have estrogen receptors and project to the MCG was thereby established; it was found to be in the nature of about 30%, although this is probably an underestimate due to the relative lack of sensitivity of the technique (Morrell and Pfaff 1982). The development of tract tracers, like pseudorabies virus that actually jump across synapses, has recently allowed us to follow multiple components of the circuitry, beginning with the nerves innervating the musculature of the back. As the number of days increases, the virus travels farther away from the site of injection, following the path of synapses. This approach has confirmed the hypothesis that the various brain regions along the neuroaxis of the lordosis reflex, i.e., the VMN, the MCG, and the spinal cord, are indeed serially connected (Daniels et al. 1999).

Probably the single biggest advance in discerning the neuroanatomical underpinnings of lordosis in recent years has been the advent of the use of Fos immunocytochemistry as a marker for neuronal excitation. This immediate early gene is quiescent under baseline conditions but is rapidly induced in many neurons following activation. The gene product is a nuclear protein that is readily visualized with immunocytochemistry and acts as an ''ON'' signal to indicate that this particular neuron has been excited (see chapter 2 for a more detailed discussion of Fos). By mapping the neurons that are turned on after the expression of lordosis behavior, researchers have been able to further refine the neural circuitry maps and can begin to identify the neurochemical profile of the individual neurons that are actively involved in the behavior.

Steroid Hormone Action in the Brain

In order for steroids to exert biological effects, they must bind to a receptor. You will recall from chapters 1 and 2 that the classic forms of these receptors are intracellular and act as transcription factors. These receptors are also specific for select hormones, making the estrogen and progesterone receptors of primary relevance to the current topic.

ESTROGEN RECEPTORS (ER)

We have already discussed the fact that estrogen acting directly in the VMN is necessary and sufficient to induce lordosis responding, and an obvious corollary of this observation is that estrogen receptors are present in abundance in the neurons of the VMN. However, this does not mean that estrogen receptors are found everywhere we look in the brain; in fact, the distribution is fairly limited. Traditionally, estrogen receptors were found restricted to the preoptic area, the hypothalamus, some components of the limbic system, and at low levels in the midbrain and spinal cord. This distribution is highly conserved phylogenetically, being essentially the same in rodents, primates, reptiles, amphibians, fish, and any other species in between (see chapter 7). This limited distribution accounted for what was considered the principle role of steroids in the control of reproductive processes. In recent years, both of these tenets—that estrogen receptors have a restricted distribution and that steroids mediate only reproduction—have been overturned by new data.

First was the stunning discovery that there is actually more than one form of the estrogen receptor. This second form is coded for by a separate gene but makes a protein that is in many ways very similar to the original estrogen receptor. In order to keep them straight, the two estrogen receptors (ER) are now referred to as ER-alpha (α) and ER-beta (β), with the α referring to the "traditional" receptor and β designating the newcomer. Establishing the function of the second estrogen receptor, ER-β, is a major challenge currently facing neuroendocrinologists.

The distribution of ER-β in the brain is both similar to and different from that of ER-α and is in many ways complimentary (Shughrue et al. 1997). As a result of this distribution pattern, the two forms are occasionally in the same cell and sometimes in separate cells. When in the same cell the two forms of the receptor can interact (dimerize) and influence each others' function (Pettersson et al. 1997). A schematic representation of the distribution of the two forms of the receptor is found in figure 4.5. There have also been extensive behavioral studies done on mice that lack both the α and the β form of the estrogen receptor, and this is reviewed in box 4.1.

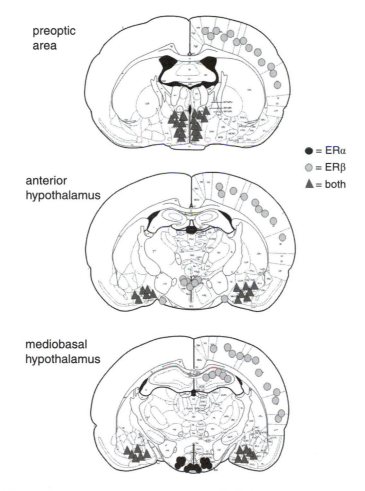

Figure 4.5 Distribution of estrogen receptors in the CNS. There are two forms of estrogen receptor, referred to as ERα and ERβ. Their distribution is largely complementary, each one occupying a unique location in relation to the other, but there are some regions in which they overlap and can be found in the same cells. This is particularly notable for the preoptic area. (Based on Shughrue et al. 1997.)

Box 4.1 ERKOs and BERKOs

The advent of transgenic mice in which the genes for estrogen receptors have been disrupted has been an important tool in determining hormonal regulation of behavior at the cellular level. ERKOs (estrogen receptor knock-out) are mice lacking the alpha form of the estrogen receptor, and BERKOs are mice in which the gene for the beta form has been disrupted (see chapter 2 for a discussion of ERα and ERβ and a review of transgenic mice). Without these animals, it would be impossible to know if estradiol is acting selectively at one or both forms of the receptor to modulate reproductive and other behaviors. Careful behavioral characterizations of ERKOs and BERKOs have been independently conducted by Emilie Rissman and colleagues at the University of Virginia and Sonoko Ogawa and Donald Pfaff at Rockefeller University. For the most part, it seems that having ERα is sufficient for normal female sexual behavior, whereas the absence of this receptor results in a total loss of lordosis responses (Ogawa et al. 1998; Rissman et al. 1997). In contrast, the lack of ERβ has little or no influence on lordosis responses in females, although there is evidence of an extension of the period of behavioral estrus (Ogawa et al. 1999). The latter observation is intriguing since it may indicate an inhibitory or antagonistic effect of ERα on ERβ.

There are several advantages to the use of ERKO and BERKO mice. First and foremost is that they have a clean ablation of the receptor, and thereby avoid confounds due to lesions, pharmacological antagonists, or even antisense oligonucleotides. However, as with any model system, there are also several important caveats (Rissman et al. 1999). One point of concern is that animals spend their entire lives without the receptor, making it difficult to discern organizational from activational hormone effects. The receptors are disrupted in all tissues in which they are normally present, which includes bone, heart, and blood vessels in addition to the organs of the reproductive tract and the brain. An additional problem is that estrogen receptors are important to negative feedback control of steroid hormone secretion. When this important link in the hypothalamic-gonadal-axis is lost, there is a dysregulation in steroid secretion so that knockout animals have abnormally high levels of estradiol and testosterone. Elevated androgens have been found to contribute to the unusual aggressiveness of female ERKOs (Ogawa et al. 1998) and may have other nonspecific effects as well. For these reasons, it is important to control for circulating levels of gonadal steroids by performing gonadectomy and hormone replacement. These issues aside, it is clear that these mice are a unique asset in the study of behavioral neuroendocrinology.

The basis for overturning the second tenet, that estrogen acts in the brain solely to mediate reproduction, is the result of a convergence of data from basic research on animals and epidemiological studies on humans. Researchers in the laboratory were collecting an increasing amount of evidence indicating that estradiol influenced nonreproductive behaviors such as learning and memory, pain perception, aggression, and even feeding. These topics are reviewed in chapters 13 to 16 in this volume. Coincident with these discoveries was the equally stunning report that estradiol exerted a protective effect against the risk of developing Alzheimer's disease in women (Henderson 1997) and that it may enhance cognition in normal women (Haskell et al. 1997). While these initial reports are still being modified and updated, they helped to focus attention on the nonreproductive effects of estrogen and have in many ways brought estrogen action in the brain into the mainstream of neuroscience.

PROGESTERONE RECEPTORS

As you are now well aware, estrogen receptors are transcription factors, meaning they interact with the DNA and influence gene expression, usually turning on a particular gene (inhibitory actions of estradiol are relatively rare, but not unheard of). One of the first genes activated by the estrogen receptor is the receptor for progesterone (PR). This sequence follows logically from the estrus cycle in which estradiol secretion precedes progesterone secretion, and as a result progesterone action is often dependent upon prior estradiol. But the progesterone receptor is also a transcription factor that presumably turns on additional genes. So we need to ask what gene products that actually change behavior are induced by estradiol and progesterone. Are one or two genes responsible, or are there hundreds? Finding the final common denominator of estradiol action to induce lordosis has been the Holy Grail for behavioral neuroendocrinologists, and as would be expected, attempts to discover it have failed. It seems increasingly likely that multiple genes are activated by estradiol to induce lordosis and that there is tremendous redundancy built in to protect the most essential of all biological functions, reproduction. The best evidence in favor of this view is the impressive list of neurotransmitter systems that are modulated by estradiol and in turn modulate lordosis responding.

The Neurochemistry of Female Sexual Behavior

We have made frequent references to information traveling up and down the neuroaxis as if they were telephone wires crackling with conversation. But of course the telephone wires are really neurons and the conversation is being conducted by neurotransmitters. These specialized chemicals released into the synapses between neurons either excite, inhibit, or modulate the postsynaptic neuron, thereby allowing the information to propagate or stop. Neuromodulators are usually peptides, and while not well understood, they generally act to enhance the action of a traditional neurotransmitter released at the same time.

GENERAL PRINCIPLES

A large number of neurotransmitters and neuromodulators regulate lordosis responding and the list can be a bit daunting. But some general principles do seem to apply. A schematic representation is given in figure 4.6 and can be summarized as follows:

1. Neuropeptides that are closely linked to the events of ovulation or are released in the CNS as a result of sensory stimulation of the genitals also facilitate lordosis. These would include GnRH, prolactin, and oxytocin.
2. Neurotransmitters that enhance neuronal excitation are increased in the mediobasal hypothalamus (where the VMN is located) by estradiol and increase lordosis. These would include norepinephrine, dopamine, acetylcholine, and oxytocin.

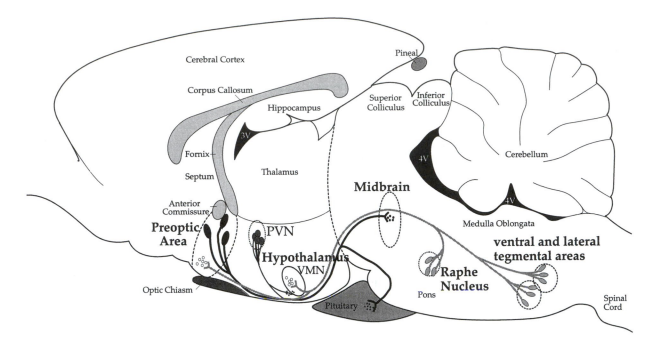

Figure 4.6 Neurochemistry of the lordosis circuitry. Myriad neurotransmitters have been identified that influence lordosis responding and just a few are pictured here. Norepinephrine and dopamine originate in the tegmental areas of the brainstem and innervate the preoptic area and mediobasal hypothalamus. Serotonin from the raphe nuclei travels along the same pathway, the medial forebrain bundle, to these regions. Oxytocin neurons from the paraventricular nucleus send collaterals to the VMN on their way to the posterior pituitary. GnRH neurons from the preoptic area do the same, as well as sending projections to the midbrain.

3. Neurotransmitters that inhibit neuronal excitation, such as opiates or serotonin, are inhibitory to lordosis.
4. Some inhibitory transmitters actually increase lordosis responding by inhibiting other inhibitors, called disinhibition. This is the case with GABA and the peptide cholecystekinin (CCK).

In trying to make further sense of these generalities, the central questions have been: what are the second messenger systems activated by the lordosis-facilitating neurotransmitters and do they have a common theme? Many neurotransmitters that facilitate lordosis increase the activity of the membrane enzyme, phospholipase C, which is a component of the phosphotidylinositol signal transduction pathway and ultimately results in an increased release of calcium from internal stores. It is this calcium that then carries on the real business of signal transduction, but in precisely what way remains unknown. Phospholipase C can also activate an additional enzyme, protein kinase C, and the activity of this enzyme is increased by estradiol as well (Ansonoff and Etgen 1998). Activation of adenylate cyclase to increase cAMP has also been implicated, but the results remain ambiguous in that some neurotransmitters increase adenylate cyclase activity while others inhibit it, but have the same effect on lordosis (Pfaff et al. 1994; Beyer et al. 1997). Recently there has been a role postulated for the gaseous neurotransmitter nitric oxide (NO) which exerts its effect via cGMP (Chu et al. 1997, 1999). It seems fair to say that at this point we have not yet elucidated a single unique signal transduction pathway by which lordosis is activated, and this goal may prove elusive for some time to come.

A DETAILED LOOK AT OXYTOCIN CONTROL OF LORDOSIS

Now let's look at the example of oxytocin, a neuropeptide made in the paraventricular and supraoptic nuclei of the hypothalamus. Many of these neurons project to the posterior pituitary and release oxytocin into the bloodstream in response to stimuli such as suckling or mating. But there are also intracranial projections of oxytocin neurons and we now know that oxytocin is a major regulator of a variety of social behaviors in females. Infusions of oxytocin into the preoptic area or hypothalamus of subthreshold hormonally primed rats increases lordosis responding. Efforts to find increased oxytocin synthesis and release in response to estradiol and progesterone treatment generally failed. However, the receptors for oxytocin are very discretely localized and are particularly dense in the ventrolateral subdivision of the VMN, the major brain area regulating lordosis.

Examination of oxytocin binding by receptor autoradiography revealed a dramatic 4-fold increase in binding in the VMN following estradiol treatment (de Kloet et al. 1986; Johnson et al. 1989). Further studies confirmed that the mRNA for the receptor was being newly synthesized by the activated estrogen receptor (Bale and Dorsa 1995). However, careful attention to detail further revealed that it was not just the number of oxytocin receptors that had increased, but the actual brain area in which the receptors were being expressed was also increased, as shown in figure 4.7.

The paraventricular nucleus is located above the VMN and the oxytocin neurons send their axons to the posterior pituitary via a sweeping descending arc that passes in the neighborhood of the VMN but doesn't actually penetrate into the nucleus. The neurons of the VMN, on the other hand, extend their dendritic trees out into the highway of passing fibers from the paraventricular neurons. In the presence of estradiol and progesterone, the VMN neurons actually transport the oxytocin receptors out into the dendritic tree so that oxytocin released by collaterals of the passing fibers can bind to and act on these receptors (Schumacher et al. 1990; Coirini et al. 1991). Oxytocin acting at these receptors then increases the neuronal excitation of the VMN neurons (Kow et al. 1991).

Thus, we have a great deal of evidence supporting the tenet that oxytocin binding to its receptor in the VMN does in fact increase lordosis responding. But if we look back on all this data we see that it is entirely in the nature of a correlation. An estradiol-induced increase in oxytocin receptor is positively *correlated* with an estradiol-induced increase in lordosis, and an increase in

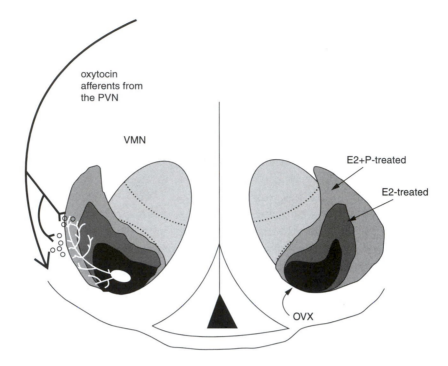

Figure 4.7 Steroid hormones increase the area covered by oxytocin receptors. The distribution of oxytocin receptors is determined by receptor autoradiography using a radioactive analog of oxytocin and exposing the brain sections to X-ray film. There is a high concentration of oxytocin receptors in the ventrolateral subdivision of the VMN in control OVX females. The region of receptor binding is increased in animals treated with estradiol (E_2) and further increased in animals receiving estradiol plus progesterone (P). This increase in receptor-binding area is due to the transport of oxytocin receptors into the distal dendrites of the VMN neurons and brings them into the vicinity of the oxytocin collateral terminals from the neurons originating in the PVN and projecting to the posterior pituitary. (Adapted from Corini et al. 1991.)

the spread of the receptor into the dendritic tree is *correlated* with an increase in lordosis.

Definitive proof for the involvement of endogenous oxytocin in the natural expression of the behavior has been obtained in two ways. One is the treatment of animals with an antagonist to oxytocin, which reduces the frequency and amplitude of lordosis (Caldwell et al. 1990; Witt and Insel 1991). In order for an antagonist to have a behavioral effect, there must by definition be activity of the endogenous ligand.

The second approach has been the use of antisense oligonucleotide technology (see chapter 2 for a detailed discussion of the use of antisense oligonucleotides) directed against the mRNA for the oxytocin receptor. By creating short stretches (18 to 22 bases) of synthetic DNA designed to be complementary to, and thereby hybridize with, the mRNA for the oxytocin receptor, the synthesis of this protein can be selectively blocked. Administration of such antisense DNA into the VMN of estrogen-primed female rats was found to reduce lordosis responding and to lower the frequency and amplitude of lordosis compared to animals that received an equal amount of synthetic DNA but in which the sequence had been scrambled and was therefore not capable of binding to the mRNA for the oxytocin receptor (McCarthy et al. 1994). Taken together, the two approaches of antagonists and antisense oligonucleotides put to rest any doubts that oxytocin is not a major player in the regulation of lordosis behavior.

OTHER NEUROTRANSMITTERS

While we have reviewed one neurotransmitter in some detail, there are many more that are equally important. Figure 4.6 reviews some of the major players but the student of behavior should always keep in mind that any diagram of this sort tends to be an oversimplification of a highly complex situation. Furthermore, even the casual reader of the literature on control of lordosis quickly gets the impression that many neurotransmitter systems have dual or mixed effects on the behavioral response. This may include having opposite effects in 2 different brain areas, in particular, the POA versus the VMN.

Another source of opposing effects by the same neurotransmitter is differential effects depending on which neurotransmitter receptor subtype is activated (box 4.2). In general, it seems there is a great deal of redundancy built into the system, but one component of this redundancy is a high degree of interrelatedness among the different neurotransmitter systems. For instance, oxytocin has its own direct effect on lordosis responding but oxytocin also increases norepinephrine release (Vincent and Etgen 1993). Norepinephrine in turn stimulates lordosis directly (see box 4.2). Similarly, GABA, which is normally an inhibitory transmitter actually facilitates lordosis when infused into the VMN (McCarthy et al. 1990), possibly by increasing norepinephrine release (Fiber et al. 1998).

As you can see, in general, agents that promote neuronal excitation, such as norepinephrine, dopamine, oxytocin, and GnRH, also promote lordosis responding. As would be predicted, those that inhibit neuronal activity will also usually inhibit lordosis. Excessive levels of opiates generally shut down reproduction, although the role of endogenous opiates in lordosis is mixed, having a facilitative effect on lordosis in some brain areas at some receptor subtypes (Pfaus and Gorzalka 1987). The major inhibitory influence on lordosis is serotonin. Simply lesioning the serotonin input to the hypothalamus is sufficient to increase lordosis responding in low-dose estradiol-treated females (Frankfurt et al. 1985). This has unfortunate clinical implications and explains why a frequently cited side effect of antidepressant drugs that elevate serotonin, such as Prozac and Zoloft, is a loss of sexual appetite.

Steroid Modulation of Gene Expression to Modulate Female Sexual Behavior

Now that we have reviewed the role of steroids and neurotransmitters in regulating female reproductive behavior, it is time to put the two systems together and ask how steroids modulate gene expression to influence neurotransmis-

Box 4.2   Neurotransmitters Do the Darndest Things

When considering the neural regulation of female sexual behavior it is important to bear in mind that neurotransmitter systems do not act in isolation. But when it comes to trying to dissect the system, most studies are designed to focus on a single transmitter. Norepinephrine is an example of one neurotransmitter that plays a major role in the regulation of lordosis and has been investigated at multiple levels. Originating in the brainstem, norepinephrine neurons innervate the preoptic area and the mediobasal hypothalamus. An increase in the activity of these neurons is a prerequisite for the LH-surge leading to ovulation, presumably via a direct activation of the GnRH neurons. Based on this observation, it was logical to ask if norepinephrine was also increased in brain areas relevant to lordosis and if blocking this increase would attenuate the lordosis response. The elegant work of Ann Etgen and colleagues (Etgen et al. 1992, 1994, 1999) indicates increased levels of norepinephrine in the VMN of sexually receptive female rats. One might expect that this is due to increased synthesis of the norepinephrine but, surprisingly, this does not seem to be the case. Instead, there is a naturally occurring brake on norepinephrine release, known as a presynaptic autoreceptor, and the inhibitory action of this receptor is inhibited by estrogen (making it a brake on a brake). An obvious mechanism would be via down regulation of the receptor by estradiol, but again this is not the case. Instead, estradiol appears to uncouple the stimulatory subunits of the receptor so that it is no longer effective at activating its second messenger. Thus, by decreasing the normal restraint on norepinephrine release, by the presynaptic autoreceptor, norepinephrine can bind to the post-synaptic receptor and increase lordosis responding.

But wait, the story doesn't end here. It turns out that there is another post-synaptic receptor for norepinephrine, only this one is actually inhibitory to lordosis. How can a single neurotransmitter act at two different receptors that have opposing effects? The answer lies in the signal transduction pathways that are activated by the receptors and the influence of estradiol and progesterone on which receptor is dominant. In this case, the receptor that inhibits lordosis is linked to the production of cAMP, and when there is no estradiol or progesterone around, it holds sway over the excitatory receptor, which is linked to the influx of calcium. The tug-of-war between the competing receptors goes in favor of the excitatory version when estradiol and progesterone are added to the line-up. By being sensitive to steroid action at multiple end points, norepinephrine can selectively modulate lordosis responding when conditions are ripe, and can actually inhibit the behavior if conditions are unfavorable to mating.

sion. The best way to get a handle on changes in the activity of a particular gene is to measure the level of mRNA. This can be achieved with several techniques, including Northern Blots, RNase protection assays, slot blots, and most commonly, in situ hybridization (see chapter 2). The advantage of the latter is that it allows for a cellular analysis by indirectly visualizing the mRNA of a particular cell, as opposed to the former techniques, which all involve homogenization of chunks of tissue. Since cells in the brain are highly heterogeneous, one can imagine that adjacent neurons may respond to steroids in a completely different manner.

We have already reviewed several examples of how steroids modulate gene expression to induce female sexual behavior. For instance, estradiol increases the mRNA for oxytocin receptors in the VMN (Bale and Dorsa 1995), which in turn increases the binding of oxytocin in this brain region and increases lordosis responding. Similarly, estradiol has been found to increase the mRNA for the rate-limiting enzyme in the synthesis of GABA, resulting in increased GABA levels in the VMN and again increasing lordosis responding (McCarthy et al. 1995). These are relatively straightforward examples of how steroids directly upregulate the transmitter system involved by increasing gene expression. However, sometimes neurotransmitters act in nontraditional ways; an interesting example of this is what is known as **ligand-independent activation** of steroid receptors.

We usually think of neurotransmitters as changing the excitatory properties of a neuron to alter behavior, but the catecholamine dopamine can take another route. When dopamine binds to its D1 receptor subtype, it actually results in activation of the progesterone receptor. The precise mechanism by which dopamine activates the progesterone receptor is unknown, but dopamine binding to the D1 receptor induces the synthesis of cAMP, and it is most likely involved in the signal transduction pathway that results in an activated progesterone receptor. Of critical importance was to establish that progesterone receptors activated in this indirect way were of functional significance. This was achieved in a series of clever experiments using antisense oligonucleotides directed against the mRNA for the progesterone receptor. By substantially reducing the synthesis of the progesterone receptor prior to administering the dopamine, it was demonstrated that the progesterone receptor is required for dopamine-induced increases in lordosis. Additional converging evidence came from the use of mice with a null mutation for the progesterone receptor, referred to as PRKOs. In these animals, both progesterone and a dopamine agonist are without effect on lordosis responding (Mani et al. 1997).

On a behavioral level, ligand-independent activation of the progesterone receptor may be important for maintaining a high level of receptivity or for pacing of mating bouts, since stimulation of the female's genital tract appears to induce dopamine release that then activates progesterone receptors (Auger, Moffatt, and Blaustein 1997). This also illustrates yet another example of the redundancy inherent in the neural control of reproductive behavior and even goes a step further in demonstrating that the failure of something as fundamental as progesterone can be compensated for. However, the lack of a progesterone receptor, cannot.

Summary

In this chapter we have reviewed the basics of the neuroendocrinology of female sexual behavior. This complex behavioral response is not easily categorized but some general conclusions can be made.

1. Female reproduction is cyclic. That is, females are not continuously sexually receptive but rather the behavioral response is coordinated with the physiological response of ovulation. The precise timing of these two events in relation to each other and whether they occur spontaneously or in response to social or environmental cues varies widely across and within species.

2. The neural circuitry mediating the lordosis response, the sexually receptive posture of the female rat, has been well mapped. It begins in the preoptic area, connecting to a key center in the ventromedial nucleus of the hypothalamus, continuing down through the midbrain central gray and ending on the motor neurons of the spinal cord innervating the back muscles.

3. Female sexual receptivity is a hormonally dependent response. Many of the neurons in this neuronal circuit contain receptors for the steroids estrogen and progesterone and they constitute a steroid-sensitive network.

4. Steroids act to induce sexual receptivity by altering the properties of neurotransmitters. This may include increasing the amount of the receptor; changing the characteristics of the receptor, increasing the amount of the neurotransmitter or altering its uptake and degradation. In some cases, steroids can also alter the distribution of neurotransmitter receptors and of synapses.

5. The full complement of female sexual behavior includes motivational aspects that are manifest as pacing behavior as well as proceptive or courtship behaviors.

6. In many species, females do not reproduce in isolation but instead interact extensively with other females in their group. These interactions may involve the suppression of reproduction by some individuals against others or a synchronization of reproductive cycles so that females produce offspring at the same time.

7. The reproductive strategy of females is also a function of their environment. Females of some species ovulate spontaneously in response to endogenous hormonal stimuli whereas females of other species only ovulate following mating, so-called reflexive or induced ovulators. Some species are opportunistic and may switch between spontaneous and induced ovulators depending on environmental conditions. In most species, female sexual receptivity is closely linked with the event of ovulation but there are notable exceptions that include humans and horses.

Study Questions

1. What are the main structural components of the ovary across the menstrual/estrus cycle and how do these influence the cyclic changes seen in circulating steroid hormone levels? Identify and describe the phases/days of the menstrual/estrus cycle.

2. Describe the relationship between GnRH, LH, and FSH, where they are synthesized and where and how they act.

3. List the main components of the neural circuitry regulating lordosis responding in the rat. What techniques were used to establish this circuitry and what is the major function of each brain region?

4. Why is lordosis a steroid-dependent behavior? How do steroids act in the cell?

5. What are some of the major neurotransmitters involved in the control of lordosis and how are they influenced by steroids? What generalizations can we make about the role of neurotransmitters in the control of lordosis?

6. What are some of the ways that females in a group can interact to influence the reproductive success of themselves and others?

References

Ansonoff, M. A., and Etgen, A. M. (1998) Estradiol elevates protein kinase C catalytic activity in the preoptic area of female rats. *Endocrinology* 139: 3050–3056.

Auger, A. P., Moffatt, C. A., and Blaustein, J. D. (1997) Progesterone-independent activation of rat brain progestin receptors by reproductive stimuli. *Endocrinology* 138: 511–513.

Bale, T. L., and Dorsa, D. M. (1995) Regulation of oxytocin receptor messenger ribonucleic acid in the ventromedial hypothalamus by testosterone and its metabolites. *Endocrinology* 136: 5135–5138.

Bandler, R., and Shipley, M. T. (1994) Columnar organization in the midbrain periaqueductal gray: Modules for emotional expression? *TINS* 17: 379–389.

Beyer, C., Gonzalez-Flores, O., and Gonzalez-Mariscal, G. (1997) Progesterone receptor participates in the stimulatory effect of LHRH, prostaglandin E2 and cyclic AMP on lordosis and preceptive behaviours in rats. *J. Neuroendocrinol.* 9: 609–614.

Caldwell, J. D., Barakat, A. S., Smith, D. D., Hruby, V. J., and Pedersen, C. A. (1990) A uterotonic antagonist blocks the oxytocin-induced facilitation of female sexual receptivity. *Brain Res.* 512: 291–296.

Chu, H.-P., and Etgen, A. M. (1997) A potential role of cyclic GMP in the regulation of lordosis behavior of female rats. *Horm. Behav.* 32: 125–132.

Chu, H. P., Etgen, A. M. (1999) Ovarian hormone dependence of alpha(1)-adrenoceptor activation of the nitric oxide-cGMP pathway: Relevance for hormonal facilitation of lordosis behavior. *J. Neurosci* 19(16): 7191–7197.

Coirini, H., Schumacher, M., Flanagan, L. M., and McEwen, B. S. (1991) Transport of estrogen-induced oxytocin receptors in the ventromedial hypothalamus. *J. Neurosci.* 11: 3317–3324.

Daniels, D., Miselis, R. R., and Flanagan-Cato, L. M. (1999) Central neuronal circuit innervating the lordosis-producing muscles defined by transneuronal transport of pseudorabies virus. *J. Neurosci.* 19: 2823–2833.

De Kloet, E. R., Voorhuis, D. A. M., Boschma, Y., and Elands, J. (1985) Estradiol modulates density of putative "oxytocin receptors" in discrete rat brain regions. *Neuroendocrionlogy* 44: 415–521.

Erskine, M. S. (1989) Solicitation behavior in the estrous female rat: A review. *Horm. Behav.* 23: 473–502.

Erskine, M. S., and Baum, M. J. (1982) Effects of paced coital stimulation on termination of estrus and brain indoleamine levels in female rats. *Pharmacol. Biochem. Behav.* 17: 857–861.

Etgen, A. M. (1990) Intrahypothalamic implants of noradrenergic antagonists disrupt lordosis behavior in female rats. *Physiol. Behav.* 48: 31–36.

Etgen, A. M. (1995) Oxytocin does not act locally in the hypothalamus to elicit norepinephrine release. *Brain Res.* 703: 242–244.

Etgen, A. M., Ungar, S., and Petitti, N. (1992) Estradiol and progesterone modulation of norepinephrine neurotransmission: Implications for the regulation of female reproductive behavior. *J. Neuroendocrinol.* 4: 255–271.

Feder, H. H. (1984) Hormones and sexual behavior. *Annu. Rev. Psychol.* 35: 165–200.

Fiber, J. M., and Etgen, A. M. (1998) Evidence that GABA augmentation of norepinephrine release is mediated by interneurons. *Brain Res.* 790: 329–333.

Frankfurt, M., Renner, K., Azmitia, E., and Luine, V. (1985) Intrahypothalamic 5,7-dihydroxytryptamine: Temporal analysis of effects on 5-hydroxytryptamine content in brain nuclei and on facilitated lordosis behavior. *Brain Res.* 340: 127–133.

Haskell, S. G., Richardson, E. D., and Horwitz, R. I. (1997) The effect of estrogen replacement therapy on cognitive function in women: A critical review of the literature. *J. Clin. Epidemiol.* 50: 1249–1264.

Henderson, V. W. (1997) Estrogen, cognition, and a woman's risk of Alzheimer's disease. *Am. J. Med.* 103: 11S–18S.

Johnson, A. E., Coirini, H., Ball, G. F., and McEwen, B. S. (1989) Anatomical localization of the effects of 17β-estradiol on oxytocin receptor binding in the ventromedial hypothalamic nucleus. *Endocrinology* 124: 207–211.

Kow, L.-M., Johnson, A. E., Ogawa, S., and Pfaff, D. W. (1991) Electrophysiological actions of oxytocin on hypothalamic neurons in vitro: Neuropharmacological characterization and effects of ovarian steroids. *Neuroendocrinology* 54: 526–535.

Kow, L.-M., Weesner, G. D., and Pfaff, D. W. (1992) α1-Adrenergic agonists act on the ventromedial hypothalamus to cause neuronal excitation and lordosis facilitation: electrophysiological and behavioral evidence. *Brain Res.* 588: 237–245.

Mani, S. K., Blaustein, J. D., and O'Malley, B. W. (1997) Progesterone receptor function from a behavioral perspective. *Horm. Behav.* 31: 244–255.

Matthews, M. K. Jr., and Adler, N. T. (1978) Systematic interrelationship of mating, vaginal plug position, and sperm transport in the rat. *Physiol. Behav.* 20(3): 303–309.

McCarthy, M. M., Kleopoulos, S. P., Mobbs, C. V., and Pfaff, D. W. (1994) Infusion of antisense oligodeoxynucleotides to the oxytocin receptor in the ventromedial hypothalamus reduces estrogen-induced sexual receptivity and oxytocin receptor binding in the female rat. *Neuroendocrinology* 59: 432–440.

McCarthy, M. M., Malik, K. F., and Feder, H. H. (1990) Increased GABAergic transmission in medial hypothalamus facilitates lordosis but has the opposite effect in preoptic area. *Brain Res.* 507: 40–44.

McCarthy, M. M., Kaufman, L. C., Brooks, P. J., Pfaff, D. W., and Schwartz-Giblin, S. (1995) Estrogen modulation of mRNA levels for the two forms of glutamic acid decarboxylase (GAD) in female rat brain. *Comp. Neurol.* 360: 685–697.

McClintock, M. K. (1971) Menstrual synchrony and suppression. *Nature* 291: 244–245.

McClintock, M. K. (1984) Estrous synchrony: Modulation of ovarian cycle length by female pheromones. *Physiol. Behav.* 32(5): 701–705.

McClintock, M. K. (1987) A functional approach to the behavioral endocrinology of rodents. In D. Crews (Ed.), *Psychobiology of Reproductive Behavior*. Englewood Cliffs, N.J.: Prentice Hall, pp. 176–203.

Morrell, J. I., and Pfaff, D. W. (1982) Characterization of estrogen-concentrating neurons by their axonal projections. *Science* 217: 1273–1276.

Ogawa, S., Chan, J., Chester, A. E., Gustaffsson, J.-A., Korach, K. S., and Pfaff, D. W. (1999) Survival of reproductive behaviors in estrogen receptor β gene-deficient (ßERKO) male and female mice. *Proc. Natl. Acad. Sci. USA* 96: 12887–12892.

Ogawa, S., Eng, V., Taylor, J., Lubahn, D. B., Korack, K., and Pfaff, D. W. (1998) Roles of estrogen receptor-α gene expression in reproduction-related behaviors in female mice. *Endocrinology* 139: 5070–5081.

Ogawa, S., Washburn, T. F., Taylor, J., Lubahn, D. B., Korach, K. S., and Pfaff, D. W. (1998) Modifications of testosterone-dependent behaviors by estrogen receptor-α gene disruption in male mice. *Endocrinology* 139: 5058–5069.

Pettersson, K., Grandien, K., Kuiper, G. J. M., and Gustafsson, J.-A. (1997) Mouse estrogen receptor β forms estrogen response element-binding heterodimers with estrogen receptor α. *Molec. Endocrinol.* 11: 1486–1496.

Pfaff, D. W., and Keiner, M. (1973) Atlas of estradiol-concentrating cells in the central nervous system of the female rat. *J. Comp. Neurol.* 151: 121–158.

Pfaff, D. W., Schwartz-Giblin, S., McCarthy, M. M., and Kow, L.-M. (1994) Cellular and molecular mechanisms of female reproductive behaviors. In E. Knobil and J. D. Neill (Eds.), *The Physiology of Reproduction*, 2nd edition. New York: Raven Press, pp. 107–220.

Pfaus, J. G., and Gorzalka, B. (1987) Opioids and sexual behavior. *Neurosci. Biobehav.* 11: 1–34.

Pfaus, J. G. (1999) Neurobiology of sexual behavior. *Curr. Opin. Neurobiol.* 9: 751–758.

Porterfield, S. P. (1997) *Endocrine Physiology*. St. Louis, MO: Mosby-Year Book.

Rissman, E. F., Early, A. H., Taylor, J. A., Korach, K. S., and Lubahn, D. B. (1997) Estrogen receptors are essential for female sexual receptivity. *Endocrinology* 138: 507–510.

Rissman, E., Wersinger, S. R., Fugger, H. N., and Foster, T. C. (1999) Sex with knockout models: Behavioral studies of estrogen receptor α. *Brain Res.* 835: 80–90.

Rubin, B. S., and Barfield, R. J. (1983) Induction of estrous behavior in ovariectomized rats by sequential replacement of estrogen and progesterone to the ventromedial hypothalamus. *Neuroendocrinology* 37: 218–224.

Schughrue, P. J., Lane, M. V., and Merchenthaler, I. (1997) Comparative distribution of estrogen receptor-α and -β mRNA in the rat central nervous system. *J. Comp. Neurol.* 388: 507–525.

Schumacher, M., Corini, H., Pfaff, D. W., and McEwen, B. S. (1990) Behavioral effects of progesterone associated with rapid modulation of oxytocin receptors. *Science* 250: 691–694.

Schwartz-Giblin, S., McEwen, B. S., and Pfaff, D. W. (1989) Mechanisms of female reproductive behavior. In F. R. Brush and S. Levine (Eds.), *Psychoendocrinology*. New York: Academic Press.

Squires, E. L. (1993) Estrous detection. In A. O. McKinnon and J. L. Voss (Eds.), *Equine Reproduction*. Philadelphia: Lea and Febiger, p. 193.

Stern, K., and McClintock, M. K. (1998) Regulation of ovulation by human pheromones. *Nature* 392: 177–179.

Vincent, P. A., and Etgen, A. M. (1993) Steroid priming promotes oxytocin-induced norepinephrine release in the ventromedial hypothalamus of female rats. *Brain Res.* 620: 189–194.

Witt, D. M., and Insel, T. R. (1991) A selective oxytocin antagonist attenuates progesterone facilitation of female sexual behavior. *Endocrinology* 128: 3269–3276.

5 Neuroendocrinology of Sexual Behavior in the Male

Michael J. Baum

The sexual behaviors of both females and males are complex, but in males the role of peripheral structures (e.g., the penis) is more obvious. As we will see, hormones may affect male sexual behavior by acting upon such peripheral structures. Pharmacological and anatomical studies indicate that hormones have distinct effects on the brain that influence male sexual motivation and performance independently. Normally there is a coordinated effort involving different metabolites of a single hormone to prepare both the brain and peripheral structures for copulation. Once again, hormones, by virtue of their widespread influence throughout the body, provide this coordination.

What are the components of male sexual behavior? Which hormones affect these components? Where do the hormones act? What are the neural mechanisms controlling male sexual behavior and which neurotransmitter systems are involved? How can we measure sexual motivation and sexual performance separately?

Introduction

As you learned in chapter 3, testosterone secreted by the testes acts during development in mammals to promote penile development and to organise neural circuits. When the animal becomes an adult, these neural circuits control male sexual motivation and mating performance. Likewise, in adulthood, testosterone or one of its metabolites act in the brain and penis to facilitate masculine sexual motivation and coital performance. A coordinated effort involving testosterone and its metabolites is needed to organize and then, later, to activate the neural and genital tissues that control copulation.

Once again, hormones, by virtue of their widespread influence throughout the body, provide this coordination. How do we measure masculine sexual motivation? What are the motoric components of the mating behavior of males of different species? Which hormones affect these two aspects of masculine sexual behavior? Finally, which parts of the nervous system and which neurotransmitter systems control sexual motivation, penile erection, and coital behavior? How do sex hormones affect the development and adult function of these neural systems? These are the questions we will address in this chapter.

As described in chapter 1, one of the first experiments of behavioral endocrinology (Berthold 1849) demonstrated that castrating a rooster inhibited its ability to mate with a hen, and this coincided with a reduction in the size of the comb. Like the rooster's comb, the nervous system is a target for **testosterone** secreted by the testes.

These early observations laid the groundwork for numerous later experiments investigating the actions of androgen on both the nervous system and other androgen-sensitive target tissues including the prostate gland and the penis. Androgens can act directly upon the brain to affect an animal's behavior. Through its action on another androgen-sensitive tissue, the penis, androgen affects masculine mating behavior indirectly.

This chapter will concentrate on the actions of androgens in the adult and fetal brain that contribute to masculine sexual motivation and the control of mating behavior in the male. We will consider the neuroendocrine mechanism that controls the secretion of the primary androgen secreted by the testes, testosterone. Then we will discuss the contribution of two neural metabolites of testosterone, **estradiol** and **5α-dihydrotestosterone** (**DHT**), which act via neural estradiol and androgen receptors, respectively, to control aspects of sexual motivation, mating, and penile erection in adult males.

Next, we will consider some of the underlying neural mechanisms that mediate the actions of androgens on masculine sexual performance. This includes inputs from the olfactory system to the medial preoptic area and outputs to the motor systems that control the pelvic movements necessary for mating in male vertebrates. The role of particular neurotransmitter systems as well as neuropeptides that modulate aspects of masculine sexual motivation, pair bonding, and coital function will be discussed.

Finally, we will examine the role of estrogen and androgen in regulating the perinatal development of neural systems that control masculine sexual motivation and performance in adulthood. Experimental findings from several vertebrate species including rat, ferret, mouse, hamster, quail, monkey, and human will be used to illustrate the relevant principles of neuroendocrine regulation.

Sexual Behavior in the Male

Definitions

A distinction between **sexual motivation** and **mating** (or **coital performance**) will be emphasized throughout this chapter. An example of this distinction is a diabetic man whose penile erectile capacity is compromised by disease-induced damage to the innervation of the erectile tissues (corpus cavernosum and corpus spongiosum) of the penis. The diabetic man's capacity to perform sexually may often not match his motivation to engage in sexual activity. Such a mismatch in sexual motivation and performance capacity has been a major source of discontent and psychological suffering in such patients. Thankfully, the recent development of drugs for treating erectile disfunction (box 5.1 describing the action of Viagra) affords new hope to diabetic men and others with this disability.

SEXUAL MOTIVATION VERSUS SEXUAL ABILITY

Much of the research using animal models has concentrated on the different neuroendocrine mechanisms that control penile erection, sexual motivation,

Box 5.1 How Viagra Works

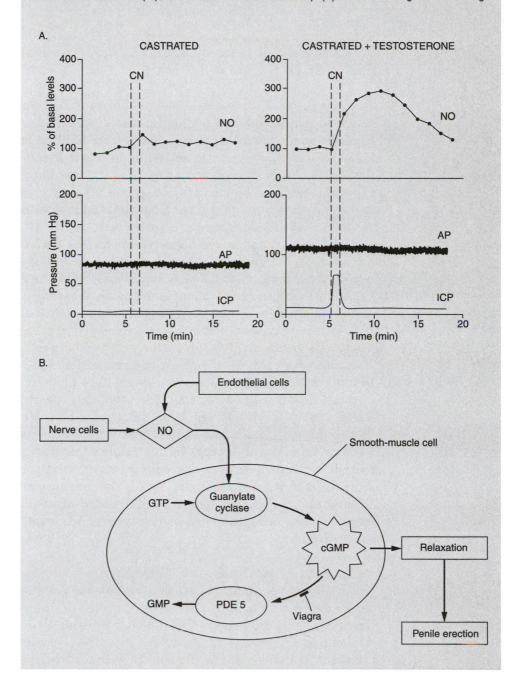

(A) Effect of electrical stimulation of the cavernosal nerves (CN; stimulation period indicated by dashed lines) in anesthetized, castrated male rats on nitric oxide (NO) release and blood pressure (ICP) in the corpus cavernosum of the penis and on arterial blood pressure (AP). Cavernosal nerve stimulation augmented NO release and ICP only in castrated males which received testosterone (reproduced from Marin et al. 1999). (B) Schematic diagram illustrating

Box 5.1   (continued)

> the mechanism whereby Viagra promotes penile erection by interfering with the breakdown of cyclic GMP (cGMP) by phosphodiesterase type 5 (PDE 5). Sexual arousal and the resulting increase in the activity of the parasympathetic innervation of the corpus cavernosum of the penis promotes the formation and release of NO. This gaseous neurotransmitter passes into adjacent smooth muscle cells lining the corpus cavernosum where it activates guanylate cyclase. This leads to the accumulation of cGMP and the relaxation of the smooth muscle wall of the corpus cavernosum which allows this vascular bed to become engorged with blood. A penile erection ensues (reproduced from Kling 1998).

and mating behavior per se. For example, studies using the male rat have analyzed penile erectile function by recording the latency (i.e., time to first occurrence) of erection as well as the number of discrete erections shown by a rat when restrained on its back with the penile sheath retracted by the experimenter. Other studies have assessed erectile function (noncontact, or psychogenic erections) shown in response to distal, mainly olfactory, signals from an estrous female and penile erections induced in anesthetized rats following electrical stimulation of the cavernosal nerves.

The most common studies observe the mating performance of a male rat during direct interactions with an estrous female. In this situation, a receptive female is placed in a chamber with the male being tested, and the observer records the occurrence of mounts with pelvic thrusting, penile intromissions, and ejaculations over time. In rats, as in many rodent species, the male displays a series of discrete mounts of the female partner that are accompanied by a very brief penile erection, pelvic thrusting, and intromission into the vagina. The male dismounts after each intromission. After 5 to 15 such mounts with intromission, the male ejaculates a **copulatory plug** composed of secretions of the prostate, seminal vesicle, and coagulating gland plus sperm from the testes. Deposition of this copulatory plug against the female's cervix ensures that sperm will pass into the uterus, thereby heightening the likelihood that fertilization of ova will occur in the female's fallopian tubes. Receipt of numerous intromissions from the male insures the activation of a neuroendocrine reflex in female rodents needed to stimulate pituitary prolactin secretion for pregnancy. Following ejaculation, a period of sexual quiescence ensues for several minutes (the postejaculatory interval or **refractory period**) until mating resumes.

VARIATION IN MALE SEXUAL BEHAVIORS

Great species variations exist in the behavioral patterns displayed by male vertebrates during mating. For example, many species of fish perform stereotyped courtship movements that entice the female to deposit eggs in a nest, whereupon the male positions himself over these eggs and deposits his sperm without ever making physically contact with the female. In avian species, the male exhibits a wide variety of courtship displays, including vocalization (crowing or singing), strutting, mounting, and deposition of sperm through direct cloacal contact with the female.

The pattern of mating displayed by the male rhesus monkey resembles that shown by the male rat described earlier. By contrast, the male ferret mates by grasping the female's neck, mounting, and exhibiting episodes of pelvic thrusting (accompanied by penile erection). Once the erect penis is inserted into the female's vagina, thrusting ceases, and the intromission is maintained for up to 1.5 hours, even after the ejaculation of sperm. This intromission activates a neuroendocrine reflex in females leading to the pituitary secretion of luteinizing hormone (LH) and subsequent ovulation. Specific patterns of masculine courtship and coital behavior have evolved in different species to maximize the chances of reproductive success. These behaviors develop within the constraints of that species' physiology, social organization, and ecological setting. Additional discussion of social, environmental, and evolutionary constraints on behavior is found in chapter 7.

Counting the incidence or timing the duration of neck grip, mounting, intromission, and ejaculation serves as a useful index of masculine coital performance. However, these parameters of sexual activity provide only partial insight into an animal's level of sexual motivation. Sexual motivation is a conceptual term that refers to the inclination of an individual to seek out and approach a partner for the purpose of mating. Masculine sexual motivation has been measured experimentally in several different ways. In an early study (Stone et al. 1935) willingness of male rats to walk across an electrified floor (which was painful) to gain access to an estrous female was assessed. More recently, the willingness of male quail to approach a window in order to see a receptive female or of a male ferret to approach an estrous female (as opposed to a nonestrous female or another male) in the arms of a T-shaped maze have been assessed.

Basic Neuroendocrine Relations in the Male

Feminine gonadal function is generally cyclic and synchronized to ensure the periodic release of ova from ovarian follicles (see chapter 4). Two steroid hormones, estradiol and progesterone, are secreted sequentially. By contrast, in males the production of both sperm and steroid hormones by the testes occurs tonically for considerable periods of time. Germ cells in the seminiferous tubules divide and differentiate into sperm. Testosterone is produced by Leydig cells located in the interstitial space between these tubules in response to the stimulatory action of the pituitary gonadotropin, luteinizing hormone (LH).

REGULATION OF TESTOSTERONE SECRETION

The secretion of LH is ultimately controlled by the neuropeptide **gonadotropin-releasing hormone (GnRH)**, which is released in a pulsatile fashion (depending on the species, one to two pulses/hour) from nerve terminals in the median eminence at the base of the brain. GnRH passes into portal blood vessels that traverse the pituitary stalk and then enter the anterior pituitary gland. Here GnRH interacts with membrane receptors in gonadotrophs, thereby stimulating the release of LH as well as follicle-stimulating hormone (FSH). Pulses of LH are detected by membrane receptors in the Leydig cells of the testes, and a pulsatile pattern of testosterone secretion results. Testosterone released from the testes influences both the expression of masculine sexual behavior in adulthood and the perinatal differentiation of brain mechanisms and genital structures destined to control masculine sexual motivation and performance.

TESTOSTERONE SECRETION DURING DEVELOPMENT

Episodes of testosterone secretion occur prenatally, within a few hours after birth, and over the first few postnatal weeks or months. The exact timing of perinatal testosterone secretion differs widely among species; it depends on the length of gestation and the speed of neural and somatic development. In all mammalian species studied to date, these episodes of perinatal testosterone exposure organize the differentiation of the male's genital structures as well as aspects of the brain circuitry destined to control masculine sexual behavior.

In addition, all vertebrates exhibit a period after birth when the reproductive neuroendocrine axis becomes relatively quiescent. Later in development this system is reactivated, whereupon puberty occurs and adult levels of testicular steroidogenesis (i.e., testosterone secretion) coupled with spermatogenesis are established.

SEASONAL VARIATION

There is considerable variation among vertebrate species in the seasonal pattern of testosterone secretion and in the sensitivity of the brain to the actions of testosterone. In many instances, the entire hypothalamic-pituitary-testis axis undergoes a yearly regression. In such seasonal breeders the output of GnRH and LH, and consequently of testosterone, is dramatically reduced as the animal passes out of breeding condition. The testicular production of mature sperm also ceases as a consequence of hormonal deprivation. In most vertebrates, the reproductive axis resumes its function as the next breeding season approaches.

There are some interesting exceptions to this rule, however, which are discussed in chapter 7. In some species, the timing of these periods of testicular regression and regrowth is linked to changes in the prevailing photoperiod (i.e., the relative duration of day and night as discussed in chapter 12). For example, in male sheep, peak testicular secretion of testosterone, spermatogenesis, and maximal breeding activity occur in the fall, in response to shortening day length. Gestation in this species lasts 5 months, and therefore lambs are born in the spring when conditions are optimal for survival of the newborn. By contrast, in male ferrets, breeding occurs in the spring, when the days are growing longer. In this species, gestation lasts only 41 days, and thus conditions are again optimal for the survival of the newborn offspring.

In addition to governing the seasonal cycle of testosterone secretion, differences in photoperiod may affect the responsiveness of the nervous system to circulating hormones. For example, castrated hamsters kept under short-day photoperiods exhibit masculine sexual behavior in response to exogenous testosterone less readily than do castrates kept under long days (Miernicki et al. 1990). In the adult male rat, however, the testicular secretion of testosterone occurs throughout the year, with pulsatile variations in output occurring on an hourly basis. Seasonal variations in behavioral responsiveness to testosterone of male laboratory rats have not been reported.

Expression of Masculine Sexual Behavior

Role of Testosterone and Its Metabolites

You will recall from chapter 3 that testosterone itself exerts some of its organizational effects by acting directly on the nervous system and on peripheral non-neural tissue (i.e., muscles, sensory receptors, and accessory sex organs). Alternatively, testosterone may be converted either in brain or peripheral tissue to a metabolite that has specific effects on the target tissue.

Two questions, therefore, must be considered regarding the role of testosterone in controlling masculine sexual behavior in adults. First, where do testosterone and its metabolites promote the expression of male sexual behavior (i.e., in the central nervous system, genital tissues, or both)? Second, what hormone(s) are necessary for expression of masculine sexual behavior? It is possible that there may be more than one active hormone and that multiple hormones acting via specific steroid receptor proteins in several types of target cells may be needed to produce the full expression of masculine sexual behavior. As we shall see, this latter scenario appears to be the case. It took a while, however, for scientists to reach this conclusion.

THE ROLE OF ANDROGENS

As stated earlier in this chapter, the castration of a male chicken reduces the expression of masculine sexual behavior. Similar results have been seen in species representing all vertebrate classes (reviewed in Meisel and Sachs 1994). Likewise, in men, hypogonadism (i.e., lack of testicular development), which results from a congenital failure of GnRH neurons to migrate into appropriate positions in the mediobasal hypothalamus, blocks the normal occurrence of puberty and attenuates the associated increments in sexual motivation and the capacity for penile erection (Davidson et al. 1979). Soon after testosterone was first synthesized, Stone (1939) showed conclusively that administration of this hormone to castrated rats reliably restored all aspects of mating behavior.

These findings, together with later demonstrations that testosterone is the primary steroid secreted by the testes in essentially all male vertebrates, provided strong evidence that testosterone activates mating behavior in adult male vertebrates. Studies carried out on male rats and dogs also showed that castration eliminated penile erections, whereas testosterone replacement restored them (Hart 1967). Thus, both erection and mating rely on the actions of testosterone.

Experiments conducted with guinea pigs (Grunt and Young 1952) and rats (Damassa et al. 1977) suggested that only a threshold concentration of circulating testosterone is required to activate masculine sexual behavior and erectile function. Typically, the plasma concentration of androgen in males of these species greatly exceeds the minimal amount sufficient to sustain the sexual motivation and coital performance of males, including penile erection. By contrast, in some other species (ferret, Baum and Tobet 1988; rhesus monkey, Michael et al. 1986) the mating performance of males varies dramatically as a function of the circulating testosterone concentrations.

Although testosterone clearly facilitates penile erection and the expression of sexual behavior, for many years it was not clear whether these effects of testosterone resulted from the action of the steroid in the central nervous system or, alternatively, in non-neural tissues including the penis. Indeed, sensory receptors on the surface of the glans penis, whose size and number are stimulated by testosterone, have been identified in several species (Phoenix et al. 1976). It seemed possible that testosterone activated erection and mating by enhancing the sensory responsiveness of these receptors. Nevertheless, effects of testosterone on sensory systems could not explain its activational effects on behavioral indices of sexual motivation such as increased approach toward an estrous female in the absence of any genital or other physical contact with a female. Indeed, Sachs (1997) showed that volatile olfactory signals from estrous female rats called **pheromones** stimulate penile erections in males, and these erections are dramatically facilitated by circulating androgens (Manzo et al. 1999).

Baulieu et al. (1968) showed that the stimulatory action of testosterone on the cells of the prostate gland as well as on those of the genital skin actually depends on its conversion by the enzyme **5α-reductase** into dihydrotestosterone (DHT). It is DHT that promotes the growth and secretory activity of target cells after interacting with specific androgen receptor proteins. Subsequently, 5α-reductase and androgen receptors were found in the brain, in the preoptic area (POA) and the hypothalamus. These brain regions are thought to participate in the control of mating behavior. For the purposes of simplifying the discussion we will use POA to indicate the entire region of the medial POA-anterior hypothalamus. The reader should be aware, however, that there may be subregions with specialized functions contained within this region. 5α-reductase and androgen receptors were also found in the corpus cavernosum of the penis where androgen has been shown to regulate the activity of the enzymes responsible for the synthesis of nitric oxide (Marin et al. 1999). This gaseous neurotransmitter (see box 5.1) has been implicated in the control of erections.

In light of these facts, it is surprising that administration of DHT to castrated rats fails to activate mating. This was true whether DHT was given systemically (McDonald et al. 1970) or implanted directly into the POA (Johnston and Davidson 1972). Interestingly, however, administration of DHT to castrated rats did activate penile erections that were displayed when rats were either restrained on their backs with the prepuce of the penis retracted (Gray et al. 1980) or placed in a chamber adjacent to an estrous female (Manzo et al. 1999). This may occur through an action of androgen receptors in the lumbar spinal cord (Breedlove and Arnold 1980) or in the corpus cavernosum of the penis itself. Systemic treatment with DHT, therefore, duplicates all the effects of testosterone on the putative sensory receptors of the glans penis and activates penile erections, yet such rats are not motivated to approach and mate with estrous females.

THE ROLE OF ESTROGEN

Testosterone (Davidson 1966), but not DHT (Johnston and Davidson 1972), when implanted directly into the POA, facilitates sexual behavior. This suggests that testosterone activates mating through a direct effect on the nervous system of male rats. At about the same time that the experiments on the behavioral effects of DHT were being conducted, it was found that administration of estrogen (given either systemically or implanted directly into the POA) strongly facilitated mounting and intromissive behavior in castrated male rats (Davidson 1969). This was surprising because estrogen had long been thought to be exclusively a "female" steroid.

It soon became apparent, however, that the enzyme **aromatase**, which converts androgen to estrogen (discussed in chapter 3), is present in the hypothalamic and limbic forebrain structures of adult males and females of all vertebrate species (Naftolin et al. 1975). Furthermore, specific receptors for estrogen are present in these same brain regions in both sexes (Vreeburg et al. 1975).

Evidence suggests that estrogen and androgen (either testosterone itself or DHT) act in different sites to activate masculine sexual activity, including penile erection in the male rat and in males of numerous other vertebrate species (Baum et al. 1987). In the ferret, for example, subcutaneous (SC) injections of either testosterone propionate (TP) or estradiol benzoate (EB) to castrated males facilitated neck gripping, mounting, and pelvic thrusting behavior to equivalent degrees (figure 5.1) (Baum 1976).

Interestingly, ovariectomized females given these same steroids showed no pelvic thrusting, very little mounting, and less neck gripping than males did. This was presumably because the neural mechanisms governing male-typical mating behaviors are less developed in females due to the lack of perinatal steroidal exposure (see chapter 3) and "Steroids and the Development of Masculine Sexual Behavior" in this chapter. At first glance, it appears that estrogen duplicates all the behavioral effects of testosterone, suggesting that estradiol, formed directly in the brain, may normally mediate all the behavioral actions of circulating androgen. Other data suggest, however, that estrogens only partially duplicate the behavioral effects of testosterone in ferrets and in other species as well.

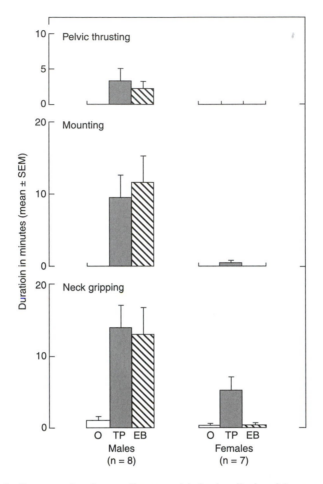

Figure 5.1 Components of masculine sexual behavior displayed by gonadectomized male and female ferrets 10 to 14 days after the onset of daily SC injections of oil vehicle (0), testosterone propionate (TP) (5 mg/kg), or estradiol benzoate (EB) (10 μg/kg). Note the similar behavioral effects of TP and EB in males and the relative ineffectiveness of either hormone in females. Data are expressed as mean ± SEM. (Adapted from Baum 1976.)

Hormones and Sexual Ability versus Sexual Motivation

A striking difference between the actions of estrogen and testosterone was observed when the masculine sexual motivation of ferrets was assessed by allowing subjects to choose between approaching and interacting with either an estrous or an anestrous female in the opposite goal boxes of a T-maze (figure 5.2) (Baum et al. 1990a). Gonadectomized male and female ferrets were tested in this situation repeatedly while receiving daily injections of oil vehicle, TP, or EB. When treated with oil vehicle, males and females both showed equivalent preferences for estrous and anestrous females. Furthermore, neither sex displayed a preference for either goal box during trials when no stimulus animals were placed in them. (i.e., extinction trials).

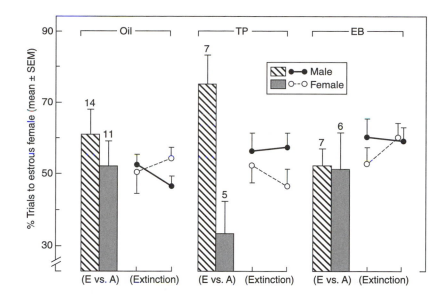

Figure 5.2 Preference for approaching and interacting with an estrous (E) versus an anestrous (A) female in a T-maze displayed by gonadectomized (Gdx) male and female ferrets tested 7 to 14 days after the onset of daily SC injections of oil vehicle, testosterone propionate (TP) (5 mg/kg), or estradiol benzoate (EB) (12 μg/kg). Stimulus females were absent from the goal boxes during the 2 days of extinction tests given under each hormone condition. TP caused males to approach an estrous female more effectively than did EB. Neither hormone caused female subjects to prefer approaching an estrous as opposed to an anestrous female. Data are expressed as mean ± SEM. (Adapted from Baum et al. 1990.)

By contrast, when treated with TP, males showed a distinct preference for the estrous female, whereas females did not. Again, preferences of both sexes for the two (now empty) goal boxes returned to chance levels during extinction trials. Finally, when given EB, neither males nor females displayed a preference for estrous or anestrous females. These results suggest that in male ferrets estrogen is unable to duplicate completely the activational effect of testosterone on the motivation to approach and interact with an estrous female. Once confronted directly with such a female, however, the estrogen-treated male readily neck grips, mounts, and exhibits pelvic thrusting behavior toward the female (see figure 5.2). Although estrogen activates these latter behaviors in castrated male ferrets as readily as testosterone, it is considerably less effective than testosterone in promoting intromission. Androgen is probably required for full erection in the ferret and in the male rat.

Estrogen activates aspects of masculine sexual behavior in several other mammalian species including hamster, pig, deer, sheep, and cow (reviewed in Baum et al. 1987), in two avian species, quail and ring dove (reviewed in Balthazart et al. 1995), and in one reptilian species, the lizard (Crews and Morgentaler 1979). In castrated male rats (Baum and Vreeburg 1973) and hamsters (DeBold and Clemens 1978), the combination of estrogen and DHT

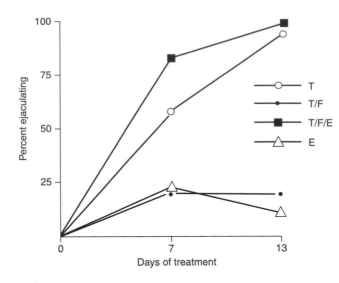

Figure 5.3 Effect of cerebroventricular infusion of the aromatase inhibitor fadrazole (F) on the occurrence of ejaculation by castrated male rats which also received SC implants of Silastic capsules filled with testosterone (T) and/or estradiol (E). Only males that showed no intromissions in tests with estrous females given two weeks after castration (test at 0 days) were used in this experiment. After treatments began, males received two more behavioral tests. Fadrazole blocked the activational effect of T on mating, and this effect was reversed by giving a low dose of E (which by itself failed to activate mating in another group of castrates) together with T. (Adapted from Vagell and McGinnis 1997.)

can duplicate all the effects of testosterone on mating behavior and erectile function.

Perhaps the most convincing evidence implicating estradiol in the control of masculine sexual behavior in the rat comes from studies (Christianson and Clemens 1975; Clancy et al. 1997; Vagell and McGinnis 1997) in which treatment with aromatase inhibitor drugs blocked the activational effect of testosterone on mating. For example, infusion of the aromatase inhibitor fadrazole into the cerebral ventricles of castrated rats that had SC testosterone capsules inhibited their ability to mate and ejaculate with an estrous female (figure 5.3). Other castrated males given Silastic capsules containing a very low dose of estradiol failed to ejaculate. However, this same dose of estradiol, when given to castrates treated concurrently with SC testosterone and intraventricular fadrazole, facilitated ejaculation up to the levels seen in castrated, testosterone-treated males. Vagell and McGinnis (1997) concluded that both androgen and estradiol are needed in the CNS to activate mating behavior in the rat.

Like ferrets (figure 5.2), castrated male rats treated with a low dose of estradiol expressed no preference to approach and interact with an estrous rather than an anestrous female, and fadrazole treatment failed to reduce the motivation of castrated, testosterone-treated males to approach an estrous female. This suggests that in rats, as in ferrets, testosterone itself makes an essential contribution to the activation of the neural circuits that control masculine sexual motivation. By contrast, in male quails, all of testosterone's stimulatory actions on sexual motivation and coital performance have been attributed to estrogenic metabolites formed in the hypothalamus (Balthazart et al. 1995).

There is controversy about whether the estrogenic metabolites of testosterone are essential for the activation of sexual behavior in male primates. Administration of estradiol to castrated rhesus monkeys failed to duplicate the effects of testosterone on mating behavior seen in other species (Michael et al. 1990). However, systemic administration of the aromatase inhibitor fadrazole significantly reduced the ability of testosterone to activate mounting and ejaculation in castrated cynomolgus monkeys (Zumpe et al. 1993). This effect of fadrazole was only partially reversed by administering estradiol concurrently, which raises the possibility that in primates, as in numerous other vertebrates, central aromatization of circulating testosterone contributes to sexual motivation and coital performance. More research will be needed to establish this unambiguously.

To summarize, there is evidence of central activation of male sexual behavior both by neural estrogenic metabolites of testosterone and by androgens (perhaps testosterone itself). Although it is well established that either testosterone or estrogen will activate masculine sexual behavior when implanted into the medial POA/anterior hypothalamic region of castrated rats, there is no agreement about the precise localization of hormone action within this brain region. More work is needed to resolve the relative contributions, and specific neural sites of action, of testosterone, DHT, and estrogen to the activation of masculine sexual motivation and the coordination of the motoric behaviors (mounts or pelvic thrusts with or without intromission) involved in mating. The role of DHT acting in the spinal cord and penis to facilitate erection is more clearly established.

Neural Integration of Masculine Sexual Behavior

Research into the neural systems mediating male sexual behavior has begun to analyze the hormonal, sensory, and neurochemical components that interact to control masculine sexual motivation and coital behaviors per se. Structures in the mediobasal forebrain, including the bed nucleus of the stria terminals, POA, and anterior hypothalamus, contain circuits which integrate these inputs and which generate outputs controlling approach behaviors, mounting and pelvic thrusting, and even penile erection.

Input from Olfactory Systems

Pheromones from estrous females motivate males to approach them and increase the sexual arousal of males and the initiation of sexual behavior in several rodent species. For example, the male hamster normally investigates the female's anogenital region and licks the viscous vaginal secretions of estrous females prior to initiating mating (Powers and Winans 1975). The male then executes a single mount with intromission and intravaginal penile thrusting that, after several minutes, lead to ejaculation.

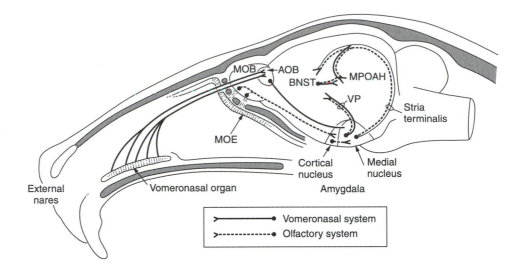

Figure 5.4 Schematic representation of olfactory and vomeronasal pathways that control male hamster mating behavior: MOB, main olfactory bulb; MOE, main olfactroy epithelium; AOB, accessory olfactory bulb; BNST, bed nucleus of the stria terminalis; MPOAH, medial preoptic area/anterior hypothalamus; VP, ventral pathway projecting from the medial amygdala to the MPOAH. (Adapted from Winans et al. 1982; drawing courtesy of S. W. Newman.)

Experimentally interfering with olfactory inputs to both the vomeronasal organs and the olfactory mucosa prevented males from mounting an estrous female. However, such interference with olfactory inputs failed to disrupt the behavior of males that had had extensive mating experience.

Critical Role for the Preoptic Area (POA) and the Bed Nucleus of the Stria Terminalis (BNST)
Neuroanatomical experiments have demonstrated that chemoreceptors in the **vomeronasal organ** project to the accessory olfactory bulb, whereas receptors in the **main olfactory epithelium** project to the main olfactory bulb (figure 5.4) (reviewed in Winans et al. 1982). Both the main and accessory olfactory bulbs project to the corticomedial nuclei of the amygdaloid complex.

These nuclei project, in turn, to the bed nucleus of the stria terminalis (BNST) and onto the POA. An extensive literature (Winans et al. 1982) shows that lesions to several different portions of this olfactory projection circuit severely disrupt both chemoinvestigative behavior (i.e., investigative behaviors initiated and sustained by odors) and mating in male hamsters.

Although the deficits are less severe, similar sites of neural destruction also reduce mating performance in male rats and mice (reviewed in Meisel and Sachs 1994). Sachs (1997) has shown that male rats display penile erections (and increased sexual motivation) in response to volatile odor cues from estrous females that are nearby but not visible or audible. These **noncontact erections** are analogous to the erections occurring in men who view erotic films or who have erections during sexual fantasy.

As shown in figure 5.5, castration of male rats eliminated their capacity to show noncontact erections, in response to the volatile body odors of females,

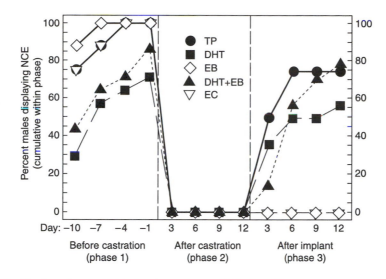

Figure 5.5 Display of noncontact penile erections (NCE) by male rats in response to distal signals (mainly pheromones) from an estrous female behind a wire mesh screen. Values are cumulative within each phase of the experiment. Males were gonadally intact in phase 1, castrated without hormone replacement in phase 2, and in phase 3 different groups of castrates received SC implants of Silastic capsules containing testosterone propionate (TP), dihydrotestosterone (DHT), estradiol benzoate (EB), a combination of EB and DHT, or empty capsules (EC). Only treatment with TP or DHT restored NCE in castrated males. (Adapted from Manzo et al. 1999.)

but SC implantation of Silastic capsules containing either testosterone, DHT, or estradiol + DHT, reinstated their capacity to show noncontact erections.

As with erections exhibited by castrated males restrained on their backs (box 5.2), estradiol alone failed to facilitate noncontact erections more than empty capsules did. From this finding, we infer that androgenic steroids prime parts of the brain circuits that receive olfactory cues so as to produce penile erections and sexual arousal. Liu et al. (1997) have shown that lesions of either the **medial amygdala** or the BNST (but not the medial POA) severely disrupted a male's ability to show noncontact erections. The medial amygdala, BNST, POA circuit has also been shown to integrate the endocrine and olfactory signals needed for mating behavior in male hamsters, as we will see below.

An early study (Michael and Keverne 1968) suggested that vaginal pheromones facilitate the motivation of male rhesus monkeys to seek out sexually receptive female partners. Occlusion of the main olfactory epithelium in male rhesus monkeys reduced their lever pressing to gain access to sexually receptive females; however, when placed together in the same chamber, these anosmic males readily mated with receptive females. The application of vaginal secretions from an estrogen-primed female rhesus onto the genital region of other ovariectomized females that had received no estrogen failed to stimulate sexual behavior in males which otherwise showed no interest in mating with these particular females (Goldfoot et al. 1976). Volatile pheromonal signals emitted from the vagina or skin of a rhesus female may, however, enhance

Box 5.2 Hormones That Control Mating Behavior and Penile Erection

Prior to castration, males show short latencies (i.e., little delay) to first intromission (in tests with estrous females) and to their first penile erection (in tests while restrained on their backs). Following castration, males receiving subcutaneous implants of Silastic capsules containing testosterone continue to show similar first intromission and erection latencies. Castrated males given empty capsules showed lengthened response latencies; in other words, it took longer before they showed the behaviors. Males given estrogen showed intromission latencies that closely resembled those of testosterone-treated males, whereas their erection latencies resembled those of males given blank capsules. Conversely, males treated with DHT showed first intromission latencies resembling those of males with blank capsules, but their erection latencies resembled those of males treated with testosterone. Systemic administration of a drug that blocks the 5α-reduction of testosterone reduced the ability of testosterone to activate penile erection in castrated rats that were tested while restrained on their backs (Bradshaw et al. 1981), suggesting that DHT is normally required for the activation of erectile function in this species.

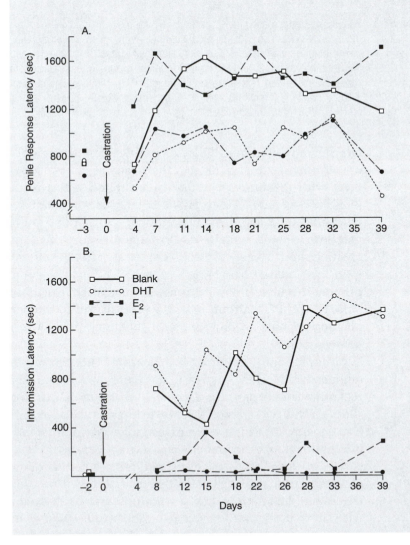

Box 5.2 (continued)

It is important to note that castrated males given estrogen managed to achieve erections that were sufficient to allow penile intromission in tests with estrous females. Thus, estrogen by itself, presumably acting in the nervous system, activates both mounting and intromission in the male rat. Meisel et al. (1984) suggest, however, that an androgenic stimulus may normally be required for full erectile function. In the rat it seems likely that this facilitation of erectile function by androgen is due to its actions in the corpus cavernosum where it stimulates nitric oxide synthesis, and to its action in motoneurons located in the spinal nucleus of the bulbocavernosus (SNB) system, which is sensitive to testosterone and DHT (see chapter 3). The SNB system is critical to the deposition of copulatory plugs containing sperm in the female's vagina and the resultant occurrence of pregnancy (Sachs 1982). It seems likely that an androgen (perhaps DHT) is also required for full penile erection in other species, including the male ferret.

In the figure above are the results of an experiment in which the effects of testosterone, DHT, and estradiol on the mating behavior and penile erection of castrated adult male rats were compared (from Meisel et al. 1984). (A) Penile response (erection) latencies of male rats tested while restrained on their backs and (B) intromission latencies of the same rats when tested with an estrous female. Groups of male rats were tested repeatedly after castration and SC insertion of Silastic capsules containing either nothing (blank), 5α-dihydrotestosterone (DHT), estradiol (E_2), or testosterone (T). The data illustrate that E_2 has little restorative effect upon reflexive erections but does facilitate actual mating, which includes seeking out an estrous female, mounting her, and having penile erections sufficient for intromission. DHT, on the other hand, facilitates reflexive erections but not mating. T, which can be metabolized to either E_2 or DHT, maintains both types of behavior (adapted from Meisel, O'Hanlon, and Sachs 1984).

a male's motivation to approach and make initial contacts which can lead to mating.

There are clinical reports of low sexual drive and erectile performance in men with congenital deficiencies in olfactory system development (Kallmann's syndrome; Federman 1967). However, these men also suffer from pituitary hypogonadism due to the inadequate development of neurons in the forebrain that synthesize and release GnRH into the pituitary portal blood vessels. It seems likely that the resulting deficit in the testicular production of testosterone, rather than deficient olfactory function per se, is responsible for the low level of psychosexual function that characterizes these patients. Indeed, administration of testosterone to hypogonadal men reversed their deficient ability to achieve penile erections in response to erotic fantasy (Bancroft and Wu 1983). This will be discussed in greater detail in the next chapter (chapter 6).

More than a half century ago Brookhart and Dey (1941) reported that large anterior hypothalamic lesions profoundly disrupted mating behavior in adult male guinea pigs without causing testicular atrophy. These observations, which suggest that different neural circuits control the expression of mating and the output of GnRH needed to stimulate pituitary gonadotropin secretion, were later confirmed using smaller lesions in the POA of male rats (Heimer and Larsson 1967) and in numerous male vertebrates, ranging from garter snakes to rhesus monkeys.

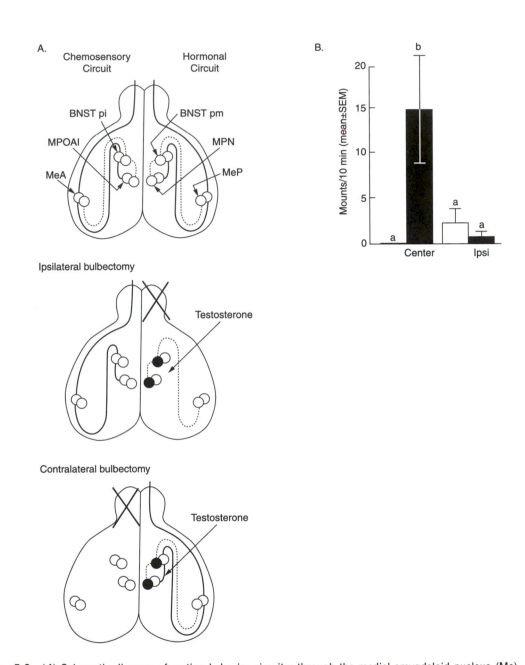

Figure 5.6 (*A*) Schematic diagram of mating behavior circuitry through the medial amygdaloid nucleus (Me), bed nucleus of the stria terminalis (BNST), and medial preoptic area (MPOA) in the male Syrian hamster brain illustrating the separate pathways for receipt of chemosensory and hormonal cues. *Top:* Normal male. Elements of the chemosensory circuit (*left*) include the anterior division of the Me, the posterointermediate subdivision of the BNST (BNSTpi), and the lateral subdivision of the MPOA. The hormonal circuit (*right*) includes the posterior subdivision of the Me (MeP), the posteromedial subdivision of the BNST (BNSTpm), and the medial preoptic nucleus (MPN). *Middle:* Testosterone stimulation of BNSTpm and MPN (solid circles) combined with removal of the ipsilateral olfactory bulb prevents communication between the chemosensory and hormonal circuits. *Bottom:* removal of the contralateral olfactory bulb does not disrupt chemosensory and hormonal integration. (*B*) Display of mounting behavior by long-term castrated male hamsters without hor-

Whereas destructive lesions disrupt sexual behavior, activation of neurons in the POA by stimulating them electrically activates mating in male rats (Malsbury 1971) and facilitates penile erection (Giuliano et al. 1996), provided that testosterone is circulating. Furthermore, localized implantation of either testosterone (Davidson 1969) or estradiol (Davis and Barfield 1979) into the POA activates mounting and intromissive behavior in castrated male rats.

As already described, implantation of the aromatase inhibitor fadrazole into the cerebral ventricles or into the POA of male rats or quails blocks the activational effects of subcutaneously administered testosterone on the expression of masculine sexual behavior. From these data we infer that in rats and quails the aromatization of androgen to estrogen in the POA contributes to the activation of masculine sexual behavior. In agreement with this idea, implantation of DHT (which cannot be aromatized to estradiol) into the POA fails to activate mating in castrated rats (Johnston and Davidson 1972) even when they received subcutaneous treatment with a low dose of estradiol (Baum et al. 1982).

Wood and Newman (1995) have provided evidence that testosterone (acting either itself or via its aromatized metabolite, estradiol) and pheromonal signals (detected via either the vomeronasal organ and/or the main olfactory epithelium) are processed by parallel subdivisions of the cortiomedial amygdaloid complex, the BNST, and the POA, and that the integration of these two inputs in the BNST and/or POA is essential for the activation of mating behavior in male hamsters. These workers took advantage of the fact that the olfactory projection circuit to the BNST/POA is restricted to each side of the brain (i.e., is primarily ipsilateral).

Different groups of sexually experienced male hamsters were castrated and then left without hormone treatment for 12 weeks, at the end of which their sexual behavior had essentially disappeared. Then these groups were given different combinations of testosterone implanted into one side of the BNST/POA and one of the olfactory bulbs, either ipsilateral or contralateral to the side of the brain with the testosterone implant, was surgically removed. In gonadally intact male hamsters, unilateral olfactory bulb removal does not disrupt mating, presumably because pheromones activate the remaining bulb and its projections to hypothalamic sites which are also exposed to circulating testosterone.

As shown in figure 5.6, when tested 12 weeks after castration males showed very little mounting behavior, as expected. A significant reinstatement of

Figure 5.6 (continued)

mone replacement (open bars) and after unilateral implantation of testosterone into the BNST/ MPOA plus removal of the olfactory bulb either contralateral (Contr) or ipsilateral (Ipsi) to the intracranial testosterone implant. Removal of the olfactory bulb on the same side of the brain as the testosterone implant blocks its ability to restore mating behavior by depriving these males of integrated chemosensory and steroidal signals. Data are expressed as mean ± SEM; different letters above the bars indicate groups that are significantly different from each other. (Adapted from Wood and Newman 1995.)

mounting was seen only in males in which the olfactory bulb was removed contralateral to the side of the BNST/POA into which testosterone was implanted. Presumably pheromones from estrous females were still being processed by the remaining intact olfactory bulb ipsilateral to the site of the testosterone implant, and the integration of these pheromonal and steroidal signals in the BNST/POA sufficed to activate mating behavior. Such integration of sensory and endocrine signals was not possible in males in which the olfactory bulb ipsilateral to the side of BNST/POA implant had been removed. As a result, they failed to mate when given access to an estrous female.

INDUCTION OF FOS
As discussed in chapter 2, in the late 1980s neuroscientists discovered that a class of "**immediate-early genes**" is expressed in specific pathways of the vertebrate brain in response to intense external sensory stimulation or homeostatic challenge. This method has been used to show that neurons present in the pathway that conveys olfactory signals to the POA also express c-*fos* after mating. Examples of increased Fos-immunoreactivity (IR) in the POA and BNST of male rats killed 90 min after the onset of a series of mounts and intromissions leading to an ejaculation are shown in figure 5.7 (Baum and Everitt 1992). Clear-cut mating-induced increments in Fos-IR occurred in the anterior olfactory bulb, the postero-dorsal portion of the medial amygdaloid nucleus, the BNST, and the POA—the same circuit that links the accessory olfactory bulbs to the hypothalamus (figure 5.4).

Mating also induced Fos-IR in the male's midbrain central tegmental field, a region which sends an afferent neuronal projection to the POA. Similar effects of mating on neuronal Fos-IR were seen in male mice, hamsters, and gerbils (Heeb and Yahr 1996). The profile of mating-induced Fos-IR seen in the anterior olfactory bulb, medial amygdala, BNST, and POA was reproduced, in part, by exposing male rats, hamsters, or mice to pheromones contained in soiled bedding from estrous females.

Likewise, exposing male rats to volatile odors from estrous females, which successfully induced noncontact erection, augmented Fos-IR in the medial amygdala, BNST, and the POA, but not in the anterior olfactory bulb, presumably because these volatile pheromones are normally detected by the main olfactory epithelium and not the vomeronasal organ (Kelliher et al. 1999). The ability of mating stimulation to induce Fos-IR in POA neurons of one side of the brain was eliminated by placing excitotoxic lesions (using the NMDA agonist, quinolinic acid) in both the medial amygdala and the central tegmental field of the same hemisphere (Baum and Everitt 1992). This suggests that olfactory and genital somatosensory signals engendered by mating with an estrous female are integrated in the POA. The fact that the majority of medial amygdaloid, BNST, and POA neurons that express Fos after mating also express androgen or estrogen receptor genes suggests that sex steroids facilitate this sensory integration.

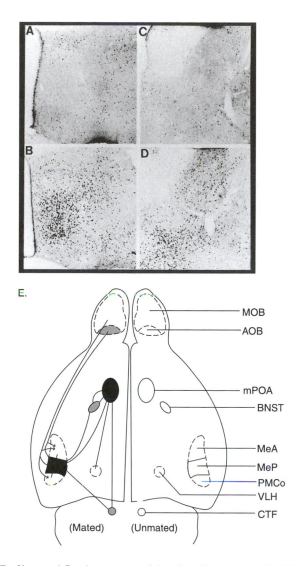

Figure 5.7 Neuronal Fos immunoreactivity (Fos-IR) in the medial POA (*A* and *B*), and posterior medial BNST (*C* and *D*), of male rats killed 1 hour after mating to ejaculation (*B* and *D*) or after spending 1 hour alone in a clean test arena (*A* and *C*). (*E*) Schematic brain diagram showing the location of clusters of Fos-IR cells (closed circles) in male rats after mating to ejaculation. Very low numbers of Fos-IR cells (open circles) were seen in males left alone in a clean test arena. AOB, accessory olfactory bulb; BNSTpm, the posteromedial subdivision of the bed nucleus of the stria terminalis; CTF, midbrain central tegmental field; MeA, medial amygdala; MeP, posterior subdivision of the medial amygdaloid nucleus; mPOA, medial preoptic area; PMCo, posterior medial subdivision of the cortical amygdaloid nucleus; VLH, ventral lateral hypothalamus; (Adapted from Baum and Everitt 1992.)

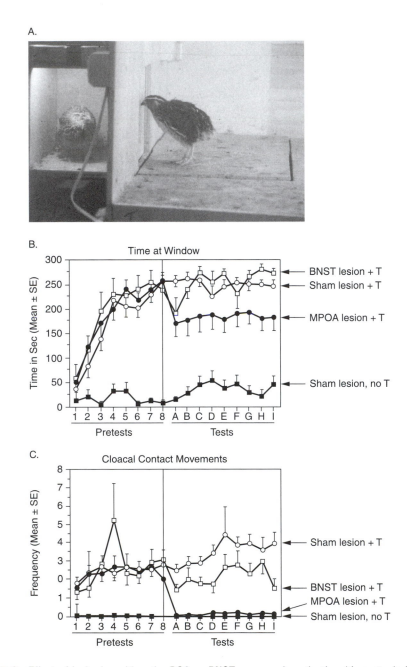

Figure 5.8 Effect of lesioning either the POA or BNST on sexual motivation (time at window) and consummatory aspects of mating (cloacal contact movements) in male quail. During pretests, castrated male quails were given Silastic capsules filled with testosterone (+T) (3 groups) or no T, and were trained to approach a window in the test apparatus that allowed them to view a receptive female in an adjacent compartment. Males were rewarded for approaching the viewing window by receiving access to the female, with which they subsequently mated. (*Top*) T-treated castrates learned to approach the viewing window whereas castrated males given no T did not. (*Bottom*) T-treated males copulated with the females after gaining access, whereas males given no T did not. Brain surgery was then carried out on the testosterone-treated groups. Males given bilateral lesions of the BNST

SEXUAL ABILITY VERSUS SEXUAL MOTIVATION

Numerous studies have assessed the effects of BNST or POA lesions on the motivation of males to seek out and approach an estrous female and on their mounting and intromissive behaviors directed toward an estrous female. There is general agreement that POA lesions disrupt a male's capacity to mount, intromit, and ejaculate with a female. This result has been obtained in species representing every terrestrial vertebrate class.

There is more controversy, however, about the effects of POA lesions on masculine sexual motivation. Hansen and colleagues (Hansen et al. 1982) first reported that male rats bearing neurotoxic lesions (made by infusing the glutamate/NMDA receptor agonist, ibotenic acid) of the cell bodies of the POA showed increased levels of anogenital sniffing and climbing over estrous females, even though after lesioning they never mated with these females. In fact, if given access to a water spout, the drinking behavior of males bearing POA lesions was dramatically increased in the presence of an estrous female. The authors argued that the frustration of not being able to convert sexual arousal into appropriate coital motor outputs was reduced as a result of the redirection of this drive.

A related observation was made of male rhesus monkeys bearing electrolytic lesions of the POA. These males stopped mounting, intromitting, and ejaculating when paired with sexually receptive females. They were, however, frequently observed masturbating to ejaculation in their home cages while watching females caged across the room. These males were clearly capable of becoming sexually aroused and were able to achieve ejaculation provided actual sociosexual interactions or coital movements were not required in the process.

A closer analysis of the possible motivational effects of POA lesions in male rodents, quails, and ferrets, using operant testing procedures in which males must move to a particular position in an apparatus in order view and/or gain access to a receptive female rather than a nonreceptive female, suggests that such lesions do reduce a male's motivation to seek out a female. For example, male rats bearing POA lesions showed a significant reduction in their preference for approaching an estrous as opposed to anestrous female tethered in different corners of a test apparatus (Edwards and Einhorn 1986). Likewise, in male quails, lesions placed in the POA, but not BNST lesions or sham surgery, significantly reduced their motivation to approach a win-

Figure 5.8 (continued)
(no destructive electric current was passed into the brain) continued to approach the window to view the female, whereas males given medial POA lesions spent less time in front of the viewing window (*top*). This latter reduction was not, however, reduced to the low level of female viewing seen in castrated males that received no T. As in other vertebrates, POA lesions eliminated cloacal contact movements (mating) in T-treated males, thereby reducing their mating performance to the level shown by castrated males that received no testosterone. T-treated males that received lesions of the BNST showed significantly less mating behavior than sham-operated control males. (Adapted from Balthazart et al. 1998.)

dow in the test apparatus which allowed them to view a sexually receptive female in an adjacent compartment (Balthazart et al. 1998; figure 5.8). Lesions of the POA also totally abolished actual mating behavior (cloacal contact movements), and lesions of the BNST partially reduced these consumatory responses. Careful anatomical analysis of the location of behaviorally effective POA lesions showed that the lesions that disrupted the sexual motivation of males most effectively were located more rostrally than lesions that disrupted mating behavior per se.

As described in chapter 3, testicular steroids have been shown to act during perinatal life to organize sexually dimorphic features of neural morphology in the POA of numerous mammalian species. In quails, the POA includes a nucleus that is larger in males than in females due to adult actions of estradiol, which is formed from circulating testosterone (Panzica et al. 1987). It is not certain whether the destruction only of this sexually dimorphic portion of the POA would differentially disrupt aspects of masculine sexual motivation and/or mating performance.

In rats and ferrets, lesions restricted to these sexually dimorphic structures of the POA had little effect on the mating performance of males (Arendash and Gorski 1983; Cherry and Baum 1990), but in gerbils (Yahr and Gregory 1993) such lesions caused very significant reductions in mating performance. No systematic study of the effects of these restricted POA lesions on sexual motivation, assessed using operant testing procedures, has been carried out in rodents. However, in the ferret, a carnivore, lesions restricted to the sexually dimorphic male nucleus of the POA made them display more female-typical motivational responses to other, sexually active males (Cherry and Baum 1990).

Neurochemistry of Masculine Sexual Behavior

The Role of Dopamine Systems

Three groups of **dopamine neurons** have been implicated in the regulation of masculine sexual arousal and coital performance. These include the **mesolimbic** dopamine neurons projecting from the midbrain ventral tegmental area to the **nucleus accumbens** and the **incertohypothalamic** dopamine neurons projecting from the dorsal-posterior hypothalmus to the POA. A third group, the **tuberoinfundibular** dopamine neurons projecting from the arcuate nucleus to the median eminence, is implicated indirectly.

LOCALIZATION OF FUNCTION

Nucleus Accumbens and Striatum
Selective destruction of the mesolimbic dopamine neurons in male rats through intracerebral injection of the catecholamine neurotoxin 6-hydroxydopamine significantly lengthened mount latencies (reviewed in Everitt 1990). However, once males had begun to mount, they proceeded to intromit and

ejaculate in a normal sequence, which suggests that the consummatory aspects of masculine coital performance were unimpaired by this treatment. These males were tested with estrous females that had been ovariectomized and made fully **proceptive** (sexually motivated) and **receptive** (displaying lordosis) through injections of estrogen followed by progesterone (as described in chapter 4). When such females were also treated with the dopamine receptor blocker cis-flupenthixol, they no longer displayed the proceptive responses characteristic of estrous rats but retained their ability to display lordosis when mounted by the male.

Interestingly, males bearing neurotoxic lesions of the nucleus accumbens rarely mounted these estrous females in which proceptive responsiveness had been largely abolished. Control males usually initiated a copulatory sequence despite the absence of overt proceptive cues from their estrous partners. Apparently other types of incentive cues (e.g., sight or smell of the female) are sufficiently arousing for most male rats to initiate mating. It seems likely that the deficits in sexual behavior observed in males with lesions of the nucleus accumbens reflect their inability to respond to the motivational cues that normally suffice to arouse the male. Everitt (1990) obtained similar results in males following infusion of dopamine receptor blockers directly into the nucleus accumbens.

Preoptic Area
Hull and co-workers (reviewed in Hull et al. 1995) have implicated dopamine projections to the POA in the control of both sexual motivation and consummatory aspects of mating in male rats. In their early research, infusion of the dopamine receptor agonist apomorphine into the POA facilitated the rate at which males achieved successive intromissions leading to ejaculation. This same treatment also stimulated penile erection in males restrained on their backs. Both the behavioral and erectile responses were blocked by pretreatment with a dopamine receptor blocker, affirming that the effects of apomorphine resulted from specific actions on dopamine receptors. Studies in which dopamine receptor antagonists have been infused directly into the POA suggest that the post-synaptic actions of dopamine facilitate masculine sexual motivation. For example, infusions of the dopamine receptor antagonist cis-flupenthixol reduced the percentage of trials on which males chose to approach an estrous female in an X-shaped maze (Warner et al. 1991) and infusions of another dopamine antagonist, haloperidol, decreased their attempts to seek out an estrous female in a bilevel testing chamber (Pfaus and Phillips 1991).

LOCALIZATION OF DOPAMINE RELEASE
Two methods allow an investigator to sample the extracellular concentrations of dopamine in the brain. These are in vivo voltammetry and in vivo microdialysis. These methods have both been used to address the question of whether dopamine release from dopamine terminals in different brain regions

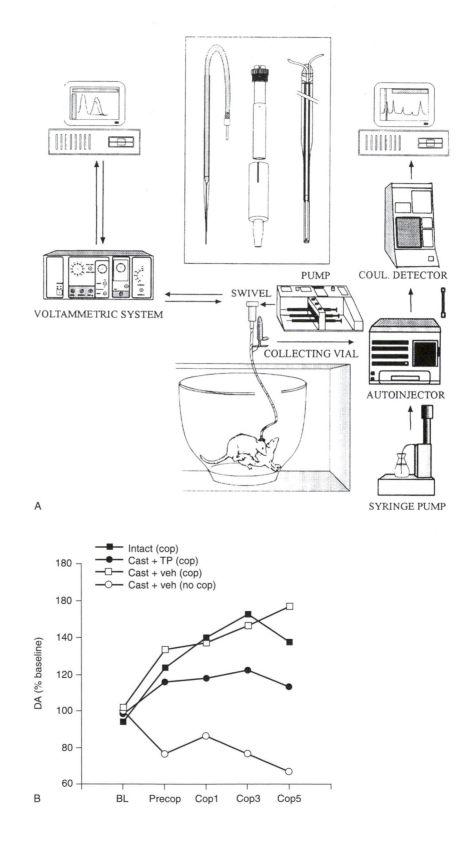

A

B

is selectively enhanced by sexual stimuli. **Voltammetry** monitors the pattern of electrical current flow at the tip of an electrode that is thought to reflect oxidation of extracellular dopamine at the electrode tip—the more dopamine there is, the more oxidation will be measured. A complementary method known as **microdialysis** measures small amounts of dopamine in extracellular fluid collected through diffusion across a semipermeable membrane at the base of a probe implanted into the brain (figure 5.9A)

Nucleus Accumbens and Striatum

Pfaus and Phillips (1991) using in vivo voltammetry and in vivo microdialysis (in different rats) found that dopamine release in the nucleus accumbens rose sharply when a male was exposed to an estrous female (the female was restrained behind a wire-mesh screen to prevent physical contract). Subsequently, when males were given access to estrous females, this dopamine signal remained elevated throughout a mating sequence, fell after ejaculation, and then rose again near the end of the post-ejaculatory period of sexual inactivity. By contrast, in vivo release of dopamine from the dorsal striatum, which receives axonal projections from dopamine neurons in the substantia nigra and is concerned with sensorimotor function (see chapter 13), was unaffected by the presentation of the estrous female.

These results confirm those of pharmacological studies implicating mesolimbic dopamine neurons in the control of masculine sexual arousal. Such findings, together with reports (Alderson and Baum 1981; Mitchell and Stewart 1989) that testosterone, as well as its metabolites estrogen and DHT, can enhance dopamine transmission in mesolimbic terminal regions further implicate this dopamine system in masculine sexual arousal. It is important to remember, however, that the mesolimbic dopamine pathway has been implicated in the control of a variety of motivated behaviors, including feeding and drinking, as well as in several types of drug-taking behaviors. Its role in governing motivated behavior is clearly not restricted to mating.

Figure 5.9 (*A*) Schematic diagram of the experimental apparatus used to determine extracellular concentrations of dopamine (DA) during microdialysis in the POA of sexually experienced male rats. (Adapted from Mas et al. 1995.) A dialysis probe (*top center*) was inserted into the POA. An aritificial cerebral spinal fluid flowed into the probe through a liquid swivel and out to be measured using high performance liquid chromatography with electrochemical detection to determine the concentration of DA in extracellular fluid. For a closer view of the dialysis probe and how it works, see chapter 13. (*B*) Extracellular levels of dopamine (DA) measured by microdialysis in the POA of sexually experienced male rats. Mean concentrations of DA (expressed as % of baseline value) (BL) are shown for different groups during a precopulatory period (precop) when an estrous female was separated from male subjects by a perforated barrier and during three intervals (cops 1–3) during which males in some group displayed mounts and intromissions leading to ejaculation. DA levels rose during the precopulatory period in all males that subsequently copulated (cop), including all nine gonadally intact males, all 7 TP-treated castrates, and nine 1-week castrates treated with oil vehicle. DA levels rose slightly more during copulation in intact males and in vehicle-treated castrates that mated. DA levels fell in all males that failed to copulate (no cop), including five 1-week castrates and four 2-week castrates treated with oil vehicle. (Adapted from Hull et al. 1995.)

Preoptic Area

Evidence that dopamine release in the POA is associated with increased masculine sexual motivation and coital performance was provided by Hull et al. (1995) who used in vivo dialysis to measure extracellular concentrations of dopamine in the POA of different groups of males which had previous mating experience (figure 5.9B). Gonadally intact males all showed a significant increase in POA dopamine levels during the pre-copulatory part of the test, when an estrous female was placed behind a screen so that the male could smell, see, and hear, but not physically contact, her. After the screen was removed, these males all mated with the estrous females and dopamine levels in the POA rose even further. Another group of males which had been castrated, given vehicle injections instead of testosterone for one week, and then tested with an estrous female showed either increases or decreases in POA dopamine levels, depending on whether or not they eventually mated with the estrous female after the barrier screen was removed. A final group of castrated males treated with testosterone (and which also mated with the female when given access) showed an intermediate rise in POA dopamine in response to distal cues from the estrous female.

Hull et al. (1995) carried out additional control experiments to rule out any association of motor activity per se (which would accompany actual mating) with the increased dopamine levels seen in males which mated. They also showed that dopamine levels declined in males for which the screen restraining the estrous female was not lifted. In these rats, dopamine levels in the POA rose immediately when the screen was eventually lifted, allowing the male to approach and mate with the estrous female.

As explained earlier, much evidence suggests that estradiol, formed in the POA via aromatization of circulating testosterone, plays an essential role in the activation of mating behavior in male rats. The results of Hull et al. (1995) suggest that female-induced increases in POA dopamine can occur at a time (1 week) after castration when no testosterone is circulating (and thus presumably no estradiol is being formed in the POA). However, a subset of such castrates will continue to mate, at least for a few weeks after castration and steroid withdrawal. It was in such males that increases in POA dopamine were seen in response to distal cues from an estrous female. This suggests that recent sex steroid exposure was needed in order for cues from the female effectively to augment POA dopamine levels. Clearly, the response of the dopamine neurons to female stimuli did not rely primarily on the concurrent action of estradiol or testosterone.

Further evidence of the independent actions of sex steroids and dopamine neurons in the control of masculine sexual behavior stems from the observation of Wersinger et al. (1997) working with male mice in which the alpha estradiol receptor was experimentally inactivated. These null mutants, in contrast to wild-type control males, did not approach or investigate odors from estrous females and their mating performance was also deficient. Surprisingly, however, administration of a dopamine agonist drug, apomorphine, activated intromission and ejaculation in estrogen receptor knockout (ERKO) null mutant mice (Wersinger and Rissman 2000), suggesting that enhanced post-synaptic activity at dopamine synapses can compensate for reduced activational effects of sex steroids on the neural circuits controlling both sexual motivation and mating performance. Thus the steroidal and dopamine systems in the POA seem to act independently to facilitate sexual motivation and performance in the male.

Serotonin

These facilitatory actions of dopamine in male rats contrast with the widely studied inhibitory action of the indoleamine serotonin on aspects of masculine sexual behavior. A large pharmacological literature (reviewed in Lorrain et al. 1997) shows that increased transmission at **serotonin** synapses inhibits both motivational and performance aspects of sexual behavior in male rats. In accordance with this view is the finding (Lorrain et al. 1997) that extracellular concentrations of serotonin in the anterior lateral hypothalamus rose after ejaculation in male rats, which is during the post-ejaculatory interval when it is difficult, if not impossible, to induce males to resume mating with an estrous female.

Some drugs used to treat depression in humans act by increasing the availability of serotonin at synapses. These drugs sometimes have the side effect of reducing libido, suggesting that serotonin suppresses sexual motivation in humans as in rats.

Prolactin

Several circulating as well as centrally formed peptides influence aspects of masculine sexual motivation, including pair bonding with specific partners and coital performance. In one instance (i.e., prolactin), the effects are primarily pharmacological and are potentially of clinical relevance. In other instances, vasopressin and endorphin are implicated in the normal physiological control of sexual motivation and mating in males.

Clinicians have long suspected that chronic hyperprolactinemia, resulting from the hypersecretion of **prolactin** (this can occur with small pituitary tumors or during chronic stress), reduces erectile function and sexual motivation in men. Studies using animals strongly support these impressions. For example, Doherty and colleagues (1986) studied adult, sexually experienced male rats in which chronic hyperprolactinemia was induced by transplanting pituitary glands from other rats under the kidney capsule. Normally the secretion of prolactin by the pituitary is restrained by the action of dopamine released from tuberoinfundibular dopaminergic neurons into the pituitary portal vessels perfusing the median eminence. Pituitary glands placed under the kidney capsule are readily vascularized and, in the absence of any inhibitory dopamine input, secrete large amounts of prolactin into the general circulation. Insertion of pituitary grafts and the resultant hyperprolactinemia significantly reduced mount and intromission rates in male rats in tests with estrous females; they also reduced erectile function in the same males tested while restrained on their backs. In a companion study, the inhibitory effect of hyperprolactinemia on erectile function was completely reversed by sever-ing the spinal cord at the thoracic level. From these results we infer that the inhibitory effect of prolactin on erection is mediated by the peptides' action at some supraspinal site in the CNS that has yet to be determined.

The physiological actions of prolactin are well established in female mam-mals. In the rat these include the promotion of lactation, enhanced maternal behavior (see chapter 9), and the stimulation of progesterone secretion by the corpora lutea during the first half of pregnancy. Prolactin is also secreted by the male pituitary gland in about the same concentrations as in females. Some evidence suggests that in males prolactin facilitates LH-induced tes-ticular steroidogenesis and increases androgen receptors in the reproductive tract. However, it is still uncertain whether prolactin plays a normal physio-logical role in the neuroendocrine regulation of masculine sexual behavior.

Endorphins

Some neurons of the arcuate nucleus produce the opioid peptide, **endorphin**, and project to the POA. These neurons seemingly inhibit the consummatory aspects of masculine sexual function, including erection. Hughes et al. (1989) showed that the infusion of β-endorphin into the POA caused dose-dependent reductions in the mating performance of males. Conversely, infusions of the opioid receptor antagonist naloxone into the same site enhanced ejaculatory performance in sexually experienced male rats. These observations comple-ment the results of an earlier study by Meyerson (1981) which showed that systemic administration of morphine inhibited mating in male rats at doses too low to affect their spontaneous locomotor activity.

The acute inhibition of masculine sexual behavior by morphine should be distinguished from the more pervasive loss of sexual motivation and erectile function that has long been known to occur in morphine and heroin addicts (Cushman 1972). In the latter instance, ingestion of opioid receptor agonists causes a long-lasting suppression of LH secretion and a resultant drop in tes-tosterone production. This withdrawal of androgen, perhaps combined with the direct effects of these drugs in POA sites, leads to a striking reduction in all aspects of sexual motivation and coital function in men.

Evidence also suggests that some opioid neurons promote sexual motiva-tion in males. Numerous studies have shown that opioid mechanisms facili-tate the consumption of sweet substances, even though they may lack any nutrient content. For example, subcutaneous injection of the opioid receptor antagonist, naloxone, significantly reduced the ingestion of saccharine solu-tion by rats (Lynch and Libby 1983). Naloxone also inhibited "sham drink-ing" of sugar water by rats implanted with esophageal fistulas that diverted the ingested fluid away from their stomachs. This type of ingestive behavior, which is especially dependent on opioid mechanisms, must be sustained by the taste of the ingested fluid rather than by any metabolic benefit.

Lieblich and co-workers (1985) asked whether analogous circumstances exist in the context of masculine sexual behavior. One such example would be the male rat that continues to mate for several weeks following androgen withdrawal due to castration. Such males quickly cease mating if tested with estrous females that display low levels of proceptive behavior (Madlafousek et al. 1976). Thus, their sexual arousal and subsequent mating performance are especially dependent on the stimulus qualities of their female partners. Subcutaneous injection of naloxone to males within 2 to 3 weeks after castration significantly inhibited mounting and ejaculation, whereas the same treatment had no effect on mating in gonadally intact male rats (Miller et al. 1987).

In another study, male rats ejaculated repeatedly with an estrous female until a criterion of sexual exhaustion was reached. If the female partner was then removed from the test cage for several minutes before being replaced, control males reliably resumed mating. In these circumstances, sexually exhausted males given naloxone were significantly less likely to resume mating, suggesting that an opioid mechanism normally facilitates sexual arousal in such animals.

Neurophysiological evidence (Gysling and Wang 1983) shows that opioid peptides activate mesolimbic dopamine neurons when infused into the ventral tegmental area. Mitchell and Stewart (1989) showed that infusion of either morphine or another opiate (dynorphin 1–13) into the ventral tegmental region of male rats stimulated orientation toward an estrous female. These findings suggest that the activation of opioid inputs to mesolimbic dopamine neurons may facilitate masculine sexual motivation.

Vasopressin and Oxytocin

Thus far we have considered the neuroendocrine regulation of masculine sexual behavior in species which are polygamous—i.e., species such as rat and ferret in which the male normally mates and sires young with many different females while providing minimal amounts of mate-guarding after mating or paternal care of newborn offspring. The vole, a small rodent that many mistake for a mouse, has provided many insights into the neuroendocrine regulation of monogamy. It turns out that some subspecies of voles are monogamous while others are polygamous. Comparisons of subspecies of vole with both monogamous and polygamous mating systems have implicated the neuropeptide **vasopressin** in the establishment of pair bonding with particular females among males of monogamous species. Parvocellular (small) neurons located in the paraventricular nuclei (PVN) of rodents project to limbic sites including the amygdala, BNST, and lateral septum, where they release vasopressin. These **parvocellular** vasopressin neurons are distinguished from the large **magnocellular** neurons of the PVN and supraoptic nuclei, which project to the posterior pituitary gland where they release neuropeptide into the bloodstream.

One indication that parvocellular vasopressin neurons may be important for pair bonding came from studies showing different distributions of vasopressin receptors in the forebrains of vole species which are monogamous (prairie voles) than in those of polygamous species (montane voles; Insel et al. 1994). Pharmacological experiments (Winslow et al. 1993) in which vasopressin itself or drugs that block vasopressin receptors were infused into the cerebral ventricles of male prairie voles established a causal link between forebrain vasopressin-receptor activation and pair bonding.

In one instance (figure 5.10A), sexually naive prairie voles were given intracerebroventroicular (ICV) infusions for 24 hours of either artificial cerebrospinal fluid (CSF; control), **oxytocin** (a neuropeptide resembling vasopressin), or arginine vasopressin while in the presence of an ovariectomized (sexually unreceptive) female. Immediately thereafter all subjects were tested for 3 hours in a three-compartment box in which each male's partner female was tethered in one compartment, a stranger female was tethered in a second compartment, and a third compartment (neutral) was left empty. Males which received ICV infusions of vasopressin spent significantly more time with their familiar partner female than with the stranger, whereas males which received either CSF or oxytocin showed an equal preference for the familiar partner and unfamiliar stranger. Results of this study showed that exogenously administered vasopressin is capable of promoting pair bonding among male prairie voles.

Evidence that endogenously released vasopressin promotes pair bonding was obtained in another experiment in which groups of sexually naive male prairie voles received ICV infusions of either CSF (control), a vasopressin antagonist or an oxytocin antagonist prior to being placed for 24 hours with a sexually receptive female vole (with whom all males mated). Immediately thereafter, the partner preferences of males were again assessed in the three-compartment box, with both the familiar and a strange female (both in estrus) tethered in different compartments (figure 5.10B). Compared with males which received cerebrospinal fluid or the oxytocin antagonist, males given the vasopressin antagonist spent significantly less time with the familiar partner and significantly more time with the unfamiliar female. These findings suggest that vasopressin, which is released from terminals of parvocellular neurons after mating, somehow promotes the formation of a pair bond with that particular female. The signals from individual females, which the male attends to in response to the activation of these vasopressin neurons, are not known; however, it seems likely that olfactory (pheromonal) cues play some role in this process.

To summarize, activity in mesolimbic and incertohypothalamic dopamine neurons facilitate sexual motivation and coital performance in the male, whereas activity in serotonergic neurons projecting to the lateral hypothalamus inhibit these functions. Certain neuropeptides are also implicated in masculine sexual behavior. Prolactin and opioids are thought to inhibit consummatory components of coital behavior, including erection and ejaculation. Paradoxically, opioid peptides like endorphin may also stimulate motivational components of male sexual behavior. In mammals with monogamous mating systems, central vasopressin neurons contribute to a special case of masculine sexual motivation, namely, the formation of pair bonds with particular females.

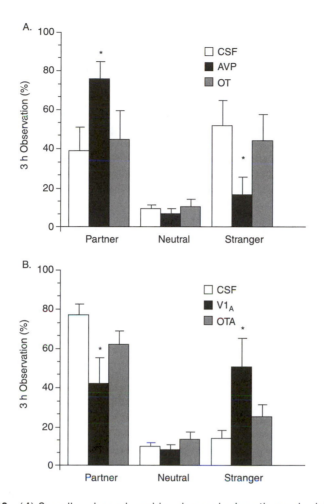

Figure 5.10 (*A*) Sexually naive male prairie voles received continuous icv infusions of either vasopressin (AVP), oxytocin (OT) or CSF vehicle in the presence of a sexually unreceptive (ovariectomized) female vole. After 24 hours of treatment, the percentage of a 3 hours observation period was measured during which males in different treatment groups spent time in each of 3 connected compartments that were either empty (neutral) or contained a tethered familiar social partner (partner) or an unfamiliar strange female (stranger). As in the initial testing, these females were not in estrus. Males that received AVP spent significantly more time with the female partner and significantly less time with the stranger. (*B*) A single, acute icv injection of vasopressin type 1 antagonist drug (V1A), oxytocin antagonist drug (OTA), or CSF vehicle was given to sexually naive male prairie voles just before they were allowed to mate for the first time with an estrous female. Then 24 hours later the percentage of a 3-hour observation period was measured during which males in different treatment groups spent time in each of 3 connected compartments that were either empty (neutral) or contained a tethered familiar sexual partner (partner) or an unfamiliar strange female (stranger). As in the initial tests, these females were all in estrus. Males that received V1A spent significantly less time with the female partner and significantly more time with the stranger. (Adapted from Winslow et al. 1993.)

Steroids and the Development of Masculine Sexual Behavior

We have considered some of the neural and endocrine mechanisms that govern masculine sexual motivation, penile erection, and the motoric patterns of mating in adult males. As shown in figure 5.1, adult male and female ferrets differ dramatically in their exhibition of masculine sexual behavior following gonadectomy and treatment with testosterone or estrogen. Likewise, adult males and females display very different responses to testosterone when allowed to choose between approaching an estrous or an anestrous female (see figure 5.2). These data from ferrets resemble results obtained in several different vertebrate species. The motivational aspects of mating, including heterosexual partner preference, and a male's capacity to perform the motoric aspects of mating are sexually differentiated. We will now consider the role of prenatal and early postnatal exposure of the nervous system to sex steroids in the differentiation of both motivational and consummatory aspects of masculine sexual behavior. We will primarily consider data from the model system of one species, the ferret. However, the relevance of these results for other mammalian species, including primates, will become apparent.

As described in chapter 3, among mammals all sex differences in the morphology of the external and internal genital organs, in portions of the central and peripheral nervous systems and in the capacity to exhibit a range of sociosexual behaviors, develop primarily because of the perinatal action of testosterone secreted by the male's testes. Ovarian steroidogenesis in female mammals is first initiated well after this perinatal period, and thus the feminine morphologic and behavioral phenotype develops in the presence of low circulating levels of ovarian hormones (although the mother's ovaries secrete considerable estrogen and progesterone during this period). As already explained, in many mammalian species, including ferrets, circulating concentrations of testosterone are significantly higher in males than in females during certain fetal periods and postnatally within hours and again for several days, weeks, or months (depending on the species). As will be illustrated, sociosexual aspects of maleness develop only after exposure of the male nervous system to testosterone or its estrogenic metabolites over the sum total of these perinatal periods.

Gestation in ferrets lasts 41 days. In males the testes begin secreting testosterone around embryonic day 24 (E24) and continue to do so during the rest of gestation. Although measurable in females, testosterone concentrations are significantly lower than in male fetuses over this entire embryonic period. At birth, plasma testosterone concentrations rise in males to even higher concentrations for a few hours, then decline to low concentrations comparable to those of females. Small though significant sex differences in plasma testosterone levels occur intermittently during the next 3 postnatal weeks (Baum 1990a). Elevations in circulating testosterone during fetal life are responsible for the differentiation of the Wolffian duct structures into the epididymis, vas deferens, seminal vesicles, and prostate glands. At the same time, DHT, formed in the genital skin, promotes the differentiation of a phallus and the fusion of the genital folds into a scrotum into which the testes descend shortly after birth (see chapter 3).

Masculine Coital Behavior

Much evidence implicates testosterone in the differentiation of both the motivational and consummatory features of masculine sexual behavior in male ferrets. Baum and Erksine (1984) showed that administration of testosterone during postnatal days 5 to 20, but not at later ages, strongly facilitated females' exhibition of male-typical sexual behaviors in adulthood. Following gonadectomy and testosterone treatment, these animals exhibited neck gripping, mounting, and pelvic thrusting behaviors when tested with estrous females.

Castration of male ferrets on postnatal day 5, but not on postnatal days 20 or 35, significantly attenuated their ability to mate with estrous females when given testosterone and tested in adulthood. From these results, it seems clear that testosterone normally acts in male ferrets during the first 20 postnatal days to promote coital masculinization. Extended prenatal exposure of female ferrets to testosterone, achieved by admininistering the steroid to pregnant ferrets from E16 to E41, failed to duplicate the coital masculinizing action of administering testosterone neonatally. At first glance, this suggests that fetal exposure of male ferrets to testosterone is not essential for coital masculinization. As will be shown below, however, this conclusion turns out to be incorrect.

For testosterone (given to females over postnatal days 0 to 20) to masculinize coital function effectively, the dose had to produce circulating concentrations of testosterone that were considerably higher than those normally found in male ferrets at these neonatal ages. Administration of a lower (more physiological) dose of testosterone produced only marginal long-term behavioral effects in females.

Are males more sensitive to the masculinizing effect of neonatal testosterone exposure than females? Baum and colleagues (1990b) showed this to be the case. Males are considerably more sensitive than females to the masculinizing action of a low dosage of testosterone given for 15 days beginning on postnatal day 5. This enhanced responsiveness to testosterone was best duplicated in females that were exposed to testosterone both prenatally and again immediately after birth for several hours (figure 5.11). This result suggests that exposure of the developing male nervous system to testosterone must occur over an extended perinatal period to achieve complete coital masculinization. Analogous data have been collected for several other mammalian species.

The role of neural estrogenic metabolites of testosterone in controlling the *activation* of sexual behavior in adult male ferrets and other species has already been discussed. Much evidence suggests that the *organizational* action of testosterone on the developing nervous system also depends, in part, on the neural conversion of circulating testosterone into estrogen. Studies conducted in several mammalian species, including rat, rabbit, ferret, and rhesus

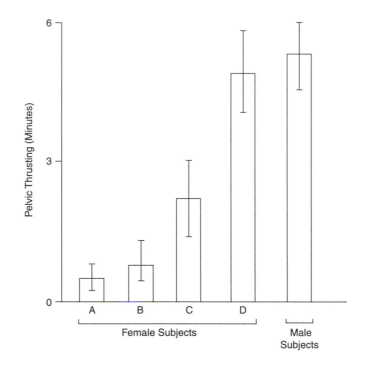

Figure 5.11 Effect of prolonged perinatal administration of testosterone (T) to female ferrets on their later display of one parameter of masculine coital behavior (pelvic thrusting) during tests with an estrous female given after treatment in adulthood with testosterone propionate (5 mg/kg). Groups of female ferrets were treated with T or vehicle either prenatally and/or within minutes after birth. All females were ovariectomized on postnatal day 5 and received T on postnatal days 5 to 20. Male subjects received vehicle prenatally and within minutes after birth; they were castrated on postnatal day 20. In adulthood, subjects were treated daily with Tp and tested with sexually receptive females. Data are expressed as mean ± SEM. (Adapted from Baum et al. 1990b.)

monkey, show that the activity of aromatizing enzyme in the nervous tissues of the preoptic area, hypothalamus, and temporal lobes is an order of magnitude higher in fetal animals than in adulthood (reviewed in Tobet et al. 1985). During the final quarter of gestation, male and female ferrets have equivalent, high levels of aromatase activity in the POA, mediobasal hypothalamus, and temporal lobes. However, males consistently have higher concentrations of circulating testosterone during this period. As a result, the nervous system of the fetal male ferret produces estrogen at a rate that exceeds that of females.

The drug ATD, like fadrazole, inhibits the aromatization of androgen to estrogen in the nervous system. When ATD was administered transplacentally to ferrets over the last quarter of gestation, it caused significant reductions in males' capacity to exhibit masculine coital behavior when they were given testosterone in adulthood and tested with estrous females (Tobet and Baum 1987). Fetal ATD treatment also blocked the formation of a sexually dimorphic POA in male ferrets (Tobet et al. 1986). Treatment of male ferrets with ATD during postnatal days 0 to 15 failed to disrupt males' later coital capacity, even though neural aromatase activity was strongly inhibited (Baum et al. 1983).

As described earlier, depriving male ferrets of endogenous testosterone by castration on postnatal day 5 or giving females a high dose of testosterone during postnatal days 5 to 20 caused a striking inhibition and facilitation, respectively, of later masculine sexual behavior. These results show that a testicular steroid, presumably testosterone, plays an important role during the first several weeks of life in masculinizing ferrets' coital potential. That testosterone itself is neonatally active is further established by the observation that neither estrogen nor DHT nor a combination of estrogen and DHT given to female ferrets during postnatal days 5 to 20 could duplicate the masculinizing action of testosterone on later mating performance (Baum et al. 1982). Thus, in male ferrets estrogen and testosterone appear to act sequentially during prenatal and early postnatal development, respectively, to masculinize coital potential.

Studies employing other mammalian species, including rat, hamster, and guinea pig, have also implicated estrogens in the differentiation of masculine sexual behavior (reviewed in Baum 1979). Whether testosterone itself also contributes to this process in these species has not been determined. Evidence of estrogenic involvement in the process of coital masculinization of male primates, however, is not as clear.

When considering the comparative data on the hormonal control of coital masculinization, it is important to note that the mechanisms controlling sexual differentiation of the gonads differ between birds and mammals. In birds the female is the heterogametic sex (has two different sex chromosomes), whereas in mammals it is the male that falls into this category (see chapter 3). Numerous experiments (reviewed in Adkins-Regan and Ascenzi 1987) using quails and zebra finches show that male-typical courtship and mating capacities will develop in both sexes unless estrogen is present at some early period (prehatching in quail; immediately after hatching in zebra finch) to block its development.

Thus, in contrast to mammals, in avian species estrogen acts to eliminate, not facilitate, the differentation of masculine coital potential. Normally, this demasculinizing action of estradiol occurs only in females. In light of this fact, it was surprising to discover (Adkins-Regan and Ascenzi 1987) that estrogen acts shortly after hatching to ensure that male zebra finches develop the capacity to form pair bonds with female conspecifics. More research is needed to specify the possible sources (gonadal or adrenal secretion; localized neural production through androgen aromatization) and timing of estrogenic stimulation prior to and shortly after hatching in both male and female birds. This information should help to explain how the same hormone (estradiol) can act in females to eliminate the capacity for displaying male-typical coital behavior while acting in males to promote heterosexual partner preference and pair bonding.

Sexual Orientation

WHICH HORMONES?

Numerous experiments using ferrets as well as other species (reviewed in Baum 1979) show that perinatal administration of androgen to females dramatically augments their later exhibition of masculine coital responses in tests with an estrous female. Far fewer studies (reviewed in Adkins-Regan 1989) have systematically explored the effects of early steroidal manipulations on later patterns of sociosexual preference.

In ferrets (Stockman et al. 1985; Baum et al. 1990b), tests of sexual-partner preference were conducted by allowing subjects to approach either a sexually active male or an estrous female in the goal boxes of a T-maze. After each approach, the animals were allowed to interact physically for 1 minute prior to a subsequent test. After gonadectomy in adulthood and treatment with estrogen, males preferred approaching estrous females rather than sexually active males. Surprisingly, when treated with testosterone, castrated male subjects showed an equal preference (i.e., no preference) for either the estrous female or the stimulus male. This ambiguous preference may have reflected the fact that testosterone-treated male subjects fought with the male stimulus ferrets after approaching them and mated with the estrous stimulus females after approaching them. Thus, both aggressive and sexual motivation were activated in males by testosterone.

When treated with either testosterone or estradiol, ovariectomized female subjects preferred to approach the sexually active stimulus male; their preference for the male stimulus was, not surprisingly, greatest when they received estradiol. Therefore, in subsequent assessments of ferrets' sexual-partner preferences, estradiol was administered to gonadectomized male and female subjects in order to assess their sexual partner preferences. This sex hormone activated sexual motivation in all groups of animals without stimulating male-typical aggressive behavior.

Baum et al. (1990b) asked whether prolonged pre-and post-natal exposure of female ferrets to malelike levels of circulating testosterone masculinize their socio-sexual partner preference? To answer this question, sexual partner preference was studied in the same groups of ferrets whose pelvic thrusting (coital performance) is shown in figure 5.11. As shown in figure 5.12, females given a low dose of testosterone over postnatal days 5 to 20 still preferred to approach a sexually active male as opposed to an estrous female in T-maze tests. Females that were also exposed to testosterone before, immediately after, and again 5 to 20 days after birth showed a preference for estrous females that was identical to that of control males. This suggests that prolonged perinatal exposure to testosterone (secreted by the testes) is normally required for male ferrets to develop a preference for a female partner, just as extensive perinatal exposure to testosterone is critical for the development of motoric elements of masculine sexual behavior.

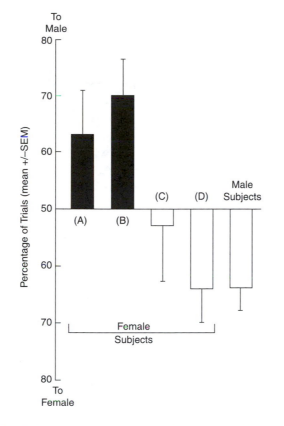

Figure 5.12 Preference for approaching and interacting with a sexually active stimulus male or an estrous female in a T-maze displayed by the same groups of female and male ferrets described in figure 5.11. Tests of sexual preference were conducted in adulthood while ferrets received daily SC injections of estradiol benzoate (15 μg/kg). As for pelvic thrusting behavior (figure 5.11), the male-typical profile of sexual-partner preference (represented by males castrated on day P20, far right bar) was best induced in females by extended perinatal treatment with testosterone (prenatally, immediately after birth, and during days 5 to 20). Data are expressed as mean ± SEM. (Adapted from Baum et al. 1990b.)

Studies with rodents (rat, mouse, hamster) have shown that testosterone secreted perinatally by the males' testes contributes to male-typical psychosexual differentiation in these species as well. In rats and mice, the neural aromatization of circulating testosterone neonatally in males is essential for the differentiation of the neural circuits that underlie males' motivation to seek out and approach an estrous female. For example, when given access to either a sexually active male or an estrous female which is tethered in opposite arms of a three-chambered box, normal male rats prefer to approach and interact with the estrous female.

By contrast, males treated with the aromatase inhibitor ATD over the first 3 weeks of life, when tested in adulthood, showed an equal preference to approach the stud male and the estrous female. These ATD-treated males displayed lordosis responses when mounted by the stimulus male and showed mounting, intromission, and ejaculation after approaching the stimulus female (Bakker et al. 1993). This suggests that the male-typical pattern of sexual partner preference is organized by the neonatal actions of estradiol, formed from circulating testosterone. Presumably, the retention of the capacity to show male-typical mating performance reflects the fact that the actions of testosterone and its estrogenic metabolite during fetal development were not affected by the neonatal inhibition of brain aromatase.

Additional evidence that is consistent with the idea that estradiol acting perinatally promotes male-typical psychosexual differentiation is derived from studies of sexual partner preference in male mice in which the estradiol receptor type α was experimentally inactivated ('estradiol receptor knock out'; ERKO (Rissman et al. 1999). Whereas gonadally intact wild-type control male mice preferred to approach and interact with a tethered female in estrus as opposed to a sexually active stud male, ERKO males had no preference for either social stimulus. Likewise, when the male and female stimulus animals were anesthetized, wild-type control males spent significantly more time investigating the genital and flank regions of stimulus females whereas ERKO males spent equivalent low amounts of time investigating the male and female stimulus animals. Both wild-type and ERKO males showed increased neuronal Fos-IR throughout the olfactory projection circuit to the hypothalamus after exposure to soiled bedding from estrous female mice, suggesting that there was equivalent sensory processing of female pheromones in both groups of males.

Wersinger and Rissman (2000) argued that functional ERα receptors are required for normal male-typical partner preferences and that the role of ER α involves the coupling of olfactory inputs and behavioral outputs leading to approach of the female-derived stimuli (especially female pheromones). Unfortunately, since the ER α gene is knocked out from the earliest stages of embryonic development and on into adulthood, it is impossible to decide whether the observed differences between ERKO and wild-type males in their sexual partner and odor preferences reflect only deficient ER α actions during perinatal development and/or in adulthood, when activational actions of testosterone may reflect, in part, the actions in the brain of estradiol derived from testosterone.

It is too early to say whether testicular steroids (and estradiol formed prenatally in the hypothalamus) contribute in a similar manner to the development of heterosexual orientation in men, or conversely, whether altered patterns of fetal or neonatal steroid secretion contribute to the etiology of homosexual orientation in human males. It is interesting to note, however, that several studies (reviewed in Zucker et al. 1996) found that women with congenital adrenal hyperplasia (CAH), which is described further in chapter 3, reported more crossgender behavior during childhood and had lower rates of exclusively heterosexual fantasies and fewer sexual experiences with men as young adults.

Other studies (reviewed in Meyer-Balburg 1995) also reported an increased incidence of self-identified bisexual orientation in women whose mothers had been given the potent synthetic estrogen DES during pregnancy. In these clinical populations, however, the majority of women (both CAH and DES-exposed) reported exclusive heterosexual orientation, both in their sexual fantasies as well as their actual romantic interests and sexual activities.

Another fascinating clinical population includes XY individuals with **complete androgen insensitivity syndrome (AIS)** due to a mutation in the gene expressing the androgen receptor. These individuals are invariably reared as girls because their external genital organs are female-typical. In adult assessments, AIS women were reported to be sexually attracted exclusively to men (Slob et al. 1993). These AIS individuals possess testes which secrete testosterone during fetal life, and their brains apparently express aromatase enzyme and estrogen receptors so that they presumably produce estradiol to which developing neurons can potentially respond. Yet the available data suggest that male-typical psychosexual development does not occur in AIS women.

We infer from such findings either that estradiol plays no role in psychosexual differentiation in men or that, as proposed earlier for the male ferret, concurrent activation of neural androgen receptors must occur in order for estrogen to promote psychosexual masculinization. Steroid hormone exposure either during development of the brain or in adulthood may not, by itself, control complex social behaviors including gender identity and sexual orientation. Instead, differential steroidal exposure of male and female fetuses (both human and animal) may affect the way the developing nervous system responds to early social experiences provided by parents and peers alike.

In male rats (Gruendel and Arnold 1969) and dogs (Beach 1968), social isolation from peers during early postnatal life disrupts later ability to exhibit masculine sexual behavior. Likewise, experimentally induced reductions in the amount of anogenital licking provided to male pups by nursing rat mothers reduced males' coital performance in adulthood (Moore 1984). Although it has been speculated about (Bem 1996), no one has studied the possible interaction between the perinatal effects of testosterone and the composition of the early social environment on the development of sociosexual orientation in humans.

WHERE IN THE BRAIN?
As discussed earlier, lesions that are restricted to sexually dimorphic portions of the POA in ferrets cause only minor deficits in masculine coital performance among castrated male ferrets treated with testosterone. By contrast, these same males, when given increasing doses of estradiol benzoate, became increasingly motivated to run to a sexually active stud male (Cherry and Baum 1990). This suggests that neurons in the sexually dimorphic POA may be important for the integration of sensory cues that determine heterosexual partner preference in the male ferret. Female-typical sexual motivation was

enhanced in males after destruction of the sexually dimorphic nucleus normally present in the POA.

As explained earlier (figure 5.12), castrated male ferrets treated with EB preferred, on average, to approach an estrous female as opposed to a stud male during a series of T-maze tests. In the minority of trials when EB-treated males did approach the stud male, they received neck grips to which they displayed a femalelike receptive posture. Estrogen-treated female ferrets strongly preferred to approach and be neck-gripped by the stimulus male. Likewise, male ferrets which received a bilateral neurotoxic lesion of the POA, including the sexually dimorphic region of the mPOA, preferred to approach a stimulus male significantly more often than did control males (Paredes and Baum 1995).

The preference profile of males with bilateral POA lesions resembled that of females which had received either sham lesions or bilateral lesions of the POA. Males with bilateral POA lesions also showed significantly less masculine coital behavior (neck gripping; mounting) in separate tests with estrous females. In a subsequent study (Kindon et al. 1996), male ferrets preferred to approach an estrous female in preoperative tests but then switched their preference to the stud male after the placement of bilateral electrolytic lesions in the POA, which again included but were not restricted to the sexually dimorphic region of the POA. The results of these two studies are summarized in figure 5.13. Male control subjects preferred to approach and interact with an estrous female, whereas female controls preferred to approach the stimulus male. Males which received bilateral lesions of the POA resembled control females in their preference to approach and interact with a stud male. Female subjects given such lesions were no different from control females in their preference for a stud male.

Interestingly, the preference of sham-operated female subjects as well as of males with bilateral medial POA lesions to approach a stimulus male was strongest in tests when they could smell, see, and hear, but not interact physically with, the stimulus animals restrained behind a wire-mesh barrier (Kindon et al. 1996). A male ferret's preference for an estrous female seems to depend on the functional integrity of neurons in the dorsal-medial POA, including those located in the sexually dimorphic region of the POA. When these neurons were absent (in normal females) or destroyed (in males by bilateral lesions), ferrets were attracted by distal cues from a stud male.

The POA has also been implicated in heterosexual partner preference in male sheep. Resko et al. (1996) screened dozens of rams to identify individuals which readily mated with estrous females (female-oriented subjects). In the course of this screening they also identified a small subgroup of rams (male-oriented) which preferred to mount other males instead of females. Aromatase activity in the POA of male-oriented rams was significantly lower than in female-oriented males. No such group difference in aromatase activity was seen in other brain regions. The authors suggested that the capacity for aromatization of circulating testosterone in the POA, especially during perinatal

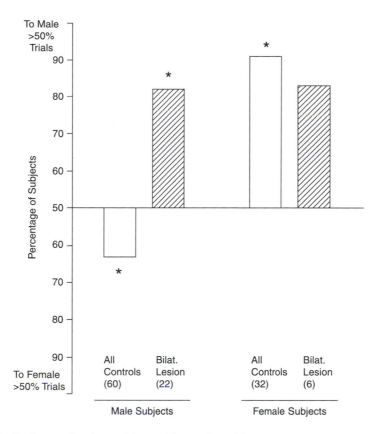

Figure 5.13 Preference for approaching and interacting with a sexually active stimulus male or an estrous female in a T-maze displayed by gonadectomized female and male ferrets given daily SC injections of estradiol benzoate (15 µg/kg). Some ferrets of each sex received bilateral excitotoxic or electrolytic lesions (Bilat. Lesion) of the POA (which included the male's sexually dimorphic nucleus) prior to testing. Control ferrets received several different brain manipulations, including bilateral sham lesions or unilateral destructive lesions of the POA. The number of ferrets in each group is given in parentheses; group means are shown. (Data taken from Paredes and Baum 1995 and from Kindon et al. 1996.)

life, may determine sexual orientation in the male sheep. This suggestion is supported by evidence from other species which we have already considered.

In several studies (Allen et al. 1989; LeVay 1991; Byne et al. 2000), the volume of a subnucleus (the third interstitial nucleus of the anterior hypothalamus; INAH-3) was reported to be larger in brains of men than of women (brains were taken during autopsies; all subjects were presumed to have been heterosexuals in the absence of reports to the contrary). In addition to establishing the existence of a sex dimorphism, LeVay (1991) reported that the volume of INAH-3 in the brains of homosexual men was significantly smaller than in heterosexual men, and thus resembled the volume of INAH-3 in a third group of women who were presumed to be heterosexual (see also chapter 3). No data were available on the size of hypothalamic nuclei from homosexual women in any of these studies.

The data presented in LeVay (1991) have been criticized on several grounds, including (as discussed in chapter 3) the possibility that the small size of INAH-3 in his sample of homosexual men was due, at least in part, to the indirect effect of an AIDS-induced suppression of testosterone secretion in these subjects, which in turn may have reduced the size of neurons in this sexually dimorphic structure. Taken at face value, however, LeVay's results demonstrate a correlation between a preference for men as sexual partners and a female-typical-sized INAH-3. As already explained, exposure of abnormally high levels of testosterone in human female fetuses with CAH has been linked to increased crossgender behavior during childhood, lower rates of exclusively heterosexual fantasies, and fewer sexual experiences with men.

It would be interesting to have data on the volume of INAH-3 in women exposed during fetal life to excessive levels of aromatizable androgen or to estrogenic drugs, with an eye to correlating further the size of INAH-3 and a subject's sexual orientation. As we have seen, results of studies with animals suggest that neurons in a male's medial POA contribute to male-typical aspects of sexual motivation, including a preference to seek out and mate with a partner of the opposite sex. Much more data will need to be collected in order to test the generalizability of this finding to humans.

Neuroendocrine Control of Penile Erection

As explained earlier, testosterone acting via its metabolite, DHT, facilitates penile erection in rats and in many other species, including humans. This effect of testosterone is demonstrated in box 5.1A (Marin et al. 1999). Male rats were castrated and implanted SC with either an empty Silastic capsule or one containing testosterone. One month later the rats were deeply anesthetized and a stimulating electrode was attached to the cavernosal nerve (CN), which innervates the corpus cavernosum of the penis. An electrode to monitor the release of nitric oxide (NO) was implanted into the corpus cavernosum, and blood pressure measuring devices were also inserted into this vascular structure of the penis and into a carotid artery.

In castrated males which received testosterone, electrical stimulation of CN augmented intracavernosal pressure (thereby causing a penile erection) at the same time that the concentration of NO rose in the corpus cavernosum. Arterial blood pressure (AP) was not affected. In long-term castrate males, electrical stimulation of CN failed to stimulate either NO release or a change in corpus cavernosum blood pressure (no erection). Other results show that testosterone, acting via DHT, upregulates the activity of NO synthesizing enzymes which convert the amino acid L-arginine into NO and citrulline in parasympathetic neurons which innervate the corpus cavernosum as well as in endothelial cells which line the corpus cavernosum. Pharmacological studies have established the critical role of NO acting in the smooth muscle cells lining the corpus cavernosum, in penile erection shown after electrical stimulation of CN or in response to more natural sexually arousing stimuli.

As shown schematically in box 5.1, NO is released from nerve endings and from endothelial cells lining the corpus cavernosum in response to sexually arousing stimuli. NO relaxes the adjacent smooth muscle cells which results in engorgement of the corpus cavernosum with blood and erection of the penis. This effect of NO depends on its activating the enzyme guanylate cyclase in smooth muscle cells, thereby catalyzing the formation of the second messenger molecule, cyclic GMP, which relaxes smooth muscles. Normally, cyclic GMP formed in the corpus cavernosum in response to NO is quickly metabolized by the enzyme phosphodiesterase type 5 (PDE 5), thereby terminating any ongoing erectile response.

The drug Viagra binds to PDE 5 and blocks its function, thereby prolonging the time that cGMP accumulates and is available to relax the endothelial muscle lining of the corpus cavernosum. When taken 30 min or so prior to planned sexual activity, Viagra facilitates penile erection in men whose testosterone secretion has declined with age or whose penile innervation has been severely damaged due to diabetes or as a side effect of surgery for prostate cancer. Few drugs have sold better than Viagra after first becoming available, which is testimony to its effectiveness against the age-old problem of impotence.

Summary

1. Masculine sexual behavior consists of both motivational and consummatory components. Motivational components include those behaviors engaged in by a male animal to gain access to a female. Consummatory components are those behaviors necessary for coitus (i.e., mounting, erection, intromission, and ejaculation).

2. In mammalian species, male sexual behavior is activated by testosterone secreted from the Leydig cells of the testes. Both spermatogenesis and testosterone secretion are under the tonic control of LH released from the pituitary in response to GnRH released from the hypothalamus.

3. Testosterone activates masculine sexual behavior through more than one mechanism:

   a. Testosterone is converted to DHT in the penis to stimulate sensory receptors, muscles, and other androgen-sensitive tissues. DHT also facilitates NO synthesis, thereby making it possible for sexually arousing stimuli to facilitate penile erection.

   b. Testosterone acts centrally in the BNST and POA to activate male sexual behavior. At least some of these effects are androgen dependent (i.e., testosterone itself or DHT acts on androgen receptors).

   c. Estrogen, formed in these forebrain regions from testosterone, also facilitates coital performance in several species. Under certain circumstances, estrogen also promotes aspects of masculine sexual motivation and even penile erection.

4. The POA is the integrative center which coordinates the actions of testosterone on both motivational and consummatory aspects of a male's sexual

behavior. In rodents, the medial amygdala, BNST, and POA integrate chemosensory and hormonal signals, which facilitates masculine sexual behavior.

5. Masculine sexual behavior is modulated by dopaminergic and peptidergic inputs to the POA. Activity in the mesolimbic and incertohypothalamic dopamine systems facilitate both motivational and consummatory aspects of male sexual behavior. Activity in serotonin neurons inhibits sexual motivation and performance in males. Opioid peptides also facilitate masculine sexual motivation. Vasopressin facilitates pair bonding with estrous females in males of monogamous rodent species.

6. Sexual differentiation of neural mechanisms which in adulthood control masculine sexual behavior in the ferret occurs through the sequential effects first of estrogen and then of testosterone, starting before birth and continuing during the first several weeks of life. These hormone actions may influence the development of sociosexual partner preference as well as mating performance, in part, by organizing morphological features of a male's POA.

Study Questions

1. Discuss how testosterone and/or its metabolites activate masculine coital behavior. Compare and contrast these effects of testosterone with its effects on sexual motivation.

2. Describe the neural systems necessary in male rodents for sexual motivation and compare with those necessary for sexual ability.

3. How does Viagra work?

4. Discuss the role of dopamine in masculine sexual motivation and in seucal ability. Where in the brain is dopamine acting in each of these roles?

5. Discuss the roles of oxytocin and vasopression in male mate preferences and pair bonding in the vole.

Acknowledgement

Preparation of this chapter was supported by an NIMH Senior Research Scientist Award (MH00392) to the author.

References

Adkins-Regan, E. (1988) Sex hormones and sexual orientation in animals. *Psychobiology* 16: 335–347.

Adkins-Regan, E., and Ascenzi, M. (1987) Social and sexual behaviour of male and female zebra finches treated with oestradiol during the nesting period. *Anim. Behav.* 35: 1100–1112.

Alderson, L. M., and Baum, M. J. (1981) Differential effects of gonadal steroids on dopamine metabolism in mesolimbic and nigrostriatal pathways of male rats. *Brain Res.* 218: 189–206.

Allen, L. S., Hines, M., Shryne, J. E., and Gorski, R. A. (1989) Two sexually dimorphic cell groups in the human hypothalamus. *J. Neurosci.* 9: 497–506.

Arendash, G. W., and Gorski, R. A. (1983) Effects of discrete lesions of the sexually dimorphic nucleus of the preoptic area or other medial preoptic regions on the sexual behavior of male rats. *Brain Res. Bull.* 10: 147–154.

Bakker, J., Brand, T., van Ophemert, J., and Slob, A. K. (1993) Hormonal regulation of adult partner preference behavior in neonatally ATD-treated male rats. *Behav. Neurosci.* 107: 480–487.

Balthazart, J., Absil, P., Gerard, M., Appeltants, D., and Ball, G. F. (1998) Appetitive and consummatory male sexual behavior in Japanese quail are differentially regulated by subregions of the preoptic medial nucleus. *J. Neurosci.* 18: 6512–6527.

Balthazart, J., Reid, J., Absil, P., Foidart, A., and Ball, G. F. (1995) Appetitive as well as consummatory aspects of male sexual behavior in quail are activated by androgens and estrogens. *Behav. Neurosci.* 109: 485–501.

Bancroft, J., and Wu, F. C. (1983) Changes in erectile responsiveness during androgen therapy. *Arch. Sex. Behav.* 12: 59–66.

Baulieu, E. E., Lasnitzki, I., and Robel, P. (1968) Metabolism of testosterone and action of metabolites on prostate glands grown in organ culture. *Nature* 219: 1155–1156.

Baum, M. J. (1976) Effects of testosterone propionate administered perinatally on sexual behavior of female ferrets. *J. Comp. Physiol. Psych.* 90: 399–410.

Baum, M. J. (1979) Differentiation of coital behavior in mammals: A comparative analysis. *Neurosci. Biobehav. Rev.* 3: 265–284.

Baum, M. J., Carroll, R. S., Cherry, J. A., and Tobet, S. A. (1990a) Steroidal control of behavioural, neuroendocrine, and brain sexual differentiation: Studies on a carnivore, the ferret. *J. Neuroendocrinol.* 2: 401–418.

Baum, M. J., Erskine, M. S., Kornberg, E., and Weaver, C. E. (1990b) Prenatal and neonatal testosterone exposure interact to affect differentiation of sexual behavior and partner preference in female ferrets. *Behav. Neurosci.* 104: 183–198.

Baum, M. J., and Erskine, M. S. (1984) Effect of neonatal gonadectomy and administration of testosterone on coital masculinzation in the ferret. *Endocrinology* 115: 2440–2444.

Baum, M. J., and Everitt, B. J. (1992) Increased expression of c-fos in the medial preoptic area after mating in male rats: Role of afferent inputs from the medial amygdala and mid-brain central tegmental field. *Neuroscience* 50: 627–646.

Baum, M. J., Gallagher, C. A., Martin, J. T., and Damassa, D. (1982) Effect of testosterone, dihydrotestosterone and estradiol administered neonatally on sexual behavior of female ferrets. *Endocrinology* 111: 773–780.

Baum, M. J., Gallagher, C. A., Shim, J. H., and Canick, L. A. (1983) Normal differentiation of masculine sexual behavior in male ferrets despite neonatal inhibition of brain aromatase or 5α-reductase activity. *Neuroendocrinology* 36: 277–284.

Baum, M. J., Kingsbury, P. A., and Erskine, M. S. (1987) Failure of the synthetic androgen, R1881, to duplicate the activational effect of testosterone on mating in castrated male rats. *J. Endocrinol.* 113: 15–20.

Baum, M. J., Tobet, S. A., Starr, M. S., and Bradshaw, W. G. (1982) Implantation of dihydrotestosterone propionate into the lateral septum or medial amygdala facilitates copulation in castrated male rats given estradiol systemically. *Horm. Behav.* 16: 208–223.

Baum, M. J., and Vreeburg, J. T. M. (1973) Copulation in castrated male rats following combined treatment with estradiol and dihydrotestosterone. *Science* 182: 283-285.

Beach, F. A. (1968) Coital behavior in dogs: III Effects of early isolation on mating in males. *Behaviour* 30: 2188–238.

Bem, D. J. (1996) Exotic becomes erotic: A developmental theory of sexual orientation. *Psych. Rev.* 103: 320–335.

Berthold, A. A. (1849) Transplantation der Hoden. *Arch. Anat. Physiol. Wissensch. Med.* 16: 42–49.

Bradshaw, W. G., Baum, M. J., and Awh, C. C. (1981) Attenuation by a 5α-reductase inhibitor of the activational effects of testosterone propionate on penile erections in castrated male rats. *Endocrinology* 109: 1047–1051.

Breedlove, S. M., and Arnold, A. A. (1980) Hormonal accumulation in a sexually dimorphic motor nucleus of the rat spinal cord. *Science* 210: 564–566.

Brookhart, J. M., and Dey, F. L. (1941) Reduction of sexual behavior in male guinea-pigs by hypothalamic lesions. *Am. J. Physiol.* 133: 551–554.

Byne, W., Lasco, M. S., Kemether, E., Shinwari, A., Edgar, M. A., Morgello, S., Jones, L., and Tobet, S. A. (2000) The interstitial nuclei of the human anterior hypothalamus: Assessment for sexual variation in volume and neuronal size, density and number. *Brain Res.* 856: 254–258.

Cherry, J. A., and Baum, M. J. (1990) Effects of lesions of a sexually dimorphic nucleus in the preoptic/anterior hypothalamic area on the expression of androgen and estrogen-dependent sexual behavior in male ferrets. *Brain Res.* 522: 191–203.

Christensen, L. W., and Clemens, L. G. (1975) Blockade of testosterone-induced mounting behavior in the male rat with intracranial application of the aromatization inhibitor, androst-1. 4,6,-triene-3,17-dione. *Endocrinology* 97: 1545–1551.

Clancy, A. N., Zumpe, D., and Michael, R. P. (1995) Intracerebral infusion of an aromatase inhibitor, sexual behavior and brain estrogen receptor-like immunoreactivity in intact male rats. *Neuroendocrinology* 61: 98–111.

Crews, D., and Morgentaler, A. (1979) Effects of intracranial implantation of oestradiol and dihydrotestosterone on the sexual behaviour of the lizard. *J. Endocrinol.* 82: 373–381.

Cushman, P. (1972) Sexual behavior in heroin addiction and methadone maintenance. *N.Y. State U. Med.* 72: 1261–1265.

Damassa, D. A., Smith, E. R., Tennet, B., and Davidson, J. M. (1977) The relationship between circulating testosterone levels and male sexual behavior in rats. *Horm. Behav.* 8: 275–286.

Davidson, J. M. (1966) Activation of male rat's sexual behavior by intracerebral implantation of androgen. *Endocrinology* 79: 783–794.

Davidson, J. M. (1969) Effects of estrogen on the sexual behavior of male rats. *Endocrinology* 84: 1365–1372.

Davidson, J. M., Camargo, C., and Smith, E. R. (1979) Effects of androgen on sexual behavior in hypogonadal men. *J. Clin. Endocrinol. Metab.* 48: 955–958.

Davis, P. G., and Barfield, R. J. (1979) Activation of masculine sexual behavior by intracranial estradiol benzoate implants in male rats. *Neuroendocrinology* 28: 217–227.

DeBold, J. F., and Clemens, L. G. (1978) Aromatization and the induction of male sexual behavior in male female and androgenized female hamsters. *Horm. Behav.* 11: 401–413.

Doherty, P. C., Baum, M. J., and Todd, R. B. (1986) Effects of chronic hyperprolactinemia on sexual arousal and erectile function in male rats. *Neuroendocrinology* 42: 368–375.

Edwards, D. A., and Einhorn, L. C. (1986) Preoptic and midbrain control of sexual motivation. *Physiol. Behav.* 37: 329–335.

Everitt, B. J. (1990) Sexual motivation: A neural and behavioral analysis of the mechanisms underlying appetitive and copulatory responses of male rats. *Neurosci. Biobehav. Rev.* 14: 217–232.

Federman, D. D. (1967) *Abnormal Sexual Development.* Philadelphia: W. B. Saunders.

Giuliano, F., Rampin, O., Brown, K., Courtois, F., and Benoit, G. (1996) Stimulation of the medial preoptic area of the hypothalamus in the rat elicits increases in intracavernous pressure. *Neurosci. Lett.* 209: 1–4.

Goldfoot, D. A., Kravetz, M. A., Goy, R. W., and Freeman, S. K. (1976) Lack of effect of vaginal lavages and aliphatic acids on ejaculatory responses in rhesus monkeys: Behavioral and chemical analyses. *Horm. Behav.* 7: 1–27.

Gray, G. D., Smith, E. R., and Davidson, J. M. (1980) Hormonal regulation of penile erection in castrated male rats. *Physiol. Behav.* 24: 463–468.

Gruendel, A. D., and Arnold, W. J. (1969) Effects of early social deprivation on reproductive behavior of male rats. *J. Comp. Physiol. Psychol.* 67: 123–128.

Grunt, J. A., and Young, W. C. (1952) Differential reactivity of individuals and the response of the male guinea pig to testosterone propionate. *Endocrinology* 51: 237–248.

Gysling, K., and Wang, R. Y. (1983) Morphine-induced activation of A10 dopamine neurons in the rat. *Brain Res.* 277: 119–127.

Hansen, S., Kohler, Ch., Goldstein, M., and Steinbusch, H. V. M. (1982) Effects of ibotenic acid-induced neuronal degeneration in the medial preoptic area and the lateral hypothalamic area on sexual behavior in the male rat. *Brain Res.* 239: 213–232.

Hart, B. L. (1967) Testosterone regulation of sexual reflexes in spinal male rats. *Science* 155: 1283–1284.

Heeb, M. M., and Yahr, P. (1996) C-fos immunoreactivity in the sexually dimorphic area of the hypothalamus and related brain regions of male gerbils after exposure to sex related stimuli or performance of specific sexual behavior. *Neurosci.* 72: 1049–1071.

Heimer, L., and Larsson, K. (1966/1967) Impairment of mating behavior in male rats following lesions in the preoptic-anterior hypothalamic continuum. *Brain Res.* 3: 248–263.

Hughes, A. M., Everitt, B. J., and Herbert, J. (1990) Comparative effects of preoptic area infusions of opioid peptides, lesions and castration on sexual behaviour in male rats: Studies of instrumental behaviour, conditioned place preference and partner preference. *Psychopharmacology* 102: 243–256.

Hull, E. M., Du, J., Lorrain, D. S., and Mtuszewich, L. (1995) Extracellular dopamine in the medial preoptic area: Implications for sexual motivation and hormonal control of copulation. *J. Neurosci.* 15: 7465–7471.

Insel, T. R., Wang, Z. X., and Ferris, C. F. (1994) Patterns of brain vasopressin receptor distribution associated with social organization in microtine rodents. *J. Neurosci.* 14: 5381–5392.

Johnston, P. Davidson, J. M. (1972) Intracerebral androgens and sexual behavior in the male rat. *Horm. Behav.* 3: 345–357.

Kelliher, K. R., Liu, Y. C., Baum, M. J., and Sachs, B. D. (1999) Neuronal Fos activation in olfactory bulb and forebrain of male rats having penile erections in the presence of inaccessible estrous females. *Neuroscience* 92: 1025–1033.

Kindon, H. A., Baum, M. J., and Paredes, R. G. (1996) Medial preoptic/anterior hypothalamic lesions induce a female-typical profile of sexual partner preference in male ferrets. *Horm. Behav.* 30: 514–527.

Kling, J. (1998) From hypertension to angina to Viagra. *Mod. Drug Discov.* 1: 31–38.

Lambert, G. M., and Baum, M. J. (1991) Reciprocol relationships between pulsatile androgen secretion and the expression of mating behavior in adult male ferrets. *Horm. Behav.* 25: 382–393.

LeVay, S. (1991) A difference in hypothalamic structure between heterosexual and homosexual men. *Science* 253: 1034–1037.

Lieblich, I., Baum, M. J., Diamond, P., Goldblum, N., Iser, C., and Pick, C. G. (1985) Inhibition of mating by naloxone or morphine in recently castrated, but not intact male rats. *Pharm. Biochem. Behav.* 22: 361–364.

Liu, Y.-C., Salamone, J. D., and Sachs, B. D. (1997) Lesions in medial preoptic area and bed nucleus of stria terminalis: Differential effects on copulatory behavior and noncontact erection in male rats. *J. Neurosci.* 17: 5245–5253.

Lorrain, D. S., Matuszewich, L., Friedman, R. D., and Hull, E. M. (1997) Extracellular serotonin in the lateral hypothalamic area is increased during the postejaculatory interval and impairs copulation in male rats. *J. Neurosci.* 17: 9361–9366.

Lynch, W. C., and Libby, L. (1983) Naloxone suppresses intake of highly preferred sacharin solutions in food deprived and sated rats. *Life Sci.* 33: 1909–1914.

Madlafousek, J., Hlinak, Z., and Beran, J. (1976) Decline of sexual behavior in castrated male rats: Effects of female precopulatory behavior. *Horm. Behav.* 7: 245–252.

Malsbury, C. W. (1971) Facilitation of male rat copulatory behavior by electrical stimulation of the medial preoptic area. *Physiol. Behav.* 7: 797–805.

Manzo, J., Cruz, M. R., Hernandez, M. E., Pacheco, P., and Sachs, B. D. (1999) Regulation of noncontact erection in rats by gonadal steroids. *Horm. Behav.* 35: 264–270.

Marin, R., Escrig, A., and Mas, M. (1999) Androgen-dependent nitric oxide release in rat penis correlates with levels of constitutive nitric oxide synthase isoenzymes. *Biol. Reprod.* 61: 1012–1016.

Mas, M., Fumero, B., and Gonzalez-Mora, J. L. (1995) Voltametric and sociosexual interactions. *Behav. Brain Res.* 71: 69–79.

McDonald, P. G., Beyer, C., Newton, F., Brien, B., Baker, R., Tan, H. S., Sampson, C., Kitching, P., Greenhill, R., and Pritchard, D. (1970) Failure of 5′-dihydrotestosterone to initiate sexual behavior in the castrated male rat. *Nature* 227: 964–965.

Meisel, R. L., O'Hanlon, J. K., and Sachs, B. D. (1984) Differential maintenance of penile responses and copulatory behavior by gonadal hormones in castrated male rats. *Horm. Behav.* 18: 56–64.

Meisel, R. L. Sachs, B. D. (1994) The physiology of male sexual behavior. In E. Knobil and J. D. Neill (Eds.), *The Physiology of Reproduction*, 2nd edition. New York: Raven Press, pp. 3–105.

Meyerson, B. J. (1981) Comparison of the effects of beta-endorphin and morphine on exploratory and socio-sexual behavior in the male rat. *Eur. J. Pharmacol.* 69: 453–458.

Meyer-Bahlburg, H. F. L., Ehrhardt, A. A., Rosen, L. R., Gruen, R. S., Veridiano, N. P., Vann, F. H., and Neuwalder, H. F. (1995) Prenatal estrogens and the development of homosexual orientation. *Devel. Psychol.* 31: 12–21.

Michael, R. P., and Keverne, E. B. (1968) Pheromones and the communication of sexual status in primates. *Nature* 218: 746–749.

Michael, R. P., Zumpe, D., and Bonsall, R. W. (1986) Comparison of the effects of testosterone and dihydrotestosterone on the behavior of male cynomolgus monkeys. *Physiol. Behav.* 36: 349–355.

Michael, R. P., Zumpe, D., and Bonsall, R. W. (1990) Estradiol administration and the sexual activity of castrated rhesus monkeys. *Horm. Behav.* 24: 71–88.

Miernicki, M., Pospchal, M. W., and Powers, J. B. (1990) Short photoperiods affect male hamster socio-sexual behaviors in the presence and absence of testosterone. *Physiol. Behav.* 47: 95–106.

Miller, R. L., and Baum, M. J. (1987) Naloxone inhibits mating and conditioned place preference for an estrous female in male rats soon after castration. *Pharm. Biochem. Behav.* 26: 781–789.

Mitchell, J. B., and Stewart, J. (1989) Effects of castration, steroid replacement, and sexual experience on mesolimbic dopamine and sexual behaviors in the male rat. *Brain Res.* 491: 116–127.

Moore, C. L. (1984) Maternal contribution to the development of masculine sexual behavior in laboratory rats. *Devel. Psychobiol.* 17: 347–356.

Naftolin, F., Ryan, K. J., Davies, I. J., Reddy, V. V., Flores, F., Petro, Z., Kuhn, M., White, R. J., Takaoka, Y., and Wolin, L. (1975) The formation of estrogens by central neuroendocrine tissues. *Recent Prog. Horm. Res.* 31: 295–319.

Panzica, G., Viglietti-Panzica, C., Calcagni, M., Anselmette, G. C., Schumacher, M., and Balthazart, J. (1987) Sexual differentiation and hormonal control of the sexually dimorphic preoptic medial nucleus in quail. *Brain Res.* 416: 59–68.

Paredes, R. G., and Baum, M. J. (1995) Altered sexual partner preference in male ferrets given excito-toxic lesions of the preoptic area/anterior hypothalamus. *J. Neurosci.* 15: 6619–6630.

Pfaus, J. G., and Phillips, A. G. (1991) Role of dopamine in the dorsal and ventral striatum. *Semin. Neurosci.* 4: 119–128.

Phoenix, C. H., Copenhaver, K. H., and Brenner, R. M. (1976) Scanning electron microscopy of penile papillae in intact and castrated rats. *Horm. Behav.* 7: 217–227.

Powers, J. B., and Winans, S. (1975) Vomeronasal organ: Critical role in mediating sexual behavior of the male hamster. *Science* 187: 961–963.

Presley, R. W., Menetrey, D., Levine, J. D., and Basbaum, A. I. (1990) Systemic morphine suppresses noxious stimulus-evoked Fos protein-like immunoreactivity in the rat spinal cord. *J Neurosci.* 10: 323–335.

Resko, J. A., Perkins, A., Roselli, C. E., Fitzgerald, J. A., Choate, J. V. A., and Storshak, F. (1996) Endocrine correlates of partner preference behavior in rams. *Biol. Reprod.* 55: 120–126.

Rissman, E. F., Wersinger, S. R., Fugger, H. N., and Foster, T. C. (1999) Sex with knockout models: Behavioral studies of estrogen receptor α. *Brain Res.* 835: 80–90.

Sachs, B. D. (1997) Erection evoked in male rats by airborne scent from estrous females. *Physiol. Behav.* 62: 921–924.

Sachs, B. D. (1982) Role of striated penile muscles in penile reflexes, copulation, and induction of pregancy. *J. Reprod. Fertil.* 66: 433–443.

Slmp, J. C., Hart, B. L., and Goy, R. W. (1978) Heterosexual, autosexual and social behavior of adult male rhesus monkeys with medial preoptic-anterior hypothalamic lesions. *Brain Res.* 142: 105–122.

Slob, A. K., van der Werff ten Bosch, J. J., van Hall, E. V., de Jong, F. H., Weijmar Schultz, W. C. M., and Eikelboom, F. A. (1993) Psychosexual functioning in women with complete testicular feminization: Is androgen replacement therapy preferable to estrogen? *J. Sex Marital Ther.* 19: 201–209.

Stockman, E. R., Callaghan, R. S., and Baum, M. J. (1985) Effect of neonatal castration and testosterone treatment on sexual partner preference in the ferret. *Physiol. Behav.* 34: 409–414.

Stone, C. P. (1939) Copulatory activity in adult male rats following castration and injections of testosterone propionate. *Endocrinology* 24: 165–174.

Stone, C. P., Barker, R. G., and Tomlin, M. I. (1935) Sexual drive in potent and impotent male rats as measured by the Columbia obstruction apparatus. *J. Genet. Psychol.* 47: 33–48.

Tobet, S. A., and Baum, M. J. (1987) Role for prenatal estrogen in the development of masculine sexual behavior in the male ferret. *Horm. Behav.* 21: 419–429.

Tobet, S. A., Shim, J. H., Osiecki, S. T., Baum, M. J., and Canick, J. A. (1985) Androgen aromatization and 5α-reduction in ferret brain during perinatal development: Effects of sex and testosterone manipulation. *Endocrinology* 116: 1869–1877.

Tobet, S. A., Zahniser, D. L., and Baum, M. J. (1986) Differentiation in male ferrets of a sexually dimorphic nucleus of the preoptic/anterior hypothalamic area requires prenatal estrogen. *Neuroendocrinology* 44: 299–308.

Vagell, M. E., and McGinnis, M. Y. (1997) The role of aromatization of male rat reproductive behavior. *J. Neuroendocrinol.* 9: 415–421.

Vreeburg, J. T. M., Schretlen, P. J. M., and Baum, M. J. (1975) Specific, high-affinity binding of estradiol in cytosols from several brain regions and pituitary of intact and castrated adult male rats. *Endocrinology* 97: 969–977.

Warner, R. K., Thompson, J. T., Markowski, V. P., Loucks, J. A., and Bazett, T. J. (1991) Microinjection of the dopamine antagonist cis-flupenthixol into the MPOA impairs copulation, penile reflexes and sexual motivation in male rats. *Brain Res.* 540: 177–182.

Wersinger, S. R., Sannen, K., Villalba, C., Lubahn, E. F., and Rissman, E. F. (1997) Masculine sexual behavior is disrupted in male and female mice lacking a functional estrogen receptor α gene. *Horm. Behav.* 32: 176–183.

Wersinger, S. R., and Rissman, E. F. (2000) Oestrogen receptor α is essential for female-directed chemo-investigatory behavior but is not required for the pheromone-induced LH surge in male mice. *J. Neuroendocrinol* 12: 103–110.

Wersinger, S. R., and Rissman, E. F. (2000) Dopamine activates masculine sexual behavior independent of the estrogen receptor α. *J. Neurosci.* 20: 4248–4254.

Winans, S. S., Lehman, M. N., and Powers, J. B. (1982) Vomeronasal and olfactory CNS pathways that control male hamster mating behavior. In W. Breipohl (Ed.), *Olfaction and Endocrine Regulation.* Oxford: IRI Press.

Winslow, J. T., Hastings, N., Carter, C. S., Harbaugh, C. R., and Insel, T. R. (1993) A role for central vasopressin in pair bonding in monogamous prairie voles. *Nature* 365: 545–548.

Yahr, P., and Gregory, J. E. (1993) The medial and lateral cell groups of the sexually dimorphic area of the gerbil hypothalamus are essential for male sex behavior and act via separate pathways. *Brain Res.* 631: 287–296.

Wood, R. I., and Newman, S. W. (1995) Integration of chemosensory and hormonal cues is essential for mating in the male Syrian hamster. *J. Neurosci.* 15: 7281–7269.

Zucker, K. J., Bradley, S. J., Oliver, G., Blake, J., Fleming, S., and Hood, J. (1996) Psychosexual development of women with congenital adrenal hyperplasia. *Horm. Behav.* 30: 300–318.

Zumpe, D., Bonsall, R. W., and Michael, R. P. (1993) Effects of the nonsteroidal aromatase inhibitor, Fadrazole, on the sexual behavior of male cynomolgus monkeys. *Horm. Behav.* 27: 200–215.

6 *Hormonal Influences on Human Sexual Behavior*

C. Sue Carter

This chapter provides an overview of a topic of interest to almost all of us: human sexual behavior. Unfortunately, there are relatively few rigorous studies of the ways in which hormones may affect human sexual relations a very difficult and demanding endeavor. Gonadal hormones do not seem to affect sexual behavior in humans or other primates as clearly or as strongly as they do in rodents, despite the expectations of many people throughout history. However, there are several indications that hormones have some influence on human sexual behavior and that some of this influence is exerted upon the brain in a manner similar to the way hormones influence the brain in other mammals.

What are the effects of castration upon the sexual behavior of humans and other primates? Which hormones appear to be responsible for hormone effects on human sexual behavior? What are some of the complicating factors that make the study of human sexual behavior difficult? Can sexual motivation or desire be dissociated from sexual performance in humans?

Introduction

In sexual reproduction, one egg and one sperm unite. The union of genetic codes from two individuals (the parents) forms another individual (the offspring). The combined genetic material from an egg and a sperm contains the blueprints needed for new life. This is sex. In a sense, all the rest is window-dressing. In spite of its essential simplicity, no aspect of human existence stirs more controversy or attracts more attention than sexual behavior.

Why Sex?

Until very recently, sex was the only mode of reproduction available to humans. However, molecular techniques have now been perfected for identifying, cloning, and otherwise manipulating existing genes. Using concepts that were considered science fiction as recently as the 1970s, it is possible to produce a new organism without a male contribution. Several years ago such procedures yielded Dolly, a Scottish ewe that was the first mammal successfully cloned from cells taken from an adult.

Does this mean that sex will soon become obsolete? Sexual reproduction is costly, dangerous, and has the potential to cause many problems. Several species, even among vertebrates, reproduce without it (see chapter 7). The value and purpose of sex are a constant source of debate. What is sex good for? Why bother?

Like all why questions, the answers to these questions are rooted in our evolutionary past. For this reason, our best guesses usually come from examining other life forms. The most common hypothesis regarding the evolution of sex is that sexual reproduction provides more genetic variation than asexual reproduction. Asexual animals replicate themselves. Sexual animals produce offspring that are genetically novel. Sexual reproduction allowed sexual creatures to have more genetic choices. In the lottery of life, many chances are better than one. Whatever the reasons for its existence, and despite the hazards and costs, sexual reproduction remains the norm in most vertebrates. Apparently sex has—at least in the long run—more benefits than costs.

In addition, the functions of sexual behavior extend well beyond reproduction. Human sexual behavior, or its absence, plays a major role in daily life and affects the behavior of both the individual and society. An enormous amount of energy goes into regulating sexual behavior, even when that behavior is not occurring for the purpose of procreation.

Why Is Sex So Hard to Understand and Control?

Anyone who lived in the era before sex education or who has kept an unneutered pet can tell you that knowledge of the biology of sex is not essential to reproduction. Research brings us to the same conclusion. Reproductive systems and sexual behavior were designed long before modern science entered the story and exist without much help from our cognitive brain.

Understanding the evolution and development of the nervous system helps us to appreciate the difficult task of managing primitive processes such as those at the core of sexual behavior. The systems responsible for sexual motivation are located, at least in part, in ancient areas of the brain stem. These areas send information to more modern (and more cognitive) areas of the brain. However, the messages generated by ancient areas of the brain are not verbal, so the message reaches the cognitive area of the brain as a vague message that is along the lines of "I need something" or "I want something."

SEXUAL BEHAVIOR IS A MOTIVATED BEHAVIOR

Drive, motivation, and related concepts have many meanings and describe complex emotions that go well beyond sex. The consequences of motivation are complicated and poorly understood, but they are also undeniable. Powerful emotions and their underlying mechanisms provide the energy for essential behaviors, of which sexual behavior is only one.

The regions of the brain that are receiving these messages are getting signals at the same time from other parts of the body and the outside world. It is the task of more recently evolved parts of the nervous system, including the cortex, to sort and label these signals. But there are limitations to the capacity of the cortex, especially when it comes to the task of telling older brain areas what to do. Thus humans, even with their complex brains, may still be vulnerable to archaic feelings and drives. Awareness of the bottom-up design of the nervous system helps to understand why drugs like cocaine or amphetamines can influence responses that were originally intended to activate and reward natural processes, such as sex or food intake. It also helps us to understand the ability of sex and sex-related functions to invade the rational worlds designed by the cortex and modern cultures.

As you will learn in this chapter, gonadal hormones are not essential for sexual behavior. However, a vast array of neurochemicals may influence the tendency of humans to engage in behaviors that lead to sex or otherwise affect sexual performance. There is no doubt that hormones can affect human behavior, although the behavioral endocrinology of human sexual behavior is not well understood, and—especially in light of its importance—receives remarkably little scientific attention.

Scientific Definitions of Sexual Behavior

Sexual behavior has many meanings. It can be argued that any behavior that increases the probability of sexual reproduction is sexual behavior. However, this definition is too broad to be useful in laboratory studies in which scientists attempt to understand the mechanisms through which the body regulates sexual activity. The terms that describe sexual behavior can be roughly grouped into those that reflect feelings or bodily states and those that depict actions or physical behaviors. For the purposes of laboratory research, scientists primarily measure actions and motor behaviors, including words, and use these to indirectly index internal states, preferences, and feelings.

Categorization of Sexual Behavior

It is common to divide sexual behavior into at least two phases. The first, the *motivational or appetitive* phase, brings the male and female together. Thus, implicit in sexual reproduction is the urge to engage in social contact, most commonly, but not always, with a member of the opposite sex. Concepts such as desire, drive, motivation, and libido may be subsumed in this phase. The second, the *mating or consummatory* phase, measures sexual ability or actions. In humans, this includes potency, intercourse, and sexual reflexes. Sensations, perceptions, and an individual's past history can influence both of these phases. There is a distinction between the ability to perform a motor act, such as approaching and mounting a female, and the desire or motivation that drives an individual to engage in the behavior (Wallen 1990).

Masters and Johnson (1966) divided the human sexual response into four phases: sexual excitement, plateau, orgasm, and sexual resolution or satiety. Even individuals with very low levels of sex steroids, for example following castration, may experience these responses, indicating that the basic physiology of the human sexual response is not dependent on gonadal hormones. However, steroid hormones may modulate human sexual behavior and, in particular, androgens and/or estrogens probably enhance sexual motivation. These ideas will be discussed later in this chapter.

Both erotic stimuli and psychological fantasy can induce sexual excitement. During the excitement phase, both male and female humans experience psychological sexual arousal and genital vasocongestion (retention of fluid). Sexually aroused individuals may reach a plateau phase, which usually lasts for a period of minutes or longer. If erotic stimulation continues, orgasm can follow.

Orgasm was described by Kinsey and his associates (1953) as "the explosive discharge of neuromuscular tensions at the peak of the sexual response.... Some, and perhaps most persons may become momentarily unconscious at the moment of orgasm." (Kinsey et al. 1953; p. 627–28) "Sexual arousal and orgasm involve the whole nervous system and, therefore, all parts of the body. Orgasm in the female matches the orgasm of the male in every physiological detail except for the fact that it occurs without ejaculation." (Kinsey et al. 1953; p. 635)

Temporal patterns of sexual response and the latency period needed before resumption of sexual responding following orgasm may be different in males and females. In general, males require a longer period of resolution before they are able to again reach orgasm (Masters and Johnson 1966). However, the basic phenomenology of the human sexual response and at least some of the fundamental neurophysiology of sexual responses appear to be similar in male and female humans.

Physiology of Genital Function

The physiology of genital function is most easily observed and thus best understood in males (Lue 2000), although parallels exist in female anatomy (Komisaruk and Whipple 1998). Vasocongestion and tumescence (swelling), penile erection (rigidity), and detumescence (return to flaccidity) are regulated by the inflow and outflow of blood. In males, well-vascularized and innervated sinusoidal chambers (cavernosa) within the penile shaft and glans penis allow penile erection. During tumescence and erection, smooth muscles are relaxed and arterioles within the penis dilate, allowing a dramatic increase in blood flow into the cavernosa. At the same time, the veins that normally carry blood from the penis are compressed and the outflow of blood is reduced. During erection, the intracavernous pressure can reach several hundred millimeters of mercury. As the penis fills with blood, it lengthens and enlarges. A similar, but less visible, shift in blood flow probably permits vasocongestion and clitoral tumescence in women (Komisaruk and Whipple 1998).

The functions of the genitalia are regulated by the central and autonomic nervous system through peripheral nerves that arise at the base of the brain (cranial nerves) and from the spinal cord (spinal nerves). It is common to divide the peripheral nerves that regulate bodily functions into somatic and autonomic (sympathetic and parasympathetic) components. The autonomic nervous system, including both cranial and spinal nerves, regulates blood flow and thus erection and detumescence. The somatic component, via neural input to the spinal cord, is responsible for sensations, including those that influence erection. Part of the autonomic nervous system enters the brainstem without going through the spinal cord. This anatomy of the autonomic nervous system accounts for the fact that following lesions of the spinal cord, and in the absence of genital sensations, it is still possible for some individuals of both sexes to experience tumescence, erection, and even orgasm (Komisaruk and Whipple 1998).

Hormone Influences on Human Male Sexual Behavior

The role of the testes in human reproduction and sexual behavior was recognized in antiquity. At puberty there is a dramatic increase in sexual activity or sexual interest. Concurrent growth in the size of the testes and penis (and other bodily changes) are readily observed, and could not have escaped the attention of any culture. It also was presumably apparent to most cultures that sexual activity by postpubertal, but not prepubertal, males was related to subsequent pregnancy. Domestication of animals and the use of castration to control reproduction and other aspects of male behavior, including aggression, date back thousands of years. Anecdotes abound, but quantitative data and controlled experiments are very rare even in the modern literature on human sexual behavior. The following discussion will examine historical and contemporary perspectives regarding the hormonal mechanisms responsible for sexual behavior.

Testicular Hormones Are Not Essential for Human Male Sexual Behavior

HISTORICAL BACKGROUND

Removal of the testes (castration) and/or external genitalia as punishment or tribute in war was common throughout history (Potts and Short 1999). Ancient drawings from Egypt and Ethiopia depict "mounds of severed genitalia gathered from enemies destroyed in battle" (Kinsey et al. 1953, 739). In Assyria, records of castration as punishment date from the fifteenth century B.C. In the fourth century B.C., Aristotle described the effects of both prepubertal and postpubertal castration.

Castration has been, and continues to be, used in attempts to control human sexual behavior (Potts and Short 1999; Abbott 2000). Castrated men (eunuchs) were preferred as harem guards, but despite expectations, many eunuchs continued to engage in sexual behavior. Some religious orders have required voluntary castration of their members in an attempt to facilitate celibacy or other aspects of spirituality. More modern attempts to subdue human male sexual behavior have involved the use of both voluntary and forced castration in the rehabilitation of sex offenders, including individuals convicted of exhibitionism, child molestation, and in some cases, homosexuality. Castration was also used to "cure" masturbation as recently as the early decades of the twentieth century. The debate over the usefulness of castration in the treatment of "excessive" or inappropriate sexual activity continues and has been supplemented by the introduction of methods of "chemical castration" (discussed later in this chapter).

THE ROLE OF THE TESTES IN ADULT SEXUAL BEHAVIOR

Adult castration is usually, but not always, followed by a decline in sexual activity. Medical records and studies of other primates indicate that castrated males may continue to show sexual behavior for years or even decades following castration. Some castrated men experience a decline or total absence of sexual activity, while others do not. Many reliable reports indicate that castrated men are capable of erections and orgasm (Kinsey et al. 1953). Castrated men are of course infertile, but they may continue to experience all other aspects of sexual behavior, although usually at lower levels than would be expected normally. Levels of circulating androgens are very low following castration or testicular failure. However, the minimal amount of testosterone needed to support the diverse components of sexual behavior has not been established.

DEVELOPMENTAL EFFECTS OF TESTICULAR HORMONES

Infants and older prepubertal males can experience nocturnal erections, indicating that mechanisms needed for erectile potency exist even under conditions when testicular activity is low. This is interesting in light of the fact that nocturnal penile erections are reportedly infrequent in hypogonadal adult men. Hypogonadism refers to various adult conditions in which the gonads are not fully functional or in which the endogenous production of testosterone falls below the normal range (usually defined in men as below 3 ng/ml of serum). In men, this condition can occur following castration for medical or other reasons, or individuals may experience testicular failure due to disease or genetic abnormalities.

A myriad of nonhormonal experiential factors confound attempts to detect the role of prepubertal hormones in subsequent adult behavior. The role of testicular secretions in childhood remains poorly understood. It has been generally assumed that prepubertal testicular failure or castration would be more detrimental to male sexual behavior than postpubertal loss of testicular function (Kinsey et al. 1953). However, as described later, testing this assumption is difficult. Overt sexual activity is usually infrequent in children. The behavioral effects of prepubertal hormones, therefore, have been examined only indirectly, in adults with a history of subnormal hormonal exposure.

AGING

A major early source of concern about the role of androgens in human male behavior, arose from the observation that sexual behavior tends to decline as men age. The testes also decrease in size, and it has been shown that testosterone levels decline somewhat with the most marked changes occurring after 60. However, various studies (Kinsey et al. 1948; Davidson et al. 1983) have indicated that even men in their 80s or older may continue to be sexually active. Correlations between levels of total testosterone and sexual activity are usually weak.

Changes in the availability of a sexual partner and concurrent declines in free testosterone (due to increased steroid hormone binding or changes in metabolism with age or illness) could influence sexual motivation and subsequent performance. A number of diseases can affect sexual function (e.g., diabetes, prostate cancer, and heart disease). Age-related changes in partner availability, declines in general health, increases in the prevalence of various diseases, and drugs or other treatments for such conditions may be more important than testosterone in determining age-related declines in sexual activity.

What Hormones Are Important?

NONTESTICULAR SOURCES OF ANDROGENS
Testicular secretions are not essential for either orgasm or potency, as measured by the ability to show a penile erection. Castrated and hypogonadal men continue to have the "ability" to perform sexually, and some may do so at high levels. These studies, however, do not prove conclusively that androgens are not involved in human sexual behavior, since the production of androgens is not limited to the testes. The adrenal glands also make androgens, although these are less potent than testicular androgens. The prostate gland, which is not usually removed with castration, is also capable of synthesizing dihydrotestosterone (DHT). In addition, adipose tissue (i.e., fat) is an important steroid hormone reservoir (in both males and females), containing concentrations of testosterone and DHT up to ten times higher than in serum. Furthermore, adipose tissue is an important site for the formation of 5α-reduced androgens, including DHT (Deslypere et al. 1985; Perel et al. 1986). Therefore, androgens from other sources in the body may contribute to the maintenance of sexual function in some individuals, and body fat may be a significant contributor to individual variations in behavior (Sherwin 1988).

EVIDENCE FROM CLINICAL STUDIES: HYPOGONADISM AND HORMONE REPLACEMENT THERAPY
One rare genetic condition, Kallman's syndrome, results from GnRH deficiency. Kallman's syndrome is especially interesting because its victims are hypogonadal from birth. Their prenatal genital development is relatively normal because testicular hormone secretion during the early developmental stages is not dependent on the fetal pituitary but is supported by the mother's gonadotropin production. Patients with Kallman's syndrome have low levels of testicular hormones during development and they do not experience puberty without medical intervention. Untreated, these individuals fail to develop secondary sex characteristics (i.e., become virilized) and they remain youthful in physical appearance, although they usually attain normal adult height.

Untreated hypogonadal adults suffering from Kallman's syndrome or related diseases are not usually homosexual. However, they do report a relative disinterest in sexual behavior, low levels of sexual activity, mild depression, and rarely experience spontaneous daytime or nocturnal penile erections. Hormone replacement therapies (either testosterone or pituitary hormones which stimulate testicular development) increase virilization. Androgenized hypogonadal men report increases in sexual interest, spontaneous daytime erections, and nocturnal penile erections. However, sexual activity, including autoerotic behavior, does not increase dramatically, at least within the first year after exposure to testosterone (Burris et al. 1991). These studies, of course, may be complicated by the unusual sexual and social histories of these men and shyness or embarrassment over their medical condition and sexual immaturity.

Sexual Performance versus Motivation
Studies of castrated men or men with adult testicular dysfunction clearly suggest that neither the testes nor high levels of androgens are essential for sexual performance when sexual stimulation is provided by a partner or intense erotic stimuli. However, the frequency of sexual activity in normal life is typically lower in men with low levels of androgens (Davidson et al. 1982; Bancroft and Wu 1983).

Until recently it was generally assumed that hypogonadal men were less able than normal men to respond with erections to erotic stimulation. However, recent laboratory studies have indicated that this is not the case. Strong erotic stimuli, including pornography or self-induced fantasy, may elicit erections with latencies similar to those seen in normal men. These studies did not attempt to examine orgasmic responses. However, self-reported frequencies (diaries) of sexual thoughts or fantasies suggest that androgens *can* stimulate this component of human behavior. Thus, it has been suggested that a major behavioral effect of testicular secretions is to increase spontaneous sexual thoughts, sexual desire, sexual interest, or libido (Alexander et al. 1997; Bancroft 1980). Erections elicited by erotic stimuli are apparently not dependent on high levels of androgens. In contrast, in hypogonadal adults spontaneous erections and sexual thoughts (not requiring external stimulation) tend to increase following androgen treatment (reviewed by Davidson et al. 1982).

Recent quantitative and experimentally controlled studies (Bancroft and Wu 1983; Davidson et al. 1982) are of theoretical importance because they suggest that testicular secretions can modulate sexual behavior by increasing thoughts or motivation, which leads to sexual activity. This hypothesis is, of course, very difficult to test. The occurrence of a thought is subject to many nonhormonal processes, including experience. The very act of requesting information could alter the frequency of sex-related thoughts. It is relatively simple to describe and measure sexual activity and erections, and much more difficult to define or assess human sexual motivation.

Problems with Assessment of Affective Behaviors
Another major problem in assessing the possible cognitive effects of any hormone relates to the behavioral specificity of hormone action. Androgens, with

their wide-ranging anabolic effects, could alter behavior at many levels and may have broad effects on human motivation and/or mood, thereby influencing sexuality secondarily. In a double-blind cross-over experiment, where hypogonadal men received different doses of testosterone or placebo at different times during the experiment, self-reports and mood questionnaires indicated that many men experience general lethargy, a loss of energy, and depression when their hormone levels are declining. These effects are seen even when the individual is not aware that he has been receiving hormone-replacement therapy (Burris et al. 1992).

Experiments in which men experience a rapid loss of androgen are also confounded by the complexity of hormone withdrawal. Like menopausal women, adult men experiencing a rapid decline in androgen sometimes have hot flashes, mood shifts, and other withdrawal symptoms. (Prepubertal boys and untreated hypogonadal adult men who have not yet experienced high levels of androgen do not experience these symptoms, suggesting that the effects of androgens or androgen withdrawal in an adult are influenced by a prior history of androgen exposure.)

In addition to cognitive or motivational interpretations of the behavioral data described here, it is possible that the perception of sensory stimuli might be altered by the presence of androgens (Davidson 1980; Davidson et al. 1982). Psychophysical techniques permit the precise analysis of human sensory perceptions. Using these methods, it was found that hypogonadal men receiving prolonged androgen exposure became progressively less sensitive to vibro-tactile stimulation of the penis (Burris et al. 1991). The ability of a hormone to modulate sensory input could be important in both sexual motivation and performance.

TESTOSTERONE, DHT, AND ESTROGEN

Early clinical studies of the effects of estrogen indicated that relatively large doses of estrogen could inhibit libido. In addition, estrogen treatment had other side effects, including mammary enlargement and female patterns of fat deposition that were not considered desirable in men. Therefore, it was traditionally assumed that estrogen was a female sex hormone, which would reduce male sexual behavior. However, more recently, the animal literature (see chapters 3 and 5) has raised the possibility that estrogens are involved in the behavioral effects of testosterone.

The possibility that low doses of estrogen may facilitate, rather than inhibit, human male sexual behavior remains largely untested. It is possible that testosterone serves as a prohormone that delivers the androgen to specific target cells, including the brain. According to this hypothesis, intracellular conversion to an estrogen would permit highly local effects of the estrogens, without the undesired feminizing actions which would follow if the entire body were exposed to high levels of estrogen. Concurrently, testosterone and its primary metabolite, DHT, would function to virilize peripheral tissues, such as accessory sex organs, genitalia, or muscle. DHT plays a role in adult patterns of body hair growth. In addition, male-pattern baldness, acne, and enlargement of the prostate gland are affected by DHT. The latter conditions may be treated by drugs or herbs (such as *propecia* or saw palmetto) that block the formation of DHT, usually through effects on the enzyme necessary for DHT production (5-alpha-reductase).

OTHER HORMONES AND HUMAN MALE SEXUAL BEHAVIOR

There has been a tendency by scientists to emphasize the effects of steroid hormones on sexual motivation and performance. However, many other hormones and neurochemicals may influence sexual behavior. Synthetic progestins, including medroxyprogesterone acetate and cyproterone acetate, have been used in the treatment of sex offenders. These "anti-androgenic" drugs provide a form of chemical castration and are reported, in uncontrolled studies, to decrease sexual motivation (Bancroft et al. 1974). In addition, oxytocin and vasopressin are released by the posterior pituitary during sexual behavior, and have actions on smooth muscle (such as the vas deferens) and blood pressure (needed for erection): both of these peptide hormones are also released into the brain and may influence sexual behavior (Carter 1992; Porges 1998).

Hormones released during stress and adrenal activation also directly or indirectly influence sexual behavior. Hormones released during chronic stress, such as the adrenal corticoids or opiates, may inhibit sexual behavior and other aspects of reproductive function. This idea is discussed further in chapter 11. However, short-term or acute stress may temporarily increase sexual arousal.

NITRIC OXIDE

One simple molecule, nitric oxide (NO), plays a pivotal role in both the central nervous system and in penile erection (Lue 2000). NO is normally released from cells in the penis and elevates the intracellular concentrations of cyclic guanosine monophosphate (cGMP); cGMP in turn produces a cascade of events that relax smooth muscle. As explained above, smooth-muscle relaxation is necessary for penile erection. In the penis, cGMP is metabolized by a selective enzyme (phosphodiesterase type 5, or PDE-5). Knowledge of this system led to the development of antagonists targeted to inhibit PDE-5, including a compound known as Viagra or sildenafil (see chapter 5, box 5.1). By blocking PDE-5, Viagra slows the metabolism cGMP and promotes erection. Because Viagra has effects at the peripheral level it may facilitate erection even in some individuals with spinal cord damage or other forms of sexual dysfunction. NO may affect and be affected by testosterone production and can promote the release of dopamine, oxytocin, and other hormones (Hull et al. 1999); thus, NO is probably important in the central control of sexual behavior in both sexes.

DRUGS AND SEXUAL BEHAVIOR

Alcohol and marijuana and a variety of other drugs are sometimes used in the context of sexual behavior. Alcohol or marijuana may reduce social inhibitions and indirectly promote sexual behavior. High doses of alcohol can directly inhibit the ability to ejaculate. Chronic use of alcohol or marijuana and many other chemicals is typically associated with gradual declines in sexual behavior. Such drugs damage the nervous system directly and may indirectly interfere with sexual behavior by inhibiting steroid hormone production. Chronic use of many drugs, especially alcohol, has also been implicated in impotence and eventual infertility.

Studies of illicit drug use or side-effects from medical treatments suggest that the chronic use of depressant drugs, including opiates (such as heroin), barbiturates, anti-anxiety drugs, anti-hypertensives, and anti-convulsants, usually reduces male sexual behavior (reviewed in Segraves et al. 1985). Conversely, acute or occasional use of stimulants such as amphetamines and cocaine reputedly can stimulate some components of sexual behavior. With chronic or repeated use of stimulants, however, sexual dysfunction may result. In addition, addicted individuals often become disinterested in both social and sexual interactions. The mechanisms of most of these phenomena remain poorly understood, but probably include effects on both peripheral systems, such as the autonomic nervous system (needed for erection and ejaculation) and the brain and endocrine systems.

Hormonal Influences on Human Female Sexual Behavior

Hormonal Effects on Performance versus Motivation

In most primates, including humans, ovarian hormones are not essential for the expression of female sexual behavior. However, to varying degrees, primate sexual behavior can be influenced by steroid hormones (Michael and Zumpe 1979; Wallen 1990). When female rhesus monkeys are tested alone with a single male in a small area, they will often show sexual behavior throughout the entire menstrual cycle, although the probability of mating may be slightly higher around the time of ovulation. In contrast, when females are tested in larger areas or in multifemale groups, most females mate primarily during the midcycle, periovulatory period. Using these data and the larger literature on primates researchers have hypothesized that ovarian hormones influence the expression of primate sexual behavior when female choice is permitted (Wallen 1990; Wallen and Tannenbaum 1997). Similar conclusions can be drawn from the literature on human females.

In rodents, both the ability (performance) and desire (motivation) to mate are hormone-dependent (Wallen 1990; Wallen and Tannenbaum 1997). In contrast, in primates, females are capable of engaging in sexual behavior without the benefit of ovarian hormones. However, the sexual motivation or desire of a female primate may vary as a function of the menstrual cycle or other endocrine events.

ESTROGEN

Estrogen has effects on every tissue of the body. Ovariectomy, which eliminates the major source of estrogen, can produce a gradual decline in female sexual behavior in rhesus monkeys and to varying degrees in other species (Wallen 1990; Wallen and Tannenbaum 1997). Estrogen, whether secreted by the ovarian follicle or given as replacement therapy, may have broad effects on primate behavior. Estrogen apparently can increase female motivation and may facilitate peripheral changes, such as the production of odors, that make the female more attractive to a male partner. In human females, estrogen increases vaginal lubrication and thus indirectly can influence sexual behavior. In addition, based on work in nonhuman primates, it is possible that estrogen alters the willingness of females to accept new males as social companions (Wallen and Tannenbaum 1997).

PROGESTERONE

During the primate menstrual cycle, progesterone is secreted around the time of ovulation, and following ovulation, the corpus luteum, formed from the follicle, is the dominant source of progesterone. There are some indications that brief exposure to progesterone can facilitate female sexual behavior in primates (Michael and Zumpe 1979). However, the most consistent effects of prolonged exposure to progesterone in primates, including humans, are inhibitory. For example, luteal phase inhibitions of sexual activity have been reported in monkeys and humans exposed to progesterone. Baum et al. (1977) have suggested that progesterone decreases female attractiveness in rhesus monkeys. Progesterone could be indirectly inhibitory, due to its capacity to act as an anti-estrogen. Progesterone could also alter the attractiveness of the female, or it could have direct inhibitory effects on female sexual motivation.

The behavioral effects of progesterone or synthetic progestins in human females remain difficult to interpret. Women taking oral contraceptives, which often contain progestins, may report either increases or decreases in sexual activity (Sanders and Bancroft 1982). These results are confounded by freedom from concern over pregnancy, which might increase sexual activity. However, a number of reports suggest declines in sexual interest in progestin-treated women. It has also been suggested that such effects could be an indirect, "anti-androgenic" action of the progestin (Sanders and Bancroft 1982). Studies of women receiving synthetic progestins, commonly administered in the postmenopausal period, also suggest that chronic exposure to progestins can have negative effects on sexual behavior.

ANDROGENS

It has been suggested that the androgens secreted by the ovary and/or adrenal during the menstrual cycle may be responsible for reported cyclic fluctuations in sexual interest (Sherwin 1988). Some women report increases in sexual activity just before and after menstruation; androgen levels also increase at this time. However, data on menstrual cyclicity in sexual behavior are rather weak (Sanders and Bancroft 1982), possibly because sexual activity involves many social factors in addition to the sexual interest of the female (Wallen 1990).

The adrenal cortex produces significant quantities of androgens, and adrenalectomy is detrimental to female sexual behavior in humans and monkeys. In monkeys, declines in sexual behavior following adrenal removal were somewhat reversed by treatment with androgen, but were not affected by treatment with estrogen. Furthermore, since the 1940s, exogenous androgen treatments have been given to human females for diverse medical purposes. Even in very low doses, androgen treatments can increase sexual motivation in some human females, and it has been suggested by Sherwin (1988) that women may be, in comparison to men, more sensitive to the behavioral effects of androgens.

The ability of exogenous androgens to promote female sexual behavior is of therapeutic interest and is being explored in medical research. However, androgenic (anabolic) hormones carry potential side effects, including sterility, virilization, male patterns of body hair growth, baldness, acne, and liver and cardiovascular damage. It should also be noted that normal men endogenously produce levels of androgens that are well above those needed to maintain high levels of sexual behavior (Davidson et al. 1982; Alexander et al. 1997). Thus, at present the usefulness of androgens as aphrodisiacs is limited to men with abnormally low levels of androgens, and other applications are potentially hazardous (Pope and Katz 1994).

Human Sexual Behavior: A Hypothesis for the Coordination of Male and Female Sexual Behaviors

As described above, there is reason to believe that both male and female humans are capable of responding to androgens with increased sexual interest. Furthermore, in the relative absence of sex steroids, at least the reflexive components of the sexual response can be elicited in males and females. Davidson et al. (1982) observed that profoundly hypogonadal men were able to experience erections as quickly as normal men if they were presented with highly erotic stimuli. In contrast, in the absence of strong stimuli, hypogonadal men typically show lower than normal levels of spontaneous sexual interest or sexual activity with a partner. In double-blind studies, androgen-replacement therapy increased sexual interest and, to a lesser degree, sexual activity in hypogonadal men (Burris et al. 1992). Such data offer further support for a role for androgens in sexual motivation, although the effects of androgens on sexual performance are less conclusive (Alexander et al. 1997).

A large pharmacological literature has implicated a variety of neurochemicals, including steroid hormones, in male sexual interest and erectile potency (Segraves et al. 1985). Apart from work on steroid hormones, very little is known regarding the pharmacology of human female sexual behavior. Presumably this is not because drugs do not effect women, but rather because women are not dependent on an erection for sexual activity. However, as argued by Kinsey and his associates (1953), the major sex difference in human behavior is based on the presence of ejaculation in the male, but not the female. "Ejaculation may constitute a spectacular and biologically significant event which is unique to the male, but it is an event which depends on relatively simple anatomic differences, rather than upon differences in the basic physiology of sexual response in the female and male" (p. 636).

NEUROPEPTIDES, OTHER NEUROCHEMICALS, AND BEHAVIOR

Neuropeptides, including oxytocin and vasopressin, may play pivotal roles in reproductive and social behavior (Carter 1992). Vasopressin is released into the bloodstream during sexual arousal and drops to low levels at the time of orgasm. Oxytocin is released during the orgasmic phase in both men and women (Carmichael et al. 1987; Murphy et al. 1987) and during ejaculation in males of several species. Through its contractile effects on smooth muscle, oxytocin could play a role in sperm transport in males. In women, uterine contractions caused by peripherally released oxytocin may facilitate sperm transport (Davidson 1980). It is also possible that centrally released oxytocin has a more direct neural role in reproduction, possibly acting both to increase social contact (appetitive behaviors) and to facilitate reflexive or consummatory components of sexual behavior (Carter 1998; Porges 1997, 1998; Komisaruk and Whipple 1998). Breast, genital, and/or cognitive stimulation can stimulate the release of oxytocin (Keverne 1988); the central release of small amounts of oxytocin may cascade (over a period of minutes) through positive feedback to cause the pulsatile release of oxytocin in the brain and also into peripheral circulation (Carmichael et al. 1987; Murphy et al. 1987). Electrical activity in the brain during the release of oxytocin could provide a substrate for the altered states of consciousness associated with orgasm (Carter 1992; Komisaruk and Whipple 1998).

These peptides do not act alone. For example, the synthesis, release, and reception of oxytocin and vasopressin can be regulated by steroid hormones, including testosterone and estrogen, as well as by a variety of other neurochemicals, such as endogenous opioids (Carter 1998) and nitric oxide (Rosselli et al. 1998; Hull et al. 1999). An inability to release or respond to oxytocin might account for some forms of sexual dysfunction.

Oxytocin is not a candidate for a perfect aphrodiasic. In animals, high or chronic doses of oxytocin inhibit sexual behavior (Carter 1992), and oxytocin has been implicated in sexual satiety (Davidson 1980). It is possible that oxytocin released during orgasm acts on the nervous system to induce a refractory state. The refractory state of the oxytocinergic system could be one component of sexual satiety. This state could vary in duration between the sexes and as a function of other hormonal or neurochemical events, such as drug treatments.

However, another argument in support of a role for oxytocin and vasopressin in the regulation of sexual behavior comes from the fact that these peptides play an important role in the autonomic nervous system. In turn, the autonomic nervous system, including its sympathetic and parasympathetic components, can affect both the appetitive and consummatory aspects of sexual behavior (Komisaruk and Whipple 1998; Porges 1998). Receptors for oxytocin and vasopressin are found in areas of the nervous system that regulate the autonomic nervous system. Both central and peripheral events surrounding the release of oxytocin and/or vasopressin might induce changes in genital blood flow, heart rate, or blood pressure which precede or follow orgasm. There is also evidence implicating oxytocin in the formation of social bonds in animals (Carter and Getz 1993; Carter 1998). Shared sexual experience may thereby facilitate social bond formation in humans. These hypotheses can be tested only indirectly, but are supported by animal research.

SOCIAL BONDS AND MONOGAMY

Social systems provide the context for sexual behavior. Humans tend to form pair bonds, which provide a social matrix for sexual activity (Carter 1998; Porges 1998). Such bonds, especially between a male and female, are at the heart of a social system termed "monogamy"—from the Greek for "one spouse." Monogamous relationships are sanctioned or even required by many religions and governments. However, in modern society, life-long sexual monogamy is rare and divorce is common. DNA fingerprinting and other methods of determining paternity have revealed that sexual monogamy is even less common than previously assumed. For these reasons, there has been a tendency to question whether humans are in fact monogamous.

To address the question of human monogamy, it is helpful to examine social monogamy and sexual monogamy separately. There are many advantages to sexual monogamy, including confidence of paternity for the male. In addition, monogamous couples have a lower likelihood of exposure to sexually transmitted diseases (Potts and Short 1999). But sexual monogamy has reproductive disadvantages as well, especially for males, who may give up opportunities to maximize their reproductive fitness.

Social monogamy and pair bonds may exist even under conditions when sexual monogamy is less than absolute. Social bonds have effects that extend beyond reproduction, and both sexes benefit from social bonds. Social bonds and social support provide a host of psychological and physiological benefits. For example, social isolation increases the risk of illness and death from all causes including cardiovascular diseases and cancer (Knox and Uvnas-Moberg 1998). Living in a socially monogamous relationship, at least if that relationship is characterized by positive experiences, can be good for your health.

Social monogamy may also be regulated by neuroendocrine systems that affect sexual behavior. Physiological systems that include oxytocin and vasopressin and their receptors are distributed throughout the nervous system in areas that integrate neuroendocrine and autonomic functions. These peptide hormones may influence both sexual behavior and the formation of social bonds (Carter 1998). In addition, the physiology of social and sexual behavior can affect autonomic functions and homeostasis, possibly accounting for the importance of social support in good health (Carter and Altemus 1997; Uvnas-Moberg 1998).

Summary

1. Human sexual behavior can occur in the absence of gonadal hormones; however, hormones and many other neurochemicals appear to modulate sexual behavior.

2. Human male sexual behavior, including erectile potency, may continue in the absence of the testes and in individuals with low levels of testosterone. However, quantitative studies suggest that reductions in testicular secretions are associated with declines in sexual interest or motivation. Testosterone may have effects on diverse processes including those responsible for spontaneous erections, mood, and sensory processing leading to sexual activity. Testosterone, within the normal biological range, is probably a true aphrodisiac. However, even androgens used in large chronic doses (for example, during anabolic steroid abuse) may inhibit sexual behavior. Anabolic steroids can also have the undesirable effect of making their users more susceptible to episodes of overreactivity and even aggression (Pope and Katz 1994), which can indirectly interfere with normal social and sexual relationships.

3. In most primates, including humans, ovarian hormones are not necessary for females to engage in sexual behavior. However, motivation or sexual desire, and possibly orgasmic responsivity, can vary as a function of the menstrual cycle. Estrogen may facilitate sexual desire and attractiveness. Progesterone is not necessary for human female sexual behavior. However, prolonged exposure to progesterone in women—for example, in the luteal phase, in pregnancy, or given as a medicine—may inhibit sexual interest. Androgen secretion in females may also vary as a function of the menstrual cycle. Although the level of androgens in women is usually much lower than that found in men, there are indications that women are more sensitive than men to androgens (Sherwin 1988).

4. The behavioral effects of androgens in both sexes may require intracellular conversion to an estrogen (see chapter 3). In contrast, several physical effects of testosterone, such as muscle development, patterns of body hair, baldness, and acne, reflect the actions of a testosterone metabolite known as DHT. Drugs commonly alter the metabolism of steroids and thus may have direct and indirect effects on behavior.

5. Oxytocin and vasopressin are released during the human sexual response in both males and females. These neuropeptides may have a direct effect on behavior; they are also affected by sex steroids and neurotransmitters like dopamine, which have been implicated in sexual behavior (see chapter 4). A variety of chemicals, including oxytocin, dopamine, and nitric oxide, might play a role in coordinating sexual excitement, orgasm, and sexual satiety with social behavior and social bonds (Carter 1992, 1998; Hull et al. 1999).

6. Most behaviorally active drugs (including many medicines) have some capacity to influence sexual behavior directly or indirectly. In general, depressants diminish sexual interest and performance. The effects of stimulants are more complicated, and may include transient facilitations of sexual behavior. Chronic drug abuse is often associated with declines in sexual behavior. Chronic stress may also inhibit sexual behavior. The effects of most drugs and the effects of stress are complex and may involve direct neural effects and indirect actions on steroid hormone production.

7. Human research in this field is rare and the cellular mechanisms of hormone actions can only be inferred from animal research. Animal studies, such as those described throughout this volume, can be used to model basic biological mechanisms and phenomena. Cross-species comparisons, including human data, facilitate an understanding of the functions, adaptive significance, and mechanisms of a particular behavioral pattern. Knowledge from diverse sources permits the development of descriptive and predictive models, which in turn may allow for the prevention and treatment of biochemically based sexual dysfunction.

Study Questions

1. Discuss the role of testosterone in sexual behavior in men. How does this differ from the role of testosterone in sexual behavior in rodents or ferrets?

2. Discuss the roles for estrogen, progesterone, and androgens in sexual behavior in women and most primates. How does this differ from the role of estrogen and progesterone in sexual behavior in rodents?

3. What is the evidence that oxytocin and vasopressin are involved in social behavior or mate choice in humans?

4. Is Viagra an aphrodisiac? Why or why not? Are there any drugs or hormones that serve as aphrodisiacs? Explain.

References

Abbott, E. (2000) *A History of Celibacy*. New York: Scribner.

Alexander, G. M., Swerdloff, R. S., Wang, C., Davidson, T., McDonald, V., Steiner, B., and Hines, M. (1997) Androgen-behavior correlations in hypogonadal men and eugonadal men. I. Mood and response to auditory sexual stimuli. *Horm. Behav.* 31: 110–119.

Bancroft, J. (1980) Endocrinology of sexual function. *Clinics Obstet. Gynaec.* 7: 253–281.

Bancroft, J., and Wu, F. C. W. (1983) Changes in erectile responsiveness during androgen replacement therapy. *Arch. Sex. Behav.* 12: 59–66.

Bancroft, J., Tennent, T. G., Loucas, K., and Cass, J. (1974) Control of deviant sexual behaviour by drugs: Behavioural effects of oestrogens and anti-androgens. *Br. J. Psychiat.* 125: 310–315.

Baum, M. J., Everitt, B. J., Herbert, J., and Keverne, E. B. (1977) Hormonal basis of proceptivity and receptivity in female primates. *Arch. Sex. Behav.* 6: 173–192.

Burris, A. S., Gracely, R. H., Carter, C. S., Sherins, R. J., and Davidson, J. M. (1991) Testosterone therapy is associated with reduced tactile sensitivity in human males. *Horm. Behav.* 25: 195–205.

Burris, A. S., Banks, S. M., Carter, C. S., Davidson, T. M., and Sherins, R. J. (1992) A long-term prospective study of the physiologic and behavioral effects of hormone replacement in untreated hypogonadal men. *J. Androl.* 13: 297–304.

Carmichael, M. S., Humbert, R., Dixen J., Palmisano, G., Greenleaf, W., and Davidson, J. M. (1987) Plasma oxytocin increases in the human sexual response. *J. Clin. Endocrinol. Metabol.* 64: 27–31.

Carter, C. S. (1992) Oxytocin and sexual behavior. *Neurosci. Biobehav. Rev.* 16: 131–144.

Carter, C. S. (1998) Neuroendocrine perspectives on social attachment and love. *Psychoneuroendocrinology* 23: 779–818.

Carter, C. S., and Getz, L. L. (1993) Monogamy and the prairie vole. *Sci. Am.* 268: 100–106.

Carter, C. S., and Altemus, M. (1997) Integrative functions of lactational hormones in social behavior and stress management. *Ann. N.Y. Acad. Sci.* 807: 164–174.

Davidson, J. M. (1980) The psychobiology of sexual experience. In J. M. Davidson and R. J. Davidson (Eds.), *The Psychobiology of Consciousness*. New York: Plenum Press, pp. 271–332.

Davidson, J. M., Kwan, M., and Greenleaf, W. (1982) Hormonal replacement and sexuality in men. In J. Bancroft (Ed.), *Clinics in Endocrinology and Metabolism* vol. II. London: Saunders, pp. 599–624.

Davidson, J. M., Chen J. J., Crapo, L., Gray, G. D., Greenleaf, W. J., and Catania, J. A. (1983) Hormonal changes and sexual function in aging men. *J. Clin. Endocrinol. Metabol.* 57: 71–77.

Deslypere, J. P., Verdonck, L., Vermeulen, A. (1985) Fat tissue: A steroid reservoir and site of steroid metabolism. *J. Clin. Endocrinol. Metab.* 61: 564–570.

Hatton, G. I. (1988) Cellular reorganization in neuroendocrine secretion. In D. Ganten and D. Pfaff (Eds.), *Current Topics in Neuroendocrinology*, vol. 9. Berlin: Springer-Verlag, pp. 1–27.

Hull, E. M., Lorrain, D. S., Du, J., Matuszewich, L., Lumley, L. A., Putnam, S. K., and Moses, J. (1999). Hormone-neurotransmitter interactions in the control of sexual behavior. *Behav. Brain Res.* 105: 105–116.

Keverne, E. B. (1988) Central mechanisms underlying the neural and neuroendocrine determinants of maternal behaviour. *Psychoneuroendocrinology* 13: 127–141.

Kinsey, A. C., Pomeroy, W. B., and Martin, C. E. (1948) *Sexual Behavior in the Human Male*. Philadelphia: Saunders.

Kinsey, A. C., Pomeroy, W. B., Martin, C. E., and Gebhard, P. H. (1953) *Sexual Behavior in the Human Female*. Philadelphia: Saunders.

Knox, S. S., and Uvnas-Moberg, K. (1998) Social isolation and cardiovascular disease: An atherosclerotic pathway? *Psychoneuroendocrinology* 23: 877–890.

Komisaruk, B. R., and Whipple, B. (1998) Love as sensory stimulation: Physiological consequences of its deprivation and expression. *Psychoneuroendocrinology* 23: 927–944.

Lue, T. F. (2000) Erectile dysfunction. *N. Engl. J. Med.* 342: 1802–1813.

Masters, W., and Johnson, V. (1966) *Human Sexual Response*. Boston: Little, Brown.

Michael, R. P., and Bonsall, R. W. (1979) Hormones and the sexual behavior of rhesus monkeys. In C. Beyer (Ed.), *Endocrine Control of Sexual Behavior*. New York: Raven Press, pp. 279–302.

Murphy, M. R., Seckl, J. R., Burton, S., Checkley, S. A., and Lightman, S. L. (1987) Changes in oxytocin and vasopressin secretion during sexual activity in men. *J. Clin. Endocrinol. Metab.* 65: 738–741.

Perel, D., Daniilescu, D., Kindler, S., Kharlip, L., Killinger, D. W. (1986) The formation of 5 alpha-reduced androgens in stromal cells from human breast adipose tissue. *J. Clin. Endocrinol. Metab.* 62: 314–318.

Pope, H. G., and Katz, D. L. (1994) Psychiatric and medical effects of anabolic-androgenic steroid use. *Arch. Gen. Psychiatry* 51: 375–382.

Porges, S. W. (1997) Emotion: An evolutionary by-product of the neural regulation of the autonomic nervous system. *Ann. N.Y. Acad. Sci.* 807: 62–77.

Porges, S. W. (1998) Love: An emergent property of the mammalian autonomic nervous system. *Psychoneuroendocrinology* 23: 837–861.

Potts, M., and Short, R. (1999) *Ever Since Adam and Eve*. New York: Cambridge University Press.

Rosselli, M., Keller, Pl J., and Dubey, R. K. (1998) Role of nitric oxide in the biology, physiology and pathophysiology of reproduction. *Hum. Reprod. Update* 4: 3–24.

Sanders, D., and Bancroft, J. (1982) Hormones and the sexuality of women—The menstrual cycle. In J. Bancroft (Ed.), *Clinics in Endocrinology and Metabolism* vol. II. London: Saunders, pp. 639–660.

Segraves, R. T., Madsen, R., Carter, C. S., and Davis, J. M. (1985) Erectile dysfunction associated with pharmacological agents. In R. T. Segraves and H. W. Schoenberg (Eds.), *Diagnosis and Treatment of Erectile Disturbances*. New York: Plenum Press, pp. 23–63.

Sherwin, B. B. (1988) A comparative analysis of the role of androgen in human male and female sexual behavior: Behavioral specificity, critical thresholds, and sensitivity. *Psychobiology* 16: 416–425.

Uvnas-Moberg, K. (1998) Oxytocin may mediate the benefits of positive social interaction and emotions. *Psychoneuroendocrinology* 23: 819–835.

Wallen, K. (1990) Desire and ability: Hormones and the regulation of female sexual behavior. *Neurosci. Biobehav. Rev.* 14: 233–241.

Wallen, K., and Tannenbaum, P. L. (1997) Hormonal modulation of sexual behavior and affiliation in rhesus monkeys. *Ann. N.Y. Acad. Sci.* 807: 185–202.

7 Diversity and Evolution of Hormone-Behavior Relations in Reproductive Behavior

David Crews

As we learned in chapter 3, each individual is bipotential. Even though adult males and females display behaviors typical of their sex, both are capable of displaying those behaviors characteristic of the other sex. To what extent are the differences observed between adult males and females due to chromosomal constitution, to differences in nongenomic yet heritable sex-typical experiences, and to evolutionary forces? It is unfortunate, but true, that we know only what we study, and we tend to study only what we know. Recent studies of species that lack sex chromosomes indicate that the organizational-activational concept does not apply to all organisms.

Because we are mammals, many people find other mammals more interesting than fishes, insects, or snakes. But some of the most fascinating variations in reproduction have arisen among the reptiles and fishes, where relations between hormones and mating behavior can be very different from those described in the previous chapters. These alternative solutions to common life problems force us to look again at mammals, including ourselves, and ask questions about the evolutionary forces that have produced the hormone-behavior relations described in the previous chapters. We also see that in spite of the variation in the ways in which hormones affect reproduction and sexual behavior, in those species of vertebrates that have been investigated, the same brain regions are important. By taking advantage of the great variety in the ways species have solved common problems, we gain insights that may not be obvious from studies of more conventional laboratory species.

Without due consideration of the neural and behavioral correlates of differences between higher taxa and between closely related families, species, sexes, and stages, we cannot expect to understand our nervous systems or ourselves.
—T. H. Bullock (1984)
We have evolved a nervous system that acts in the interest of our gonads, and one attuned to the demands of reproductive competition.
—M. Ghiselin (1974)

Introduction

Through televised documentaries we have been to the poles and everywhere in between observing the lives of animals. The episodes captured on film usually focus on sexual or aggressive behaviors and adaptations to life's perils. What stands out is the incredible diversity of the behaviors exhibited. Each species engages in some behaviors that are characteristic of and unique to that species. These are referred to as species-typical behaviors. From reading the first few chapters, you have probably already realized that there is also great diversity in the ways in which hormones can affect an animal's nervous system and behavior. To the student, this diversity might seem like an unwanted complexity, something else to complicate the story and your studying. It is the object of this chapter to convince you that as you gain an appreciation of the diversity in hormone-behavior relations, you will begin to understand more completely the basic mechanisms mediating these processes. In addition, you will gain a greater understanding of and appreciation for the evolution of hormone-brain-behavior relations.

At the most fundamental level, the study of diversity provides us with a different perspective from which to view hormone-brain-behavior relations (Bartholomew 1982; Bern 1972; Bullock 1984; Crews and Moore 1986; Diamond 1983; Prosser 1988). There has been a tradition in modern times to specialize: the study of the causes and development of behavior is usually separated from the evolution and ecological patterns of behavior. There has also been a trend toward reductionistic investigations of behavior. In other words, scientists have been inclined to investigate the molecular changes in the brain that are correlated with a behavior rather than to study the actual behavior itself. However, it is important to keep in mind that there are many levels of biological organization and that molecules always function within cells, cells within organs, organs within animals and, ultimately, animals within environments. The cellular and molecular aspects of hormonal action (that is, proximate causation) are important for our understanding of these processes. But they tell us very little about the behavior itself, especially about why the behavior is exhibited. For this, we must turn to studies of the whole animal and questions of ultimate causation. To learn about the evolution of behavior, we must turn to ecological and evolutionary analyses.

Those scientists interested in immediate causes of behavior tend to be unaware of the great advances that have been made in evolutionary biology. Similarly, most scientists interested in ecological and evolutionary questions ignore advances in neuroendocrinology and molecular biology. Quite simply, "reductionists see little to be gained from holistic studies, and whole organism biologists do not recognize the value of molecular analysis" (Prosser 1986). This philosophical gap and lack of communication between these two approaches to the study of brain-behavior relations make it difficult to be a generalist. Yet to understand behavior, we must attempt to integrate the different levels of biological organization. If done with insight, it can lead to new discoveries in evolution, ecology, physiology, and molecular biology.

This chapter emphasizes an interdisciplinary approach to behavioral analysis, including an evolutionary approach. Obviously, a scientist can apply Darwinian thinking to behavioral questions without being an evolutionary biologist, as is evident in the now-vibrant field of human evolutionary psychology. For readers who might be encountering an evolutionary or ecological approach for the first time, it is important *not* to assume that evolutionary thinking is confined to a particular discipline. Indeed, modern Darwinian theory can be a powerful tool for molecular, anatomical, physiological, and behavioral research regardless of your formal disciplinary home.

The general principles that should guide you in considering behavioral endocrinology from an evolutionary and ecological perspective will be discussed next. These principles will be illustrated by describing some of the modes and patterns of reproduction in animals. A variety of evolutionary forces have led to various behavior-controlling mechanisms. These will be discussed first and will be followed by examples of the diversity in hormone-behavior relations that have been observed to date. These and other studies are at the interface of ecological physiology, evolutionary biology, and behavioral endocrinology. Next, several nonconventional animal model systems will be described in detail to illustrate how these three fields might be integrated. Finally, some thoughts are offered about why complementarity is a fundamental aspect of biological organization, whether a principle tenet of behavioral endocrinology encompass all vertebrates, and how hormone-brain-behavior relations might have evolved. We will conclude with some thoughts about the evolution of sex versus the evolution of sexual behavior.

Overview of General Principles

Modes of Reproduction

In the preceding chapters, the discussion of sexual behaviors has focused on species with two sexes. In the animal kingdom, however, this is not the only way species propagate. We tend to focus on mammals because their mode of reproduction is like ours and employs internal fertilization of the egg in a female by a male, with the female giving birth to live young. But this is only one mode of reproduction, and a remarkable array of reproductive modes has evolved.

Animals can be classified according to (1) the division across individuals according to egg or sperm production (or both), (2) the method of production of the young, and (3) the method of fertilization (table 7.1). Most vertebrates have two sexes, male and female. As you have already learned, this means that during development, the fetal gonads become testes in males and ovaries in females. This separation of the gonads into separate-sexed individuals is called gonochorism. On the other hand, in some species the same individual has both types of gonad and can produce both eggs and sperm. These individuals are called hermaphrodites. In some hermaphroditic species (e.g., earthworms and sea bass), the production of eggs and sperm occurs simultaneously. In others (e.g., coral reef fish), the production of eggs and sperm occurs sequentially. It is important to keep in mind that these two forms of hermaphroditism are fundamentally different. In the former instance, individuals are two sexes at the same time, whereas in the latter instance, individuals are only one sex at a time.

Table 7.1 Different Modes of Reproduction

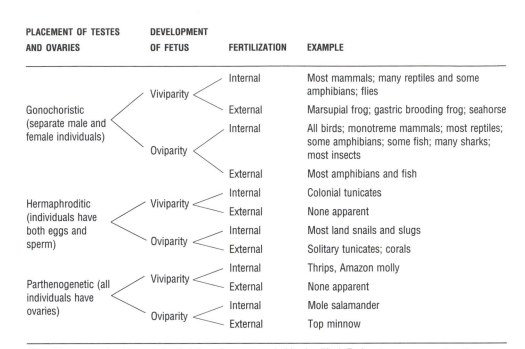

PLACEMENT OF TESTES AND OVARIES	DEVELOPMENT OF FETUS		FERTILIZATION	EXAMPLE
Gonochoristic (separate male and female individuals)	Viviparity		Internal	Most mammals; many reptiles and some amphibians; flies
			External	Marsupial frog; gastric brooding frog; seahorse
	Oviparity		Internal	All birds; monotreme mammals; most reptiles; some amphibians; some fish; many sharks; most insects
			External	Most amphibians and fish
Hermaphroditic (individuals have both eggs and sperm)	Viviparity		Internal	Colonial tunicates
			External	None apparent
	Oviparity		Internal	Most land snails and slugs
			External	Solitary tunicates; corals
Parthenogenetic (all individuals have ovaries)	Viviparity		Internal	Thrips, Amazon molly
			External	None apparent
	Oviparity		Internal	Mole salamander
			External	Top minnow

Note: The reader should recognize that the scheme presented is simplified. Each category represents extremes on what is really a continuum, and intermediate forms exist. Furthermore, some animals may actually exhibit different reproductive modes at different stages of their life cycle. The interested reader should consult Blackwelder and Shepard (1981) for a more complete survey of the diversity of animal reproduction.

Finally, there are some species where all individuals have only ovaries and produce only eggs. This is called parthenogenetic reproduction. (The word comes from the Greek words *parthenos*, meaning virgin, and *genesis*, meaning birth.) In some of these all-female species, such as the Amazon molly, the popular aquarium fish, sperm from the male of another species is required to activate development, although the sperm's genome is not incorporated into the genome of the offspring. In other parthenogenetic forms (e.g., aphids and whiptail lizards), sperm are not required for complete and normal development.

Still another important distinction in modes of reproduction is the method by which the young are reproduced—viviparity or oviparity. Basically, viviparity ("live-bearing") exists when the young develop within the body of the mother, as in mammals. An important component of viviparity is that nutrients and waste products are exchanged between the mother and the fetus. Oviparous animals are egg-layers. Eggs may be ovulated and laid singly or by the thousands and may or may not have protective shell coverings. Still another reproductive mode, which is believed to have led to viviparity, is called ovoviviparity. In this instance, the fertilized eggs are retained within the body, but there is a reduction in the placental membranes, compared with viviparous animals, and no nutrients are exchanged.

The last distinction to be made is whether fertilization occurs internally or externally. Mammals, birds, and reptiles all practice internal fertilization. The mode of fertilization in amphibians, fish, and sharks and rays varies from species to species. This distinction is important because hormones can have opposite effects in these two modes of fertilization. It is also important because male and female reproductive behaviors, including mating behaviors, can vary dramatically depending whether fertilization is internal or external.

Patterns of Reproduction Among Seasonal Breeders

Multiple patterns of seasonal reproduction exist even within species that have two sexes. As discussed in chapters 4, 5, and 12, many species of animals are seasonal breeders. One important distinction among reproductive patterns depends on whether the animal mates in relation to its seasonal gonadal cycle. If the animal produces and releases its sperm or eggs during the mating season, this is known as an associated reproductive pattern (figure 7.1). If a species produces sperm and eggs at some time other than during the mating season and then stores them until mating occurs, this is known as a dissociated reproductive pattern. A third possibility is when the gonads are maintained continually at or near maximum development, which is known as a constant reproductive pattern; these are the opportunistic breeders referred to in later chapters.

Humans have developed ways to modify the environment and so have become emancipated from many of the factors that have led to seasonal reproduction in other animals. There is evidence, though, of some vestiges of seasonality in humans, which were imposed by periodic variations in food availability and high temperatures (Bronson 1995). For example, there is a seasonal variation in birth rates, and hence in the rate of conception, in Hong Kong, where the low temperatures in January are correlated with a peak in conceptions.

The animal model systems most widely used in behavioral endocrinology are those of the rat, guinea pig, mouse, and hamster. These species, as well as many other mammalian and avian species, exhibit associated reproductive patterns. That is, the periods of sexual behavior are restricted to the periods when the gonads are active. In species exhibiting an associated reproductive pattern, sexual behavior in the male is activated by elevated serum concentrations of testicular steroid hormones (see chapter 5). In the female, it is the pattern and amount of estrogens and progestins produced by the ovary that regulate the periods of sexual receptivity (see chapter 4). In species with dissociated reproductive patterns, breeding activity occurs when the gonads are small and not producing gametes or steroid hormones. In these species, sexual behavior is independent of steroid hormone control but is activated by some other stimulus. Species exhibiting a constant reproductive pattern are always ready to breed, waiting only for a specific environmental cue. In the

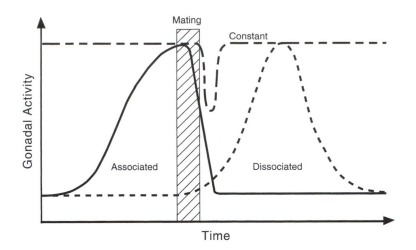

Figure 7.1 Vertebrates display a variety of reproductive patterns. Here gonadal activity is defined as the development of eggs and sperm and/or increased sex steroid hormone secretion. Individuals exhibiting the associated reproductive pattern (solid line) live in temperate regions where seasonal cycles are regular and prolonged; in such species, the gonads are fully developed at the time of mating and circulating levels of sex hormones are maximal. Individuals exhibiting the dissociated reproductive pattern (dashed line) live in extreme environments in which seasonal changes are regular, but the length of time available for breeding is limited; in such species, the gonads are small and sex steroid hormone levels are low at the time of mating. Individuals exhibiting a constant reproductive pattern (hatched line) live in harsh environments where breeding conditions are completely unpredictable; in such species, the gonads are maintained at nearly maximal development so that when breeding conditions do arise, breeding can occur immediately. Just as the reproductive cycles have adapted to the environment, so too have the neuroendocrine mechanisms subserving breeding behavior. The temporal uncoupling of sexual behavior and gonadal recrudescence in vertebrates exhibiting these different reproductive patterns is reflected in the dynamics of their hormone-brain-behavior relationship. *NB*: The dimension of reproductive pattern is depicted as mutually exclusive extremes only for the sake of argument; intermediate forms are known to exist. (Adapted from Crews 1984.)

Australian outback, the zebra finch will begin to court and build nests within minutes of the first drops of rain.

Another pattern of reproduction is determined by whether ovulation is spontaneous or induced (conaway 1971). In many animals, gonadal activity is initiated by environmental changes that occurred many weeks or months earlier (see later discussion). Once initiated, the eggs develop and are released spontaneously at a particular time regardless of whether or not mating occurs. This is known as spontaneous ovulation. In other animals, however, mating activity actually induces ovulation or, in some, gonadal growth. Cats and rabbits are examples of animals that are behaviorally receptive during the breeding season but do not ovulate unless mated. As discussed in chapter 4, experiments have shown that the act of copulation in cats and rabbits enables a neuroendocrine reflex that results in luteinizing hormone (LH) release by the pituitary and consequently ovulation. Other animals show even more extreme variations. In the ferret and the mink, the eggs do not undergo final maturation nor does ovulation ever occur unless the female experiences the violent precopulatory behavior of the male in which he energetically throws her about. In the musk shrew and the red-sided garter snake, ovarian activity is not even initiated unless the female is first courted and mated.

Some of the Evolutionary Forces Leading to the Reproductive Modes and Patterns Displayed by Animals Today

A successful approach to investigating and making sense of diversity in the neuroendocrinology of reproduction is to look for generalities across species. The comparative method is the traditional approach in biological investigations. It has been shown repeatedly that a comparison of various organisms leads to discoveries of themes or traits that recur throughout all animals. Traits are any property of the organism that a scientist is interested in measuring. When closely related species are compared, it becomes possible to trace the progressive specialization of traits and thus illuminate the course of evolution.

But simply comparing various species, populations, individuals, and even genes without concern for their shared history is not scientifically or statistically valid. New statistical methods known as evolutionary or phylogenetic analyses make it possible to estimate these historical relationships among any set of morphological, behavioral, or molecular data, and then depict these relationships in the form of a branching diagram, known as a phylogenetic tree (Hillis et al. 1996; Ryan 1996; Thorton 2001). For example, DeVoogd et al. (1993) compared the song and the structure of certain brain areas involved in song production (see chapter 8) among 41 species of songbirds. They found a significant correlation between the relative volume of a song-control nucleus known as the high vocal center (HVC) and the size of the species' song repertoire. Further, their analysis suggested that behavioral changes preceded brain changes; that is, selection for an enhanced song repertoire augmented the volume of the HVC.

While it is important to know what is present, it is equally important to know what might occur but is not present. For example, in table 7.1, we see that there apparently are no examples of hermaphroditic or parthenogenetic viviparous species practicing external fertilization. What is absent usually reflects a basic and sometimes insurmountable conflict among constraints or limitations inherent in the environment, development, or evolutionary history of an organism. When we understand such constraints, we can account for observed differences and, whatever the cause, predict what might be found in certain circumstances. Such an understanding can also suggest what is unlikely or has not evolved in our world.

Four concepts can guide you as you learn about these evolutionary forces. The first considers the evolutionary underpinnings of sexual behavior: did they emerge from forces that facilitated reproduction between individuals or from forces that prevented individuals from breeding? The second concerns the distinction between natural selection and sexual selection. The third describes the nature of the constraints that have shaped the evolution of reproductive processes. The fourth is the importance of individual variation and the concept of phenotypic plasticity.

REPRODUCTIVE SYNERGISM VERSUS REPRODUCTIVE ISOLATION

In an evolutionary sense, reproduction is the single most important element in an individual's life. It is more important even than the length of an individual's survival. Simply put, and with rare exceptions, if an individual does not reproduce, its genes will not be represented in future generations.

Reproduction has been host to the evolution of many specialized behaviors. Detailed analyses indicate that in many species, behaviors associated with reproduction tend to be highly ritualized, stereotyped, and characteristic of a species. We assume that individuals exhibiting these behaviors left more offspring. However, although they have both focused on sexual behaviors, behavioral endocrinologists and evolutionary biologists have traditionally viewed the function of sexual behaviors differently. Traditionally, behavioral endocrinologists have emphasized the fact that reproductive behaviors serve to coordinate the events that lead to successful reproduction, and evolutionary biologists have emphasized the fact that reproductive behaviors serve to isolate a species. This gulf has narrowed recently as we have learned more about mating and its consequences.

The position that reproductive behaviors have evolved to coordinate hormonal, gonadal, and behavioral events is known as *reproductive synergism*. Proponents of this position point out that reproduction is a carefully regulated process. Each successive phase of reproduction is dependent upon preceding events. At the same time, each phase sets the stage for what follows (figure 7.2). Reproduction occurs only when the participants send and receive appropriate visual, auditory, chemical, seismic, ultrasonic, or electrical signals (see chapter 8). This results in the appropriate coordination of the maturation and release of each individual's gametes (eggs and sperm) in an effort to increase their reproductive success.

The position that reproductive behaviors evolved to keep species from interbreeding is known as *reproductive isolation*. Proponents of this position hold that species-typical sexual behaviors serve as reproductive isolating mechanisms to maintain species boundaries. If individuals from different species do mate, fertilization will not occur. If fertilization does occur, viable offspring often will not result because the egg lacks the necessary sets of compatible chromosomes required for normal growth and development. Even when the species are closely related, indicating a recent (in an evolutionary time scale) divergence, the young produced tend to be sterile.

Recently there has been a shift in evolutionary biology away from the isolationist perspective (Carson 1987). The argument is that if evolution favors reproductive success, then it is more in the individual's interest to focus on selecting the best mate than to avoid mating with the wrong species. Further, the act of mating is only the beginning of a complex process in which the

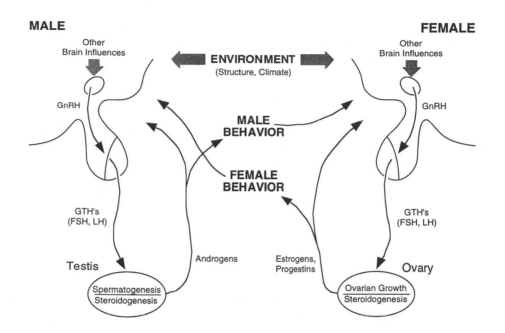

Figure 7.2   Dynamic relationship between the internal and external environments in the control of mating behavior in vertebrates. The complementary behavior of the male and the female help to synchronize the maturation and release of the sperm and eggs so that fertilization occurs. Changes in climate, ecology, or behavior of other members of the species initiate and modulate gonadal and hormonal changes during reproduction. Thus, hormones regulate behavior in the individual animal and are themselves affected by other stimuli, including the behavior and, indirectly, the physiology of its mate. In such reciprocal systems, each successive phase of reproduction depends upon preceding events and, at the same time, sets the stage for the following phase. (See figures 1.9 and 1.10 for details of hypothalamus-pituitary-gonadal axis.)

male's intromission and insemination induce behavioral and physiological responses in the female that increase the likelihood that his sperm will fertilize her eggs (Eberhard 1996).

NATURAL SELECTION VERSUS SEXUAL SELECTION

Darwin considered natural selection and sexual selection as different processes. Both are primary forces driving the evolution of traits. For our purposes, natural selection results in traits that are adaptational responses to changes in the environment. The resulting variation in traits between and within species is shaped by differential survivorship. In other words, animals that survive are those with traits that are adaptive to their environment (Williams 1966).

Sexual selection, in its simplest form, states that males compete for females and females choose between them. Most of the research in this field today focuses on how females choose males on the basis of the morphological and/or behavioral characteristics they display. Female choice continues after intromission with a host of physiological, morphological, and behavioral hurdles that continue to evaluate male quality, enabling the female to maximize the genetic contribution of desirable mates. It is, of course, even more complicated in that females compete among themselves for males as well as for resources. Natural selection and sexual selection often act in opposite directions on male traits, favoring, for instance, drabber plumage (natural selection) on the one hand and showier plumage (sexual selection) on the other.

Sexual selection has led to the evolution of extravagant sex-linked coloration, ornamentation, and behaviors with no apparent function in the struggle for survival. Such traits are often sexually dimorphic. Males tend to develop specific traits that are involved in courtship or mating and occur during the breeding season. In this instance, individual variation in these traits is sculpted by differential reproductive success (Clutton-Brock 1988). Indeed, we will see how this variation can reflect different neuroendocrine mechanisms or even serve as the substrate for the evolution of novel mechanisms. The number of offspring an individual produces during its lifetime will determine whether this trait is continued in the species. Thus, "Sexual selection is responsible for most of the morphological, physiological, and behavioral characters that are observed as subserving the efficiency of the reproductive act as an important monitor of fitness" (Carson 1987, 598).

Darwin conceived of sexual selection as arising from aggressive interactions between males (male-male competition) and the female's selection of a mate (mate choice). Males compete among themselves for access to females. A variety of traits, such as antlers, horns, and tusks, have evolved as a result of male-male antagonism as they compete for access to a female's eggs.

Aggression between males can have a direct effect on female reproduction. It will prevent other breeding males from having access to a female or from harming the female. Aggression among males can also have an indirect effect. It can inhibit or suppress the normal reproductive physiology of the female (figure 7.3) or even terminate a pregnancy. Mate selection may also be based on the availability of a particular resource such as food. Thus, in many species, females choose real estate and males compete to control access to that real estate.

At least three competing variants of the natural selection hypothesis have been offered for the evolution of female preference (Kirkpatrick and Ryan 1991), each of which emphasizes that females choosing optimally will produce young whose viability and survivorship are enhanced by the choice. The "good genes" explanation suggests that a female benefits by mating with a particular male that has traits that enhance survivorship, thereby imparting these benefits to her young. In this case, the quality of the male's displays is assumed to reflect the individual male's genetic constitution. A second variant of the natural selection hypothesis is the "handicap principle," which postulates that females favor males with "expensive" traits. These are traits that put the male at greater risk of predation or have greater energetic cost. It is reasoned that males that can exhibit elaborate traits have a greater handicap and therefore must be more fit than males with less developed traits.

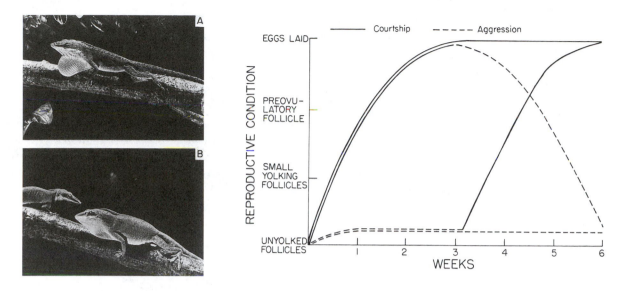

Figure 7.3 Different behaviors can stimulate or inhibit reproduction. In the left panel are pictures of male green anole lizards performing a courtship display (*A*) and an aggressive display (*B*). Note the differences in body posture. In the right panel, we see how the courtship display facilitates ovarian growth in female green anoles, whereas the aggressive posture inhibits ovarian growth. In this experiment, females were exposed to the courtship or aggression stimulus for the entire 6 weeks, or for 3 weeks and then the stimulus switched for the next 3 weeks.

Finally, a relatively recent variant is the "parasite load" idea. If a male is parasitized, the breeding plumage is dull rather than brilliant. This idea suggests that brighter coloration or some other elaborate trait is associated with a genetic resistance to deleterious parasites. Thus, females choose brighter, more colorful males because this coloration indicates heritable disease resistance that can be passed on to their young. In all three forms of the natural selection hypothesis, male traits are regarded as being indicative of high genetic quality. Female preference is thought to evolve because of advantages her offspring acquire as a result of the female mating with these males.

The sexual selection hypothesis has two main variants. One is Fisher's runaway sexual selection hypothesis. In this paradigm, male traits that influence mate choice become genetically correlated with female preference by virtue of the mating system; that is, the gene(s) for the trait is linked to the gene(s) for the preference. As the traits increase in frequency, the preference for the trait passively increases in the female. Thus, females do not gain directly from choosing particular males. Rather, the preference evolves as a correlated response to selection of the male trait.

A more recent variant of the sexual selection hypothesis that attempts to account for the evolution of female preferences is that of sensory exploitation. Ryan (Ryan 1990; Ryan et al. 1990) has pointed out that sensory systems are predisposed to specific stimuli. For example, as you will see in chapter 8, the frog auditory system is tuned to certain frequencies and female frogs prefer certain qualities in the call of males. The sensory exploitation hypothesis postulates that males have evolved calls to exploit preexisting sensory biases in the female that evolved for reasons independent of female mate choice.

The latter two hypotheses present different scenarios for the evolution of behavior-controlling mechanisms. Fisher's runaway selection hypothesis presumes a genetic linkage between male traits and female preferences, so that changes in the female are a passive function of changes in the male. The sensory exploitation hypothesis predicts that preference in the female is determined by various constraints and that male behavior has changed to maximize stimulation of the female's sensory systems. Whatever the evolutionary reason, the act of choosing the correct mate is of utmost importance. We will see how in birds the compatibility of mates has a dramatic effect on whether or not young are produced.

CONSTRAINTS ON REPRODUCTION

You have learned that sexual behavior in vertebrates is dependent on gonadal steroid hormones for its activation. However, as we will see, this conclusion stems primarily from the species that have been studied. It does not reflect a universal truth. Indeed, species differences in hormone-behavior relations can often be traced to adaptational responses to the physical and social environments. This is because reproduction is constrained by (1) the immediate environment, (2) limitations inherent in developmental and physiological processes, (3) the social and behavioral context, and (4) evolutionary history.

Environmental Constraints

The evolution of reproductive seasons is determined by factors selecting against those individuals bearing young during times of food scarcity or other adverse environmental conditions. Individuals that produce young during optimum conditions have been favorably selected. In other words, these individuals were most likely to reproduce and pass on their genes to the next generation. This has been termed the *ultimate* cause of breeding seasons. Ultimate factors that determine the timing of breeding seasons include adequate food, availability of nesting materials, and predation pressure. *Proximate* causation refers to those stimuli used by the organism to actually initiate and terminate breeding. Well-known examples of proximate factors are seasonal fluctuations in day length, temperature, moisture, and so on. The responsiveness of the neuroendocrine system to proximate cues may vary seasonally. This seasonal variation probably reflects endogenous circadian and circannual rhythms (see chapter 12).

Environmental constraints on reproduction are especially severe when the environment is harsh. For animals living in a harsh environment there is only a brief favorable period for reproduction. Under these conditions, animals must respond rapidly and directly to physical changes in order to mate. The female must respond rapidly in order to reproduce. The young must grow sufficiently to survive the upcoming harsh conditions. These species exhibit an explosive or opportunistic pattern of reproduction in which all breeding activity is compressed into a few days or weeks.

Developmental and Physiological Constraints

Developmental and physiological processes may also dictate when animals breed. These processes can shape the mechanisms controlling reproduction. For example, mature sperm in most species cannot be produced in less than 6 weeks. Although some mice and ground squirrels can produce mature sperm in as little as 31 days, they appear to be the only exceptions to this rule. A similar time constraint applies to the production of eggs, although some small rodents are capable of generating eggs in less than a week. In cold-blooded vertebrates, it is common for egg maturation to take many months or even years.

A second constraint is the temperature-dependence of gonadal activity. Gamete production and steroid hormone secretion will not occur at cold temperatures. This presents a problem for many animals that live at high altitudes or latitudes. For these animals, mating must occur as early in the spring as possible so that young can be born and grow enough to survive the next winter. Some species produce sperm during the summer and then store them through the winter. In this way, the male is able to inseminate females immediately on emergence from hibernation. In many bats, sperm storage lasts for several months, but in some reptiles it can be as long as 17 years. Seasonally high temperatures can also inhibit reproduction, which occurs in humans living in equatorial regions where spermatogenesis is sufficiently suppressed to influence the incidence of fertilization (Bronson 1995).

In many mammals, including some species of bears, the western spotted skunk, and kangaroos, implantation of the embryo is delayed. The embryo goes into a kind of suspended animation called embryonic diapause that can last for as little as one week or as long as several years. At the end of diapause, the embryo implants and development resumes. In other species, particularly cold-blooded vertebrates, there simply is not enough time available in one season for gametes to grow, adults to mate, and the young to develop. Cold-blooded animals, or ectotherms, rely more on the external environment for temperature regulation, whereas mammals and birds, often called warm-blooded animals or endotherms, rely on metabolic energy to produce and maintain an elevated body temperature. This can be an arbitrary distinction, however, as many ectotherms, such as honeybees and lizards, can maintain elevated body temperatures by behavioral means.

Warm-blooded animals living at high altitudes or latitudes typically migrate to warmer areas or hibernate for the duration of the cold months. In those species that hibernate, such as small rodents, it was long a puzzle how males could enter hibernation with small testes but emerge with large testes. Recently, it has been discovered that animals such as Turkish hamsters periodically arouse from hibernation, warming up for a few hours or days. It is during these arousals that the gonads grow. Cold-blooded animals living in extreme environments, however, do not exhibit periodic arousals, nor do they show any signs of gonadal growth during the cold winter months. In these animals, it is common for gamete growth and steroid secretion to be temporally dissociated from breeding activities.

The embryonic environment may also represent a constraint, shaping an individual's physiology, body, and even intellect. In some mammals, the position of the fetus relative to siblings in utero or its intrauterine position can mold morphology, reproductive physiology, and sociosexual behavior in adulthood (Clark and Galef 1995). In gerbils, mice, and rats, female fetuses located between two males (2M females) are exposed to higher levels of androgens produced by the neighboring males than female fetuses located between two females (2F females) (see chapter 13). As adults, 2M females have lower estradiol and higher testosterone levels in the circulation, have a masculinized phenotype, and are less attractive to males and more aggressive to females. 2M females also produce litters with more male-biased sex ratios relative to 2F females. Additionally, 2M females have later onsets of estrous cycles, longer estrous cycles, shorter reproductive lives, and fewer litters. Differences in phenotype due to intrauterine position are also evident in males. Males positioned next to two males (2M males) are more aggressive and more sexually active than are males positioned next to two females (2F males). It should be noted, however, that the pattern of intrauterine effects is not necessarily consistent across species. For example, in gerbils 2M males outcompete their 2F counterparts in reproductive success, whereas in mice 2F males are more sexually active than are their 2M brothers.

A mechanism by which intrauterine position may affect or constrain reproduction is by altering brain metabolism in specific brain areas. A convenient measure of metabolic activity of brain nuclei is cytochrome oxidase histochemistry.[1] In gerbils, the metabolic capacity in the sexually dimorphic area of the preoptic area (SDA-POA) and the posterior portion of the anterior hypothalamus is greater in 2M than 2F females. In gerbils, the SDA-POA is responsible for copulatory behavior in males, and the posterior portion of the anterior hypothalamus is an area replete with neurons containing gonadotropin-releasing hormone. These differences in metabolic capacity may explain, respectively, the behavioral and hormonal masculinization of 2M females relative to 2F females.

First noted by Aristotle, the female spotted hyena in many ways resembles the male; in fact, it is larger, more aggressive, and more dominant. Most remarkable, however, is that the female's clitoris is so hypertrophied that it resembles the male's penis. This unique pattern of female urogenital development results from the increased production of androstenedione from the mother's ovaries during pregnancy, which in turn is transformed to testosterone in the placenta and subsequently transported to the fetus (Glickman et al. 1997).

There is no doubt that the early environment plays a profound role in health in humans. It has long been recognized that malnutrition during pregnancy influences the subsequent growth, cognitive ability, and immune system of offspring, dictating even the length of life. For example, the circulating levels of androgen and sex hormone binding globulin during the mother's pregnancy may also have an organizing effect on both the hormone profiles and psychosocial test scores of young adult women (Udry et al. 1995). In this remarkable study, a substantial portion of the variance in the women's "gendered" behavior was accounted for by measurements of androgen exposure during only the mid-trimester of development and of the circulating levels of androgen as adults. Then there is the curious property of the cochlea whereby it produces spontaneous otoacoustic emissions. In general, human females produce more emissions than males (McFadden 1997). The prenatal environment influences the frequency of these emissions. The sexual dimorphism is not evident in the female of opposite-sex fraternal twins, suggesting that the hormonal environment created by the male fetus decreases these emissions in the female co-twin. Finally, through meta-analysis of published twin studies, it was demonstrated that the environment in utero might play a significant role in the heritability of IQ (Devlin et al. 1997).

What about animals that lay eggs rather than gestate the young internally? The yolk produced by the female that supports embryonic development is full of hormones (Bern 1990). In birds, the hormonal profile of the female is reflected in the yolk; hence, during the early stages of follicular growth, when androgens and estrogens are the dominant steroid hormones in the systemic circulation of the female, these hormones occur in the highest concentrations in the initial layers of yolk deposition. During the final stages of follicular growth and immediately after ovulation as the egg enters into the oviduct to get its shell coat, progesterone levels are highest, and this hormone is in higher concentrations in the outer layers. Thus, how the yolk is utilized by the growing embryo—from the outside in, or from the inside out—becomes an important question.

Hormone content can also change through egg laying. In canaries and zebra finches, eggs laid later have higher testosterone levels than eggs laid earlier; this, in turn, correlates positively with the subsequent growth and social rank of the individual. This is believed to be a way in which the younger, weaker hatchlings can compete with their older nestlings. In the cattle egret, however, it is the earliest egg that has the highest level of testosterone. In this instance, the oldest chick will evict the younger, weaker chick from the nest when resources are limited.

Females also appear to be able to control the amount of hormones in their eggs. Female zebra finches prefer to mate with males that have red leg bands (as discussed earlier, this appears to be related to the fact that the intensity of the male's red beak is related to his circulating concentration of androgens). Females that chose males with red leg bands had greater amounts of androgens in their eggs. Since more androgens in the yolk result in more aggressive offspring, a female's mate choice may indirectly (via hormones) influence the reproductive success of her offspring.

Finally, the experiences of the female while pregnant or even the behavior of the mother toward the neonate can influence how the individual grows and behaves. Indeed, 40 years ago it was discovered that the adverse effects of crowding mice during pregnancy can continue to be detected in the physiology and behavior of the following two generations of progeny. Handling pregnant females or housing them in socially unstable conditions can induce similar stress effects. The attention paid by the mother to her young is also important in behavioral development. For example, mother rats behave differently toward male and female pups; furthermore these differences reinforce and accentuate subsequent sex differences when the pup reaches adulthood (Moore 1995).

Social and Behavioral Constraints

As described in chapter 11, stress can have a profound negative effect on reproduction. Crowding, social domination, and captivity can effectively inhibit reproduction. On the other hand, specific social conditions or behaviors can also stimulate reproduction. Research with species representing every vertebrate class has shown that certain behaviors are necessary for the proper stimulation of the physiological changes that must occur in reproduction. For example, in ring doves and in green anole lizards (figure 7.3), the courtship behavior of the male is required if the ovaries of the female are to grow. Indeed, the rate of ovarian growth is determined by how much male courtship behavior the female sees. The male's aggressive behavior has the opposite effect and inhibits ovarian growth (Crews 1975).

Evolutionary Constraints

The evolutionary history, or phylogeny, of the species is another constraint predisposing the evolution of certain mechanisms and not others. Simply put, what has come before determines to a large extent what will follow. We might predict, therefore, that closely related species sharing a similar reproductive pattern but living in different environments will exhibit similarities in the neuroendocrine mechanisms underlying their modes of reproduction.

An example of this can be found in the garter snake (*Thamnophis*), a large genus believed to have radiated into the New World after crossing the Bering Strait. All garter snake species that have been examined to date, even those living in Mexico, exhibit a dissociated reproductive pattern and probably exhibit the same neuroendocrine mechanisms controlling mating behavior. We might also predict that distantly related species living together and facing similar challenges would have similarities in the neuroendocrine mechanisms controlling mating behavior. For example, most vertebrates that originated in the tropics but presently live in temperate regions exhibit an associated reproductive pattern. Thus, constraints imposed by both the external and internal environments of a species influence its social displays and their physiological consequences.

GENETIC RECOMBINATION AND PHENOTYPIC PLASTICITY

We are all individuals and, ultimately, evolution is the consequence of the behavior of individuals. Individuality is a product of sexual recombination; in all instances, with the single exception of the blue-green algae or cyano-bacteria, present-day asexual organisms arose from sexual organisms. But sex is costly compared to asexual reproduction. There are a number of reasons for this (Maynard Smith 1978), but in terms of the growth of a population, meiotic recombination can disrupt co-adapted combinations and, in organisms where eggs and sperm combine, *halves* the rate of reproduction. Why then is sex so common? Recent studies on sexual and asexual populations of yeast reveal that the sexual yeast are more efficient at removing deleterious mutations than asexual yeast (Zeyl and Bell 997).

The "selfish gene" hypothesis posits that the fundamental struggle of evolution takes place not among individuals but at the level of the gene, and that behavior, physiology, morphology, and indeed every somatic cell exist only to promote the successful maintenance and dispersal of an individual's genes (Dawkins 1976). Genes, however, require a vehicle, the organism, to go through time. Genetic replication is accomplished in virtually all organisms (but see below for instructive exceptions) by sexual reproduction. Reproductive success can be defined as the successful reproduction of offspring, or grandchildren. Thus, it is not so much survival of the individual organism as the continuity of its genes that matters in evolution.

Phenotype is a concept that describes the constellation of morphological, physiological, and behavioral traits that, when considered together, characterize the individual. Thus, the phenotype refers to aspects of an individual's behavior, brain, body parts, physiology, or organs at any given time. We have come to appreciate that the phenotype can change throughout different stages of an individual's life history and that every genotype can yield a variety of phenotypes.

Phenotypic plasticity refers to the process by which the internal and external environments induce different phenotypes from a given genotype (Piglucci 1996). An example of phenotypic plasticity can be found in amphibians (Denver 1997). Probably the most important environmental variable for a tadpole is water availability, and frogs living in deserts accelerate metamorphosis as the ponds created by seasonal rains dry up. This is an adaptive response to the risk of mortality. As the water level falls, the brain produces corticotropin-releasing hormone, the primary vertebrate stress neurohormone. This in turn activates the thyroid and interrenal endocrine systems that control metamorphosis.

Survey of Diversity in Hormone-Behavior Relations

The Importance of Mate Compatibility

Making the correct choice of a mate can have a definite impact on a female's reproductive success. This is seen particularly well in long-lived species where it has been possible to monitor an individual's lifetime reproductive success. For example, for the past 35 years, Coulson has studied a colony of kittiwake gulls. These gulls nest on the windowsills of a riverside warehouse in Northumberland, England. In many instances, they pair for life. Other kittiwakes, however, choose a different mate the next breeding season. In about half of the pairs that break up, mates are changed because the original partner has died. In the other half, pairs of kittywakes "divorce." The cause of divorce can be traced to the failure of the pair to hatch at least one egg the preceding year. Not only do successful pairs fledge more young, but they also produce eggs faster, indicating that females in these pairs reach breeding condition earlier (Thomas and Coulson 1988).

Bluhm (1985) has studied the reproductive consequences of pair incompatibility using canvasback ducks. The reproductive success of females that were allowed to stay with their self-chosen partner was compared with the reproductive success of females that were separated from their self-chosen partner and paired with another male chosen at random. The results were clear-cut. Only females from pairs with self-selected males laid eggs. A similar situation was found in the cockatiel where reproductive success was enhanced if females were allowed to choose a mate as opposed to being forcibly paired with a male (Yamamoto et al. 1989).

Bluhm also pioneered an exciting new area of research in behavioral endocrinology that includes the endocrine correlates of mate compatibility. She has found that the female canvasbacks from forced pairings lack specific hormone changes (Bluhm et al. 1984). We know from research with other vertebrates, including humans, that copulation can trigger changes in circulating hormone levels, which can promote sperm transport and implantation. Courtship stimulation can result in more rapid ovarian growth in animals such as ring doves and green anole lizards. Thus, behavior-physiology interactions are an important aspect of neuroendocrine relations. You will learn more about this subject in chapter 18.

Mixed Reproductive Strategies

If environmental, physiological, social, and phylogenetic constraints can influence reproductive processes (like when the gametes are produced), it is likely that the neuroendocrine mechanisms controlling each of these processes must have undergone corresponding adaptations. What evidence is there for this?

First, recall the associated and dissociated reproductive patterns described earlier. Although we know a good deal about the neuroendocrinology of sexual behavior in species exhibiting associated reproductive patterns, we know next to nothing about these mechanisms in species that exhibit dissociated reproductive patterns. This deficit has occurred because scientists have concentrated almost exclusively on species which have associated reproductive patterns. Indeed, even in those species in which we know that gonadal growth is associated with mating, we often do not know whether it is the cause or the

Table 7.2 Reproductive Strategies in Gonochoristic Vertebrates

		MALE	
		Associated	*Dissociated*
FEMALE	*Associated*	Many laboratory and domesticated mammals; most birds; many temperate and tropical lizards, crocodilians	Most temperate turtles and tortoises, Indian lizard, timber rattlesnake, rough earth snake; tiger salamander; pike
	Dissociated	Musk shrew; Arctic fulmar; Mexican spiny lizard, Australian skink, mole skink, leaf-toed gecko, European viper, eastern coral snake; shiner perch, catfish	Hibernating bats; several rattlesnake spp., cobra, and harmless North American snakes; plaice, common carp

Gonadal activity may be temporally associated or dissociated from mating behavior in each sex. The result is a reproductive strategy in which the sexes have the same or different reproductive patterns.

consequence of the mating behavior. The importance of this point should not be underestimated. As you have already learned, in a variety of species, mating can initiate gonadal activity in the female or in the male. In other species, copulatory stimuli are known to be responsible for the final stages of gamete development or for successful fertilization or implantation of the fertilized embryo.

If we consider just these two patterns alone, it is possible to discern four basic reproductive patterns in vertebrates (table 7.2). In most domesticated species, both the male and the female have an associated reproductive pattern. There also are a number of species in which both sexes exhibit a dissociated reproductive pattern. However, there are some species in which the sexes exhibit a mixed reproductive pattern. In these species, one of two things can happen. The male can produce sperm before breeding and store them until mating occurs. Alternatively, mating occurs and the female stores the sperm in her reproductive tract for later use. In this instance, the act of mating initiates gonadal growth in the female.

Those species that have mixed reproductive patterns hold great promise for untangling ecological and evolutionary forces on reproductive behavior. That is, in species exhibiting mixed reproductive patterns, different selection forces must have caused the sexes to differ in fundamental ways in the organization and activation of behavior-controlling mechanisms. For example, Rissman (1995) discovered that in the Asian musk shrew, mating behavior in the male coincides with testicular growth and is activated by increasing testicular androgen secretion. In the female, however, receptivity precedes ovarian growth and is independent of estrogen from the ovary. Instead of a behavioral estrus cycle such as occurs in rodents, female musk shrews become receptive and allow mating within minutes of their encounter with a male. The female's receptivity is regulated by testosterone secreted by the adrenal glands and the ovaries and which, in turn, is converted in the POA to estrogen in the neurons that produce the enzyme aromatase.

Different reproductive strategies can also be found within the same sex of a single species. A recent discovery suggests that individuals within a species may differ fundamentally in neuroendocrine-controlling mechanisms. For example, in several rodent species, researchers have found that individuals within a population may utilize different proximate cues for regulating gonadal activity. Photoperiod may be important in some individuals; in others, it may be temperature or food (Bronson 1989; Prendergast 2001). Individual differences in the required proximate cue can be adaptive, resulting in a fine-tuning of reproduction in the population in response to its environment.

A recent discovery in behavioral ecology is that individuals within a given population may adopt distinctly different physiologies, morphologies, or behaviors. These are termed alternative life-history strategies. In some species these alternative life history strategies are heritable, whereas in others they appear to arise from social or environmental conditions. For example, there are three types of male bluegill sunfish: a large colorful male that defends territories and solicits females, a small male that sneaks matings when the territorial male is otherwise occupied, and a large but drab male that mimics females in appearance (Gross 1984). The sneaker steals fertilizations by streaking in to release sperm as the female releases her eggs. The female mimics effectively insert themselves between a courting territorial male and the female he is courting; in this manner the female is courted by the male but it is the mimic that fertilizes the eggs. Developmental and genetic studies indicate that sneakers grow up into female mimics, whereas territorial males produce male young that are large and brightly colored. Circulating concentrations of androgens differ in the different types of male bluegill sunfish, with androgen levels being higher in territorial males than in sneakers or in female-mimics (Kindier et al. 1989).

Many fish are hermaphroditic. Some have testicular and ovarian tissue simultaneously and trade behavioral roles during the spawning act (simultaneous hermaphrodite). Others undergo a sex change during life (sequential hermaphrodites). There are two basic types of sequential hermaphrodites. Protogynous individuals mature and reproduce first as females and then, as they age, turn into males. Protandrous individuals develop and reproduce first as males, and then later turn into females. A third type, continual sex change, was recently described in the Okinawan goby. In this species the individual functions first as a female, changes into a functional male, and then reverts to a female, repeating this process over and over again. This latter pattern is functionally equivalent to simultaneously hermaphroditic species in that individuals alternate their behavior and the type of gamete that is shed in successive matings. How they differ is that in continual sex change, the gonads undergo a complete morphological change, producing exclusively the gonad-typical gamete during each successive phase, whereas in simultaneous hermaphroditism, the gonads are ovotestes.

Behavioral endocrinologists have begun to study these unusual reproductive systems. It was believed originally that the behavioral changes observed in sex-changing fish were a consequence of the changes in the gonads or their hormonal products. Yet experiments with a variety of protandric and protogynic coral reef fish consistently yielded negative results. That is, while administration of steroid hormones will cause a morphological sex change, it takes weeks for this transformation to be completed. Yet in nature, sex change is primarily under social control and can be induced experimentally by removing the dominant TP males from small reef populations. Within minutes of removal of the dominant male, the largest female will begin to behave as a male, aggressively defending the coral head and soliciting other females. It is only many days later that the morphological changes in the gonad are observed and some days after that, the physiological changes. In other words, approximately two weeks after a female takes over the male role, the ovaries are transformed into testes.

Recently this assumption that the gonads drive sex change has been turned on its head. The protogynous bluehead wrasse has two alternative male mating morphs. Females and one adult male morph are light yellow with a dark dorsal stripe (initial phase or IP coloration) and are not territorial or aggressive. Terminal phase males (TP males) are brightly colored with blue heads, green over most of the body, and a vertical white bar bordered by black bars just posterior to pectoral fin insertion. TP males exhibit territorial aggression in defense of spawning sites, as well as distinctive courtship behaviors. During an afternoon spawning period, females travel to spawning sites, usually coral heads. If the site is defended, the TP male will court the female and the pair will mate. If the spawning site is undefended, the female will mate with a group of IP males. Mating consists of a rapid ascent called a "spawning rush"; eggs are released at the apex of this rush, and the fish quickly return to the bottom. Females spawn approximately two out of every three days, while successful TP males spawn 30 to 50 times per day on average.

Godwin et al. (1996) conducted a study in which the largest bluehead female in a group was ovariectomized and the dominant male was removed all in the same morning. Surprisingly, the female would still exhibit all of the behavioral and color changes that typically follow the removal of the dominant male. Indeed, even though these neutered females do not shed gametes, they entice other females to spawn with them. In almost all instances, this occurred immediately, just as they would occur when an intact female assumed the dominant role and defended a coral head. Further studies indicate that the transcript of the gene coding for arginine vasotocin changes in parallel with these behavioral changes. When considered together with the experiments with the unisexual whiptail lizard that will be detailed later, it is clear that sexuality resides in the brain and not in the gonad.

If the social or environmental stimuli are transduced in the brain, how then is the information transferred to the gonads? There are afferent and efferent neural connections between the gonad and the brain in vertebrates, including hermaphroditic fish, that are important to reproduction. Electrical stimulation of these circuits in a simultaneous hermaphroditic sea bass results in sperm or egg release, whereas in some other species, denervation leads to atrophy of the gonads. Further, the steroidogenic cells in the gonad are themselves directly innervated, and electrical stimulation of appropriate brain regions can either increase or decrease gonadal steroid secretion. That sex steroid hormones will functionally sex-reverse fish (albeit over a prolonged time period) and that the steroidogenic cells are in close proximity with the gonial cells in the gonad suggest that an individual's perception or psychology, combined with a fundamental requirement of behavioral complementarity (see below), mediate the behavioral role an individual adopts (in a simultaneous hermaphrodite) or drives the process of sex-change (in a sequential hermaphrodite) (Crews 1993).

Proximate Stimuli Activating Sexual Behavior

We know that for a number of vertebrates the steroid hormones secreted by the active gonads are necessary for sexual behavior. This elevated concentration of gonadal steroid hormones is required if proximate stimuli such as the behavior or scent of another individual or some change in the environment are to release sexual activity. In these animals, the sex hormones are altering the perceptions of the individual and stimuli take on new meanings (Beach 1983). Other organisms, however, have circumvented this reliance on gonadal steroid hormones. Instead, they rely solely on various proximate cues to activate sexual behavior. Here we will mention some examples of this by considering first the environment as a source of critical stimuli. We will then consider animals in which the behavior or tactile stimuli provided by members of the opposite sex initiate sexual behavior. Finally, we will learn how chemical signals, or pheromones, can trigger complex sexual behavior in vertebrates.

ENVIRONMENTAL STIMULI

If mating behavior can occur when the circulating concentrations of sex steroid hormones are low, does another stimulus activate sexual behavior? In species inhabiting extreme environments and that are opportunistic breeders, the use of other stimuli is apparent. Physiological constraints have led to specific stimuli being co-opted as proximate triggers for sexual behavior. We have mentioned the desert-dwelling zebra finch in which the male maintains mature sperm and high androgen levels throughout the year. Similarly, the female's ovaries contain developed ova at all times. In the deserts of western Australia, rain may occur only once in a three-year period. The falling rain initiates reproductive behavior in the zebra finch. Within 10 minutes after rain begins falling, the zebra finch begins copulating. Nest are built within 4 hours. Eggs are laid within a week. Thus, although the androgen-dependence of sexual behavior in adult male zebra finches is well established, androgens may play only a permissive role. That is, the ability of rainfall to activate sexual behavior depends upon the priming effect of androgen. While considerable research has been conducted on the reproductive behavior and biology of zebra finches, in all the studies on their mating behavior, water has been freely available. Thus, although it is likely that the specialized adaptation to water in the zebra finch will be reflected in the neuroendocrine-controlling mechanisms, this water hypothesis remains to be tested experimentally.

SOCIAL STIMULI

Wingfield has shown that endocrine profiles associated with mating are specific to the social system of a number of species of birds (Wingfield et al. 1990). This probably reflects important differences in the neuroendocrinology of these birds. For example, in species of birds in which one male pairs with one female to help to feed its young (monogamy), the male exhibits only a brief period of high levels of testosterone when territories are being established in the spring. In species in which males pair with two or more females and do not help feed the offspring (polygyny), the male maintains high testosterone levels and remains aggressive throughout the breeding season. When testosterone was administered to males so that high testosterone levels were maintained, males from monogamous species became polygynous in their behavior.

Social context is also important in sexual behavior and its consequences. Behaviorists interested in mating systems focused initially on male sexual and aggressive behaviors. This was supplanted by investigations of female choice of males and, most recently, has developed into studies of how a female's social rank relates to her reproductive success. For example, dominant female chimpanzees have a disproportionate share of quality resources and, in turn, tend to reproduce more frequently and wean their offspring faster (Pusey et al. 1997).

CHEMICAL STIMULI

Another example of diversity in the hormone-behavior relations concerns the relationship between hormones and chemical signals or pheromones. The original definition of hormones emphasized internal communication and the definition of pheromones emphasized external communication. However, this distinction is blurring as scientists discover that some hormones may also function as pheromones. A well-known example is found in pigs (Signoret 1976). Two metabolites of androgen play an integral part in the courtship and copulatory sequence. When the boar faces the sow, he positions himself in front of her and forcefully breathes into her face. The air current picks up the molecules of sex attractant secreted by submaxillary salivary glands in the male's mouth, which has a distinctive odor. If the female is receptive, one whiff of the male will cause her to stand immobile, arching her back in lordosis, and allow the boar to mount and copulate. Application of this discovery to animal husbandry has resulted in the manufacture of an aerosol preparation containing these androgen metabolites called Boar Mate, which is used to immobilize sows for artificial insemination.

Another example of hormones serving as pheromones can be found in goldfish (figure 7.4). Research by Sorenson and Stacey (1991) has revealed that the female produces two hormones that have specific, separate actions on the physiology and behavior of the male. One hormone is a progestin produced by the preovulatory follicle. This hormone is involved in the final maturation and ovulation of the oocyte. It is also excreted into the water in which the fish are swimming and has a profound influence on the male's endocrine physiology (figure 7.4). The presence of this hormone in the water leads to increased circulating concentrations of pituitary gonadotropins and testicular progestins, which in turn stimulate sperm production.

Another group of hormones found to activate species-typical reproductive behaviors are the prostaglandins. Administration of prostaglandins elicits female-typical spawning behavior in goldfish and other fishes with external fertilization. During ovulation, prostaglandins are released and receptive behavior is stimulated in the female. In the water, prostaglandins then trigger sexual behavior in males.

It is of interest that in species with internal fertilization, prostaglandins have very different effects. For example, in crickets, lizards, red-sided garter snakes, and guinea pigs, prostaglandins stimulate rejection behavior and the loss of sexual receptivity. If prostaglandins are given to female or to male Tamara wallabies (small kangaroos), they will crouch and behave as if they were giving birth.

Studies of fish hormonal pheromones may force us to reconsider some basic concepts of pheromonal function. For example, it is doubtful that the hormonal pheromone system of goldfish functions in true chemical "communication." There is no evidence that the female chemical signal is either specialized or released in such a way as to increase female reproductive success directly. Rather, it appears more likely that goldfish hormonal pheromones function in "chemical spying" in a manner consistent with the sensory exploitation interpretation of sexual selection. In other words, males have evolved the ability to detect these chemicals in response to intense competition among males for access to ovulated females. Such chemical spying almost certainly represents an early stage of pheromonal evolution. This association would be expected to lead to chemical communication when increasing the efficiency of signaling could increase the reproductive success of the signaler.

We have sampled just a portion of the diversity in hormone-behavior relations found in animals. Regardless of the mechanics of reproduction, the coordination of individuals leads to a synchronization of reproductive processes. This is true even in species that do not reproduce sexually. As men-

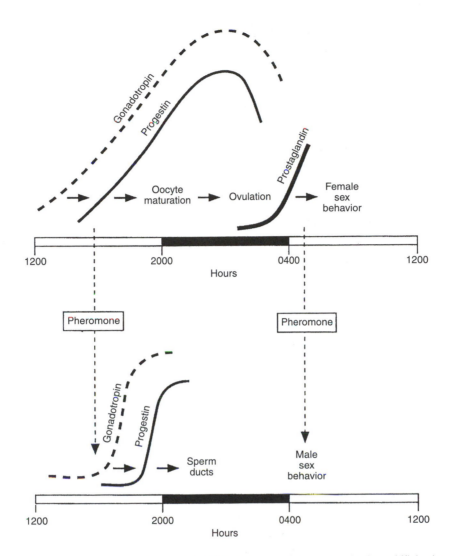

Figure 7.4 Example of how released hormones can function as pheromones. In the goldfish, the ovulating female sequentially releases two hormones with distinct pheromonal effects on male physiology and behavior. This dual pheromone system is set in motion when environmental cues (warm water temperature and appropriate spawning substrate) trigger a preovulatory surge of gonadotropin release from the pituitary. The gonadotropin surge rapidly stimulates ovarian follicle cells to synthesize a progestin, $17\alpha,20\beta$-dihydroxy-4-pregnen-3-one, which acts hormonally on the oocyte to promote maturation (resumption and completion of meiosis). When released to the water, this progestin acts via sensitive and specific male olfactory receptors to rapidly increase plasma gonadotropin, which in turn increases the numbers of sperm in the sperm ducts by stimulating testicular synthesis of this same progestin. Males that detect the progestin pheromone are believed to benefit by being able to release more sperm during the highly competitive spawning. When ovulation occurs, the presence of the oocytes in the reproductive tract stimulates synthesis of a prostaglandin, $PGF_2\alpha$, which triggers female spawning behavior. At the same time, the prostaglandin is released to the water and stimulates males to court the ovulated female.

tioned in the beginning of this chapter, some species consist only of female individuals that reproduce parthenogenetically; no males exist. There are two forms of parthenogenesis in vertebrates. In gynogenetic reproduction, the female mates with males of another species and his sperm induce the development of the embryo. In obligate parthenogenesis, sperm are not required to induce embryogenesis but, as we will see, the presence of male-like behavior is still important. Thus, individuals of even all-female species must coordinate their reproductive states to insure successful reproduction.

Particularly in birds and mammals, the freedom to choose a mate is an essential element in successful reproduction. It is evident from this survey that males and females can vary in ways other than by producing sperm or eggs. When the gametes are produced relative to when mating occurs and whether the gametes are stored or used immediately varies according to the constraints outlined above. Males and females need not respond to these pressures in the same way. This conclusion is clearly evident in species in which one sex exhibits an associated reproductive pattern and the other sex has a dissociated reproductive pattern. Comparative studies reveal that the "exceptional cases" are less rare and more widespread than is generally realized. Finally, the trigger for sexual behavior can vary from species to species. In some it is a change in a particular physical factor in the environment such as rainfall or even the color green, which signify new growth of vegetation. In other species it can be the sight, sound, or smell of other individuals. In these instances, hormones are affecting the perceptions of the individual.

Insights into the Evolution of the Process and Mechanisms of Reproduction

Nongenetic Transmission of Traits

We all learned in introductory biology that traits are inherited by the transmission of genes. Some may also have heard about Lamarck, a contemporary of Darwin. A keen observer of animal behavior, he suggested that traits might also be transmitted to the next generation if the organism was exposed to, or engaged in, certain activities. Lamarkianism, or the inheritance of acquired characteristics, was discredited early this century. However, like many things, there was an element of truth that only in recent years has been recognized. We now know that traits can be transmitted from parent to offspring both by nongenomic means as well as by the inheritance of genes. As we have seen, social context, the architecture of pregnancy, and the physiological state of the female as she deposits yolk prior to laying can all play a role in the nongenetic transmission of traits across generations. For example, one of the more interesting aspects of the effects of intrauterine position is *how* phenotypes can be transmitted across generations. As stated above, 2M females tend to have litters with more male-biased sex ratios. This means that the female offspring of such females are more likely to be 2M females than are the female offspring of 2F females. The same is true for male offspring (i.e., males are more likely to have male fetuses as neighbors). Therefore, through hormonal effects in utero, the life histories of females may be transmitted nongenomically.

TEMPERATURE-DEPENDENT SEX DETERMINATION

In species with genotypic sex determination, such as mammals, the inheritance of specific chromosomes, whether in type or in number, fixes the sex of the individual at the moment of fertilization (figure 7.5). Scientists have known for many years that in certain plants and invertebrates, the sex ratio can be skewed by environmental conditions, so much so that only female or male young may result. However, it has only been in the last two decades that we have come to realize that many vertebrates also exhibit environmental sex determination. You just read about one type of environmental sex determination, behavior-dependent sex determination, in which the individual's perception of its social environment establishes gonad type. Another type is temperature-dependent sex determination (TSD), in which the temperature experienced by the embryo determines whether it becomes a male or a female.

Temperature-dependent sex determination occurs in all alligators and crocodiles, most turtles, and many lizards (figure 7.6); in snakes and in the tuatara (spiny-backed reptiles), gonadal sex is determined by sex chromosomes as in mammals and in birds. Species with TSD lack sex chromosomes and have little or no genetic predisposition to respond to temperature in particular ways. Research with the red-eared slider turtle indicates that the physical stimulus of temperature is transduced in the midtrimester of development to modulate expression of the genes coding for steroidogenic enzymes and sex steroid hormone receptors (Crews 1996).

Unlike the fish just discussed, reptiles are gonochoristic. Thus, in TSD species each individual has an equal ability to become a male or a female. Temperature serves as the trigger, activating one sex-determining cascade while suppressing the complementary sex-determining cascade; that is, being a male also means not being a female. Environmental sex-determining mechanisms, of which TSD is one, are believed to be the evolutionary precursor to the genotypic sex-determining mechanisms characteristic of birds and mammals (figure 7.7) (Crews 1994). A still unanswered question is whether females select a particular ground temperature when excavating the nest. That is, gravid females may use temperature in choosing the place or depth to place their eggs. Given what we know already, both the sex ratio and the phenotype of the offspring would be altered by such a choice. If such nest-site selection occurs, is it influenced by the temperature which the female herself experienced as an embryo?

What do we know about the sexual differentiation process in TSD species? To date only one species, the leopard gecko, has been studied (Crews 1997; Crews et al. 1998). In the leopard gecko, only females result if eggs are incubated at 26 °C (= low-temperature females); above 34 °C (= high-temperature

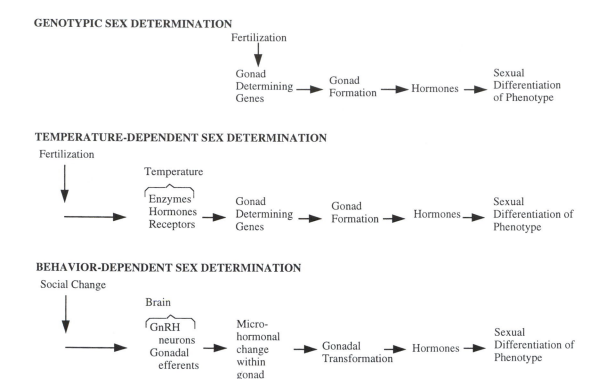

Figure 7.5 Different mechanisms of sex determination in vertebrates. In vertebrates with sex chromosomes (male or female heterogamety), gonadal sex is fixed at fertilization by the union of specific chromosomes. Only after the gonad is formed do hormones begin to exert an influence, sculpting specific structures that eventually will differ between the sexes. Research on fish with behavior-dependent sex determination suggests that social stimuli encountered by the adult leads to sex change via the brain, acting first on hypothalamic neurons that secrete arginine vasotocin and gonadotropin-releasing hormone which, in turn, act on neurons that project to the gonads. The activity of these neurons modifies the endocrine environment within the gonad, bringing about gonadal transformation. Research on reptiles with temperature-dependent sex determination indicates that sex determination in such species is fundamentally different in at least one way. Gonadal sex is not irrevocably set by the genetic composition inherited at fertilization, but rather depends on which enzymatic and hormone receptor genes are activated during development by temperature. Incubation temperature modifies both the temporal and spatial sequence of steroidogenic enzymes and hormone receptors so that sex-specific hormone milieus created in the urogenital system of the developing embryo determine gonad type. In such species, an alternative form of sexual differentiation may exist. (From Crews 1993.)

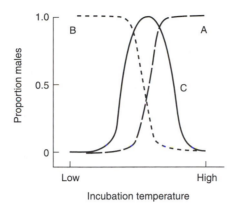

Figure 7.6 Response of hatchling sex ratio to incubation temperature in various egg-laying reptiles. These graphs represent only the approximate pattern of the response and are not drawn according to any single species. The three patterns recognized presently are (*A*) only females produced from low incubation temperatures, males at high temperatures, (*B*) only males produced from low incubation temperatures, females at high temperatures, and (*C*) only females produced at the temperature extremes, with male production at the intermediate incubation temperatures. Genotypic sex determination also occurs in other reptiles with the result that the hatchling sex ratio is fixed at 1:1 despite incubation conditions. (From Crews 1994.)

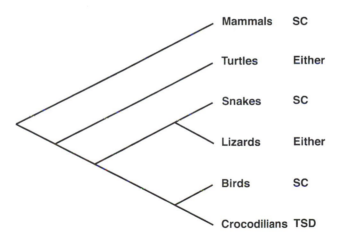

Figure 7.7 Phylogeny of sex-determining mechanisms in amniote vertebrates. In lizards and turtles both SC and TSD have been documented. SC, sex chromosomes determine sex; TSD, temperature-dependent sex determination. (From Crews 1994.)

females) only about 5% of the hatchlings are male. Incubation at 30 °C produces a female-biased sex ratio, and 32.5 °C produces a male-biased sex ratio. This becomes important because we have found that by incubating eggs at various temperatures and then following individuals as they age, much of the phenotypic variation seen among adults, both between and within the sexes, can be accounted for by the individual's incubation temperature. For example, adult leopard geckos are sexually dimorphic, with males having open secretory pores anterior to the cloaca. In low-temperature females these pores are closed, whereas in females from a male-biased temperature they are open. Head size is also sexually dimorphic, with males having wider heads than females, yet within females, those from a male-biased temperature have wider heads than do those from a low temperature. Similarly, although males are the larger sex, incubation temperature has a marked effect on growth within a sex. Females from a male-biased temperature grow faster and larger than females from a female-biased temperature, and become as large as males from a female-biased temperature.

TEMPERATURE DEPENDENCE OF OTHER TRAITS
Circulating concentrations of testosterone in adult males are approximately 100 times higher than in adult females. However, the endocrine physiology of the adult varies in part due to the temperature experienced during incubation (figure 7.8). For example, plasma estrogen levels are significantly higher in males from a female-biased temperature than in males from a male-biased temperature. Among females, circulating estrogen levels are significantly higher, and androgen levels significantly lower, in low-temperature females than in females from a male-biased temperature.

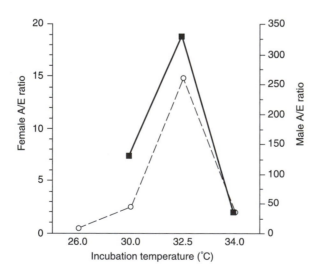

Figure 7.8 Ratio of the plasma levels of total androgens (A) and estrogens (E) in adult female (dashed line) and male (solid line) leopard geckos, *Eublepharis macularius*, from different incubation temperatures. (From Crews et al. 1997.)

Aggression
Incubation temperature also has a major influence on the nature and frequency of the behavior displayed by the adult leopard gecko. For example, females usually respond aggressively only if attacked, whereas males will posture and then attack other males but rarely females. However, males from a female-biased temperature are less aggressive than males from the higher, male-biased temperature and, although not as aggressive as males from that same incubation temperature, females from a male-biased temperature are significantly more aggressive toward males than are females from a low or female-biased temperature. These same females show the male-typical pattern of offensive aggression. Incubation temperature also influences the ability of exogenous testosterone to restore aggression. Following ovariectomy and testosterone treatment, low-temperature females do not exhibit increased levels of aggression toward male stimulus animals, whereas females from male-biased temperatures return to the high levels exhibited while gonadally intact. This suggests that incubation temperature influences responsiveness to steroid hormones in adulthood in males.

Courtship
This is a male-typical behavior. In a sexual encounter, the male will slowly approach the female, touching the substrate or licking the air with his tongue. Males also have a characteristic tail vibration, creating a buzzing sound, when they detect a female. Intact females have never been observed to exhibit this tail-vibration behavior, regardless of their incubation temperature. However, if ovariectomized females are treated with testosterone, they will begin to tail-vibrate toward female, but not male, stimulus animals; males appear to regard such females as male because they attack them.

Attractiveness
This is a female-typical trait and is measured by the intensity of a sexually active male's courtship behavior toward the female. Females from a male-biased temperature are less attractive than females from lower incubation temperatures. Long-term castrated males are attractive and initially courted by intact males, presumably because of their odor, but on further chemosensory inspection they are attacked. This suggests that both sexes can produce both a female-typical attractiveness pheromone and a male-typical recognition pheromone, as the red-sided garter snake does (see below).

Brain Morphology
It stands to reason, therefore, that the morphological, physiological, and behavioral phenotypes we have discovered in the leopard gecko might be reflected in neural phenotypes. The first (and surprising) discovery was that at temperatures that produce both sexes, the volume of the POA and the VMH do not significantly differ between males and females (figure 7.9). There are, however, consistent differences across incubation temperatures. The volume of the POA is larger both in males and in females from the male-biased

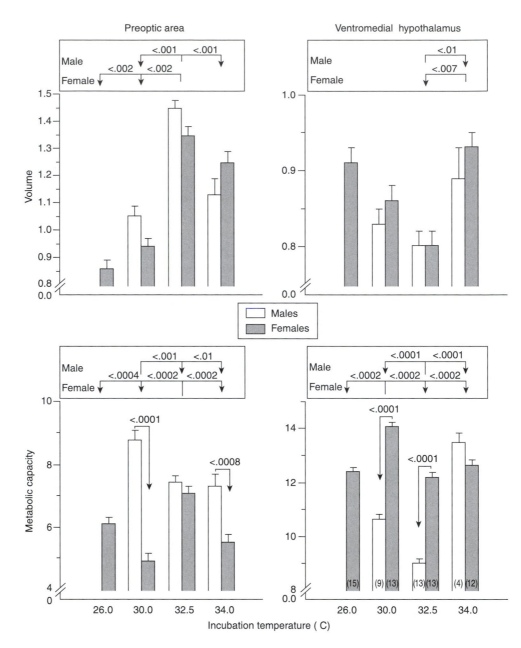

Figure 7.9 Effect of incubation temperature and gonadal sex on the volume (*top panels*) and cytochrome oxidase (COX) activity (*bottom panels*) of the preoptic area (POA) (*left panels*) and ventromedial hypothalamus (VMH) (*right panels*) in the leopard gecko, *Eublepharis macularius*. Volumes are normalized by entire forebrain volume. Significant differences (entries are p values) within each sex are illustrated in box above each panel, indicating the effect of incubation temperature. Significant differences between the sexes are illustrated *above bars*, indicating the effect of gonadal sex. Sample sizes in parentheses. Means depicted with vertical bars representing standard error. (From Crews et al. 1997.)

temperature than in animals from the female-biased temperature. Similarly, the volume of the VMH is larger in low-temperature females than in females from the male-biased temperature. This suggests that the incubation temperature of the embryo directly organizes the size of these brain areas independent of its effect on gonadal sex.

Thus, experiences before birth arising out of the hormonal and physiological milieu during embryogenesis can have a profound effect on the adult phenotype. Experiences accumulated over a lifetime as well as during a reproductive season set the stage for how individuals respond to these immediate stimuli. Indeed, experience needs to be viewed broadly to include the genetic history of the individual, the population, and the species, as well as the environment in which the individual develops.

Hormone Independence of Courtship Behavior in the Red-Sided Garter Snake

As discussed in chapter 1, Berthold demonstrated in 1849 that the testes of the rooster produced a chemical that dramatically changed the animal's behavior. Since that experiment, there have been thousands of studies on a variety of vertebrate species that have yielded similar results. Yet with rare exceptions, all the species studied exhibited an associated reproductive pattern (Crews and Moore 1986) (figure 7.1 and table 7.2). The consistency of the data has led many to presume that gonadal steroid hormones activate mating behavior in all vertebrates. Here the dissociated reproductive pattern provides us with a natural experiment. In the Candian red-sided garter snake, a basic conflict between environmental and physiological constraints has created novel neuroendocrine mechanisms (Crews 1990). As we will see, the neuroendocrine mechanisms controlling courtship behavior in adult male red-sided garter snakes does not rely on the activational effects of sex steroid hormones.

The red-sided garter snake is found in the northern United States and in Manitoba, Canada. In these regions winters are usually severe, and the snakes may spend as long as 9 months in hibernation in subterranean limestone caverns (figure 7.10). With the spring thaw, the animals emerge, and there is a brief 3- to 4-week breeding season. After this there is a summer feeding phase that can last 2 to 3 months. During this time the females also gestate and give birth. Beginning in late August, animals start returning to the caverns from which they emerged the previous spring.

Increasing ambient temperatures stimulates the emergence from winter dormancy in the spring. Males emerge en masse while the females emerge singly beginning about 1 week later (figure 7.11). As each female emerges, males in the immediate vicinity approach her. A pheromone on the female's back elicits a vigorous response in the male called "chin-rubbing." Chin-rubbing consists of the male coursing up and down the back of the female rapidly and repeatedly with his chin, all the time rapidly flicking his tongue on the female's back. The male next aligns his body along the female's body and attempts to intromit a hemipenis. (All male lizards and snakes have two

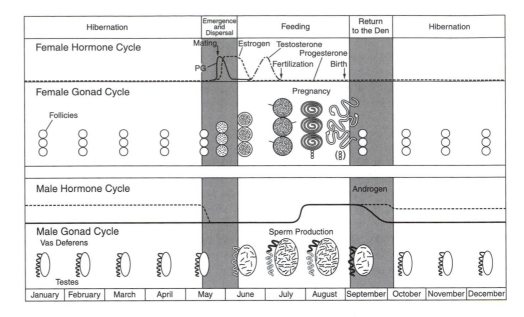

Figure 7.10 The major physiological and behavioral events in the annual reproductive cycle of the red-sided garter snake in Canada. Animals spend most of the year underground. In the spring, they emerge and mate before dispersing to summer feeding grounds. In the female, mating initiates gonadal growth as well as changes in the hormone profile. Young are born in late summer. Since all metabolic processes slow down during the cold months, androgen levels in the male will be elevated in the spring if he entered hibernation with elevated levels (dotted lines); however, androgen levels are usually basal on emergence (solid line). Sperm are produced during the summer after mating and are stored in the vas deferens (heavy squiggle line next to testis) over winter.

penises rather than one and alternate their use in successive matings.) Since one hundred or more males may be attracted to a single female, a writhing mass of snakes results, called a "mating ball" (figure 7.11). After the female mates, usually with only one of the males, she immediately leaves the den area. Approximately 3 weeks after the first emergence, virtually all the females have emerged from hibernation. Males then leave the area and disperse to their feeding grounds, not to return until the fall when the weather cools.

All these events can be duplicated in the laboratory simply by cooling animals, during the fall, to a body temperature of 2° to 4 °C and maintaining animals at this temperature for 17 weeks. In the laboratory, males typically do not court the first few days after emergence, but then show intense courtship which wanes 3 to 4 weeks following emergence. Only prolonged periods of cold temperatures can restimulate male behavior. Indeed, captive males will never again exhibit this same intense and synchronous courtship behavior unless they are hibernated.

SPERM IS STORED OVER WINTER IN MALES

Males emerge from hibernation with regressed testes and epididymides enlarged with stored sperm (figure 7.10). The sperm that a male uses in mating are produced during a testicular growth cycle the previous summer. In the adult male, spermatogenesis begins about 6 weeks after emergence in the spring and continues for 10 to 12 weeks. Associated with spermatogenesis is an increase in the circulating concentrations of androgens. Testicular collapse occurs when males return to begin hibernation. If the winter is early, they may enter hibernation while androgen levels are still elevated. If the androgen titer is high in the fall, it will be elevated initially on emergence in the spring due to the slow metabolic clearance rates during hibernation.

FEMALES DO NOT STORE MATURE OVA

Females also emerge with regressed ovaries and low serum estrogen. Unlike sperm, mature ova cannot be stored successfully over a winter. However, females are attractive and receptive on emergence and quickly mate. As soon as the female mates, she becomes unattractive and unreceptive to males. Mating stimulates a neuroendocrine reflex that culminates in ovarian growth and ovulation 6 weeks later. Immediately after mating, or perhaps initiated during copulation, there is a significant rise in circulating concentrations of prostaglandins. This is followed shortly by a surge in the circulating concentrations of estrogen, which remains elevated for several days before declining to basal level. Estrogen remains low until 3 to 6 weeks later, when the ovarian follicles enlarge.

This mating-induced neuroendocrine reflex is essential for ovulation. Specific sensory stimulation received during mating initiates this neuroendocrine reflex. It begins with the male's intromission into the female's cloaca. (The word *cloaca* in Latin means "sewer"; it refers to the fact that in all vertebrates except mammals there is a single urogenital opening.) Anesthetization of the cloaca or spinal cord prior to copulation prevents the transmission of sensory information essential for the reflex (Mendonça and Crews 1990, 2001). Females so manipulated do not show the surge in hormones associated with mating and their follicles do not grow.

A question that immediately comes to mind is how can red-sided garter snakes mate when their gonads are regressed and sex steroid hormone concentrations are low? As we might expect, the neuroendocrine mechanisms controlling reproduction in the red-sided garter snake are different from those of more commonly studied species that mate when their gonads are fully active. In this species the circulating concentrations of androgen are low during courtship, and testicular steroidogenesis does not occur until after all courtship behavior has ended.

COURTSHIP BEHAVIOR

Chin-rubbing behavior in the male red-sided garter snake is elicited by the tongue-flick delivery of the female attractiveness pheromones to the vomeronasal organ (VNO). The VNO projects to the nucleus sphericus, which in turn projects to the POA. As in other vertebrates, this brain area is involved in the display of the male's courtship behavior. 2-deoxyglucose (2DG) uptake in the POA is increased in males that are courting females. If the POA is

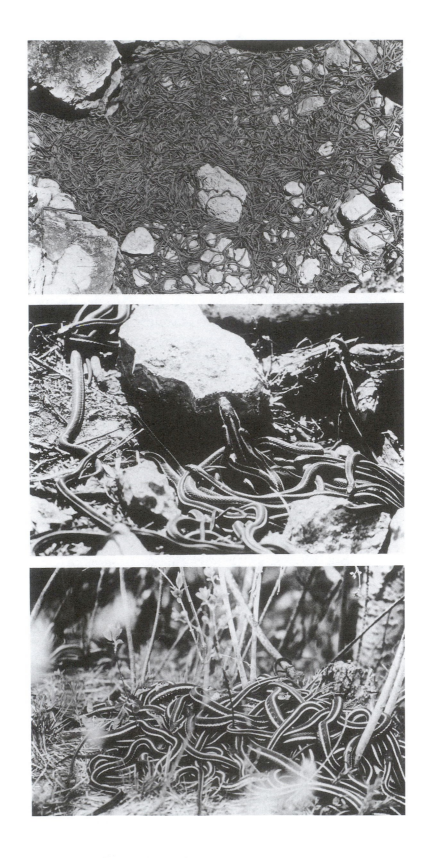

destroyed in males shortly after they have emerged, they will immediately stop courting. Even if the lesions are produced before entering hibernation, males with damage in the POA will not court. The deficits in courtship behavior that result following lesions of the POA are not due to the destruction of hormone-concentrating neurons in the POA. We know this because courtship behavior is not activated by increased concentrations of testicular androgens. It probably has something to do with the ability of lesioned animals to detect temperature, since in addition to abolishing male mating behavior, POA lesions also disrupt thermoregulatory behavior. Research with mammals indicates that this brain area is the final common pathway in temperature regulation.

Temperature then appears to be the key requirement for courtship in male red-sided garter snakes. As long as males have undergone a period of low-temperature dormancy, they will display courtship behavior on emergence into warm temperatures and in the presence of an attractive female. Photoperiod plays no role in the activation of courtship, which is unlike most homeotherms; males housed in complete darkness for a year will court as long as they have been through hibernation. Nor do testicular androgens play a role in the activation of courtship behavior. Adult males castrated on emergence from hibernation will still court females with the same intensity and duration as intact males; indeed, such castrates will again court the following spring if they undergo hibernation. Significantly, androgen treatment neither maintains courtship behavior in castrated males in the spring nor will it stimulate courtship in males in the summer (when courtship does not occur). Even if androgen is implanted directly into the POA, males fail to court. Administration of other sex hormones also fails to elicit courtship behavior.

It is not the case that male red-sided garter snakes are insensitive to androgens. Androgen is concentrated in the same brain areas as observed in other vertebrates, including the POA. Further, if males are castrated and then maintained in the laboratory and hibernated at the normal time for several years, then the frequency and intensity of their courtship behavior gradually declines (Crews 1991). After the third emergence, castrates respond to females at very low levels. If they then receive a testosterone implant during the summer when their testes would normally recrudesce and are hibernated the following fall, they will once again exhibit vigorous courtship behavior the following spring. Thus, testicular androgens organize the nervous system during the summer in such a way that the male will respond to the appropriate stimuli the following spring rather than activating male courtship behav-

Figure 7.11 Emergence of male red-sided garter snakes at hibernaculum entrance during the spring. (*Top*) Males emerge first and en masse. (*Middle*) Females then emerge singly over a 3-week period, resulting in the formation of mating balls. The female is the snake with the large head in the center of the figure; the rest are courting males. In garter snakes, the females are about three times larger than males. Unlike in most mammals, the testes inhibit body growth in male garter snakes. (*Bottom*) A mating ball of red-sided garter snakes, there is only one female.

ior in the spring. The long latency (8 months) between the androgen exposure in the summer and the consequent behavioral response the following spring suggests that the hormone-mediated organization of the brain is occurring on a seasonal basis, a process that can be regarded as seasonal organization. But if brain organization occurs on a seasonal basis in red-sided garter snakes, then it is of a fundamentally different nature than that for early organization effects described for species exhibiting an associated reproductive pattern. In this respect it is not surprising that unlike in other species, there are no statistical differences between male and female red-sided garter snakes nor are there differences across seasons in the size of those limbic nuclei involved in the control of sexual behavior (Crews et al. 1993).

Chapter 12 will describe how the pineal gland, via its hormone melatonin, is a major neuroendocrine transducer of photoperiod in birds and mammals, affecting the circadian rhythmicity of various locomotor, feeding, and drinking activities, as well as seasonal reproductive cycles. In cold-blooded vertebrates, such as reptiles, the pineal transduces changes in temperature as well as photoperiod. Since the only manipulation known to stimulate courtship in male red-sided garter snakes is exposure to prolonged periods of low temperatures followed by subsequent warming, we decided to investigate to see if the pineal is somehow involved in the control of male sexual behavior. Male garter snakes will not exhibit courtship upon emergence if their pineal is removed in the fall before they enter hibernation, yet the same operation will have no effect on courtship behavior if performed in the spring when they emerge from hibernation (figure 7.12, top panel) (Crews et al. 1988; Mendonça et al. 1996a, b). Thus, it appears an intact pineal is necessary for proper interpretation of the temperature cue but once the cue is transduced, the pineal gland per se is unnecessary in maintaining the behavior.

The day/night, or diel, cycle of melatonin secretion varies seasonally (Mendonça et al. 1995). Melatonin levels are approximately 5-fold higher in the night than in the day during the summer and fall, but during hibernation, melatonin cannot be detected in the circulation. On emergence, melatonin levels rise rapidly and precipitously and, within an hour of emergence, are at least 20-fold higher than levels seen in the fall. This surge in melatonin secretion lasts only about 24 hours, and thereafter the typical day/night difference is evident. Removal of the pineal disrupts the diel cycle of melatonin secretion, suggesting that the reestablishment of a normal diel cycle may function to synchronize and modulate courtship behavior in male red-sided garter snakes.

Some male red-sided garter snakes never court when they emerge from hibernation. What was surprising was the effect of pinealectomy on these noncourting males. In each of the three years of our experiments, pinealectomy of noncourting males increased their courtship activity; that is, they suddenly begin to court frequently and vigorously (figure 7.12, bottom panel) (Mendonça et al. 1996b). This is remarkable because it is the first experimental manipulation besides hibernation that has been found to stimulate a non-

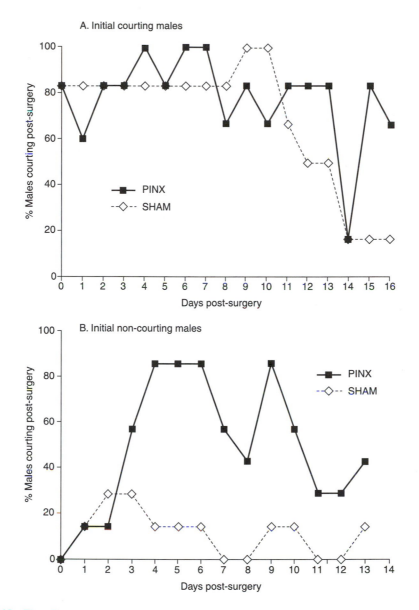

Figure 7.12 The effect of pinealectomy on courtship behavior in courting and noncourting male red-sided garter snakes, *Thamnophis sirtalis parietalis*. (*Top*) The percentage of male snakes that courted vigorously in the spring on emergence from hibernation. (*Bottom*) The percentage of male snakes that initially failed to court in the spring on emergence from hibernation. PINX, pinealectomized; SHAM, sham operation. (From Mendonca et al. 1996.)

courting male garter snake to exhibit courtship behavior. It is possible that males that court in the spring have a different neuroendocrine mechanism controlling courtship behavior than noncourting males. Intact noncourting males lack a normal diel pattern of melatonin secretion when sampled either just a few days or 10 days after emergence (when the mating period is about half over). It may be that these animals are not able to process the temperature change that occurs at emergence and stimulates courtship.

TERMINATION OF MATING BEHAVIOR

Why do male garter snakes stop courting females about 1 month after emergence from hibernation? This decline in courtship behavior is not due to the males becoming used to females. Males that have had daily exposure to females exhibit courtship behavior equal to that of males kept isolated after emergence and only tested later with attractive females. The answer may lie in the natural sequence of events. Even after spending many months without food, recently emerged male red-sided garter snakes do not feed. This is not due to a lack of food, because males will refuse food if it is offered. Females, on the other hand, begin to feed soon after they emerge and leave the den areas. Males leave the den to forage for food 3 to 4 weeks after emergence, at the same time courtship begins to decline. The remainder of the summer is spent feeding. Males do not court attractive females during the summer feeding phase. This voluntary abstinence from food is common in species inhabiting marginal habitats. In ground squirrels, pinnipeds, Emperor pigeons, the arctic fulmar, and the red-sided garter snake, feeding and mating behaviors are mutually exclusive events in at least one of the sexes. The hormone neuropeptide Y (NPY) is known to play a role in the regulation of both feeding and sexual behavior and, as in mammals, infusion of NPY into the brain of male red-sided garter snakes will cause them to temporarily cease courtship of females and begin to eat.

We have seen how environmental and endocrine factors influence specific reproductive functions and behaviors in the red-sided garter snake. Some conclusions that can be drawn include the following: (1) gonadal growth and sexual behavior are not necessarily temporally associated, (2) sexual behavior can be independent of gonadal steroid hormones, (3) the initiation, maintenance, and termination of sexual behavior are independent of each other and are controlled by different cues, and (4) behavioral differences between the sexes can occur without corresponding sex differences in the size of the brain areas that regulate these behaviors.

Evolution of the Neuroendocrine Control of Sex-Typical Behaviors

Most whiptail lizard species are gonochoristic, having both male and female individuals that reproduce sexually. However, one-third of the 45 species of whiptail lizards are unisexual, consisting only of individuals that reproduce by true parthenogenesis. We know that the parthenogenetic species arose from the hybrid mating of two sexual whiptail species and, in many instances, we know which species were involved. For example, the parthenogen *C. uniparens* arose from the hybrid union of *C. inornatus* and *C. burti*. Furthermore, we know that *C. inornatus* is the maternal ancestor of *C. uniparens* and *C. burti* is the paternal ancestor. Thus, two-thirds of the triploid genome of *C. uniparens* is derived from *C. inornatus*.

Just as the research on the red-sided garter snake has led to new information about neuroendocrine adaptations, the study of unisexual vertebrates has proved useful for understanding how these neuroendocrine adaptations may have evolved. This is because these species allow the investigator to study brain-behavior evolution in a manner impossible with conventional species. That is, parthenogenetic whiptail lizards and their related sexual species present a "snapshot" of evolution. Here we have an opportunity to compare the neuroendocrine mechanisms that control reproductive behaviors in the descendant species with those of the ancestral species. This ability in turn allows us to address two fundamental issues from a new perspective. First, do the neural circuits that subserve male-typical and female-typical sexual behaviors differ or are they similar? Second, how might the cellular mechanisms that control sexual behaviors have evolved?

PSEUDOSEXUAL BEHAVIOR IN THE PARTHENOGENIC LIZARD

As pointed out earlier, reproductive behaviors tend to be unambiguous, characteristic of the species, and critical to the individual's reproductive and evolutionary success. Twenty years ago I made the serendipitous observation that unisexual whiptail lizards exhibit behaviors remarkably similar to the courtship and copulatory behavior of related sexual species (figure 7.13). In gonochoristic whiptail lizards (e.g., *C. inornatus*), the male approaches and investigates the female with his bifid (split) tongue, an action that presumably indicates involvement of chemical senses. If the female is sexually receptive, she stands still for the male, allowing him to mount her back. Usually just before the male mounts the female, he grips with his jaws either a portion of the skin on the female's neck or her foreleg. As the male rides the female, he scratches her sides and presses her body against the substrate. The male then begins to maneuver his tail beneath the female's tail, attempting to appose their cloacal regions. During mating, one of two hemipenes is intromitted into the female's cloaca. With intromission, the male shifts his jaw-grip from the female's neck to her pelvic region, thereby assuming a contorted copulatory posture I have termed the *doughnut*. This posture is maintained for 5 to 10 minutes, after which the male rapidly dismounts and leaves the female.[2]

This same sequence of events is observed in at least five species of unisexual whiptail lizards (figure 7.13). That is, one individual will approach and mount another individual and, after riding for a few minutes, the mounting (male-like) individual will swing its tail beneath that of the mounted (female-like) individual, apposing the cloacal regions. At the same time, the mounting individual will shift its jawgrip from the neck to the pelvic region of the

C. inornatus   *C. uniparens*

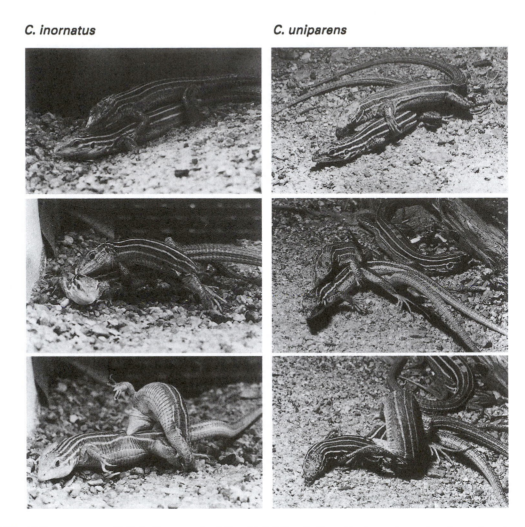

Figure 7.13 Mating sequence (*left*) in the gonochoristic whiptail lizard, *Cnemidophorus inornatus*, the maternal ancestor of the parthenogenetic whiptail, *C. uniparens*. Pseudosexual behavior (*right*) in the all-female parthenogenetic whiptail lizard, *C. uniparens*. Note the similarity in the behavioral sequence to that of its gonochoristic ancestor. (From Crews 1987.)

mounted individual, forming the doughnut posture. Since parthenogens are morphologically female, there are no hemipenes, and intromission does not occur. Two weeks later these roles reverse and the mounting individual is now mounted.

How do we know whether pseudosexual behavior in a unisexual lizard is not just a trivial discovery? (Every scientist should ask himself or herself this kind of question whenever an unusual behavior or phenomenon is discovered.) First, we know that pseudosexual behavior is not peculiar to *C. uniparens*. Pseudosexual behavior has been observed in at least five other species of parthenogenetic whiptail lizards as well as in the parthenogenetic morning gecko. Furthermore, behaviors similar to pseudosexual behavior have been described in other unisexual or asexual vertebrate and inverte-brate species. So this is not an isolated occurrence of the behavior. Second, pseudosexual behavior facilitates ovarian development. Studies show that parthenogens are more likely to lay eggs and will lay more clutches if they engage in pseudosexual behavior (Crews et al. 1986). This indicates that the behavior has an adaptive function.

Is pseudosexual behavior simply the result of the development of par-thenogenesis? If this were true, one would not expect females of sexually reproducing species to exhibit male-typical behaviors or males to exhibit female-typical behaviors. This is clearly not the case. Females mounting and males allowing mounting are a normal part of sexual activity in many spe-cies. Importantly, females of the ancestral species *C. inornatus* have occa-sionally been observed to mount other females. Thus, pseudocopulatory behavior is not a newly evolved trait in unisexual whiptails. Rather, the neu-ral circuits underlying these behaviors have been retained from their sexual ancestral species. This reflects, in part, the brain organization of the sexual behavior in vertebrates.

Could pseudosexual behavior be a consequence of captivity? Is this an un-usual behavior induced by the stress of the laboratory? If this were the case, we would not expect *C. uniparens* to reproduce at normal levels in the labo-ratory. Reproduction is an extremely complex process that is sensitive to the organism's environment. Even slight perturbations in certain variables can result in captive animals failing to reproduce, a fact evident in many zoos. In my laboratory, however, both unisexual and sexual whiptail lizards re-produce as frequently as they do in nature. That is, they typically lay three clutches of eggs, each containing three-to-four eggs, during the course of a reproductive season. Also, it is clear that stress does occur in these animals, as evidenced by the fact that in cages containing three or four individuals, there is always one dominant individual who lays many clutches and one subordinate individual who does not lay eggs.

Since our original observations, pseudocopulation has been observed in nature in *C. uniparens* and other parthenogenetic whiptail lizards as well as in other all-female species of fish, fruit flies, and geckos. This behavior in whiptails has been quantified using indirect evidence, namely the incidence of copulatory bite marks on the back (Crews and Young 1991). These are caused by the jaw-grip of the mounting animal, which leaves a distinct black V-shaped scar on the lateral abdominal area of the mounted animal. We found copulation marks in over three-quarters of adult females of the sexual ances-tral species, *C. inornatus*, but only on about half of the descendant parthe-nogen, *C. uniparens*. Since in our study the animals were collected at the beginning of the reproductive season, we predicted that only half of the par-thenogens would bear copulation marks initially since these animals assume complementary roles and the mounting animal would not be mounted until it was about to ovulate.

HORMONE DEPENDENCE OF PEUDOSEXUAL BEHAVIOR

Do parthenogenetic whiptails have high levels of male-typical androgens when displaying male-like behavior? No. Radioimmunoassay of the circulating androgens revealed uniformly undetectable plasma concentrations at all stages of the reproductive cycle. Not only is there no evidence of transient surges in these androgens during the course of the ovarian cycle, but post-ovulatory animals exhibiting male-like pseudosexual behavior are no more likely to have detectable androgens than are preovulatory parthenogens exhibiting female-like pseudosexual behavior. Also, the nature and pattern of sex steroid hormone secretions in females of the sexual species and in the parthenogens are virtually identical. Taken together, this indicates that the evolution of parthenogenesis has not been accompanied by an alteration of the usual pattern of endocrine changes.

The reproductive cycles of both female sexual whiptails and unisexual whiptails are very similar. Both consist of a series of 3 to 4 discrete ovarian cycles that are 3 to 4 weeks long. The ovaries simultaneously ovulate from 1 to 3 eggs each. After ovulation the ova pass into the oviducts, where shell deposition occurs. Shelled eggs are usually laid 7 to 10 days after ovulation. Production of the next clutch may be initiated within several days of egg laying.

The temporal patterns of ovarian hormone secretion are also remarkably similar in the ancestral and descendant species. In both, the circulating concentrations of estradiol increase as the follicle grows, peaking around the time of ovulation (figure 7.14). Progesterone levels begin to increase during the latter stages of follicular maturation and are at their peak after the time of ovulation. In both female whiptails and parthenogenetic whiptails, circulating concentrations of androgens are uniformly low and not detectable by radioimmunoassays.

Although the unisexual whiptail descended directly from a sexual whiptail, the two species differ in an important aspect of their reproductive biology; namely, circulating concentrations of estradiol in reproductively active parthenogenetic whiptails are approximately five-fold lower than in reproductively active female sexual whiptails (Young and Crews 1995) (figure 7.15). Since changes in the circulating concentrations of sex steroid hormones can have dramatic effects on endocrine physiology and behavior, one might expect that the several-fold difference in estradiol between the parthenogenetic whiptail and the sexual whiptail would be accompanied by species differences in estrogen-dependent phenomena. Comparisons of estrogen receptor (ER)-mRNA content in the brains of whiptail lizards indicate that parthenogenetic whiptails have higher concentrations of ER-mRNA expression in the POA than do females of the ancestral sexual species. These species differences in circulating concentrations of estradiol and ER-mRNA are accompanied by differences in sensitivity to estradiol. Dose-response studies reveal that lower dosages of estradiol benzoate are required to induce receptive behavior as well as changes in gene expression in the POA and VMH of parthenogenetic

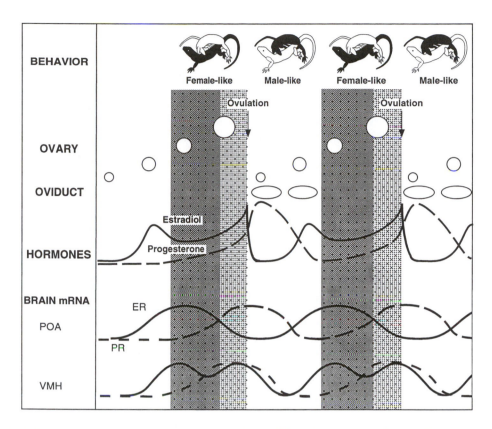

Figure 7.14 Relation among malelike and femalelike pseudosexual behavior, ovarian state, and circulating levels of estradiol and progesterone during different stages of the reproductive cycle of the parthenogenetic whiptail lizard. The transition from receptive to mounting behavior occurs at the time of ovulation (arrow). Also shown are the changes in the expression of genes coding for estrogen receptor (ER)-mRNA and progesterone receptor (PR)-mRNA in the preoptic area (POA) and the ventromedial hypothalamus (VMH), two brain areas involved in the regulation of pseudosexual behavior. (Redrawn from Crews 1996.)

whiptails than in sexual whiptails (figure 7.15). As in other vertebrates, the VMH is involved in the hormonal induction of receptive behavior in whiptail lizards. Thus, species differences in reproductive physiology (e.g., brief follicular phases, as in the rat and mouse, rather than extended follicular phases, as in whiptail lizards and rabbits) may explain species differences in neuroendocrine-controlling mechanisms.

Female *C. inornatus* are receptive to the courtship displays of the male only in the vitellogenic or yolking stage. Females are highly aggressive to courting males prior to ovulation or during pregnancy. Removal of the ovaries abolishes sexual receptivity, whereas estradiol replacement therapy will restore receptivity. Interestingly, postovulatory female *C. inornatus* have been observed to exhibit the heterotypical or male-typical mounting behavior, and there is some evidence that progesterone will stimulate female-female mounting in the sexual whiptail.

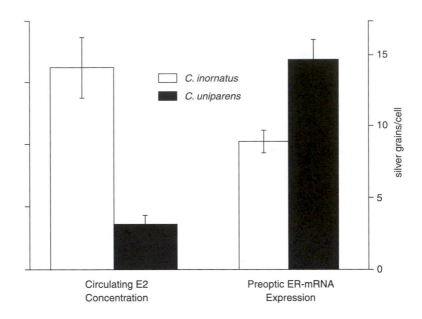

Figure 7.15 Circulating estradiol concentrations and estrogen receptor ER-mRNA expression in the preoptic area of the vitellogenic female whiptail (*Cnemidophorus inornatus*) and the parthenogenetic whiptail, (*C. uniparens*). (From Young and Crews 1995.)

Pseudosexual behavior in parthenogenetic whiptails is also related to the ovarian state. Female-like receptive behavior is limited to the preovulatory stage of the follicular cycle, whereas expression of male-like mounting behavior occurs most frequently during the postovulatory stages of the cycle (figure 7.14). These behavioral roles during pseudocopulations in the unisexual species are paralleled by differences in the circulating levels of sex steroid hormones. That is, individuals show primarily female-like behavior during the preovulatory stage when estradiol concentrations are relatively high and progesterone concentrations relatively low. Just the opposite is seen during the display of male-like behavior in the postovulatory phase, when concentrations of estradiol are low and concentrations of progesterone have increased.

It appears that ovarian hormones trigger pseudocopulatory behaviors in unisexual whiptails. In support of this idea, pseudocopulatory behaviors have never been observed in reproductively inactive or ovariectomized individuals. This means that in the absence of hormones, pseudocopulation does not occur. In addition, female-like receptivity is almost completely restricted to the yolk deposition phase. Male-like pseudocopulatory behavior, on the other hand, is most frequent in postovulatory or pregnant animals. Also, individuals alternate female-like and male-like pseudosexual behaviors as they progress through the ovarian cycles during the course of the breeding season.

When investigating the causal basis of any behavior, the place to begin is with those physiological events that are in transition at the onset of the behav-

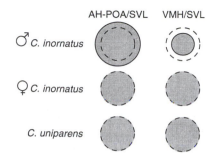

Figure 7.16 Schematic representations of the volumes of the sexually dimorphic areas in the brain relative to body size in sexual and parthenogenetic whiptails. To aid in comparison, the volume of the AH-POA and the VMH of a female *C. inornatus* is represented as a dashed outline in other drawings.

ior. It is clear that the transition from female-like to male-like pseudosexual behavior occurs when hormone concentrations in the blood are changing. At ovulation, estradiol concentrations decrease and progesterone concentrations increase (figure 7.14). Is it possible that this shift in hormone concentrations plays a crucial role in controlling the expression of pseudosexual behavior? To test this, animals were ovariectomized and then treated with progesterone, estradiol, or with a sham (control) operation. The results were clear-cut. Pseudocopulations occurred only in pairs in which both individuals were hormone-treated, but in a complementary fashion. In other words, animals treated with estradiol exhibited the female-like role and the progesterone-treated parthenogen assumed the male-like role.

NEURAL BASIS OF PSEUDOSEXUAL BEHAVIOR

The greatest advantage of unisexual vertebrates, in my opinion, is that they enable us to address the fundamental question of the neural basis of sex-typical behaviors from a new perspective. The idea that there are dual neural circuits in the brain of all vertebrates, one mediating mounting and intromission behavior and the other mediating receptive behavior, is not new. Researchers have long commented on males that exhibited female-typical sexual behaviors or, conversely, females that exhibited male-typical sexual behaviors. The bulk of modern research, however, has focused on the neuroendocrine mechanisms controlling homotypical behaviors, namely mounting behavior in gonadal males and receptive behaviors in gonadal females. In other words, each neural circuit has been studied extensively, but almost always in isolation from its complement. The parthenogenetic whiptails allow us to study these circuits operating together. Comparison studies will allow us to say what is common to both and what is specific to each.

An opportunity to study sexually dimorphic dual neural circuits together in the same individual is provided in the whiptail lizard. We find complementary sexual dimorphisms in two hypothalamic regions of the ancestral species, *C. inornatus* (figure 7.16). The POA is larger in males than in females whereas the VMH is larger in females than in males. Other research has shown that the POA is involved in mounting behavior whereas the VMH controls sexual receptivity, as in rodents and other mammals (see chapters 4 and 5). During hibernation or following castration, the POA shrinks and the VMH enlarges (that is, these brain areas become femalelike); in the female *C. inornatus* these areas show no change across seasons or after the female is treated with exogenous androgen. These results clearly indicate that in the ancestral sexual species structural dimorphisms develop in the adult and, further, that testicular androgens control the seasonal growth of these areas.

Given that the parthenogen exhibits both male-like and female-like pseudosexual behaviors, it would seem reasonable to expect the brain of the parthenogen to be bisexual, resembling both the male and the female of the ancestral sexual species. After all, the same brain areas are involved in the regulation of these behaviors. Implantation of androgens into the POA elicits, and lesioning this area abolishes, mounting behavior in both the sexual and unisexual whiptails. Implants of androgens into the VMH fail to elicit mounting behavior and have no effect on receptive behavior. Conversely, implantation of estrogen in the VMH activates receptivity in both species, but estrogen implants in the POA have no effect on receptive or mounting behavior. Lesion damage in the dorsolateral VMH, the area containing ER, abolishes estrogen-dependent receptivity. Finally, using 2DG uptake as a measure of metabolic activity, researchers found that parthenogenetic whiptails displaying male-like pseudosexual behavior had a 6-fold greater uptake in the medial POA than parthenogens displaying female-like receptivity (Rand and Crews 1994). In contrast, the VMH showed significantly greater 2DG accumulation in receptive parthenogens than in courting parthenogens.

To my great surprise, we found that the size of the POA and VMH of the parthenogenetic whiptail did not resemble both males and females of the sexual ancestral species (Crews et al. 1990; Wade et al. 1993). Even in individuals exhibiting male-like or femalelike pseudosexual behavior naturally or under hormone treatment, the POA and the VMH were similar in size, as is characteristic of female whiptails. A similar relationship exists at the level of individual neurons located in these brain regions. Further, there was no difference in neuron somata size in those individuals exhibiting malelike pseudosexual behavior than in those exhibiting femalelike pseudosexual behavior. Even if the parthenogen is treated with androgen so that it exhibits only male-like behavior and coloration, the brain remains unchanged.

Does this reflect the genetic sex or the gonadal sex of the individual? There is some evidence that the genetic basis for male-typical sexual behavior may be distinct and separate from that for female-typical sexual behavior, and further, that the genetic mechanisms of sex determination may influence the brain directly (reviewed in Arnold et al. 1995; Crews et al. 1998). But this important question cannot be addressed with conventional animal models. As outlined in chapter 3, the Y chromosome-linked gene initiates the genetic cascade leading to testicular development, thereby causing individuals to develop a male-typical phenotype. Female development is generally believed to be a default mode, resulting from the absence of this gene. Thus, in species with sex chromosomes, the sexes differ in genetic constitution and hence, genetic sex and gonadal sex are inextricably linked.

The whiptail lizards provide a unique opportunity to circumvent this problem. The male is the heterogametic sex (XY) in the ancestral sexual species, and the descendant parthenogenetic species is triploid (XXX). We have found that administration of the aromatase inhibitor Fadrazole early in embryogenesis results in hatchlings being gonadally male with fully developed hemipenes and vasa deferentia; on achieving sexual maturity, their testes even produce motile sperm. This ability to create normal-appearing males in an otherwise all-female species is further evidence that each individual possesses all of the genetic machinery to produce the male phenotype and lacks only a hormone-mediated trigger for activating the male-determining cascade and suppressing the female-determining cascade. Thus, we now have an animal model that allows us to distinguish the effects of genetic sex from gonadal sex on sexually dimorphic traits. That is, we can ask if the sexual dimorphisms evident in brain and behavior in the ancestral species are also evident when we compare female parthenogens and "created male" parthenogens.

We have discussed how the parthenogens and females of the sexual species have a smaller AH-POA volume and a larger VMH volume as well as a greater increase in PR-mRNA in the VMH in response to estrogen treatment than males of the sexual species, all of which can serve as a marker for the female-like brain. Developmental studies indicate that this latter sex difference, namely the ability of estrogen to increase abundance of PR-mRNA in the VMH, is observed in hatchlings of the sexual species, but not in the parthenogenetic species. This is consistent with other research and indicates that there can be a significant genetic sex component in sexually dimorphic traits.

EVOLUTION OF PSEUDOSEXUAL BEHAVIOR

How have the cellular mechanisms subserving pseudosexual behaviors evolved? Again, unisexual organisms provide an unusual opportunity for study of this question because we can compare the ancestral with the descendant species to discover how the neuroendocrine mechanisms regulating behavior might have changed. Specifically, we want to know how the progesterone activation of male-like pseudosexual behavior in the parthenogen evolved from the ancestral sexual species in which male-typical sexual behavior is androgen-dependent.

Whiptail lizards are seasonal breeders, with male *C. inornatus* courting and copulating only during the spring and early summer months. At this time, the circulating concentrations of androgens in males are elevated. The circulating concentrations of progesterone during this period are low and unchanging. Estradiol is undetectable. As in other vertebrates exhibiting an associated reproductive pattern, the courtship and copulatory behaviors of the male *C.*

inornatus depend upon testicular steroid hormones. Castrated males court females significantly less often than do intact, sexually active males and, as expected, treatment of castrates with exogenous androgens reinstates courtship and copulatory behaviors. However, administration of exogenous progesterone also restores the complete repertoire of sexual behavior in about one-third of castrated males. Indeed, these progesterone-sensitive males actively court and copulate with females with an intensity equal to that shown by castrates treated with androgen. While not all exogenous androgen-sensitive males are sensitive to progesterone, all progesterone-sensitive individuals are sensitive to both progesterone and exogenous androgens, suggesting that progesterone-sensitive males are a subset of exogenous androgen-sensitive males.

It is always possible that progesterone is being converted to another hormone and its metabolites produce the results described above. To test whether progesterone was acting directly to activate mounting behavior, we used various ligands, or synthetic agonists and antagonists that bind to the hormone receptors. In mammals, R5020 acts as an agonist and simulates the effect of progesterone at its receptor, whereas RU486 acts as an antagonist and prevents receptor activation. In castrated male *C. inornatus*, administration of R5020 stimulates sexual behavior in a similar proportion of castrated males as does progesterone, while RU486 prevents sexual behavior in castrated, progesterone-treated males. Other work revealed that (1) progesterone synergizes with testosterone as well as dihydrotestosterone to stimulate sexual behavior in males (Lindzey and Crews 1992), much like estradiol and progesterone synergize to elicit sexual receptivity in female rodents, and (2) that the androgen receptor (AR) of the sexual species is similar to that of mammals in its specificity and kinetics (Lindzey and Crews 1993). Taken together, these data suggest that progesterone is probably exerting its stimulatory action as a progestagen and not via conversion to other sex steroid hormones. These data also suggest that progesterone acts via the progesterone receptor (PR) and not via AR. This conclusion is further supported by the finding that implantation of progesterone directly into the POA induces courtship and copulatory behavior in progesterone-sensitive, but not in progesterone-insensitive, males; the pattern of regulation of AR- and PR-mRNA in progesterone-sensitive and progesterone-insensitive males is also different (Crews et al. 1996).

Is this behavioral responsiveness to progestin in males specific only to reptiles? Initially this was an odd question, as progesterone has long been believed to be a "female hormone." Recent studies, though, on the physiology of progesterone in males points to a functional role. For example, dihydroxyprogesterone stimulates spawning behavior in castrated rainbow trout. In male rats there is a pronounced diurnal rhythm in progesterone secretion, with the peak in progesterone levels coinciding with the period of greatest copulatory activity. When administered in physiological dosages (rather than the pharmacological dosages usually used), progesterone causes some castrated male rats to mate with receptive females; when combined with subthreshold dosages of testosterone, all the males respond (Witt et al. 1995).

Further, this progesterone response is blocked if the progesterone antagonist RU486 is administered either systemically or directly into the brain. Thus, although progesterone has long been known to be involved in the control of female-typical sexual behavior, new evidence points to a previously unsuspected role of progesterone in the control of male sexual behavior. Indeed, progesterone and androgen appear to synergize in the control of male courtship behavior much as progesterone and estrogen synergize in the control of female sexual receptivity.

As discussed in chapters 2 and 4, progesterone need not be present for the PR to be activated. How might this occur? Sex hormone receptors and neurotransmitters are found in limbic nuclei such as the POA and the VMH and can even be located in the same neuron, suggesting that there are various signaling pathways in behaviorally relevant neurons. We have already learned in chapters 4 and 5 that sex steroid hormones can act directly or indirectly by altering neurotransmitter biosynthesis. Neurotransmitters and neuropeptides such as norepinephrine, GnRH, oxytocin, and GABA facilitate, whereas CRF, ACTH, and NPY inhibit, sexual behavior. Serotonin and dopamine are interesting in that depending upon the receptor type occupied, they can either stimulate or suppress sexual behavior. For example, dopamine can induce receptivity in estrogen-primed female mice as effectively as progesterone. This ligand-independent activation of PR by dopamine and its agonists occurs through the D_1 subtype receptor. Other studies indicate that dopamine is released in the POA in male rats during sexual interactions, and that the amount of dopamine produced is positively correlated with the intensity of sexual behavior an individual male displays (Hull et al. 1997).

We have used the PRKO male mouse as a model to study the role of PR in androgen-dependent male sexual behavior (Phelps et al. 1998). We first found that PRKO males were much more sensitive to the effects of castration than were wild-type males. They were also less responsive to androgen-replacement therapy. This effect may be mediated by dopamine, because administration of a selective dopamine agonist elicits sexual behavior in wild-type male mice, but not in their PRKO counterparts (Woolley et al. 1999). Taken together, these results indicate that progesterone and its receptor are as much a part of the hormonal mediators of sexual behavior in males as in females. In other words, progesterone is as much a "male" hormone as it is a "female" hormone.

How might this evolution from an androgen-dependent, male-typical behavior in the sexual ancestral species to a progesterone-dependent, male-like behavior in the unisexual descendant species have occurred? Gould and Vrba (1982) have pointed out that two distinct historical processes can produce existing features. One of these is adaptation, or the gradual selection of traits that results in improved functions. Some traits, however, evolved from features that served other roles or had no function at all, and only later were co-opted for their current role because they enhance current fitness. The latter process, in which a useful feature is not built by selection for its current role, may be termed exaptation. The difference between the two is that in adaptation, traits are constructed by selection for their present functions. Exaptations are co-opted for their present use. In the present case, the variation in sensitivity to progesterone in the sexual ancestral species may be the substrate on which selection operated. This resulted in the novel hormone-brain-behavior relationship observed in the parthenogen. That is, because reproduction requires reciprocal behavioral stimulation, the elevation of progesterone following ovulation presented a reliable and appropriately timed stimulus that, given the low circulating concentrations of androgens, was coopted to trigger mounting behavior in the parthenogen. Evidence that this, indeed, has occurred is indicated by the finding that exogenous estradiol upregulates PR-mRNA in the POA of the parthenogen, but not in females of the ancestral sexual species (figure 7.17).

Thus, in the sexual ancestral species, individual variation in the sensitivity to progesterone appears to have served as the substrate for the evolution of the novel hormone-brain-behavior relationship observed in the parthenogen. That is, the elevation of progesterone following ovulation presented a reliable stimulus that, given the low circulating concentrations of androgens, was coopted to trigger mounting behavior in the parthenogenetic whiptail. Further, the ability of the parthenogen to express malelike pseudocopulatory behaviors is not because it has developed a morphologically masculinized POA, but because it has coopted a naturally occurring progesterone surge to

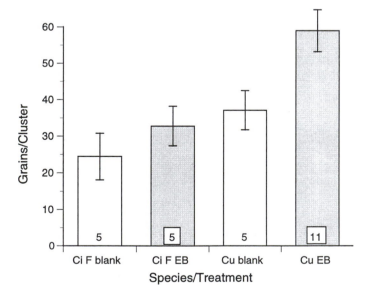

Figure 7.17 Evolution of a novel neuroendocrine mechanism controlling male-typical mounting and copulatory behavior. Depicted is the abundance of progesterone receptor-mRNA measured as average number of silver grains per cluster in the preoptic area (POA) of the ancestral sexual female (F), *Cnemidophorus inornatus*, (Ci), and descendant parthenogenetic, *C. uniparens*, Cu, whiptail lizards receiving no hormones (blank) or estradiol benzoate (EB). (Redrawn from Crews 1996.)

trigger the masculine behavioral potential remaining in a feminized brain. This is an important point because it shows again how behavioral differences need not be paralleled by structural differences in the brain.

We have seen how species can be compared to dissect the neuroendocrine mechanisms underlying sexual behavior and how the study of individual variation can be used to trace the evolutionary sequence that gave rise to alternative forms. This comparative approach can in turn lead to new concepts that may help to explain species differences in endocrine physiology and behavior. In this regard at least three factors appear to be important: (1) sensitivity to sex steroid hormones, (2) hormone-dependent regulation of sex steroid hormone receptor gene expression, and (3) neuroanatomical distribution of steroid receptor gene expression, especially in nonlimbic structures.

How Study of Diversity Raises New Questions About Old Answers

The Principle of Complementarity

Evolution of a species, a behavior, or a hormone does not occur in a vacuum. Complementarity, or the combination of parts required for completion, is evident at all levels of biological organization (table 7.3). Animals and plants have evolved in the presence of other plants and animals and their survival has become dependent upon, or is modulated by, the presence or behavior of others within the environment. For example, figs depend on fig wasps for pollination; the fig wasps oviposit in the fig and the resulting young feed on the fruit. Herbivores depend on plants for sustenance. Plants depend upon animals to disperse seeds. Sexual reproduction requires two kinds of complementary gametes, eggs and sperm. During mating, two individuals must interact in a complementary fashion if fertilization is to occur. In reproductive physiology, there are complementary feedback relationships among hormones and the complementary interaction of hormones and their receptors such as those discussed in chapter 1. Thus, complementarity is fundamental to biological systems.

Table 7.3 Examples of the Principle of Complementarity in Behavioral Biology

LEVEL OF BIOLOGICAL ORGANIZATION	COMPLEMENTARY PROCESS	EXAMPLE
Species	Coevolution of plants and animals	Figs and fig wasps
Organism	Sexual behaviors	Intromission and receptive behaviors
Physiology	Signal-receiver	Feedback control in neuroendocrinology
Molecule	Hormone-receptor	Steroid hormones and their receptors

At every level of biological organization there are fundamental complementary processes.

This perspective is useful when considering complex systems such as reproduction. Anyone who has ever watched carefully how animals mate will be struck by the complementary nature of copulation and of the actions that lead up to it. Normally, copulation is a behavior made possible only by mutual consent. This consent is a reflection not only of the satisfactory nature of the external stimuli provided, but also of the internal milieu that motivates each individual to seek a partner. Beach (1979) referred to this as "the principle of stimulus-response complementarity." According to this principle, successful mating will occur only if both partners are in the appropriate physiological and behavioral condition and if the behaviors of each partner elicit the appropriate behavioral response from the other. This can be restated as two simple sentences: Mounting will not be successful if the mounted animal is not receptive. A receptive animal will not be mounted unless there is a willing partner.

The principle of stimulus-response complementarity has broad implications. For example, it can be applied to all animals, regardless of their mode of reproduction and of the genetic or gonadal sex of the participants. Female-associated responses tend to evoke masculine responses in both males and females. Similarly, male-associated responses tend to evoke feminine responses in both females and males.

This principle may also have an impact on our understanding of sexual selection. Just as there is variance in male displays, there is variance in female preference. Indeed, if we examine any morphological, physiological, or behavioral trait, we will find that females are more variable than males—an important phenomenon waiting to be investigated. As Bluhm (1985) has documented, female canvasback ducks forced into pairs with males they did not select fail to lay eggs. Could this phenomenon be generalized to other species? If we refer to a successful pairing as a "resonance" between the preference behaviors of the partners, may this reflect a similar "resonance" at a physiological level? That is, when females choose their mating partners, are they selecting males whose physiology will stimulate maximum reproductive success? As Bluhm has shown, such a hypothesis is relatively easy to test. The answer should reveal itself best in those species exhibiting strong mate preference or giving evidence of assortative mating.

The concept of complementarity in biological systems is also useful because it encourages investigators to think of units rather than single elements. In biology it is often said that the whole is more than the sum of its parts. This is readily seen in mating behavior where two individuals must coordinate and synchronize reproductive processes. Only from such interactions will reproduction be successful. This logic can be extended to all levels of biological organization. Still, the trend in behavioral endocrinology is to focus on a single sex, a single behavior, or a single hormone. This is evident in studies where the investigator may spend years determining the reproductive cycle in the male (or female) while ignoring the potential contribution of the partner.

On the other hand, at the genetic level, individuals are far from being complementary. Differences in reproductive interests lead to something very different from harmony and mutual coordination in courtship and mating behavior. In fact, another descriptor for male-female relations is the conflict of reproductive interests. Put simply, no two sexually reproducing individuals, other than monozygotic twins, share identical genetic (reproductive) interests. In this framework, courtship behavior by males and mate choice by females may represent "salesmanship" and "consumerism," respectively.

Can the Organizational Concept Apply to Vertebrates Lacking Sex Chromosomes?

The organizational concept has had great heuristic value and aided our understanding of the fundamental elements of sexual differentiation in mammals, birds, and other vertebrates. But can it be applied to vertebrates that exhibit other modes of reproduction? In its present formulation the organizational concept appears to be restricted to gonochoristic vertebrates that have genotypic sex determination (Crews 1993). In reptiles with TSD, such as leopard geckos, the environment during development plays a major role in shaping the adult phenotype. In hermaphroditic fish where sex changes in the adult organism, can there even be an organizing or neutral sex? In parthenogenetic lizards only female individuals exist, yet each individual exhibits both male-like and female-like pseudosexual behaviors. Can the organizational concept be redefined and still account for the evidence at hand (figure 7.18)?

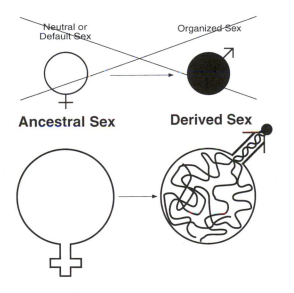

Figure 7.18 The organizational concept (*top*) postulates that the female is the neutral or the default sex, whereas the male is the organized sex. This paradigm emphasizes how males and females differ. Yet the organizational concept does not apply to vertebrates lacking sex chromosomes. An alternative paradigm (*bottom*) called the Evolutionary Concept, focuses more on the common origin of females and males, namely a single fertilized egg. Since males evolved only after the evolution of self-replicating (i.e., female) organisms, the female can regarded as the ancestral sex, whereas the male is regarded as the derived sex. (From Crews 1993.)

There can be little doubt that males evolved only after the evolution of self-replicating (i.e., female) organisms. Males have repeatedly been gained and lost, but females have remained. Speaking in terms of mechanisms, and not outcomes such as the presence of male and female individuals, the female may be considered as the ancestral sex and the male as the derived sex. This is not inconsistent with some of the original interpretations of the evidence of organization in mammalian sexual development. Such a perspective which I call the Evolutionary Concept accounts for the observation that maleness appears to be imposed upon a female phenotype, not vice versa. This formulation is independent of which sex is the heterogamete (XY or ZW) in those species with genetic sex determining mechanisms. This in turn suggests the intriguing possibility that males may be more like females than females are like males. In mammals the relative ease of masculinizing individuals compared to the difficulty of defeminizing individuals would be a case in point. Thus, Professor Higgins may have posed the wrong question in *My Fair Lady* when he asked rhetorically "Why can't a woman be more like a man?" A more interesting (and perhaps more accurate) question may be "Why can't a male be more like a female?"

The Evolutionary Concept perspective affords several problems worthy of study. First, at a basic level, the above question can only be answered by a study of the *similarities* of the neuroendocrine mechanisms subserving female-typical and male-typical sexual behavior. This would be a departure from the present focus on sex *differences* and the emphasis on studying mounting in gonadal males and receptivity in gonadal females. Is there any evidence that the Evolutionary Concept would yield new insights? One well-documented instance concerns the role of estrogen in the control of sex behavior. In most species of female vertebrates, estrogen activates sexual receptivity. Circulating testosterone is aromatized to estrogen in the brain of sexually active males and, in some species, estrogen is the active molecule in males as well as in females. Another example already discussed is role of progesterone in facilitating hormone-induced sexual behaviors in both sexes.

Hypothetical Steps in the Evolution of Behavioral Controling Mechanisms

Evolution is the cumulation of successful outcomes. We have already seen how a steroid hormone–dependent neuroendocrine mechanism might change. But how could such a complex and delicate system have evolved (table 7.4)? There appears to be an ancient functional relationship between gamete (i.e., sperm and or eggs) production and gonadal steroid secretion (Kanatani and Nagahama 1980). Gametes are never produced without a concomitant rise in gonadal steroid production. It is often the case, however, that gonadal steroid hormones are secreted without the production of sperm or eggs. It is clear that the sex steroid hormones have come to serve as activators of sexual behavior in a wide variety of vertebrate species.

How might hormone-brain-behavior relations have evolved in vertebrates? As a first step, the nervous system might have become responsive to hor-

Table 7.4 Hypothetical Scenarios in the Evolution of Hormone-Brain-Behavior Relationships in Vertebrates

1. Functional association between gametogenesis and steroid hormone production.
2. Functional association between steroid hormones and nervous system responsiveness.
3. Functional association between higher neural centers, the pituitary, and gonadal activity.
4. Functional association of gonadal steroid production and the development and later activation of gamete delivery systems.
5. Recruitment of integrative (limbic) areas influencing behavior via expansion of steroid-sensitive hypothalamic areas involved in the control of pituitary gonadotropin secretion.
6. Functional association of specific sexual signals and the secretion of gonadal steroids.

The first four major steps are probably shared by all vertebrates and hence are more ancient than the last two, which probably vary between species.

mones during development. This could have been followed by the development of a structure to regulate gonadal activity—in vertebrates, the anterior pituitary gland. Because the anterior pituitary is situated directly beneath the hypothalamus, a second step would involve the hypothalamic modulation of pituitary activity. As the animal perceives changes in its environment, this information could have been integrated at the level of the hypothalamus.

Development of a feedback control system involving the hypothalamus, the pituitary, and the gonads is the foundation of the functional association between gonadal hormone secretion and reproductive behavior. An expansion of the brain regions involved in the feedback control of pituitary function, including adjacent behavioral and integrative areas, could have mediated the development of these mechanisms. A further step in the evolution of hormone dependency of sexual behavior is seen in some species in which specific sexual signals elicit the secretion of reproductive hormones.

However, it should be emphasized that the presence of sex steroid hormone–concentrating neurons in behavioral integrative areas is not evidence a priori of a functional association between sex steroid hormones and sexual behavior. As pointed out earlier, neither female red-sided garter snakes nor female Asian musk shrews exhibit hormone-dependent sexual receptivity, yet sex steroid hormone–concentrating neurons have been identified in both species. As described earlier, species exhibiting dissociated reproductive patterns appear to have evolved alternative neuroendocrine mechanisms.

Another chicken-and-egg puzzle concerns the evolution of hormones and their receptors. For example, what came first, hormones or their receptors? How can a hormone evolve unless there is a receptor present to recognize it? Alternatively, how could a receptor evolve without hormones being already present? One popular scenario is that the common biochemical pathway in steroid metabolism, with progesterone being the precursor to androgens, which, in turn, give rise to the estrogens, reflects the evolutionary sequence for steroid hormones and their receptors. In this paradigm new receptors evolved with the emergence of each new class of steroid hormone. Hence, progesterone receptor (PR) would be the most ancient steroid hormone receptor and estrogen receptor (ER) the most recently evolved steroid hormone receptor. Attractive as it is, Thornton (2001) has provided an elegant and convincing challenge to this hypothesis.

The gene sequences of the steroid hormone receptors have been determined for several dozen species. Using bioinformatics and statistical techniques, Thornton reconstructed the gene sequence of the ancestral hormone receptor at the root of the steroid receptor evolutionary tree. Analysis of that sequence indicates that the ancestral steroid hormone was an ER (figure 7.19A). Thus, estrogen, the last hormone in the steroid biosynthetic pathway, appears to have been the first hormone to function through a steroid receptor. Thus, ER appears to have been the first steroid hormone receptor and coopted estrogen as a signaling molecule. Since estrogen synthesis and maturation of the egg is linked (for reasons as yet unknown), this union served as a reliable indicator to the brain to coordinate the reproductive process. In so doing, all of the intermediate steroid molecules in the steroidogenic pathway leading to estrogen became available as possible chemical signals for receptors that emerged by gene duplication (figure 7.19B). Thornton (2001) calls this co-evolutionary dance ligand exploitation, noting its similarity to the already discussed sensory exploitation model for the evolution of sexual signals. It is also possible that after the initial estrogen–estrogen receptor signaling system had evolved, subsequent receptors created by gene duplication were shaped by the intermediates themselves. That is, the fixed molecular structure of the steroid intermediates shaped through selection the gene sequence to render receptors having the greatest affinity/specificity for these intermediates. PR was the next steroid receptor to evolve, and its ancestral function may have been in the control of ovulation because it is associated with the ovulation. The role of androgen in development of a sexually dimorphic phenotype in males was a relatively recent evolutionary novelty, requiring the later emergence of the androgen receptor by gene duplication. The more ancient nature of estrogen receptors would explain the seeming paradox of why estrogen is the active molecule that "masculinizes" the brain in male mammals and birds.

Reconstructing evolutionary scenarios is useful because they help place systems in a larger context. Such scenarios can also lead to predictions or point the investigator toward potential areas of research. For example, a complete understanding of the role of the pituitary in vertebrate reproduction is aided by studies of primitive chordates in which the pituitary is exposed directly to the environment through a hole in the roof of the mouth. Reconstructed scenarios also help to place in perspective such apparent anomalies as dissociated reproductive patterns or environmental sex determination. Are these phenomena specialized adaptations or are they representative of more primitive conditions?

Similarly, the union of phylogenetic systematics and molecular genetics not only suggests solutions to questions of when and how molecules evolved, but also broadens our understanding of existing problems. For example, the

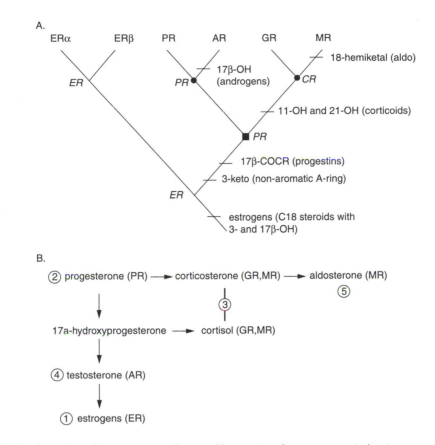

Figure 7.19 Evolution of hormone-specific steroid receptors from an ancestral estrogen receptor by ligand exploitation. (*A*) Phylogenetic tree of vertebrate steroid receptors, inferred from amino acid sequences of extant receptors. Branching points represent gene duplications; dark circles indicate a genome expansion after the divergence of lamprey from jawed vertebrates, and the dark square indicates a genome expansion before this divergence. Ancestral receptors at each node are shown based on reconstructions of ancestral sequences and characteristics. Bars on branches show the emergence of each receptor's capacity to bind ligands with the specific chemical structures. (*B*) The terminal hormone in the synthesis pathway for steroid hormones was the first for which a receptor evolved. A simplified form of the biochemical pathway for synthesis of mammalian steroid hormones is shown. The receptor bound by each hormone is shown, and the circled numbers shows the order in which those receptors emerged during evolution. Natural selection for estrogen-ER signaling also selected for the synthesis of progesterone and testosterone as intermediates, before there were receptors for these steroids. Subsequent gene duplications created novel receptors, which evolved high affinity for these steroids, transforming them into bona fide hormones. ER, estrogen receptor; PR, progesterone receptor; CR, corticoid receptor; GR, glucocorticoid receptor; MR, mineralocorticoid receptor; AR, androgen receptor; aldo, aldosterone.

conclusion that estrogen is the most ancient steroid hormone would account for its apparent endocrine role in a wide variety of taxa, from sea stars and amphioxus to vertebrates. This in turn would account for why so many species are profoundly affected when exposed to estrogenic pesticides and industrial organochlorines early in development.

Conclusions

With the great variety of animals, particularly their behaviors and their physiologies, are there any generalities? With the establishment of evolutionary theory, evidence that there is "unity in diversity" has come with discoveries of common anatomical features, the cell cycle, conservation of intermediary metabolism, and the genetic code, to name but a few. To this can be added that in vertebrates there is a conservation of the neural circuits underlying sexual behavior. Based on the examples in this chapter alone, it does not appear that the same can be said of the hormonal mechanisms underlying behavior.

This particular chapter has documented how some widely held assumptions are generalities only in a very restricted sense. I have shown how much of our conceptual understanding of the behavioral endocrinology stems from extensive studies on relatively few species. According to Beach (1979), there are

two cardinal rules that should govern not only the construction of animal models for human behavior, but for all interspecific comparisons regardless of the behavior and the species involved. The first rule is that meaningful comparisons are based not upon the formal characteristics of behavior, but upon its causal mechanisms and functional outcomes.... The second rule is that the validity of interspecific generalization cannot exceed the reliability of intraspecific analysis. Significant comparison of a particular type of behavior in two different species is impossible unless and until the behavior has been adequately analyzed in each species by itself. Only after independent, intraspecific analysis is achieved can we properly interpret the nature and degree of interspecific similarities and differences." (pp. 113–114)

To these two rules, a third and a fourth might be added. Third, make the consideration of the organism's natural history the first and last step in any biological study of behavior. Fourth, open the way to new insights by questioning traditional paradigms.

Applying an evolutionary perspective to behavioral endocrinology challenges the breadth and validity of assumptions about the mechanisms that control species-typical behaviors. This is not the same thing as saying that no unitary explanations apply to all mammals (versus nonmammals), endotherms (versus ectotherms), or even vertebrates (versus invertebrates). As this volume testifies, we have gathered considerable information about the neuroendocrine bases of behavior in a few species. To uncover truly broad generalizations, however, we must begin looking with equal intensity and rigor at other organisms.

Thus, the ecological and evolutionary perspective points the way to a variety of natural experiments or "experiments of nature." The pattern of evolution is best illustrated in the diversity of organisms. By studying closely related species that live in different habitats, we see how each has become adapted. By studying distantly related species that live in the same habitat, we can see if the solutions to similar problems are different or analogous.

The unique qualities of each species also give us a deeper understanding of the constraints and the potential for change in fundamental processes. Where basic conflicts exist, control mechanisms adapt or the species goes extinct. To echo the beginning admonition of Bullock, to ignore comparative research would greatly limit our understanding of the evolution of hormone-brain-behavior relations.

Summary

1. The timing of reproduction is subject to various constraints, including environmental, developmental, physiological, social and behavioral, and evolutionary factors.
2. These constraints have resulted in some animals in a dissociation between gonadal activity and sexual behavior in one or both of the sexes. In other animals they have led to the development of alternative mating strategies in males.
3. The behavioral interactions between the mating partners are important in facilitating and synchronizing the respective physiologys and advancing through the reproductive cycle.
4. There are a variety of sex-determining mechanisms in vertebrates, including genotypic, temperature, and behavioral sex determination. This means that the factors controlling the development of sexual dimorphisms may vary in fundamental ways in animals exhibiting different mechanisms of sex determination.
5. Sexuality resides in the brain, not in the gonad.
6. The adult phenotype results from a combination of hormonal and nonhormonal stimuli both early in development and later in adulthood. These might include the hormones or temperature experienced by an embryo or the behavior of the mother toward the young. Later in life these stimuli may include the behavioral experiences of the individual.
7. The neural circuits in the limbic forebrain the regulate social and sexual behavior are ancient and conserved among vertebrates.
8. Species differences in the distribution of sex steroid hormone–concentrating neurons are rare, but species differences in the abundance and regulation of sex steroid hormone receptors are common.
9. Progesterone and its receptor are important in the regulation of sexual behavior in male vertebrates.

10. Androgen and progesterone synergize in the control of the copulatory behavior of males much as estrogen and progesterone synergize in the control of the sexual receptivity of females.

Study Questions

1. Behavior and the neuroendocrine mechanisms that underlie it are subject to selection pressures. What environmental constraints shape the timing of reproductive behavior?
2. What is sexual selection and how might it be a factor in shaping the brain mechanisms that govern species-typical courtship behaviors?
3. What is phenotypic plasticity and what are some of the factors that influence it?
4. Reproduction requires behavioral and physiological synchronization of the participating animals. Explain what this means and give examples.
5. The organizational concept was developed from research on organisms that possess sex chromosomes. Does it apply to organisms that lack sex chromosomes? Discuss.

Acknowledgments

Preparation of this chapter was supported by the National Institute of Mental Health.

Notes

1. Energy metabolism in the brain can be mapped using several techniques two of which are: 2-deoxyglucose uptake determines acute changes in tissue metabolic activity due to energy use over a period of minutes, and cytochrome histochemistry which assesses the chronic alteration in tissue metabolic capacity resulting from sustained metabolic demands over a period of weeks or months.
2. The fundamental difference between sexual and unisexual organisms makes it important to have subtle but necessary semantic rules. (i) Strictly speaking, it is inaccurate to refer to "male sexual behavior" (i.e., mounting and intromission behavior) and "female sexual behavior" (i.e., receptive behavior); each individual usually displays the behaviors characteristic of its gonadal sex (or homotypical behaviors), but has the capacity to exhibit behaviors characteristic of the opposite gonadal sex (or heterotypical behaviors). Thus, it is more accurate to refer to male-typical and female-typical sexual behaviors. (ii) Although parthenogenetic whiptails have only ovaries and lack male genitalia, it is not appropriate to refer to them as females. The term "female" only has meaning in the context of "male." (iii) Parthenogenetic whiptails exhibit behaviors seen commonly in sexually active male whiptails during mating. (These I term "pseudosexual" behaviors.) Since male-typical and female-typical sexual behaviors can only refer to those behavioral displays associated with males and females in gonochoristic species (e.g., intromission and receptive behaviors, respectively), it is not appropriate to use this terminology when describing the pseudosexual behaviors of parthenogenetic species. Therefore, because two sexes usually do not occur in unisexual organisms, the terms "male-like" and "female-like" rather than "male-typical" and "female-typical" are used to refer to the appropriate pseudosexual behaviors.

References

Arnold, A. P., Wade, J., Grisham, W., Jacobs, E. C., and Campagnoni, A. T. (1996) Sexual differentiation of the brain in songbirds. *Devel. Neurosci.* 18: 124–136.

Bartholomew, G. A. (1982) Scientific innovation and creativity: A zoologist's point of view, *Am. Zool.* 22: 227–235.

Beach, F. A. (1979) Animal models for human sexuality. In R. Potter and J. Whelan (Eds.), *Sex, Hormones and Behaviour*. Ciba Foundation Symposium 62, Amsterdam: Excerpta Medica, pp. 113–143.

Beach, F. A. (1983) Hormones and psychological processes. *Can. J. Psych.*, 37: 193–210.

Bern, H. A. (1972) Comparative endocrinology—the state of the field and the art. *Gen. Comp. Endocr. Suppl.* 3: 751–761.

Bern, H. A. (1990) The new endocrinology: Its scope and its impact. *Am. Zool.* 30: 877–885.

Bluhm, C. K. (1985) Social factors regulating avian endocrinology and reproduction. In B. K. Follett, S. Ishii, and A. Chandola (Eds.), *The Endocrine System and the Environment*. Tokyo: Japanese Sci. Soc. Press, Berlin: Springer-Verlag, pp. 247–264.

Bluhm, C. K., Phillips, R. E., Burke, W. H., and Gupta, G. N. (1984) Effects of male courtship and gonadal steroids on pair formation, egg-laying, and serum LH in canvasback ducks (*Aythya valisineria*). *J. Zool. Lond.* 204: 185–200.

Bronson, F. H. (1989) *Mammalian Reproductive Biology*. Chicago: University of Chicago Press.

Bronson, F. H. (1995) Seasonal variation in human reproduction: Environmental factors. *Quart. Rev. Biol.* 70: 141–164.

Bullock, T. H. (1984) Comparative neuroscience holds promise for quiet revolutions. *Science* 225: 473–478.

Carson, H. L. (1987) The contribution of sexual behavior to Darwinian fitness, *Behav. Genet.* 17: 597–611.

Clark, M. M., and Galef, B. G. (1995) Prenatal influences on reproductive life history strategies. *Trends Ecol. Evol.* 10: 151–153.

Clutton-Brock, T. H. (1988) *Reproductive Success. Studies of Individual Variation in Contrasting Breeding Systems*. Chicago: University of Chicago Press.

Conaway, C. H. (1971) Ecological adaptation and mammalian reproduction, *Biol. Reprod.* 4: 239–247.

Crews, D. (1975) Psychobiology of reptilian reproduction, *Science* 189: 1059–1065.

Crews D. (1984) Gamete production, sex hormone secretion, and mating behavior uncoupled, *Horm. Behav.* 18: 22–28.

Crews D. (1987) Diversity and evolution of behavioral controlling mechanisms. In D. Crews (Ed.), *Psychobiology of Reproductive Behavior*. Englewood Cliffs, N.J.: Prentice Hall, pp. 88–119.

Crews, D. (1990) Neuroendocrine adaptations. In J. Balthazart (Ed.), *Hormones, Brain and Behaviour in Vertebrates*. Basel: S. Karger AG, pp. 1–14.

Crews, D. (1991) Trans-seasonal action of androgen in the control of spring courtship behavior in male red-sided garter snakes. *Proc. Natl. Acad. Sci.* 88: 3545–3548.

Crews, D. (1993) The organizational concept and vertebrates without sex chromosomes. *Brain Behav. Evol.* 42: 202–214.

Crews, D. (1994) Temperature, steroids, and sex determination. *J. Endocr.* 142: 1–8.

Crews, D. (1996) Temperature-dependent sex determination: The interplay of steroid hormones and temperature. *Zool. Sci.* 13: 1–13.

Crews, D. (1997) On the organization of individual differences in sexual behavior. *Am. Zool.* 38: 118–132.

Crews, D., and Moore, M. C. (1986) Evolution of mechanisms controlling mating behavior. *Science* 231: 121–125.

Crews, D., and Young, L. J. (1991) Pseudocopulation in nature in a unisexual whiptail lizard. *Anim. Behav.* 42: 512–515.

Crews, D., Godwin, J., Hartman, V., Grammar, M., Prediger, E. A., and Shephard, R. (1996) Intrahypothalamic implantation of progesterone in castrated male whiptail lizards (*Cnemidophorus inornatus*) elicits courtship and copulatory behavior and affects androgen- and progesterone receptor-mRNA expression in the brain. *J. Neurosci.* 16: 7347–7352.

Crews, D., Grassman, M., and Lindzey, J. (1986) Behavioral facilitation of reproduction in sexual and parthenogenetic whiptail (*Cnemidophorus*) lizards. *Proc. Natl. Acad. Sci. USA* 83: 9547–9550.

Crews, D., Hingorani, V., and Nelson, R. J. (1988) Role of the pineal gland in the control of annual reproductive behavioral and physiological cycles in the red-sided garter snake (*Thamnophis sirtalis parietalis*). *J. Biol. Rhythms* 3: 293–302.

Crews, D., Robker, R., and Mendonça, M. (1993) Seasonal fluctuations in brain nuclei in the red-sided garter snake and their hormonal control. *J. Neurosci.* 13: 5356–5364.

Crews, D., Sakata, J., and Rhen, T. (1998) Developmental effects on intersexual and intrasexual variation in growth and reproduction in a lizard with temperature-dependent sex determination. *Comp. Biochem. Physiol. (Part C)* 119: 229–241.

Crews, D., Wade, J., and Wilczynski, W. (1990) Sexually dimorphic areas in the brain of whiptail lizards. *Brain Behav. Evol.* 36: 262–270.

Dawkins, R. (1976) *The Selfish Gene.* Oxford: Oxford University Press.

Denver, R. J. (1997) Proximate mechanisms in phenotypic plasticity in amphibian metamorphosis. *Am. Zool.* 37: 172–184.

Devlin, B., Daniels, M., and Roeder, K. (1997) The heritability of IQ. *Nature* 388: 468–471.

DeVoogd, T. J., Krebs, J. R., Healy, S. D., and Purvis, A. (1993) Relations between song repertoire size and the volume of brain nuclei related to song: Comparative evolutionary analyses amongst oscine birds. *Proc. Roy. Soc. Lond. B*, 254: 73–82.

Diamond, J. (1983) Laboratory, field, and natural experiments. *Nature* 304: 586–587.

Eberhard, W. G. (1996) *Female Control: Sexual Selection by Cryptic Female Choice.* Princeton: Princeton University Press.

Francis, D., Diorio, J., Liu, D., and Meany, M. J. (1999) Nongenomic transmission across generations of maternal behavior and stress responses in the rat. *Science* 286: 1155–1158.

Ghiselin, M. T. (1974) *The Economy of Nature and the Evolution of Sex.* Berkeley: University of California Press.

Glickman, S. E., Zabel, C. J., Yoerg, S. I., Weldele, M. L., Drea, C. M., and Frank, L. G. (1997) Social facilitation, affiliation, and dominance in the social life of spotted hyenas. In C. S. Carter, I. I. Lederhendler, and B. Kirkpatrick (Eds.), *The Integrative Neurobiology of Affiliation.* New York: Annals New York Academy of Sciences, pp. 175–185.

Godwin, J., Crews, D., and Warner, R. R. (1996) Behavioral sex change in the absence of gonads in a coral reef fish. *Roy. Soc. London B*, 263: 1683–1688.

Gould, S. J., and Vrba, E. S. (1982) Exaptation—a missing term in the science of form, *Paleobiology* 8: 4–15.

Gross, M. R. (1984) Sunfish, salmon, and the evolution of alternative reproductive strategies and tactics in fishes. In G. W. Potts and R. J. Wooten (Eds.), *Fish Reproduction: Strategies and Tactics.* New York: Academic Press, pp. 55–75.

Hillis, D. M., Moritz, C., and Mable, B. K. (1996) *Molecular Systematics*, 2nd edition. Sunderland, Mass.: Sinauer.

Hull, E. M., Lorrain, D. S., Du, J., Matuszewich, L., Bitrand, D., Nishita, J. K., and Scaletta, L. L. (1998) Organizational and activational effects of dopamine on male sexual behavior. In L. Ellis, and L. Ebertz (Eds.), *Males, Females, and Behavior: Towards Biological Understanding.* Wesstport, Conn.: Praeger Press, in press.

Kanatani, H., and Nagahama, Y. (1980) Mediators of oocyte maturation. *Biomed. Res.* 1: 273–291.

Kindler, P. M., Philipp, D. P., Gross, M. R., and Bahr, J. M. (1989) Serum 11-ketotestosterone and testosterone concentrations associated with reproduction in male bluegill (*Lepomis macrochirus: Centrachidae*). *Gen. Comp. Endocr.* 75: 446–453.

Kirkpatrick, M., and Ryan, M. J. (1991) The evolution of mating preferences and the paradox of the lek. *Nature* 350: 33–38.

Lindzey, J., and Crews, D. (1992) Interactions between progesterone and androgens in the stimulation of sex behaviors in male little striped whiptail lizards, *Cnemidophorus inornatus. Gen. Comp. Endocr.* 86: 52–58.

Lindzey, J., and Crews, D. (1993) Effects of progesterone and dihydrotestosterone on stimulation of androgen-dependent sex behavior, accessory sex structures, and *in vitro* binding characteristics of cytosolic androgen receptors in male whiptail lizards (*Cnemidophorus inornatus*). *Horm. Behav.* 27: 269–281.

McFadden, D. (1997) Sex differences in the auditory system. *Develop. Neuropsych.* (in press).

Mason, R. T., Fales, H. M., Jones, T. H., Pannell, L. K., Chinn, J. W., and Crews, D. (1989) Sex pheromones in garter snakes. *Science* 245: 290–293.

Maynard Smith, J. (1978) *The Evolution of Sex.* Cambridge, UK: Cambridge University Press.

Mendonça, M. T., and Crews, D. (1990) Effect of fall mating on ovarian development in the red-sided garter snake, *Am. J. Physiol.* 26: R1548–R1550.

Mendonça, M. T., and Crews, D. (2001) Control of attracturty and receptivity in the female red-sided garter snake, *Thamnophis sirtalis parietalis. Horm. Behav.* (in press).

Mendonça, M. T., Tousignant, A. J., and Crews, D. (1995) Seasonal changes and annual variability in daily plasma melatonin in the red-sided garter snake (*Thamnophis sirtalis parietalis*). *Gen. Comp. Endocr.* 100: 226–237.

Mendonça, M. T., Tousignant, A. J., and Crews, D. (1996a) Pinealectomy, melatonin and courtship behavior in male red-sided garter snakes (*Thamnophis sirtalis parietalis*). *J. Exp. Zool.* 274: 63–74.

Mendonça, M. T., Tousignant, A. J., and Crews, D. (1996b) Courting and noncourting male garter snakes, *Thamnophis sirtalis parietalis*: Plasma melatonin levels and the effects of pinealectomy. *Horm. Behav.* 30: 176–185.

Moore, C. L. (1995) Maternal contributions to mammalian reproductive development and divergence of males and females. In P. J. B. Slater, J. S. Rosenblatt, C. T. Snowdon, and M. Milinski (Eds.), *Advances in the Study of Behavior*. New York: Academic Press, pp. 47–118.

Phelps, S. M., Lydon, J., O'Malley, B. W., and Crews, D. (1998) Regulation of male sexual behavior by progesterone receptor, sexual experience and androgens. *Horm. Behav.* 34: 294–302.

Pigliucci, M. (1996) How organisms respond to environmental changes: From phenotypes to molecules (and vice versa). *Trends Ecol. Evol.* 11: 168–173.

Prendergast, B. J., Kriegsfeld, C. J., and Nelson, L. J. (2001) Photoperiodic polyphenisms in rodents: Neuroendocrine mechanisms, costs and functions. *Q. Rev. Biol.* (in press).

Prosser, C. L. (1986) *Adaptational Biology: Molecules to Organisms*. New York: Wiley.

Prosser, C. L. (1988) Comparative physiology and biochemistry: Challenges for the future. *Comp Biochem Physiol.* 93A: 309–312.

Pusey, A., Williams, J., and Goodall, J. (1997) The influence of dominance rank on the reproductive success of female chimpanzees. *Science* 277: 828–831.

Rand, M. S., and Crews, D. (1994) The bisexual brain: Sex differences and sex behaviour differences in sexual and parthenogenetic lizards. *Brain Res.* 665: 163–167.

Rissman, E. (1995) An alternative animal model for the study of female sexual behavior. *Curr. Directions Psychol. Sci.* 4: 6–10.

Ryan, M. J. (1990) Sexual selection, sensory systems, and sensory exploitation, *Oxford Survey Evol. Biol.* 7: 157–196

Ryan, M. J. (1996) Phylogenetics in behavior: Some cautions and expectations. In E. P. Martins (Ed.), *Phylogenies and the Comparative Method in Animal Behavior*. New York: Oxford University Press, pp. 1–21.

Ryan, M. J., Fox, J. H., Wilczynski, W., and Rand, A. S. (1990) Sexual selection for sensory exploitation in the frog *Physalanaemus pustulosus*. *Nature*, 343: 66–67.

Signoret, J. P. (1976) Chemical communication and reproduction in domestic mammals. In R. L. Doty (Ed.), *Mammalian Olfaction, Reproductive Processes, and Behavior*. New York: Academic Press, pp. 243–256.

Sorensen, P. W., and Stacey, N. E. (1991) Identified hormonal pheromones in the goldfish: The basis for a model of sex pheromone function in teleost fish. In D. MacDonald, D. Muller-Schwarze and R. M. Silverstein (Eds.), *Chemical Signals in Vertebrates V*. Oxford: Oxford University Press, pp. 302–311.

Thomas, C. S., and Coulson, J. C. (1988) Reproductive success of kittiwake gulls, *Rissa tridactyla*. In T. H. Clutton-Brock (Ed.), *Reproductive Success*. Chicago: University of Chicago Press, pp. 251–262.

Thornton, J. (2000) *Pandora's Poison: Chlorine, Health and a New Environmental Strategy*. Cambridge, Mass.: MIT Press.

Thornton, J. W. (2001) Evolution of vertebrate steroid receptors from an ancestral estrogen receptor by ligand exploitation and serial genome expansions. *Proc. Natl. Acad. Sci. USA* 98: 5671–5676.

Udry, J. R., Morris, N. M., and Kovenock, J. (1995) Androgen effects on women's gendered behavior. *J. Biosoc. Sci.* 27: 359–368.

Wade, J., Huang, J.-H., and Crews, D. (1993) Hormonal control of sex differences in the brain, behavior, and accessory sex structures of whiptail lizards (*Cnemidophorus* species). *J. Neuroendocrinol.* 5: 81–93.

Williams, G. C. (1966) *Adaptation and Natural Selection: A Critique of Some Current Evolutionary Thought*. Princeton: Princeton University Press.

Wilson, E. O. (1975) *Sociobiology: The New Synthesis*. Cambridge, Mass.: Belknap Press of Harvard University Press.

Wingfield, J. C., Hegner, R. E., Dufty, A. M., and Ball, G. F. (1990) The "challenge hypothesis": Theoretical implications for patterns of testosterone secretion, mating systems and breeding strategies of birds. *Am. Nat.* 136: 829–846.

Witt, D. M., Young, L. J., and Crews, D. (1995) Progesterone modulation of androgen-dependent sexual behavior in male rats. *Physiol. Behav.* 57: 307–313.

Yamamoto, J. T., Shields, K. M., Millam, J. R., Roudybush, T. E., and Grau, C. R. (1989) Reproductive activity of force-paired cockatiels (*Nymphicus hollandicus*). *Auk* 106: 86–93.

Young, L. J., and Crews, D. (1995) Comparative neuroendocrinology of steroid receptor gene expression and regulation: Relationship to physiology and behavior. *Trends Endocr. Metabol.* 6: 317–323.

Zeyl, C., and Bell, G. (1997) The advantage of sex in evolving yeast populations. *Nature* 388: 465–468.

8 Hormonal Influences on Courtship Behaviors

Darcy B. Kelley and Eliot Brenowitz

Almost all vertebrates engage in some sort of courtship as part of mate selection. This chapter examines the neural and hormonal control of courtship in three different groups: electric fish, clawed frogs, and songbirds. Electric fish use unusual kinds of signals, brief electrical discharges from modified muscle cells, as sexual advertisements. Electrical discharges propagate well in turbid underwater habitats where visual signals, for example, would be hard to distinguish. Another very beautiful, to human ears, example of courtship is birdsong. In temperate zones, seasonal song is produced only by males, while in the tropics both sexes sing highly synchronized duets. The springtime chorus of croaking frogs also functions as a courtship song to attract potential mates and to advertise the qualities of the signaler. These complex behaviors are strongly affected by gonadal hormones and provide an opportunity for behavioral endocrinologists, to explore how steroidal effects on the nervous system influence behaviors.

What are courtship displays, what are their functions, and why are they more often performed by males than females? How do hormones influence the development and adult function of courtship signals? These themes underlie our exploration of three fascinating courtship systems.

Introduction

Courtship behaviors are critical for successful reproduction. During courtship a member of one sex produces a series of signals that induces a member of the other sex to mate. In addition to attracting and stimulating potential mates, courtship signals convey information that can be used in selecting a reproductive partner. Some examples of the sorts of information conveyed are the species to which the signaler belongs, the sex of the signaler, his or her readiness to mate, the size and age of the signaler, and the kind of territory he or she holds.

Evolution of Courtship Behavior

Identifying the sex of a potential mate is obviously critical, and courtship behaviors that differ markedly between males and females can function in this way. However, the signaling systems used in courtship displays are often much more elaborate than would be required simply to tag the signaler as male or female. Charles Darwin attempted to account for these and other features of courtship behaviors through his theory of sexual selection (described in chapter 7). Sexual selection operates when individuals of a species differ in their ability to compete for resources critical for successful reproduction. Darwin believed that sexual selection accounted for some extreme differences between the sexes, such as the peacock's tail. These extreme effects are balanced by natural selection. Natural selection favors the integration of reproductive behavior and physiology with physiological adaptations (e.g., metabolism) and other sorts of behavior (e.g., foraging) that are essential for survival.

In most species, courtship is initiated by males. Robert Trivers (Trivers 1985) helped to explain why males usually compete for access to females while females usually choose among males. His explanation involves the relative investment of energy and time made in reproduction by each sex. First, each sex produces different gametes. Males produce sperm and females produce eggs. Females make a greater energetic investment in the production of their gametes, because in addition to containing the female's chromosomes, eggs generally contain a high-energy nutritive substance, the yolk. The yolk sustains the early development of the fertilized embryo. Each sperm cell of a male, on the other hand, is small and therefore energetically much cheaper to produce than an egg. Sperm consist simply of the male's chromosomes surrounded by a protein coat with an attached flagellum to provide mobility (figure 8.1).

The large difference in energy invested in gamete production between males and females is reflected in a sex difference in the number of gametes produced over a lifetime. Females usually produce mature eggs in numbers that range from tens to thousands (egg numbers for human females are a few

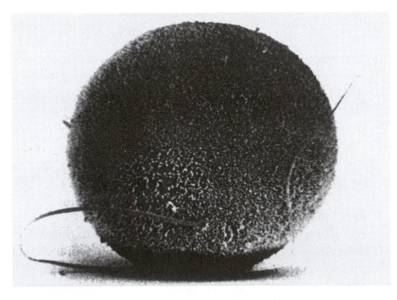

Figure 8.1 Hamster sperm fertilizing a hamster egg. Note the size difference between the sperm and the egg (magnification ×1640). (Photograph by David M. Phillips, reprinted with permission.)

hundred). Males, however, produce sperm in nearly astronomical numbers. During a single ejaculation, for example, a human male releases about 100 million sperm cells. Differences in investment by males and females are not confined to the gametes. Once the egg is fertilized by a male's sperm, females of many species continue to make a greater investment in the offspring than males do. For example, in mammals the female nourishes the developing embryo throughout a gestational period that may last many months. In addition, female care of offspring may persist after birth or hatching until her progeny become fully independent. The role of hormones in parental behavior will be discussed in greater detail in chapter 9.

Thus, in most animal species, females make a greater investment of energy and time in the production of offspring than males do. A consequence of this difference in investment is that males and females differ fundamentally in the strategies that will maximize reproductive success over their entire lifetimes. Since sperm are relatively cheap for the male to produce, his reproductive success is not limited by the numbers of sperm that he can make. Instead, the male's reproductive success will be determined by the number of eggs that he can fertilize. Males will usually maximize the number of eggs fertilized by mating with as many females as possible. We therefore expect males to compete fiercely for access to females.

The number of offspring that a female can produce during her lifetime will be severely limited by the costs of making eggs and rearing young. Each egg, then, is of relatively greater importance to a female's reproductive success than each sperm is to a male. A female can maximize her reproductive investment by ensuring that each egg fertilized has a good chance of producing an offspring that will itself survive to reproduce. The female's best means of accomplishing this is to mate only with males of high genetic quality or with males that contribute through care or territorial defense to the survival of offspring. Consequently, females will tend to be choosy about which males they allow to fertilize their eggs. By choosing among competing males, females in effect force males to demonstrate their relative quality. This selective force has led to the evolution of courtship behavior by males.

Production of Courtship Behavior

How then is a particular courtship behavior produced? Usually the behavior is triggered by a specific stimulus, for instance, hearing the song produced by a member of the opposite sex. Stimuli are detected by sensory receptors and conveyed into the central nervous system by sensory neurons. Because some stimuli are very complex, different components of the stimulus (for instance, sound pitch, rate, and rhythm) are processed by separate groups of interneurons (neurons whose processes are confined to the CNS) working in parallel. Different sensory stimuli evoke activity in different brain nuclei; this activity then affects interneurons dedicated to producing patterned motor output. The final step is a change in the activity of motoneurons, resulting in contraction and relaxation of the muscles that produce the courtship behavior. Synaptically interconnected brain nuclei that participate in producing courtship behavior have been identified for the three courtship systems discussed in this chapter.

When males are responsible for courtship, brain nuclei and muscle groups involved in the behavior can differ dramatically in structure and function from those found in females (Kelley 1988). In some insects, house flies and moths, for example, sensory receptors and neurons associated with detecting sexual signals are different in males and females. In some birds, the brain nuclei that affect motor patterning also differ. In certain frogs, the motoneurons and muscles that produce attraction calls are different in the sexes. These sensory, neural, and muscular behavioral effector systems are thus sexually dimorphic (different in form in males and females), as are the behaviors they produce.

The hormonal and neural bases of sexually dimorphic courtship behavior will be the focus of this chapter. We will concentrate on three model courtship systems spanning various vertebrate classes and sensory modalities of communication. These are electric communication in fish, vocalizations in frogs, and song production in birds. Hormones influence the production of courtship signals by acting at different levels of the nervous system in these three groups. In electric fish, hormones act directly upon cells at the most peripheral level of the neuromuscular circuits involved in the production and reception of electric mating signals. Hormones are essential for the organization of the sexually dimorphic vocal organ in clawed frogs and play an important role in the activation of regions of the hindbrain in the central nervous system that control advertisement calling. In songbirds, hormones are critical in both the organization and activation of nuclei in the forebrain that regulate song behavior. In considering these systems, we will also see that hormones act on the nervous system as the proximate agents for sexual selection.

Sex Electric: Courtship in Electric Fish

Freshwater fish that use electric signals for orientation and for courtship displays occur in the American and African tropics. These fish are called weakly electric because, unlike electric eels, their discharges are not strong enough to stun prey. They are nocturnal and often live in murky water, conditions that favor nonvisual forms of communication. Two groups of fish use these weak electric signals: the South American gymnotiforms and the African mormyriforms (figure 8.2). In both groups, courtship is triggered by environmental changes associated with the onset of the breeding season (Hagedorn 1986; Zakon 1993). In some species, courtship is triggered when the male detects the electrical signals generated by females. Subsequent pairing involves changes in the electrical signals of both sexes much like the duets that characterize pair bonds in tropical birds (see the last section in this chapter).

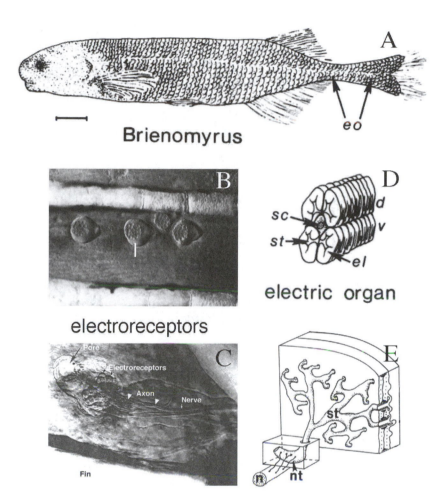

Brienomyrus

electroreceptors

electric organ

Figure 8.2 Overview of electric organs and electroreceptors. (*A*) Line drawing of *Brienomyrus* (a mormyrid) showing the electric organ, located in the tail; scale bar: 1 cm. (Modified from Bass and Volman 1987.) (*B*) Electrosensory organs from the anal fin of the glass catfish. Each organ contains a cluster of electroreceptors (white line). These ampullary electroreceptors are similar to the tuberous electroreceptors used in electric communication. (*C*) Each organ communicates with the environment via a pore. Clusters of electroreceptors send information to the central nervous system via sensory nerve axons. (Photograph by Michele Bever, reprinted with permission.) (*D*) A magnified view of the electric organ surrounding the spinal cord (sc). The electric organ consists of columns of serially stacked, disk-shaped cells, the electrocytes (el). A stalk (st) lies on the anterior side of each electrocyte. (*E*) Line drawing showing a cut away view of one-half of a *single* electrocyte. The three action potential-generating membranes of the electrocyte are the anterior and posterior faces and the stalk. The stalk is innervated in a restricted zone by nerve terminals (nt) that arise from axons of the electromotor nerve (n). The entire cell is enclosed in a compartment containing a gelatinous matrix. (Modified from Bass, A. H. 1986b.)

It has been difficult to study electrical courtship in the wild because mormyrids and gymnotids are nocturnal and elusive. Fortunately, electric fish can be successfully bred in the laboratory by mimicking the natural conditions (pH, water electrical conductivity, rain, and water depth) that characterize the start of the breeding season. Hagedorn and Heiligenberg (1985) used this method to observe the mating behavior of the glass knife fish, *Eigenmannia virescens*, in laboratory aquaria. Hagedorn (1986) observed,

The night of spawning is an electrical extravaganza, males will fight for many nights for dominance in the mating hierarchy, the females defend spawning territories (floating plants) and the dominant male will spawn only with the dominant female. The female hangs almost vertically in the plants, while the male courts her with a barrage of electrical "chirping" (60 to 80/minute) that may last all night. As the female lays her eggs, she produces low amplitude chirps; then the male rubs through the plants fertilizing the eggs. Peripheral, subordinate females try to sneak their eggs into the spawning territory, often turning off their EOD [electric organ discharge] as they rush towards the plant, only to be driven away by the dominant pair. (Hagedorn and Heilenberg 1985).

The electrical signal is so powerful in reproductive behavior that gravid females will lay eggs in response to a recording of male chirping.

As might be expected, the electrical signals given by mature males differ from those of mature females and juveniles that are not yet reproductively mature. In this section, we will consider how sex differences in the EOD are generated and detected. As is the case for frog and bird song (see below), much evidence implicates sex-specific hormones in electrical signaling during courtship. In some cases we are beginning to understand the cellular bases for these hormone effects. So far, the effects of hormones on electrical signaling appear to be purely activational; male/female differences reflect sex-typical patterns of hormone secretion during the breeding season.

The Electric Channel of Communication

Some electrogenic fish (like *Torpedo*) are capable of delivering sizeable electric shocks of up to 600 volts to stun their prey. The gymnotids and mormyrids, however, generate much weaker signals, in the range of a few millivolts to a few volts. In most species, electrical discharges are produced by modified muscle cells called electrocytes (figure 8.3) located in the fish's tail; electrocytes are innervated by a specialized type of motoneuron, the electromotoneuron. In some species (the Apternotids), the EOD is produced by the axons of electromotoneurons directly (Bennett 1971). Electric signals are detected by electroreceptors, a type of sensory organ located in the fish's skin. The electroreceptors contain a group of sensory cells. The electroreceptor is contacted by an afferent fiber of a sensory neuron that sends its axon into the brain.

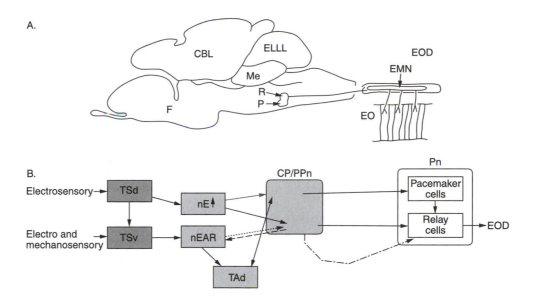

Figure 8.3 (*A*) Side view of a mormyrid brain illustrating the electromotor pathway. CBL, cerebellum; ELLL, nucleus electrosensorius; EMN, electromotor neurons; F, forebrain; Me, midbrain; P, pacemaker nucleus; R, relay nucleus. (Modified from Bass et al. 1986.) (*B*) Brain regions involved in responding to conspecific electric signals. EOD, electric organ discharge; CP/PPn, prepacemaker nucleus; nEAR, nucleus electrosensorius; TAd, dorsal anterior tuberal nucleus; TSd,v, dorsal and ventral torus semicircularis of the midbrain. (Modified from Metzner 1999.)

How far away from another electric fish can a signal producer be and still have its electric organ discharges detected? In other words, how big is the signaling fish's active space? The answer depends somewhat on the type and size of fish and the electrical characteristics of the water; best estimates are in the range of 70 to 100 cm (Hopkins 1986). As the water's electrical conductivity is lowered (as would happen, for example, when it rained), the active space of the electric signal increases dramatically (Squire and Moller 1982). On the receptive side, a noisy electrical environment (lightning, for example) can interfere with another fish's ability to locate the source of a signal. Thus, electrical signaling is a short-range form of communication; the fish generally have to be within 100 cm (several feet) of each other to interact using this modality. Unlike vision, in which the receptor organs have to be oriented toward the signal source, electroreception does not require directed attention to be effective. The electroreceptors will be stimulated, although to varying degrees, no matter what the orientation of the receiving fish with respect to the signaler.

INFORMATION COMMUNICATED IN ELECTRIC SIGNALS
The basic unit of electrical signaling is the EOD. The EOD is made up of individual pulses that can have a simple or a complex waveform, depending on the geometry of the electrocyte that generates them (reviewed in Bass 1986b).

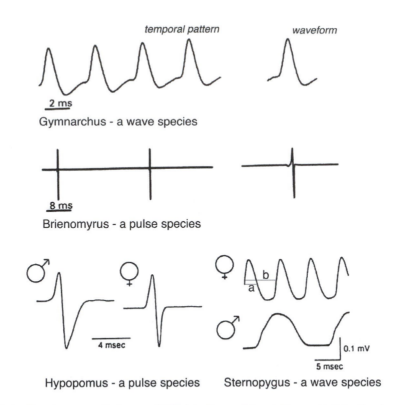

Figure 8.4 Electric organ discharges (EODs) in Gymnotid and Mormyrid fish. If pulse duration is long compared to the interval between pulses, then the signal is called a wave EOD (*Gymnarchus* is a wave species). If the pulse duration is short compared with the interval between pulses, then the signal is called a pulse EOD (*Brienomyrus* is a pulse species). (Modified from Bass 1986.) In both wave (*Sternopygus*) and pulse (*Hypopomus*) species, the EOD can be sexually dimorphic. The duty cycle of the EOD (a/b) is illustrated for *Sternopygus*, a wave species. (Modified from Zakon 1993.)

Individual pulses can be strung together in trains with particular rhythms. If pulse duration is long compared to the interval between pulses, then the signal is called a wave EOD. If the pulse duration is short compared with the interval between pulses, then the signal is called a pulse EOD (figure 8.4).

During the first phase of courtship, EODs are used to locate a conspecific of the other sex. The other fish is easy to locate because most electric fish continually discharge at low rates. In addition to location, these spontaneous EODs convey information about the age and sex of the signaler because, in many species, the EOD is different for adult males, females, and juveniles. For example, in *Sternopygus macrurus*, a wave discharging species (figure 8.4), mature males discharge at a characteristic rate of 50 to 90 Hz (cycles per second), mature females at 100 to 150 Hz, and juveniles are intermediate between these two (Hopkins 1972). Since the EOD is correlated with the breeding condition of the animal, it can also convey information about its reproductive state.

Some fish use specific EOD discharges as courtship signals. A good example is the "chirp" used in the courtship of male glass knife fish (*Eigenmannia virescens*). Chirps consist of brief and rapid increases in the EOD rate. There is no audible component to this electrical signal, but when it is played through a loudspeaker it sounds like a chirp. In some species males do most of the chirping. In others, females also chirp as eggs pass through their reproductive tract. In *Sternopygus*, adult males respond to female (but not to male) EOD rates by chirping (Hopkins 1974). Thus, in different species of electric fish EODs can be used to attract and stimulate females, to synchronize reproductive behaviors of males and females, and to convey information about the sex of the signaler.

METHOD OF GENERATION AND RECEPTION OF ELECTRIC SIGNALS

As mentioned earlier, electric signals (with rare exceptions) are produced by specialized muscle cells called electrocytes. The electric organ is located in the tail and consists of stacks of disclike electrocytes (figure 8.3). The electrocyte has two sides or faces: anterior and posterior. In addition, the electrocyte has a thin protrusion, the stalk, which in many species passes through the main body of the electrocyte and connects the anterior and posterior faces. These morphological elements are believed to contribute to the EOD waveform (Bennett and Grundfest 1961; Bass and Volman 1987). Electrocytes generate electrical signals in response to activity in their motoneurons. In mormyrids, these electromotor neurons in the spinal cord discharge synchronously in response to a command signal emanating from a nearby relay nucleus (figure 8.3). The relay nucleus is synaptically connected to an adjacent command nucleus which in turn is driven by nuclei in the midbrain (Bell and Szabo 1986). In gymnotiforms, pacemaker and relay cells are located in the same nucleus (Dye and Meyer 1986).

Electrical signals used in courtship are detected by specialized sensory receptors that are located just below the skin surface. Electrical current gains access to these electroreceptors through a canal that is open to the external water. Electroreceptors are modified hair cells, a type of sensory receptor found also in the vertebrate ear. When electrically stimulated, electroreceptors release a neurotransmitter that stimulates sensory neurons. Axons of these sensory neurons form the lateral line nerve. Incoming lateral line axons terminate on sensory interneurons located in a nucleus of the hindbrain (the electrosensory lateral line lobe), which in turn projects to a midbrain nucleus (the torus semicircularis).

Sex Differences in Electroproduction and Reception

Sex differences in the form and function of electrocytes have been described in both mormyriforms and gymnotiforms. In many species, the EOD waveform differs in males and females (figure 8.4). Typically, the waveform is longer in males. Sex differences in EOD waveform are correlated with the thickness and complexity of the electrocyte membrane, which is greater in males than in females. Increases in membrane thickness should increase the ability of the electrocyte to store electrical charges and thus prolong the EOD waveform. In addition, the properties of the ion channels that control the electrical activity of electrocytes differ in the sexes (Zakon 1993).

In addition to the waveform itself, the EOD rhythm can be sex specific. For example, male *Sternopygus macrurus* discharge at much lower rates than females (figure 8.4) (Hopkins 1972). Sex differences in pulse rhythms are a result of sex differences in the command signals coming from the brain. We do not yet have a clear understanding of how such sex differences in pulse rhythms and rates are generated by brain interneurons dedicated to producing patterned motor output.

Each fish's electroreceptors are most sensitive (tuned) to specific characteristics of electrical stimuli, typically those associated with the fish's own EOD. This is because the EOD is also used for orientation, and the fish must monitor how EOD transmission is affected by nearby objects. When the EOD is different in males and females, the tuning of the electroreceptors is also different in the sexes (Zakon 1987). Note that even though the fish's receptors are most sensitive to its own frequencies for weak (low amplitude) signals, they can also detect the frequencies used by the opposite sex if signals are stronger (higher amplitude).

How does the sensitivity of the electroreceptor come to match the fish's own EOD? The EOD could tune the receptor, or receptor tuning could be achieved independently. These alternatives have been studied by removing a piece of skin containing the original electroreceptors in *Sternopygus* and following the tuning of the new receptors that appear as the skin regenerates (Zakon 1986). Even if the fish experiences no electrical field at all during regeneration, the new receptors become tuned to the same frequency as the fish's EOD. This result implies that receptor tuning occurs independently of external stimulation by a particular EOD. However, the actual mechanism that produces receptor tuning is not known. In mormyrids, retuning does depend on intact electric organ discharges (Bass and Hopkins 1984).

HORMONAL CONTROL OF THE EOD AND ELECTRORECEPTORS
Several lines of evidence suggest that sex differences in EODs are controlled by hormones. The primary clue is that the EODs of males and females differ; in many vertebrates, such sex differences are controlled by sex differences in circulating gonadal hormones during the breeding season. However, field observations of EOD variation by sex often failed to find any sex differences at particular times of the year, suggesting that hormone effects are of the transitory or activational variety (Bass 1986a; Hopkins 1988). When steroid hormones are given to adult fish, both the waveform of the EOD and its temporal pattern are affected (Dunlap et al. 1997; Dunlap and Zakon 1998).

In the mormyrid *Brienomyrus brachistius* (triphasic), either of two major androgenic steroids, testosterone (T) and dihydrotestosterone (DHT), will broaden the EOD of adult females or juveniles to a form resembling that of the adult male (Bass and Hopkins 1984). In the gymnotid *Sternopygus macrurus*, dihydrotestosterone will prolong the EOD pulse duration and decrease the rate at which the pulses are given (Meyer 1983; Mills and Zakon 1987). In *Eigenmannia virescens* (a gymnotid), androgens (T and DHT) decrease EOD rate. Another androgen that is very active in fish, 11-ketotestosterone, also increases pulse duration without affecting duty cycle (see figure 8.4), duration of negative and positive phases, or EOD frequency composition (Dunlap and Zakon 1998). The changes produced by androgens are in the male direction for each species.

Changes in the opposite direction are observed following castration. In male *B. brachistius*, castration causes a shortening of the EOD pulse (Bass 1986a). Gonadectomy of adult *S. macrurus* causes the EOD rate to increase in males and decrease in females (Meyer 1983). (Recall that both the waveform of individual EOD pulses and the temporal pattern with which pulses are produced can differ in males and females.) The effect of ovariectomy on EODs of adult female fish suggests that hormones secreted by the female gonad also contribute to the EOD. In *Sternopygus*, administration of estradiol induces an increase in the rate at which pulses are given (Meyer 1983; Dunlap et al. 1977). The amounts of hormones given in these experiments produced serum concentrations roughly comparable to those measured in individual fish during the breeding season (Zakon et al. 1991). It is thus reasonable to suppose that changes in circulating hormone concentrations that are experienced by adult fish are responsible for sex differences in electric organ discharges.

Are sex differences in the tuning of electroreceptors also attributable to gonadal hormones? In *Sternopygus*, DHT has been shown to shift sensitivity of individual electroreceptors in females to lower frequencies (Meyer and Zakon 1982). A similar effect is seen in *Brienomyrus* (Bass and Hopkins 1984). These androgen effects shift the tuning of electroreceptors in the masculine direction. It is not known whether individual differences in circulating hormone levels contribute to the individual differences in the electroreceptor tuning described earlier.

How do steroid hormones change the characteristics of EODs? Intracellular recording from electrocytes under current and voltage clamp conditions (together with the use of drugs that block specific channels) has allowed us to determine what ion channels are active as the EOD is being generated and how channel activity is affected by hormones. In *Sternopygus*, androgens increase EOD pulse duration by slowing down the inactivation of the sodium current. Estrogen shortens EOD pulse duration by accelerating sodium current inactivation (Dunlap et al. 1997). Some nuclei of electrocytes in this species express androgen and estrogen receptors, as determined by immunocytochemistry (Dunlap et al. 1997; Dunlap and Zakon 1998). Since steroid hormone receptors are transcription factors, hormones could act directly on the electrocytes themselves to control the expression of ion channel characteristics, perhaps via regulation of ion channel isoforms (different genes or differently spliced mRNAs from the same gene) with different inactivation characteristics.

How hormones control the frequency of EOD discharges is still a mystery. The rhythm and rate of EOD discharges are controlled by a dedicated motor circuit in the brain. The prepacemaker nucleus expresses androgen receptor in *Brienomyrus* (Bass et al. 1986) and *Sternopygus*, but neither the pacemaker nucleus nor the electromotoneurons themselves express androgen receptor; where estrogen might act in the CNS is unknown.

RETUNING OF ELECTRORECEPTORS AFTER HORMONE EXPOSURE
Androgenic hormones change both the EOD and the sensitivity of the electroreceptor. If, as was suggested in the study of regenerating electroreceptors in a gymnotid fish, the tuning of receptors is independent of changes in the EOD, then electroreceptors in hormone-treated fish should retune even without exposure to an altered EOD. To test this possibility, male fish were given DHT and their EOD was silenced by removing neural input to the electromotoneurons or by lesioning the medullary nucleus that drives the EOD. The sensitivity of electroreceptors was shifted downward by the androgen treatment, as would have occurred in an intact, electrically discharging fish (Keller et al. 1986; Ferrari and Zakon 1989). It is not clear what cellular mechanisms are responsible for this hormone-induced change in receptor tuning. One hypothesis is that the sensory receptor cells themselves contain intracellular receptors for steroid hormones that are capable of changing the cell's electrical properties through changes in membrane ion channels (Bass and Volman 1987).

Summary

Thus we see that gonadal hormones have very powerful effects on the generation and reception of electric courtship signals in electric fish.

1. All the hormonal effects observed are reversible and can be readily obtained in adult animals. These two characteristics suggest that the effects are "activational" because they are not permanent and are not confined to a particular developmental period.

2. Many of the effects of hormones on the form of individual pulses in the EOD are closely related to changes in the morphology and excitability of the electrocytes themselves. Some of these changes reflect alterations in sodium channel kinetics that could be due to the direct action of steroids via nuclear receptors.

3. The rate of EOD discharge is also hormone sensitive. EOD discharge patterns are determined by the rate at which neurons in the motor pattern generator fire.

4. Because some neurons that appear to be part of this circuit concentrate androgenic steroids, hormones could exert effects on the EOD by acting on brain nuclei that produce the EOD motor pattern (Bass et al. 1986).

5. Understanding how hormones affect electroproduction and electroreception could yield important insights into the cellular and molecular basis of steroid actions.

Vocal Courtship in Frogs

In temperate zones frog songs are the vocal harbingers of spring. These songs are acoustic signals from males to females and to other males. Why do frogs use sounds rather than visual displays, for example, in their courtship activities? What kinds of information are sent and received? How are the sounds produced and heard? Are acoustic signals different in males and females and how are these differences generated? These questions form the focus of this section on frog courtship behavior.

The Acoustic Channel of Communication

At the start of the breeding season, males and females are often far from each other and from the breeding site. A problem that such dispersal poses is how to bring the sexes together at a good site for tadpole development while conditions are favorable. The choice of a breeding site is dictated by the physiological limitations of anurans (frogs and toads): tadpoles usually require fresh water in order to survive and develop. Some species have developed strategies to transcend this limitation. Some anuran groups (such as *Xenopus*) never leave the water. In some tropical species the male carries the developing tadpoles on his back from pond to pond. In other species (*Pipa pipa*), the male presses the fertilized eggs into the spongy back of the female where the tadpoles develop before "hatching" as miniature frogs. These unusual strategies are largely confined to the tropics with their potentially longer breeding seasons. The great majority of anurans, particularly those in temperate zones, face the problem of locating a body of water and a potential mate during a short time period, a few days or weeks.

Frog songs attract members of the same species to the breeding site. Why do frogs sing rather than, for example, flash a visual signal? Sound has many advantages as a communication signal. Songs are broadcast; the auditory receptors do not need to be in a certain orientation relative to the sound source in order to receive stimulation. Loud songs, particularly those made by choruses of frogs calling together, can travel long distances and thus attract distant frogs. Sounds travel around large obstacles. These advantages are not found in the visual modality, where the receiver must be attentive and have its visual receptor apparatus oriented in the right direction. Further, most frogs and toads breed at night when light levels are low but sounds can be easily localized. We can conclude that the auditory channel of communication is utilized by frogs and toads because it can be effective over long distances at night.

INFORMATION COMMUNICATED IN FROG SONG

Male frogs do most of the courtship calling. Other male frogs can respond by adding their voices to form a calling chorus. Male frogs can also vocalize to each other as part of aggressive displays. Aggressive calls can be distinct from the advertisement calls used to attract females. Females can respond to male songs by moving toward the sound source or by selecting certain males as reproductive partners. In some species females also respond to males by calling; receptive pairs can even duet (Tobias et al. 1998b). Predators may also cue in on calling frogs as potential prey (Ryan 1985).

Frog songs contain several potentially important pieces of information about the calling male. First, sound amplitude can indicate the size of the individual that is calling. Since many frogs exhibit indeterminate growth (i.e., they keep getting bigger as they get older), size is a good predictor of relative age. In many species, call amplitude is increased by specialized vocal sacs that can enlarge as the animal grows; thus, older frogs produce louder calls. The male's age matters to the female because older frogs have successfully survived the environmental hazards that the offspring they sire will soon be facing. Amplitude can also convey information on how far away the calling frog is or, for choruses, how many frogs are calling together. An intensely vocalizing chorus may indicate a particularly favorable breeding site. Sound amplitude (subjectively: loudness) can be an ambiguous cue for a female, however. A very intense sound can indicate an old male at some distance or a younger male that is close. A close, small chorus could be confused with a louder chorus that is further away.

Sound frequencies (or pitch) can also convey information about the calling male because the vocal apparatus grows larger as the frog grows older. A larger vocal apparatus is capable of producing lower frequency sounds. In some frogs, the pitch of individual sounds varies with age, so that older and larger males give lower-pitched calls. Sound pitch is affected by temperature; small males can mimic the lower pitch of larger, older males by calling from colder locations. Finally, the length of time that an individual male can afford to spend calling is a good indicator of his health. Many frogs invest considerable energy in calling, both because they do not feed and because it is a physically demanding behavior that relies on rapid muscular contractions of the vocalization apparatus. This effort can be debilitating in a male frog that is not in top physical condition. Calling in tree frogs is said to be the most energetically expensive behavior yet measured in any vertebrate (Taigen and Wells 1984).

Sound frequencies and the overall temporal pattern of the song can also reveal the species of the calling male. The frequencies of frog sounds and their temporal patterns (rhythm and rate) are species-specific. The species of a potential mate is extremely important to the female. Females that choose to mate with members of another species risk losing the energy invested in their eggs because the hybrid offspring will usually not survive and reproduce.

The complexity of a frog song can also affect how attractive it is to a female. The songs of male Tungara frogs (*Physaelemus pustulosus*), for example, can consist simply of short ''whines'' (notes that descend in pitch) or of whines followed by several ''chucks'' (Ryan 1985). More females approach loudspeakers playing whines plus chucks than whines alone. Producing attractive songs, however, also has disadvantages: the chucks attract bats that eat the frogs!

We can see that taken together, the information present in a male frog's song could serve as an advertisement of his reproductive state. A male that calls rapidly, in a deep pitch, and for many hours is likely to be a large, old, physically fit male in a location without many predators or other rivals. A short, higher pitched series of calls might be given by a smaller male who may frequently be chased away from an attractive breeding site by predators or other males.

Not all species have evolved systems for mate choice. In some frogs, the environmental conditions favorable for breeding may be present for such short periods of time that females have no chance to be picky. In such "explosive breeders," the main job is just to find the breeding site and a member of the other sex to mate with so that the resulting tadpoles can develop before the pond dries up (Wells 1977). The evolution of mate-choice strategies will be discussed in the next chapter.

METHOD OF GENERATION AND RECEPTION OF ACOUSTIC SIGNALS

The vocal organ for frogs and toads is the larynx, a muscular and cartilagenous structure located in the airway, just before the trachea branches into the two bronchi that enter the lungs. Sounds are produced in most frogs by interposing muscular or membranous elements into the air flow. As air moves through the larynx during expiration, air expulsion can be shaped (altered in frequency or temporal pattern) by sound-producing elements. However, in some frogs (including *Xenopus laevis*, the species discussed below), sounds are produced in a simpler way. The larynx has developed into a cartilaginous "clicker" (figure 8.5). When the muscles that flank the laryngeal cartilages contract, they pull on tendons connected to the sound discs. These discs then pop apart, producing a click (Ridewood 1898; Yaeger 1982). Repeated click trains make up the trills that male and female *Xenopus* use in courtship signaling.

Male and female frogs have externally located ears; there is no ear canal as in mammals. Sounds are detected by transducers or hair cells located in two organs, the amphibian and the basilar papillae. Nerve cells convey information from the hair cells into the central nervous system (figure 8.6). The first relay station is a nucleus in the hindbrain, the dorsal medullary nucleus (DMN). Sound information is sent to the auditory midbrain (laminar nucleus of the torus semicircularis (LTOR) and then on, via synaptic relays, to specific nuclei in the forebrain (auditory thalamus: TH, preoptic area: POA and basal forebrain: BF). Similar brain pathways for receiving auditory information are present in all vertebrates. Auditory input to basal forebrain nuclei is thought to be responsible for endocrine stimulation in males. In a chorusing frog species *Hyla cinerea*, exposure to male advertisement calls maintains testicular hormone production while exposure to altered calls results in decreased

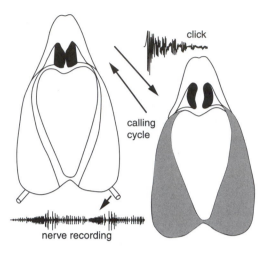

Figure 8.5 Click production by the larynx of male *Xenopus laevis*. When laryngeal muscles contract, the arytenoid disks (black structures) open producing a single click. Activity of the laryngeal motor neurons is conveyed via its axons (nerve recording) to laryngeal muscle. Nerve activity drives the production of alternating fast and slow clicks that comprise the male's advertisement call.

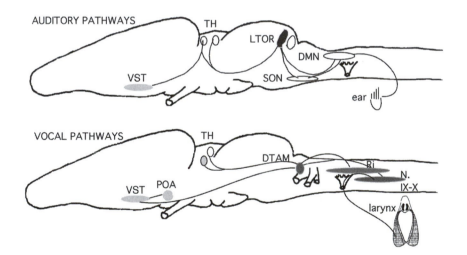

Figure 8.6 Auditory and vocal pathways in the brain of *Xenopus laevis*. *Auditory pathways*: Auditory information enters the brain via the VIIIth nerve and axons synapse in the dorsal medullary nucleus (DMN). From the DMN, auditory information travels to the superior olive (SON) and the laminar nucleus of the torus semicircularis (LTOR) in the dorsal midbrain. LTOR, in turn, sends information to auditory nuclei of the thalamus (TH) and ventral forebrain (VST). Many of these connections are reciprocal. *Vocal pathways*: Motor neurons in cranial nerve nucleus (N.) IX-X exit via the caudal root of n. IX-X and travel to synapse on muscle fibers in the larynx. Input to n. IX-X derives from adjacent reticular formation (Ri) and nucleus DTAM of the anterior medulla. DTAM, a pattern generating nucleus for vocalizations, receives input from the thalamus, and ventral forebrain. Many of the connections shown are reciprocal.

hormone levels (Brozska and Obert 1980). In the frog *Rana pipiens*, exposure to advertisement calls increases testis size and plasma androgen levels (Chu and Wilczynski 1997).

Sex Differences in Song Production and Reception

The vocal repertoire is different in male and female frogs. How are sex differences in vocal behaviors established and maintained? In theory, there are four ways to produce sex differences in vocal behaviors: (1) the sexes might differ in whether or not they can perceive the stimulus responsible for evoking song (sex differences at the level of the sensory receptor or sensory neuron), (2) the brain circuitry responsible for processing the incoming sensory information and producing the vocal pattern might differ between males and females (sex differences at the level of brain interneurons), (3) perhaps the vocal producers—motoneurons and musculoskeletal effectors—are so different in males and females that males can sing while females cannot (sex differences at the level of the motoneurons and muscles), and (4) all the above could be the same in both sexes, but the system might require a sex-specific hormone to function (Kelley 1988).

The cellular and molecular bases for sex differences in vocal circuitry have been explored through the songs of the African clawed frog, *Xenopus laevis*. These anurans are native to the southern part of Africa where they inhabit muddy ponds, lakes, and even sewers. *Xenopus* is a member of the Pipid family that includes the frog described earlier (*Pipa pipa*) in which the mother incubates the tadpoles in her back.

Clawed frogs become dormant during the dry season by burrowing into the mud. When the rainy season starts, shallow pools of water fill up, and the male frogs emerge (and submerge) and start to call. All calls are produced while the frogs are underwater. The water is typically murky and frogs call at night, good conditions for vocal/acoustic communication. Males interact with each other at the beginning of the breeding season to establish vocal hierarchies (Kelley et al. 1999). The vocal repertoire is a complex one and all male calls are used in interactions with other males. The male's courtship song, the advertisement call, is a metallic-sounding trill with alternating slow and fast phases. The male advertisement call attracts females to the vicinity of the calling male. If a sexually receptive female (one about to lay eggs) cannot locate the calling male, she produces her own song, rapping. Rapping is an acoustic aphrodisiac for the male: it stimulates him to call rapidly for long periods and to approach the calling female (Tobias et al. 1998b). Unreceptive females produce another vocal behavior, ticking. If ticking is played to a male while he is calling, he becomes silent (figure 8.7). Ticking and rapping are simple trills that differ only in click rate: rapping is fast (80 ms between clicks) and ticking is slow (230 ms between clicks).

Once the male locates a female, he attempts to clasp her. If the female is sexually receptive, she tolerates his clasp (directed toward her "waist" region). The pair remain in this clasping position while the female extrudes her

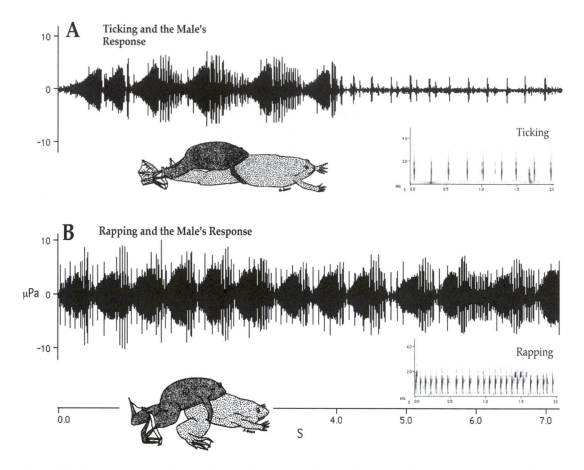

Figure 8.7 Vocal responses of male *Xenopus laevis* to female vocal behaviors: ticking, an unreceptive call, and rapping, an acoustic aphrodisiac. (*A*) Ticking silences males, while (*B*) rapping stimulates males to call. Both ticking and rapping evoke the answer call, a modified advertisement call in which the fast trill is lengthened, the slow trill is shortened and amplitude modulation is enhanced.

eggs and the male fertilizes them by spraying the eggs with sperm as they leave her cloaca. If the female is sexually unreceptive, she ticks and the male releases her (figure 8.7).

The advertisement calls of the male are loud and so is rapping. The loudness of these calls and their ability to travel long distances underwater suggest that they serve as advertisements that help potential mates locate each other. Ticking is a much quieter vocal behavior, suggesting that it is a close range, relatively private channel of communication between two frogs.

If one male clasps another, the clasped male will tick or growl (a slow trill) and be released. Thus both males and females can and do tick. A normal female, however, never produces the alternating faster and slower trills of the advertisement call. Why? To answer this question the Kelley laboratory has examined the way the larynx produces calls and the way the central nervous system controls the larynx.

CENTRAL AND PERIPHERAL MECHANISMS OF CALL PRODUCTION

Laryngeal muscles contract and relax in response to activity of the laryngeal motoneurons located at the very end of the hindbrain in cranial nerve nucleus IX to X. The axons of these motoneurons travel to the vocal organ as the laryngeal nerve (figure 8.5). Because laryngeal motoneurons control only vocal muscles, we can identify other brain regions that participate in calling by identifying nuclei whose interneurons synapse on laryngeal motoneurons (figure 8.6). These brain regions include two nuclei in the hindbrain (the dorsal tegmental nucleus or DTAM and the nucleus reticularis inferior or Ri.) Nucleus DTAM is probably responsible for generating the advertisement call pattern in frogs (Schmidt 1974, 1976). DTAM receives input from auditory nuclei in the thalamus (dorsal forebrain) and from interneurons in the laryngeal motor nucleus (N. IX–X). Recordings from axons of laryngeal motoneurons reveal that male and female brains generate sex-specific vocal patterns including advertisement calling and growling in males and ticking in females (Yamaguchi and Kelley 2000).

SEX DIFFERENCES IN VOCAL NEUROEFFECTORS IN THE CLAWED FROG

Are there any differences in the vocal organ or in the brain that can help to explain why females rap and tick while males growl and advertise? Yes; in fact, at both levels the sexes differ in ways that reflect differences in their vocal repertoires. For example, the male larynx contains a large number of muscle fibers that are capable of contracting and relaxing at very rapid rates (up to 100 times/second). The muscle fibers in the female larynx are fewer in number; furthermore, most of them can only contract and relax slowly (up to 40 times/second).

In the brain, males have more laryngeal motoneurons and vocal interneurons (Kelley et al. 1988; Kelley and Dennison 1990). The vocal pattern generator (DTAM) appears to be more active metabolically in males than in females. Axonal connections from N. IX to X to DTAM are robust in males but weak in females (Wetzel et al. 1985). Do these sex differences in circuitry and muscle fibers contribute to differences in behavior?

To separate the contributions of sex differences in the brain from those of the vocal organ, we devised a way to produce mate calls from the larynx while it is isolated from the brain (Tobias and Kelley 1987). If the nerves that control laryngeal muscle contractions are stimulated in a male with a pattern that mimics the advertisement call, actual sounds very similar to those of intact males are produced. If the same pattern of stimulation is applied to the laryngeal nerves in the female, advertisement calls are not produced because the muscles cannot contract and relax rapidly enough. The larynx produces only the temporal pattern that is supplied to it (if it can). The temporal patterns for sex-specific songs are produced by the brain (Yamaguchi and Kelley 2000).

When a male hears a rapping female, he switches from the somewhat lackadaisical advertisement call to an intense answer call. One of the hallmarks of the answer call is the extreme amplitude enhancement of the fast trill: clicks become louder as the trill progresses (figure 8.7). Amplitude enhancement reflects two processes. First, as the brain generates the fast trill pattern, more and more laryngeal motoneurons are drawn into activity (recruitment) (Yamaguchi and Kelley 2000). Second, as the motoneurons fire repeatedly, the male's normally weak neuromuscular synapses become stronger (facilitation) (Ruel et al. 1998) and can evoke muscle action potentials and contraction. Amplitude enhancement thus reflects recruitment of motoneurons in the CNS and facilitation of the laryngeal synapse at the vocal neuromuscular synapse.

Why amplitude enhancement? Fast trills that become progressively louder are more attractive to females than trills whose clicks are of equal loudness. Why females prefer amplitude-enhanced trills is not clear. Amplitude enhancement may help females localize males. It is also possible that females can use amplitude enhancement to select males with particularly well-masculinized and robust vocal organs (i.e., many neurons are available for recruitment and muscle fibers for facilitation).

HORMONAL CONTRIBUTIONS TO SEX DIFFERENCES IN VOCAL BEHAVIOR
What other factors contribute to sex differences in the vocal behavior of clawed frogs? In adult males, mate calling depends upon the presence of the testes; castrated males that have stopped mate calling will resume it if treated with androgen (testosterone and dihydrotestosterone) (Wetzel and Kelley 1983). Perhaps exposure to high levels of androgen could induce adult females to give mate calls. However, even after many months of androgen treatment, adult females still do not mate call (Hannigan and Kelley 1986). Why doesn't androgen work in females? One reason is that it is very difficult to masculinize the larynx in adult females. As we have seen, without a masculine larynx, a female cannot generate the rapid trills of mate calling (no matter what her brain produces). In males, the larynx is masculinized by the secretion of testicular androgens during the first 6 months after metamorphosis (Tobias et al. 1991a,b; Marin et al. 1990). If a female is supplied with the appropriate hormones during this period (via a testis transplant), she will later generate mate calls under appropriate behavioral circumstances. Her larynx is almost fully masculinized in terms of muscle fiber number and has the right kind of fast-twitch muscle fibers (Marin et al. 1990; Tobias et al. 1991b), thus permitting the vocal expression of the masculine call patttern produced by her brain.

The adult male vocal organ does not require the continued presence of androgen in order to produce advertisement calls. The developing male larynx, on the other hand, has an absolute requirement for androgen if it is to undergo postmetamorphic masculinization. Thus, during postmetamorphic development, androgen organizes the sexual differentiation of the vocal organ in clawed frogs.

What determines the developmental period for sexual differentiation of the vocal system? Why do gonadal steroids act during certain periods and not others? For the larynx, masculine muscle fiber addition begins just after metamorphosis is over and ends 6 months later (Marin et al. 1990). The process is androgen dependent and perhaps androgen or its receptor are only available during this period. But this is not the case; androgen is secreted beginning early in tadpole life and the androgen receptor gene is expressed as the larynx is forming in the tadpole (Kelley 1996). It turns out that the ability of the male's androgen to cause cell division in muscle precursors (competency) depends on another hormone, thyroxine (Cohen and Kelley 1996). Thyroxine rules metamorphosis and also turns on androgen competency. Thyroxine initiates the synthesis and release of the pituitary hormone, prolactin. Prolactin is responsible for androgen-controlled muscle-fiber type switching. Without a pituitary, the male never acquires enough fast muscle fibers to produce the rapid trills of advertisement calling (Edwards et al. 1999).

MASCULINIZATION OF BRAIN REGIONS THAT GENERATE MATE CALLS
We have identified a number of brain regions that participate in the production of vocal behaviors. Many of these regions are different in males and females (reviewed in Kelley 1996). For example, males have more laryngeal motoneurons and interneurons in the vocal motor nucleus than females do. This difference is established late in tadpole life via the prevention of ontogenetic cell death as a result of androgen secretion in males (Kay et al. 1999). Certain connections between vocal nuclei, such as the reciprocal connection between DTAM and N. IX–X (shown in figure 8.6) are missing in females (Wetzel et al. 1985). We assume that these and other CNS sex differences are responsible for generating sex differences in vocal output from the brain (Yamaguchi and Kelley 2000); how is not yet clear.

All the brain regions that affect vocal behavior contain cells that have intracellular receptors for sex steroid hormones (testosterone, dihydrotestosterone, and estradiol) (figure 8.6). Expression of steroid hormone receptors characterizes the neurons in the calling circuit. Castrated males do not mate call even though their larynx is fully capable of producing this vocalization (Wetzel and Kelley 1983; Tobias and Kelley 1987). We suspect that the action of androgen on the brain is necessary for it to produce the male vocal pattern in the adult. If true, the *activational* effects of androgen on song would be accomplished in the brain. What about ovarian hormones such as estradiol to which males are never exposed? Estradiol is responsible for the strong vocal neuromuscular synapses of females (Tobias et al. 1998a). Since the effects of estradiol are not apparent until females are fully mature (2 years after metamorphosis is complete) and are readily reversible, estrogen effects on synaptic strength fit into the activational category. It is likely that steroid hormones also masculinize and/or feminize the brain circuitry that produces vocal patterns, much as they masculinize the larynx. The sexual dimorphism seen in brain vocal circuits is compatible with this idea.

Summary

In *Xenopus*, the clawed frog, sex differences in brain vocal circuitry and the peripheral vocal organ, the larynx, make important contributions to sex differences in courtship song.

1. The female does not have as many fast-twitch muscle fibers as a male does, so she cannot produce the fast, prolonged trills of male advertisement calling. The female produces short, slower trills of ticking and rapping.

2. The masculine pattern of muscle fiber number and type is established during early postmetamorphic development under the influence of androgens secreted by the testes. If a female is provided with a testis transplant during this period, her larynx is permanently masculinized and she can produce advertisement calls.

3. Once masculinized, the larynx does not become demasculinized if deprived of androgens. Thus, masculinization of the vocal organ in *Xenopus laevis* is a clear example of the **organizational** effects of hormones secreted early in development.

4. The neural pathway for vocal behavior is also different in male and female frogs. Males require androgens to mate call even though their larynx remains masculinized. So it seems likely that androgen action on the brain is responsible for activating male-specific vocal behavior.

5. It is also likely that androgens organize the neural circuitry for mate calling. Because females given testis transplants during early postmetamorphic development can mate call, this time period may be essential for organizing the effects of androgen on vocal circuitry in the central nervous system.

6. In contrast to androgen, estrogen effects on the laryngeal synapse are **activational** and may affect whether or not the female raps.

Vocal Courtship in Songbirds

There are approximately 8,700 species of birds living in the world today. The great majority of these species produce vocal sounds. Vocal behavior is most elaborate among members of the oscine suborder of the Passeriform birds, more commonly known as the songbirds. More than half of all living species are found in this successful suborder.

The most distinctive trait of songbirds, as the common name suggests, is their ability to produce complexly structured songs. Songs generally consist of a series of syllables, or brief sounds, arranged in a rhythmic sequence that lasts for seconds to minutes (figure 8.8). Successive renditions of a particular type of song are usually stereotyped; i.e., they are very similar in structure. The songs produced by each species have a unique structure that sets them apart from the songs of other species found in the same location. A consequence of this species-specific nature of song is that there is tremendous diversity in the structure of songs produced by the different species of birds found around the world. In addition, species often differ in the complexity of their song behavior. For example, the white-throated sparrow produces only

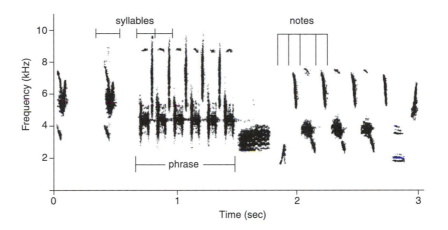

Figure 8.8 Sound spectrogram of a single song produced by a male song sparrow, showing a frequency vs. time representation. The simplest individual sounds in the song are *notes*. A sequence of one or more notes that occurs together in a regular manner in song is a *syllable*. A series of one or more syllables that is repeated in song is a *phrase*. The entire combination of phrases is a song *type* that is sung repeatedly. An individual male song sparrow has a *repertoire* of several different song types.

one very simple song, whereas the rock wren has been estimated to have a repertoire of over 100 song types (Kroodsma 1977). Such extreme interspecific diversity provides excellent opportunities for comparative studies of the adaptive function and physiological control of song behavior.

Functions of Song

Song serves two main functions in birds. It can play an important role in aggressive behavior, usually between members of the same sex. This function of song is most often seen in defense of a territory. The second main function of song occurs in the context of courtship. In most songbird species, males use song to attract females to their territories. Females may select among many potential mates on the basis of individual song characteristics (Payne 1983). The male's song may directly stimulate reproductive behavior in females (Kroodsma 1976). In addition to these two main functions, song may act in other behavioral contexts. For example, song may be important in mediating dominance behavior among members of a social group.

SONG AND THE SEASONS

Breeding occurs seasonally in most species of birds that live in temperate and subtropical latitudes. It generally occurs at times of the year when the resources necessary for successfully rearing offspring are most abundant. In such species, song is also seasonal in occurrence. Males sing at high rates early in the breeding season when they first establish territories. Once males have mated with one or more females, who then lay eggs in nests, the rate of song production drops considerably. Outside the breeding season, males may sing only occasionally or not at all.

In tropical latitudes (23.5°N to 23.5°S), seasonal cycles in environmental factors are not as pronounced as at other latitudes. The availability of critical resources for rearing young birds, therefore, does not vary as much with seasons in the tropics. A consequence of this relative lack of seasonality is that breeding in many tropical species may occur at almost any time of the year. Birds of such species may defend territories and attempt to attract new mates throughout the year. Therefore it is not surprising that in tropical species, song production is often much less seasonal in occurrence than in temperate and subtropical species.

SONG AND THE SEXES

In most temperate and subtropical species, only the male normally sings. There are, however, numerous exceptions to this observation. In the red-winged blackbird, females produce a relatively simple song that is used in aggressive behavior directed at other females (Beletsky 1983). In the cardinal, late in the breeding season females sing a song similar to that sung by males during the breeding season (Lemon 1968). Among tropical species of birds there is much greater diversity in sexual patterns of song production. Females of many species normally sing. The most complex form of female song is heard in tropical species in which the male and female join together to produce elaborate song duets. Duets are distinguished by precise temporal coordination between the songs of males and females. To a naive listener, these duets may sound as though they are produced by only one bird. Among duetting birds there is more interspecific variability in the complexity of female song than in that of conspecific males. In an African species, the white-browed robin chat, males produce about eight times as many song syllables in duets as do females (Todt et al. 1981). On the other hand, in the bay wren of Central America, females produce as many different types of songs in duets as males do (Levin 1988).

SONG LEARNING

Songbirds learn how to sing. If a young bird is raised in isolation from other birds, he will never produce a normal song (Thorpe 1958; Marler 1970). Some species of birds learn to sing only if they are exposed to song (either from a live tutor or from a tape recorder) during their first year of life. We refer to these species as **age-limited learners**.

One age-limited learner is the swamp sparrow. Male sparrows must hear song between 10 and 60 days after hatching (Marler and Peters 1982). With repeated exposure to the tutor song, males form a sensory memory or template of the song. At about 8 months of age males first start to translate this sensory template into a motor program during the sensorimotor phase of song learning. Initially, male sparrows emit sounds that bear only a remote resemblance to the tutor song. This first phase of subsong is marked by the production of crude sounds that are highly variable in structure. The young male improves his vocal performance during the next few months. With practice, he comes to produce more polished sounds that bear a closer resemblance to the tutor song. This period of **plastic song** begins at about 10 months of age and is marked by variability in the order in which song syllables are combined. Over the next 1 to 2 months, the male continues to improve his performance so that by 12 months of age he produces a **crystallized song** that has a well-defined, invariant structure. This progressive improvement in the performance of singing depends upon the bird being able to hear himself sing. If a bird is deafened before the onset of subsong, he will never develop the ability to produce normal song (Konishi 1985). If deafened after he has developed crystallized song, however, he continues to be able to sing.

In contrast to age-limited learners, other bird species are able to learn new songs beyond their first year. These species are referred to as **open-ended learners**. An example is the canary. A young male canary begins to produce subsong about 40 days after hatching (Nottebohm 1987). Plastic song begins at about 60 days. A male starts to produce stereotyped adult song by about 8 months of age. Throughout the first breeding season, song remains stable in structure. After the breeding season ends, however, the song becomes extremely variable. In the late summer and early fall, the adult male's vocalizations are similar to those of juvenile subsong. During this period, some song syllables are lost from the bird's repertoire, others are modified, and new syllables may be added. The result is that by his second breeding season, the number of song syllables in a male's repertoire may have increased by up to 40%.

We should note that vocal learning is not restricted to the songbirds. Parrots (order Psittaciformes) show highly developed vocal behavior, which plays an important role in the complex social behavior observed in many parrot species. As known by anyone who has taught a pet parrot to speak, members of this order excel at learning to modify their vocal behavior. Hermit hummingbirds (order Trochiliformes) also learn to vocalize (Baptista and Schuchmann 1990).

HORMONAL INFLUENCES ON THE DEVELOPMENT OF SONG-CONTROL REGIONS OF THE BRAIN

Song behavior, in songbirds, is controlled by a discrete network of interconnected nuclei in the forebrain. Two pathways that are involved in song learning and production are illustrated in figure 8.9. The motor pathway controls song production and is also presumed to participate in the sensorimotor phase of song learning. This circuit consists of projections from the neostriatal nucleus HVc (also known as the high or higher vocal center) to the robust nucleus of the archistriatum (RA) in the telencephalon. RA projects both to the dorsomedial part of the intercollicular nucleus (DM) in the midbrain (not shown in figure 8.9) and to the tracheosyringeal part of the hypoglossal motor nucleus in the brainstem (nXIIts). Motor neurons in nXIIts send their axons to the muscles of the sound-producing organ, the syrinx. Neuronal activity in HVc and RA is synchronized with the production of sound by

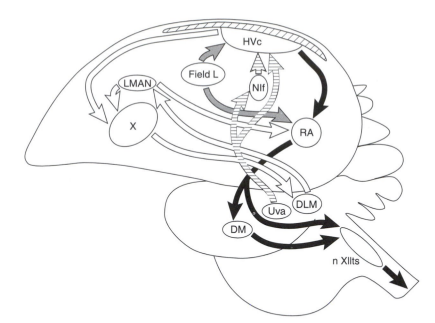

Figure 8.9   A schematic sagittal drawing of the songbird brain showing projections of major nuclei in the song system. The descending motor pathway (black arrows) controls the production of song and consists of projections from HVc in the neostriatum to RA in the archistriatum and thence to the vocal nucleus nXIIts in the medulla. Motor neurons in nXIIts innervate the muscles of the syrinx, the sound-producing organ. The white arrows indicate the anterior forebrain pathway that is essential for song learning. It indirectly connects HVc to RA, via area X in the parolfactory lobe, DLM in the thalamus, and lMAN in the neostriatum. LMAN also projects to area X. Field L is an auditory region in the neostriatum that projects to HVc (gray arrow). DLM, medial portion of the dorsolateral nucleus of the thalamus; lMAN, lateral portion of the magnocellular nucleus of the anterior neostriatum; RA, robust nucleus of the archistriatum; V, ventricle; X, Area X; nXIIts, tracheosyringeal part of the hypoglossal nucleus.

the syrinx. If nuclei in this motor pathway are inactivated, a bird is unable to produce song.

RA also projects to nucleus retroambigualis (RAm) and nucleus ambiguus (Am) in the medulla. RAm contains respiratory-related neurons that fire in phase with expiration. Am contains neurons that innervate the larynx. This pattern of descending projections from RA may be critical for the coordination of syringeal, respiratory, and laryngeal muscle activity during song production. Birds produce song only during expiration, and the larynx may filter the sound frequencies produced by the syrinx.

A second, anterior forebrain pathway is thought to be necessary for song learning and recognition (figure 8.9). This pathway consists of projections from HVc to area X, then to nucleus DLM in the thalamus, from DLM to the lateral portion of the magnocellular nucleus of the anterior neostriatum (lMAN), and finally to RA. lMAN neurons that project to RA also send collaterals to area X, thus providing the potential for feedback within this pathway. Inactivation of lMAN, DLM, or Area X in adults seems to have no effect on previously crystallized song, whereas the same lesions in juveniles prevent the development of normal song. Nuclei in this pathway may continue to play an important role in adults of species that develop new songs beyond the first year. Lesions of lMAN made in adult male canaries in mid-September, when song is seasonally plastic in structure, lead to a progressive decline in structural complexity.

Gonadal steroid hormones and their metabolites influence the development of the song-control system. Cells that contain receptors for androgenic hormones are present in all the song-control nuclei except area X. Receptors for estrogenic hormones are found in HVc and ICo, but not in the other song-control regions. Gurney (1981) demonstrated that when newly hatched female zebra finches are treated with estrogen, the structure of their song-control system is masculinized. Such estrogenized females will produce male-typical song if they receive testosterone implants as adults. Hormones influence the incorporation of newly generated neurons into song-control nuclei. As you will remember from chapter 3, we can identify newly born neurons by injecting animals with a radioactive form of the nucleotide thymidine. Female zebra finches implanted with estradiol soon after hatching and injected with radioactive thymidine show many more newly generated neurons in HVc and area X than do females that do not receive hormone implants (Nordeen and Nordeen 1989). We do not yet know whether hormones affect the birth of new neurons, the migration of these neurons from the ventricular zone where they are born, or the survival of these cells in developing zebra finches. In adult female canaries, however, hormones do not alter the incorporation of thymidine into dividing cells in the ventricular zone, but do increase the migration and/or survival of new neurons (Brown et al. 1993; Rasika et al. 1994; Hidalgo et al. 1995).

The masculinization of the female song system induced by treatment with estrogen may involve an androgen-dependent step. In juvenile male zebra finches that are castrated and implanted with flutamide, an anti-androgenic agent, the song nuclei lMAN and area X are smaller than in normal males (Bottjer and Hewer 1992). Treatment of developing male zebra finches with an inhibitor of 5-α reductase, the enzyme that catalyzes the conversion of testosterone to 5-α dihydrotestosterone, reduces the number of neurons in the song region RA (Grisham et al. 1997). Nordeen and colleagues (1986) found that early estrogen treatment of female zebra finches causes them to have more androgen-accumulating cells in song-control brain regions. Bottjer (1987) showed that in normal male zebra finches, the proportion of cells that accumulate androgen in two song-control nuclei, HVc and lMAN, increases during the time when song becomes crystallized. If hatchling female zebra finches implanted with estradiol are also treated with the anti-androgen flutamide, the song-control pathways are not masculinized as they would normally be by the estrogenic hormone (Grisham et al. 1999).

If estradiol is responsible for masculinization of the song system in young male zebra finches, then we might predict that males would have higher plasma levels of estradiol than females early in development. One group of investigators (Hutchison et al. 1984) reported that male zebra finches do in fact have much higher levels of estradiol in their plasma than females during the first week after hatching. They also reported that the sexes do not differ in plasma levels of androgens at this time. Two other studies, however, failed to detect sex differences in the plasma levels of estrogens during the first week after hatching (Adkins-Regan et al. 1990; Schlinger and Arnold 1992). These studies also did not observe a sex difference in plasma androgen levels. The explanation for this difference between studies is not yet clear. It is possible that the levels of gonadal steroid hormones in the plasma may not accurately reflect the levels present in the brain. Indeed, the brain appears to be the primary source of estradiol for the entire body in young male zebra finches (Schlinger and Arnold 1991). While additional work will be necessary to resolve the apparent dilemma over the lack of sex differences in gonadal hormone levels in the plasma, this question does not invalidate the model that estrogenic and androgenic hormones interact to masculinize the song system of young birds.

Gonadal steroids interact with neurotrophic factors to regulate the development of the song-control regions. Lesions of lMAN in young zebra finches result in the death of neurons in RA that receive synaptic input from lMAN. If neurotrophins are infused into RA just after lMAN is lesioned, however, the death of RA neurons is completely suppressed (Johnson et al. 1997). Brain-derived neurotrophic factor (BDNF) is present in HVc, RA, area X, and lMAN during the development of the song system in juvenile male zebra finches, but is nearly absent from these regions in adult birds (Akutagawa and Konishi 1998). The gene for BDNF is normally expressed at high levels in HVc of male, but not female, zebra finches starting 30 to 35 days after hatching. If males are implanted with estradiol 15 to 25 days after hatching, the BDNF gene expression increases within 24 hours (Dittrich et al. 1999). Treatment of adult female canaries with testosterone increases the size of their song-control nuclei. This hormone treatment increases the level of BDNF in HVc. Infusion of an antibody that neutralizes BDNF blocks the testosterone-induced growth of HVc (Rasika et al. 1999).

These studies indicate that steroid hormones are important in the masculinization of song-control brain regions. Furthermore, these hormones are accumulated by receptors in the nuclei of target cells in these regions. Therefore, hormones may act directly upon target cells in song regions through a classic steroid-receptor mechanism (see chapters 1 and 2). However, masculinization of song-system anatomy may also occur through indirect actions of steroid hormones. As an example, area X in the forebrain of female zebra finches is masculinized in size by early systemic treatment with testosterone or estradiol. But autoradiographic and immunocytochemical studies indicate that area X itself lacks receptors for these hormones. We can hypothesize that the size increase in area X occurs in response to afferent input to this nucleus from HVc (figure 8.9). According this model, early exposure to testosterone or estradiol increases the number of neurons in HVc. This in turn may lead to an increase in the number of HVc neurons that successfully form synapses with area X neurons early in development. The increase in synapse number may result in survival of a greater number of postsynaptic neurons in area X. In support of this hypothesis, area X fails to develop in juvenile female zebra finches in which HVc is lesioned just before the birds receive implants of estradiol (Herrmann and Arnold 1988). It is a general principle of neural development that the survival of many neurons in vertebrate brains depends upon the formation of a trophic relationship with other neurons (Purves and Lichtman 1985).

HORMONAL INFLUENCES ON THE DEVELOPMENT OF SONG BEHAVIOR

Hormones are important for the acquisition of song. This has been studied in swamp sparrows by Marler and his colleagues (1987, 1989). As we discussed above, swamp sparrows are age-limited song learners. During the first 60 days after hatching, male sparrows learn a sensory model of their species' song. Starting at about 8 months of age, males go through a process of sensorimotor learning in which they translate the sensory template of song to a motor program. Marler and his colleagues measured circulating concentrations of steroid hormones in young male sparrows during different phases of song learning. They found that there are two periods of high-circulating testosterone concentration. These testosterone peaks coincide with the times of the sensory and sensorimotor leaning phases of song development. Estradiol levels are also high during the sensory learning phase.

To test whether steroids are necessary for song learning, males were castrated at 3 weeks and then tutored with tape-recorded song. The surprising result of this study was that castrated males acquired a sensory model of song and subsequently produced subsong and early plastic song. However, these castrated males did not produce crystallized song unless they received implants of testosterone. Within 3 weeks of receiving testosterone, castrates achieved crystallized song. Apparently testosterone is not necessary for the sensory and early motor phases of song learning but is essential for the final motor phase. Marler and his co-workers observed that while castration eliminated testosterone in males, estradiol continued to be present during the early phases of song learning. Such estradiol must arise from nontesticular sources in castrates and may play a role in the sensory acquisition of song.

Gonadal steroids also play a role in song development in zebra finches. If young males are castrated and treated with the anti-androgenic agent flutamide, the order in which syllables are produced in their songs fails to become stereotyped as the birds mature (Bottjer and Hewer 1992). Subsequent exposure of these males to testosterone induces the production of crystallized song. Chronic exposure to testosterone during juvenile development severely impairs song learning in males (Korsia and Bottjer 1991).

Circulating concentrations of sex steroids are also correlated with song development in open-ended learners. Remember that male canaries are able to learn new songs even as adults. The development of songs by adults occurs in a seasonal manner. Rates of song production are highest in the spring, when testosterone concentrations are highest. When the breeding season ends, testosterone concentrations drop and song becomes unstable. Starting about one month after testosterone concentrations reach their lowest yearly level, male canaries show pronounced plasticity of song behavior. Song syllables are modified or replaced at a high rate, resulting in a net increase in song repertoire size. Testosterone concentrations begin to rise during this period of greatest song learning. When testosterone concentrations rise to their highest point, the male's song repertoire stabilizes and new syllables are no longer acquired. This cycle repeats itself each year (Nottebohm 1987).

The studies of swamp sparrows and zebra finches suggest that the sensory memorization phase of song learning requires low testosterone and perhaps high estradiol levels. Males go through the initial stages of sensorimotor learning while testosterone levels remain low. They are unable to achieve stereotyped adult song, however, until circulating tesosterone levels rise at puberty. This association between low testosterone levels and vocal plasticity followed by high testosterone levels and vocal stereotypy is repeated in a seasonal manner in open-ended learners.

HORMONAL INFLUENCES ON ADULT SONG BEHAVIOR

Like other reproductive behaviors, song is strongly influenced by circulating hormone levels. In seasonal breeders, hormones provide a proximate mechanism to restrict song production to appropriate times of year. For such species, production of song outside the breeding season may waste much-needed energy and expose the bird to an unnecessary risk of predation. In temperate zone species there is generally a correlation between circulating hormone levels and the degree of song activity (Prove 1974).

Arnold (1975) demonstrated that the rate of song production by male zebra finches is dependent upon the presence of steroid hormones derived from the testes (figure 8.10). Castration of a male greatly reduces his rate of song production. If this male then receives an implant of a pellet that releases testosterone propionate, his rate of singing increases again. Removal of this hormone pellet results in another decline in his song production. These results indicate that song is directly influenced by circulating hormones.

Harding (1983) asked what specific hormones regulate song production. Testosterone may act upon target cells either directly or through one or more of its metabolites. For example, testosterone may be metabolized to several different androgens or may be aromatized to various estrogens (see chapter 3). Harding castrated male zebra finches and implanted them with different combinations of testosterone metabolites. She found that only males receiving hormone treatments that provide both estrogenic and α-androgenic metabolites (testosterone, androstenedione, or estradiol plus 5 α-dihydrotestosterone) sing to females. Estradiol or 5 α-dihydrotestosterone, by itself, cannot reinstate song behavior to its precastration level.

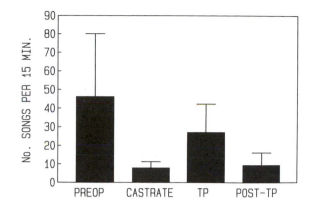

Figure 8.10 The rate of song production by male zebra finches before castration (preop), after castration, after receiving implants of testosterone propionate (TP), and after removal of the TP implants (post-TP). Note that song is produced at a much lower rate following castration, and the rate of singing in castrated males is increased by the hormone implant. (Modified from Arnold 1974 with permission.)

It is interesting that estrogen is necessary for song in males. As we will discuss below, estrogen is also necessary to masculinize song-control regions in the brain of juvenile female zebra finches. Together, these observations suggest that estrogen plays an important role in both the organization and activation of the song system.

Up to this point we have considered only species in which courtship behavior is directly activated by circulating steroid hormones. There are, however, bird species in which courtship behavior is dissociated from the hormonal state. For example, white-crowned sparrow males will attempt to mate with females even if they have been castrated (Moore 1984). In the African stonechat, seasonal patterns of reproductive behavior may not be reflected in seasonal changes in circulating levels of gonadal steroid hormones (Dittami and Gwinner 1985). For such species, other cues may activate courtship behaviors such as song (Crews and Moore 1986). These cues could be environmental stimuli, such as the arrival of seasonal rains, or social stimuli, such as the sight of a member of the opposite sex. Under these conditions, we might expect that the activation of song behavior will not be directly dependent upon steroid hormones (see chapter 7).

HORMONAL INFLUENCES ON THE SONG-CONTROL REGIONS OF THE BRAIN IN ADULTS

As we noted above, song behavior in temperate-zone bird species varies seasonally in correlation with changes in circulating hormone levels. There are also seasonal changes in the structure of the song-control regions of the brain in adult birds. HVc, RA, area X, and nXIIts increase in volume by as much as 300% during the breeding season. The HVc of breeding birds may contain approximately 100,000 more neurons than in nonbreeding birds (reviewed by Tramontin and Brenowitz 2000). The seasonal change in HVc is regulated primarily by changes in circulating testosterone levels (Smith et al. 1997). The growth of RA and area X in the breeding season, however, is regulated by trophic input from HVc and therefore represents another indirect effect of gonadal steroids on song-control regions.

Factors other than gonadal steroids also contribute to seasonal changes of the song-control nuclei. Receptors for the pineal hormone melatonin are found in HVc, RA, and area X. Melatonin is released from the pineal mostly at night and therefore can act as a physiological marker of seasonal changes in day length. Treatment of European starlings with exogenous melatonin reduces the growth of HVc and area X in response to photoperiod cues typical of the breeding season (Bentley et al. 1999). Social cues provided by other birds also contribute to the seasonal growth of the song-control regions. HVc and RA in male white-crowned sparrows housed in a breeding photoperiod with females in reproductive condition were about 20% larger than in males housed in the absence of females (Tramontin et al. 1999). The role of these other cues in seasonal growth is secondary compared with the dominant role played by gonadal steroids.

Hormones can produce dramatic changes in the behavior and song-control brain nuclei of adult female canaries. Females normally do not sing. Treatment of adult females with testosterone, however, causes them to sing (Nottebohm 1980). In response to such testosterone treatment, HVc and robust nucleus of the archistriatum (RA) increase in size by about 90% and 50%, respectively. The increase in the size of HVc may be due at least partly to an increase in the number of neurons.

Gonadectomized females that have received implants of testosterone have a greater number of newly generated neurons in HVc than do females implanted with estradiol, dihydrotestosterone, estradiol plus dihydrotestosterone, or blank pellets (Nottebohm 1989). Part of the increase in RA is due to an increase in the length of female dendritic fibers to a value comparable with that seen in male canaries. This leads to the formation of new synapses (DeVoogd and Nottebohm 1981; DeVoogd et al. 1985). Despite this androgen-induced growth of RA, the volume of this nucleus in adult females does not reach male values. Also, the songs produced by testosterone-treated adult females are much simpler in structure than those of males. These observations indicate that hormones may also need to act during the juvenile organization of the song system to produce complete masculinization of song nuclei in the brain and of song behavior.

SEX DIFFERENCES IN SONG BEHAVIOR

In 1976 Nottebohm and Arnold overturned the long-held view that sexual dimorphisms in brain structure would be subtle (see chapter 3). They reported that in bird species in which only males sing, such as the zebra finch, and species in which males sing much more than females, such as the canary, there are pronounced sex differences in the size of the forebrain song nuclei HVc, RA, and area X. (Nottebohm and Arnold 1976). Comparable patterns of sexual dimorphism were subsequently observed in the brains of other species in which only males sing (MacDougall-Shackleton and Ball 1999). A logical explanation for these large anatomical differences is that they are related to sex differences in the ability to sing. As compelling as this hypothesis is, however, it cannot be directly tested by studying species in which only males sing. A comparative approach can be of value in this regard. As noted above, there is great diversity among songbird species in sex patterns of song behavior. Such pronounced interspecific variation allows us to test the hypothesis that the degree of sexual dimorphism in the size of the song nuclei is related to the extent to which the sexes differ in the complexity of their song behavior.

The strongest comparative analyses take into consideration the evolutionary history of the species being compared (MacDougall-Shackleton and Ball 1999). Closely related species, for example, might share a given trait because they inherited it from their common ancestral species and not as an evolutionary response to similar selective factors. Conversely, unrelated species may differ in that same trait because they are the descendents of different ancestral species rather than having diverged in response to different selective factors. If we compare closely related species that differ in the degree of sex differences in the occurrence and complexity of song behavior, then we can have confidence that any differences observed in the magnitude of sexual dimorphisms in the song-control system were not the result of these species having different ancestors. An example of such a comparative analysis is illustrated in figure 8.11. It shows the male:female ratios of the volume of HVc in four species of wrens in the same taxonomic family (*Certhiidae*). In the marsh wren, only males sing. Female rufous-and-white wrens of Central America routinely sing in duets with males, but males sing about twice as many different types of songs as females do. In two other species of Central American wrens that sing duets, the bay wren and buff-breasted wren, there are no sex differences in the number of song types produced. As we proceed from the marsh wrens to the bay and buff-breasted wrens in this group we find, therefore, a decreasing incidence of sex differences in song behavior (Brenowitz et al. 1994; Brenowitz 1997).

Several interesting observations emerge from comparisons of the neural song-control systems of these four species. In the marsh wren, the nonsinging females have a much smaller HVc (and RA), and do not have a well-defined area X. In the other three wren species, in which females are normally capable of singing, we find the same network of song-control nuclei in the female brain as we observe in males. In the rufous-and-white wren we see an intermediate degree of sexual dimorphism in the size of HVc and the other song nuclei, which parallels the intermediate degree of sex difference in song behavior. In the bay and buff-breasted wrens, we find no sex differences in

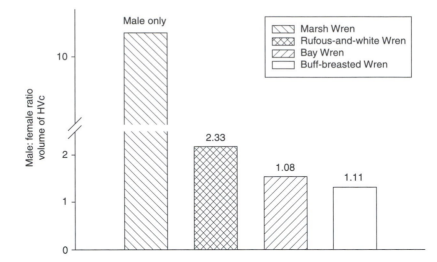

Figure 8.11   Male : female ratios for the volume of the song control nucleus HVc in the marsh wren, rufous-and-white wren, bay wren, and buff-breasted wren. The text and numbers above the bars refers to sex differences in song behavior for each species. In the marsh wren, only males sing. The numbers above the bars for the other three species indicates the male : female ratio in the number of song types produced. The more alike the sexes of a species are the volumes of HVc and song behavior, the smaller the male : female ratio. This figure demonstrates that the extent of sexual dimorphism in the size of HVc is correlated with the extent to which the sexes of a species differ in the complexity of song behavior.

either the song nuclei of the brain or song behavior. The same pattern is observed for the number of neurons in these regions. This and other comparative analyses thus support the hypothesis that the degree of sexual dimorphism present in the neural song-control system is related to the extent to which the sexes differ in the complexity of their song behavior.

The sex patterns of hormone accumulation by cells in song-control brain nuclei also vary across species. This pattern has been examined in the zebra finch, the canary, the rufous-and-white wren, and the bay wren using steroid autoradiographic techniques; recall that female zebra finches do not sing and male canaries sing much more than females. Birds are gonadectomized and injected with radioactively labeled testosterone. Cells that accumulate the radioactive testosterone or its metabolites are referred to as testosterone target cells. Comparison of these species shows that the more alike the sexes are in song behavior, the more alike they are in the number of testosterone target cells in the song-control nucleus HVc (figure 8.12) (Brenowitz 1997).

These comparative studies indicate that singing females develop song-control systems in their brains that are similar in basic structure and hormone sensitivity to those of males of their species. This observation suggests that the network of brain regions has been conserved during the evolution of new species of songbirds. As you can see, comparative studies provide a

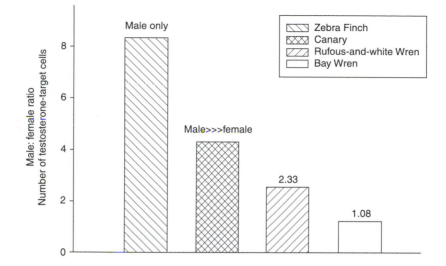

Figure 8.12 Male : female ratios for the number of cells in HVc that accumulate testosterone or its metabolites in the zebra finch, canary, rufous-and-white wren, and bay wren. The text and numbers above the bars refers to sex differences in song behavior for each species. Only male zebra finches sing. Female canaries can sing, but do so less often and with less complexity than males. Females of the two wren species routinely sing in duets with males, and numbers above the bars indicate the male : female ratios in the number of song types produced. The more alike the sexes of a species are in the complexity of vocal behavior, the smaller the difference between the sexes in the number of testosterone target cells in HVc.

powerful means of testing hypotheses about the relationship between neural function and behavior.

Summary

1. Song is a learned behavior that plays a critical role in courtship by birds.
2. The production of song is regulated by a network of discrete nuclei in the brain. The organization and activation of the neural song-control system are both strongly affected by gonadal steroid hormones. Both androgenic and estrogenic hormones play a role. Cells in several song nuclei have receptors for these steroids.
3. There is extensive interspecific diversity in the degree of sexual dimorphism in song production. Comparative studies indicate that this behavioral variation is accompanied by concomitant variation between species in the neural and hormonal control of song.

General Chapter Summary

1. During courtship, members of one sex produces a series of signals that induces members of the other sex to mate. These courtship behaviors are interesting for three reasons: First, in species in which individuals are widely

dispersed at the beginning of the breeding season, courtship signaling brings the sexes together. Second, in closely related species that share similar territories, courtship rituals can aid in species recognition. And finally, courtship is also a way for individuals to assess or influence each other's reproductive readiness.

2. Courtship signals are not produced to the same extent by both sexes. Typically, males initiate courtship and engage in showy and energetic courtship behaviors, songs, or visual displays. This behavior occurs because for males of many species, the resource most critical to their reproductive success is access to females. In terms of energy expenditure, sperm are relatively cheap to produce, whereas eggs are expensive. Males compete for access to eggs and, in mammals and birds, for the maternal care that increases the chances of survival of their offspring. In an attempt to attract females, males of many species have evolved courtship behavior. This behavior involves production of a communication signal. In this manner, sexual selection has repeatedly led to the evolution of sexually dimorphic communication behavior in animals.

3. Male courtship signals can be read for signs of vigor or longevity, desirable attributes that may be transmitted to the young. Females can also use male courtship signals to assess possible paternal contributions to survival of their offspring through direct paternal care protection from predators, and maintenance of a feeding territory. Females maximize their reproductive success by selectively mating with males of high genetic quality or with males that contribute care or resources to the survival of offspring.

4. Hormone secretion can alter the development of brain pathways and muscles that are involved in the production of courtship signals. In males, androgens and their metabolites can permanently change the structure and function of neurons and muscles that produce courtship signals. These changes reflect the *organizational* actions of steroid hormones.

5. The organizational effects of hormones on sexually dimorphic courtship behavior can be due to the direct effects of hormones on the brain, the indirect effects of hormones on target muscles, which result in sexually dimorphic innervation (*target-derived effects*) OR–BOTH.

6. Hormones also strongly control the production of courtship signals in adult animals. Hormone effects in adulthood typify the *activational* effects of androgens.

7. The production of communication signals in diverse sensory modalities is regulated by discrete circuits of brain nuclei. In species in which communication behavior is sexually dimorphic, the associated brain nuclei also differ in structure and function between the sexes. In fact, the most dramatic sex differences yet observed in vertebrate brain structure are found in nuclei involved in the production of courtship behavior in various species. Steroid hormones play a crucial role in establishing these sexual dimorphisms in brain structure. These hormones provide a proximate mechanism for the organization and activation of neural circuits associated with the production of communication signals. Studies of disparate animals such as electric fish,

clawed frogs, and songbirds point to the dominant role of androgenic hormones and their metabolites in the development and adult production of male courtship. This is a striking example of evolutionary conservatism.

8. Closely related species with differing social systems may show pronounced variation in the pattern of courtship behaviors. Such behavioral variation may result from subtle differences between species in the balance of steroid hormones secreted.

9. Species differences may also result from the timing of hormone secretion, both during critical stages of early development and seasonally in adults. The presence of such extensive interspecific variation in the neural and hormonal bases of courtship shows that there is considerable evolutionary flexibility in the interaction between hormones and the nervous system. Thus, comparative studies of courtship systems provide rich opportunities to integrate behavioral, endocrinological, and neurobiological approaches.

Study Questions

1. What are some courtship behaviors? Discuss proximal and ultimate reasons for the roles that reproductive hormones play in induction of these behaviors.

2. Why do males of most species tend to engage in more showy and energetic courtship behaviors?

3. Female clawed frogs produce a courtship song, rapping. What factors might have led to production of courtship song in females of this species?

4. Discuss the 3 different mechanisms through which hormones can cause sex differences in courtship behavior.

5. Discuss the differences among the electric fish, the clawed frog, and the songbird in the roles that gonadal hormones play in sexual differentiation of courtship behavior.

6. Compare and contrast the differences among the electric fish, clawed frog, and songbird in the activational effects of gonadal hormones in courtship behaviors.

References

Adkins-Regan, E., Abdelnabi, M., Mobarak, M., and Ottinger, M. A. (1990) Sex steroid levels indeveloping and adult male and female zebra finches. *Gen. Comp. Endocrinol.* 78: 93–109.

Akutagawa, E., and Konishi, M. (1998) Transient expression and transport of brain-derived neurotrophic factor in the male zebra finch's song system during vocal development. *Proc. Natl. Acad. Sci. USA* 95: 11429–11434.

Arnold, A. P. (1975) The effects of castration and androgen replacement on song, courtship, and aggression in zebra finches. *J. Exp. Zool.* 191: 309–326.

Baptista, L., and Schuchmann, K. (1990) Song learning in the Anna's hummingbird (*Calypte anna*). *Ethology* 84: 15–20.

Bass, A. H. (1986a) A hormone-sensitive communication system in an electric fish. *J. Neurobiol.* 17: 131–156.

Bass, A. H. (1986b) Electric organs revisited: Evolution of a vertebrate communication and orientation organ. In T. Bullock and W. Heiligenberg (Eds.), *Electroreception*. New York: Wiley, pp. 13–70.

Bass, A. H., Denziot, J.-P., and Marchaterre, M. A. (1986) Ultrastructural features and hormone dependent sex differences of mormyrid electric organs. *J. Comp. Neurol.* 254: 511–528.

Bass, A. H., and Hopkins, C. (1984) Shifts in frequency tuning of electroreceptors in androgen-treated mormyrid fish. *J. Comp. Physiol. [A]* 155: 713–724.

Bass, A., Segil, N., and Kelley, D. (1986) A steroid-sensitive electromotor pathway in mormyrid fish: Autoradiography and receptor biochemistry. *J. Comp. Physiol.* 159: 535–544.

Bass, A. H., and Volman, S. (1987) From behavior to membranes: Testosterone-induced changes in action potential waveform duration in electric organs. *Proc. Natl. Acad. Sci. USA* 84: 9295–9298.

Beletsky, L. D. (1983) Aggressive and pair-bond maintenance songs of female red-winged blackbirds. *Z. Tierpsychol.* 62: 47–54.

Bell, C., and Szabo, T. (1986) Electroreception in mormyrid fish: Central anatomy. In T. Bullock and W. Heiligenberg (Eds.), *Electroreception*. New York: Wiley, pp. 375–422.

Bennett, M. (1971) *Electric Organs in Fish Physiology*, vol. V (W. Hoar and D. Randall, Eds.). New York: Academic Press, pp. 347–481.

Bennett, M., and Grundfest, H. (1961) Studies on morphology and electrophysiology of electric organs III. Electrophysiology of electric organs in mormyrids. In C. Chagas and A. Paes de Carvalho (Eds.), *Biogenesis*. Amsterdam: Elsevier, pp. 113–115.

Bentley, G. E., Van't Hof, T. J., and Ball, G. F. (1999) Seasonal neuroplasticity in the songbird telencephalon: A role for melatonin. *Proc. Natl. Acad. Sci. USA* 96: 4674–4679.

Bottjer, S. W. (1987) Ontogenetic changes in the pattern of androgen accumulation in song-control nuclei of male zebra finches. *J. Neurobiol.* 18: 125–139.

Bottjer, S. W., and Hewer, S. J. (1992) Castration and antisteroid treatment impair vocal learning in male zebra finches. *J. Neurobiol.* 23: 337–353.

Brenowitz, E. A. (1997) Comparative approaches to the avian song system. *J. Neurobiol.* 33: 517–531.

Brenowitz, E. A., Nalls, B., Kroodsma, D. E., and Horning, C. (1994) Female marsh wrens do not provide evidence of anatomical specializations of song nuclei for perception of male song. *J. Neurobiol.* 25: 197–208.

Brown, S. D., Johnson, F., and Bottjer, S. W. (1993) Neurogenesis in adult canary telencephalon is independent of gonadal homrone levels. *J. Neurosci.* 13: 2024–2032.

Brzoska, J., and Obert, H.-J. (1980) Acoustic signals influencing hormone production of the testes in the grass frog. *J. Comp. Physiol.* 140: 25–29.

Chu, J., and Wilczynski, W. (1997) Conspecific social signals influence testes size and androgen levels in the southern leopard frog. *Soc. Neurosci. Abstr.* 23: 1088.

Crews, D., and Moore, M. C. (1986) Evolution of mechanisms controlling mating behavior. *Science* 231: 121–125.

Cohen, M., and Kelley, D. B. (1996) Androgen induced proliferation in the developing larynx of *Xenopus laevis* is regulated by thyroid hormone. *Devel. Biol.* 178: 113–123.

DeVoogd, T. J., Nixdorf, B., and Nottebohm, F. (1985) Synaptogenesis and changes in synaptic morphology related to acquisition of a new behavior. *Brain Res.* 329: 304–308.

DeVoogd, T. J., and Nottebohm, F. (1981) Gonadal hormones induce dendritic growth in the adult avian brain. *Science* 214: 202–204.

Dittami, J. P., and Gwinner, E. (1985) Annual cycles in the African stonechat and their relationship to environmental factors. *J. Zool. (Lond.) [A]* 207: 357–370.

Dittrich, F., Feng, Y., Metzdorf, R., and Gahr, M. (1999) Estrogen-inducible, sex-specific expression of brain-derived neurotrophic factor mRNA in a forebrain song control nucleus of the juvenile zebra finch. *Proc. Natl. Acad. Sci. USA* 96: 8241–8246.

Dunlap, K., and Zakon, H. (1998) Behavioral actions of androgens and androgen receptor expression in the electrocommunication system of an electric fish, *Eigenmannia virescens*. *Horm. Behav.* 34: 30–38.

Dunlap, K., Mcanelly, M., and Zakon, H. (1997) Estrogen modifies an electrocommunication signal by altering the electrocyte sodium current in an electric fish, *Sternopygus*. *J. Neurosci.* 17: 2869–2875.

Dye, J., and Meyer, J. (1986) Control of the electric organ discharge. In T. Bullock and W. Heiligenberg (Eds.), *Electroreception*. New York: Wiley, pp. 71–102.

Edwards, C. J., Yamamoto, K., Kikuyama, S., and Kelley, D. B. (1999) Prolactin opens the sensitive period for androgen regulation of a larynx-specific myosin heavy chain gene. *J. Neurobiol.* 41: 443–451.

Ferrari, M., and Zakon, H. (1989) The medullary pacemaker nucleus is unnecessary for electroreceptor tuning plasticity in Sternopygus. *J. Neurosci.* 9: 1354–1361.

Grisham, W., Lee, J., McCormick, M. E., Yang-Stayner, K., Kakar, N. R., and Arnold, Arthur P. (1999) Antiandrogen substantially blocks the estrogen-induced masculinization of the song system in female zebra finches. *Soc. Neurosci. Abst.* 25: 865.

Grisham, W., Tam, A., Greco, C., Schlinger, B. A., and Arnold, A. P. (1997) A putative 5α-reductase inhibitor demasculinizes portions of the zebra finch song system. *Brain Res.* 750: 122–128.

Gurney, M. E. (1981) Hormonal control of cell form and number in the zebra finch song system. *J. Neurosci.* 1: 658–673.

Hagedorn, M., and Heilgenberg, W. (1985) Court and spark: Electric signals in the courtship and mating of gymnotid fish. *Anim. Behav.* 32: 254–265.

Hagedorn, M. (1986) The ecology, courtship and mating of gymnotiform electric fish. In T. Bullock and W. Heiligenberg (Eds.), *Electroreception.* New York: Wiley, pp. 497–527.

Hannigan, P., and Kelley, D. (1986) Androgen-induced alterations in vocalizations of female *Xenopus laevis*: Modifiability and constraints. *J. Comp. Physiol. [A]* 158: 517–528.

Harding, C. F. (1983) Hormonal specificity and activation of social behavior in the male zebra finch. In J. Balthazart, E. Prove, and R. Gilles (Eds.), *Hormones and Behaviour in Higher Vertebrates.* Berlin: Springer-Verlag, pp. 275–289.

Herrmann, K., and Arnold, A. P. (1988) Effect of HVc lesions on estradiol-induced masculinization of zebra finch song system. *Soc. Neurosci. Abstr.* 14: 289.

Hidalgo, A., Barami, K., Iversen, K., and Goldman, S. A. (1995) Estrogens and non-estrogenic ovarian influences combine to promote the recruitment and decrease the turnover of new neurons in the adult female canary brain. *J. Neurobiol.* 27: 470–487.

Hopkins, C. (1972) Sex differences in signalling in an electric fish. *Science* 176: 1035–1037.

Hopkins, C. (1974) Electric communication in the reproductive behavior of *Sternopygus macrurus*. *Z. Tierpsychol.* 35: 518–535.

Hopkins, C. (1986) Behavior of mormyridae. In T. Bullock and W. Heiligenberg (Eds.), *Electroreception.* New York: Wiley, pp. 527–576.

Hopkins, C. (1988) Neuroethology of electric communication. *Annu. Rev. Neurosci.* 11: 497–536.

Hutchison, J. B., Wingfield, J. C., and Hutchison, R. E. (1984) Sex differences in plasma concentrations of steroids during the sensitive period for brain diffeentiation in the zebra finch. *J. Endocrinol.* 103: 363–369.

Johnson, F., Hohmann, S. E., DiStefano, P. S., and Bottjer, S. W. (1997) Neurotrophins suppress apoptosis induced by deafferentation of an avian motor-cortical region. *J. Neurosci.* 17: 2101–2111.

Kay, J. N, Hannigan, P., and Kelley, D. B. (1999) Trophic effects of androgen: Development and hormonal regulation of neuron number in a sexually dimorphic vocal motor nucleus. *J. Neurobiol.* 40: 375–385.

Keller, C., Zakon, H., and Sanchez, D. (1986) Evidence for a direct effect of androgens upon electroreceptor tuning. *J. Comp. Physiol. [A]* 158: 301–310.

Kelley, D. (1988) Sexually dimorphic behaviors. *Ann. Rev. Neurosci.* 11: 225–251.

Kelley, D. (1996) Sexual differentiation in *Xenopus laevis*. In R. Tinsley and H. Kobel (Eds.), *The Biology of Xenopus.* Oxford: Oxford University Press, pp. 143–176.

Kelley, D., and Dennison, J. (1990) The vocal motor neurons of *Xenopus laevis*: Development of sex differences in axon number. *J. Neurobiol.* 21: 869–882.

Kelley, D., Fenstemaker, S., Hannigan. P., and Shih, S. (1988) Sex differences in the motor nucleus of cranial nerve IX–X in *Xenopus laevis*: A quantitative study. *J. Neurobiol.* 19: 413–429.

Kelley, D. B., Tobias, M. L., and Horng, S. (1999) Producing and perceiving frogs songs; dissecting the neural bases for vocal behaviors in *Xenopus laevis*. In M. Ryan and S. Rand (Eds.), *Anuran Communication.* Washington, D.C.: Smithsonian Institution Press, in press.

Konishi, M. (1985) Birdsong: From behavior to neuron. *Annu. Rev. Neurosci.* 8: 125–170.

Korsia, S., and Bottjer, S. W. (1991) Chronic testosterone treatment impairs vocal learning in male zebra finches during a restricted period of development. *J. Neurosci.* 11: 2362–2371.

Kroodsma, D. E. (1976) Reproductive development in a female songbird: Differential stimulation by quality of male song. *Science* 192: 574–575.

Kroodsma, D. E. (1977) Correlates of song organization among North American wrens. *Am. Nat.* 111: 995–1008.

Lemon, R. E. (1968) The relation between organization and function of song in cardinals. *Behaviour* 32: 158–178.

Levin, R. N. (1988) The adaptive significance of antiphonal song in the Bay wren, *Thryothorus nigricapillus.* Ph.D. dissertation, Cornell University, Ithaca, New York.

MacDougall-Shackleton, S. A., and Ball, G. F. (1999) Comparative studies of sex differences in the song-control system of songbirds. *TINS* 22: 432–436.

Marin, M., Tobias, M., and Kelley, D. (1990) Hormone-sensitive stages in the sexual differentiation of laryngeal muscle fiber number in *Xenopus laevis*. *Development* 110: 703–12.

Marler, P. (1970) A comparative approach to vocal learning: Song development in white-crowned sparrows. *J. Comp. Physiol.* Psychol. 71(Suppl.): 1–25.

Marler, P., and Peters, S. (1982) Subsong and plastic song: Their role in the vocal learning process. In D. E. Kroodsma and E. H. Millers (Eds.), *Acoustic Communication in Birds*, vol. 2. New York: Academic Press, pp. 25–50.

Marler, P., Peters, S., Ball, G. F., Dufty, A. M., and Wingfield, J. C. (1989) The role of sex steroids in the acquisition and production of birdsong. *Nature* 336: 770–772.

Marler, P., Peters, S., and Wingfield, J. (1987) Correlations between song acquisition, song production, and plasma levels of testosterone and estradiol in sparrows. *J. Neurobiol.* 18: 531–548.

Metzner, W. (1999) Neural circuitry for communication and jamming avoidance in gymnotiform electric fish. *J. Exp. Biol.* 202: 1365–1375.

Meyer, J. H. (1983) Steroid influences upon the discharge frequency of a weakly electric fish. *J. Comp. Physiol.* 153: 29–38.

Meyer, J. H., and Zakon, H. (1982) Androgens alter the tuning of electroreceptors. *Science* 217: 635–637.

Mills, A., and Zakon, H. (1987) Coordination of EOD frequency and pulse duration in a weakly electric fish: The influence of androgens. *J. Comp. Physiol.* 161: 417–430.

Moore, M. C. (1984) Changes in territorial defense produced by changes in circulating levels of testosterone: A possible hormonal basis for mate-guarding behavior in white-crowned sparrows. *Behaviour* 88: 215–226.

Nordeen, E. J., and Nordeen, K. W. (1989) Estrogen stimulates the incorporation of new neurons into avian song nuclei during adolescence. *Devel. Brain Res.* 49: 27–32.

Nordeen, K. W., Nordeen, E. J., and Arnold, A. P. (1986) Estrogen establishes sex differences in androgen accumulation in zebra finch brain. *J. Neurosci.* 6: 734–738.

Nottebohm, F. (1980) Testosterone triggers growth of brain vocal control nuclei in adult female canaries. *Brain Res.* 189: 429–436.

Nottebohm, F. (1987) Plasticity in adult avian central nervous system: Possible relation between hormones, learning, and brain repair. In F. Plum (Ed.), *Higher Functions of the Nervous System*. Section 1, *Handbook of Physiology*. Baltimore: Williams and Wilkins, pp. 85–108.

Nottebohm, F. (1989) Hormonal regulation of synapses and cell number in adult canary brain and its relevance to theories of long-term memory storage. In J. M. Lakoskin, J. R. Perez-Plo, and D. K. Rassin (Eds.), *Neural Control of Reproductive Function*. New York: Liss, pp. 583–601.

Nottebohm, F., and Arnold, A. (1976) Sexual dimorphism in vocal control areas of the songbird brain. *Science* 194: 211–213.

Payne, R. B. (1983) Bird songs, sexual selection, and female mating strategies. In S. K. Wasser (Ed.), *Social Behavior of Female Vertebrates*. New York: Academic Press, pp. 55–90.

Prove, E. (1974) Der Einfluss von Kastration und Testosteronsubstitution auf das Sexualverhaltern mannlicher Zebrafinken. *J. Ornithologie* 115: 338–347.

Purves, D., and Lichtman, J. W. (1985) *Principles of Neural Development*. Sunderland, Mass.: Sinauer.

Rasika, S., Alvarez-Buylla, A., and Nottebohm, F. (1999) BDNF mediates the effects of tesosterone on the survival of new neurons in an adult brain. *Neuron* 22: 53–62.

Rasika, S., Nottebohm, F., and Alvarez-Buylla, A. (1994) Testosterone increases the recruitment and/or survival of new high vocal center neurons in adult female canaries. *Proc. Natl. Acad. Sci. USA* 91: 7854–7858.

Ridewood, W. (1898) On the structure and development of the hyobranchial skeleton and larynx in *Xenopus* and *Pipa*; with remarks on the affinities of the aglossa. *Linn. Soc. J. Zool.* 26: 53–128.

Ruel, T., Kelley, D., and Tobias, M. (1998) Facilitation at the sexually differentiated laryngeal synapse of *Xenopus laevis*. *J. Comp. Physiol.* 182: 35–42.

Ryan, M. J. (1985) *The Tungara Frog—A Study in Sexual Selection and Communication*. Chicago: University of Chicago Press.

Schlinger, B. A., and Arnold, A. P. (1991) Brain is the major site of estrogen synthesis in the male zebra finch. *Proc. Natl. Acad. Sci. USA* 8: 4191–4194.

Schlinger, B. A., and Arnold, A. P. (1992) Plasma sex steroids and tissue aromatization in hatchling zebra finches: Implication for the sexual differentiation of singing behavior. *Endocrinology* 130: 289–299.

Schmidt, R. (1974) Neural correlates of frog calling: *Trigeminal tegmentum. J. Comp. Physiol.* 92: 229–254.

Smith, G. T., Brenowitz, E. A., and Wingfield, J. C. (1997) Roles of photoperiod and testosterone in seasonal plasticity of the avian song control system. *J. Neurobiol.* 32: 426–442.

Squire, A., and Moller, P. (1982) Effects of water conductivity on electrocommunication in the weak-electric fish *Brienomyrus niger* (mormyriformes). *Anim. Behav.* 30: 375–382.

Taigen, T., and Wells, K. (1984) Energetics of vocalization by an anuran amphibian, *Hyla versicolor. J. Comp. Physiol. [B]* 155: 163–170.

Thorpe, W. H. (1958) The learning of song patterns by birds, with especial reference to the song of the chaffinch, *Fringilla coelebs. Ibis* 100: 535–570.

Tobias, M., and Kelley, D. (1987) Vocalizations by a sexually dimorphic isolated larynx: Peripheral constraints on behavioral expression. *J. Neurosci.* 7: 3191–3197.

Tobias, M., Marin, M., and Kelley, D. (1991a) Development of functional sex differences in the larynx of *Xenopus laevis. Devel. Biol.* 147: 251–259.

Tobias, M., Marin, M., and Kelley, D. (1991b) Temporal constraints on androgen directed laryngeal masculinization in *Xenopus laevis. Devel. Biol.* 147: 260–270.

Tobias, M., Tomasson, J., and Kelley, D. B. (1998a) Attaining and maintaining strong vocal in female *Xenopus laevis. J. Neurobiol.*, 37: 441–448.

Tobias, M. L., Viswanathan, S., and Kelley, D. B. (1998b) Rapping, a female receptive call, initiates male/female duets in the South African clawed frog. *Proc. Natl. Acad. Sci. USA* 95: 1870–1875.

Todt, D., Hultsch, H., and Duvall, F. P., III (1981) Behavioral significance and social function of vocal and non-vocal displays in monogamous duet-singer *Cossypha heuglini. H. Zool. Beitr.* 27: 421–448.

Tramontin, A. D., and Brenowitz, E. A. (2000) Seasonal plasticity in the adult brain. *TINS.*, in press.

Tramontin, A. D., Wingfield, J. C., and Brenowitz, E. A. (1999) Contributions of social cues and photoperiod to seasonal plasticity in the adult avian song control system. *J. Neurosci.* 19: 476–483.

Trivers, R. L. (1985) *Social Evolution*. Menlo Park, Calif.: Benjamin/Cummings Publishing.

Wells, K. (1977) The social behavior of anuran amphibians. *Anim. Behav.* 25: 666–693.

Wetzel, D., Haerter, U., and Kelley, D. (1985) A proposed efferent pathway for mate calling of male South African clawed frogs, *Xenopus laevis. J. Comp. Physiol. [A]* 157: 749–761.

Wetzel, D., and Kelley, D. (1983) Androgen and gonadotropin control of the mate calls of male South African clawed frogs, *Xenopus laevis. Horm. Behav.* 17: 388–404.

Yaeger, D. (1982) A novel mechanism for underwater sound production in *Xenopus borealis. Am. Zool.* 122: 887.

Yamaguchi, A., and Kelley, D. B. (2000) Generating sexually differentiated vocal patterns: Laryngeal nerve and EMG recordings from vocalizing male and female African clawed frogs (*Xenopus laevis*). *J. Neurosci.* 20: 1559–1567.

Zakon, H. H. (1986) The electroreceptive periphery. In T. Bullock and W. Heiligenberg (Eds.), *Electroreception*. New York: Wiley, pp. 103–156.

Zakon, H. H. (1987) Hormone mediated plasticity in the electrosensory system of weakly electric fish. *Trends Neurosci.* 10: 416–421.

Zakon, H. H. (1993) Weakly electric fish as model systems for studying long-term steroid action on neural circuits. *Brain Behav. Evol.* 42: 242–251.

Zakon, H. H., Thomas, P., and Yan, H.-Y. (1991) Plasma steroids, reproductive state and electric organ discharge in a natural population of the weakly electric fish *Sternopygus macrurus. J. Comp. Physiol. [A]* 169: 493–499.

9 Hormones and Parental Behavior

Larry J. Young and Thomas R. Insel

After courtship, copulation, and fetal development have ended, successful reproduction hinges upon whether the offspring will ever reach reproductive age. In response to this requirement, parental behavior has evolved in many species, especially among the mammals and birds. Once again, hormones, perhaps as a result of their preexisting roles in sexual physiology and behavior, have come to coordinate these efforts by preparing the nervous system to display nurturing and defensive behaviors.

What are the varieties of parental behavior, and why do most mammals require extensive maternal care? What are the hormones supporting pregnancy and lactation, and how do these hormones affect behavior? What parts of the nervous system mediate these hormonal influences upon parental behavior?

Introduction

In his 1948 book, *Hormones and Behavior*, Frank Beach provided three important guides to the study of how endocrine factors influence behavior (Beach 1948). First, he emphasized the need for a careful description of the behavior, including a detailed study of what initiates and what terminates the behavior. Second, he stressed the importance of understanding that hormones do not cause behavior but serve a permissive or modulatory role. And finally, he pointed out that most reproductive behavior is overdetermined, regulated by redundant physiological mechanisms. More than half a century later, these guides are still useful, with the added insight, because we have learned more about the cellular and molecular mechanisms of hormone action, that hormones initiate a cascade of events that result collectively in behavioral change.

In this chapter we will follow Beach's suggestions by focusing first on the behaviors that comprise parental care. Then we will review the major factors implicated in the initiation and expression of parental care, including experience, sensory stimuli, and hormones. These factors will lead us to examine the neurobiology of parental care, with consideration of the likely targets of hormone action and the relevant neural circuits involved in parental care. As Beach suggested, the story will be complex, with multiple hormones and several neural systems involved. Adding to the complexity, there are marked species differences, not only in the quality and quantity of parental care but also in its neuroendocrine or neurobiological basis. We will consider the neuroendocrine basis of rat maternal care in detail, looking for basic principles that should help us to understand parental care in other species. The study of parental care has provided one of the best opportunities to investigate how molecular and cellular changes in specific neural circuits influence behavior. Species differences in parental care, while adding to the complexity, also suggest the opportunity for comparative studies to identify how species differences in behavior are associated with differences in neuroendocrine organization. Finally, we will examine parental care in human and nonhuman primates, with some thoughts about how primates are similar to, and different from, other mammals.

Parental Behavior

Evolution requires reproduction, but reproduction is more than mating. For reproduction to be successful in an evolutionary sense, mating must result in offspring and these offspring must survive to reproduce themselves. Parental behavior is any behavior that contributes to the survival of the offspring. It follows then that parental behavior is essential for the evolutionary fitness of many species and one might therefore expect parental behavior to be shaped by various selection pressures.

When does parental behavior first emerge in phylogeny? The vast majority of invertebrate species as well as many fishes, amphibia, and reptiles lay eggs in great numbers and then abandon them to fate, a strategy referred to as an r-selected pattern of reproduction. But even among invertebrates, there are some stunning exceptions in which parents care for the young either by selective feeding or protection of the brood (Trumbo 1996). For instance, the mosquito *Trichosprosopon digitatum* tends her eggs for as many as 30 hours on floating rafts within water-holding fruit husks to protect them until hatching. In some earwig species, the mother cares for her eggs in the burrow until hatching; she then leaves the burrow and provisions the nest with prey. In burying beetles, *Nicrophorus orbicollis*, both males and females prepare and maintain a nest of decomposing carrion, even feeding offspring by regurgitation. E. O. Wilson (Wilson 1971) has written at great length about elaborate parental care in eusocial insects in which cooperative brood care is common. However for most invertebrates, parental care is either nonexistent or brief and nonselective.

Parental Care in Nonmammalian Vertebrates

There are examples of elegant parental care in all vertebrate classes. Among teleost fish, parental care is fairly common and ranges from guarding the nest and fanning the eggs to, in the case of mouthbreeders, carrying the fertilized eggs or even the hatchlings in the mouth for transport or protection. Interestingly, parental care in teleost fish is more prevalent in males than females, possibly as an extension of male territoriality. An example of extensive parental care among amphibia is found in spotted poison frogs, *Dendrobates vanzolinii* (Caldwell 1997). In many *Dendobates* species, parents nourish their tadpoles with unfertilized eggs. In the spotted poison frog, males and females pair bond and rear a single tadpole in a small water-filled cavity. Males will transport newly hatched tadpoles to a safe cavity, and then vocalize to guide the female to follow. Once the female arrives, pairs cooperate to feed their tadpole unfertilized, nutritive eggs. Among reptiles, the most spectacular instances of parental care are found in crocodylians, in which the parents often guard the nest, respond to vocalizations of the hatchlings, and retrieve offspring by carrying them in their mouths (Gans 1996).

But the most completely developed forms of parental behavior are observed in birds and mammals, species that, relative to other vertebrates, usually give birth to fewer offspring and have offspring that develop more slowly. The most important feature of parental behavior that needs to be addressed at the outset of our discussion is the remarkable diversity among species in the quality and quantity of parental care. This diversity is an opportunity for comparative studies that has not yet been fully realized. In the next section we will describe a few of the dimensions of this diversity with an eye to areas for future study.

Diversity of Parental Care Patterns

UNIPARENTAL VERSUS BIPARENTAL

Species can generally be classified as uniparental or biparental, depending on who is taking care of the young. Approximately 90% of bird species are biparental, meaning that both males and females participate in the care of the offspring. Although one might assume that the offspring in the nests of biparental species are the offspring of the parents, DNA fingerprinting has demonstrated that this is often not the case. That is, the offspring may be the result of females copulating with males other than their mates, even among species that appear to be socially monogamous. Within biparental species, males and females may have different roles. Parental care in birds includes nest building, incubation of the eggs and, following hatching, a later phase of brooding behavior with foraging and feeding the young until the offspring fledge. There is great variation in how species divide these tasks between males and females, but a general rule is that the demands of protecting and feeding the young have made biparental care highly adaptive for birds (Buntin 1996).

In contrast to birds, over 90% of mammals are uniparental. Indeed, the uniquely female specialization of nursing partly defines mammals. Incidentally, one possible exception to the rule that only female mammals nurse is the Dayak fruit bat, *Dyacopterus spadiceus*, in which males have been discovered to lactate although never observed to nurse young (Francis et al. 1994). But even among mammals, there are several monogamous species that provide biparental care. Paternal care can include all aspects of care of the young except for nursing and may involve specialized forms of grooming or defense. It should also be noted that in many species (especially primates), alloparenting, that is parental behavior from kin or even unrelated conspecifics, is an important adjunct to either uniparental or biparental care.

PRECOCIAL VERSUS ALTRICIAL YOUNG

Parental care can also be classified by the maturity of the infants at birth. Altricial infants are helpless, blind, deaf, and deficient in both motor control and temperature regulation at birth. The offspring of most rodents as well as dogs, cats, and rabbits fall into this category. About 80% of bird species are altricial, including the ring dove, which has been studied extensively as a model for the hormonal regulation of parental care (Lehrman 1961). Parental care in species with altricial offspring must include nest building and retrieval and may even require anogenital licking or grooming to facilitate urination and defecation by the offspring. Marsupials, such as kangaroos and opossums, have exceedingly short gestations that may be no longer than a normal estrus cycle (Sharman 1970). Their newborn offspring are among the most altricial of mammalian neonates. In most marsupial species, rather than inhabiting a terrestial or arboreal nest, newborn offspring crawl into a pouch on the mother's ventrum where they develop for several months. This pouch serves the thermoregulatory and protective role of a nest while keeping the altricial offspring attached to an active mother.

By contrast, species with precocial infants have offspring that are born with more developed motor and sensory systems and may be able to move independently and thermoregulate within hours of birth. They require feeding and protection, but do not need a nest for warmth. Among the precocial mammals are the ungulates (e.g., sheep, goats, horses, and cattle) and marine mammals, species that live in large social groups and forage over a wide range rather than having a specific nest site. About 10% of birds are precocial (e.g., chickens and geese). Parental care for precocial species involves what Rosenblatt (Rosenblatt 1993) has called a leading-following pattern. Because many mammalian precocial species live in herds, parental behavior may require individual, selective maternal-infant bonds, which are usually absent in altricial species. As infants may join the herd on the first day postpartum, these bonds are formed within the first few hours after birth. While the following behavior of goslings and chicks has been the prototype of imprinting behavior, precocial mammalian offspring may also develop a selective bond to a caretaker.

Most primates and some birds (e.g., gulls and terns) are not clearly precocial or altricial. At birth the young can thermoregulate and their eyes and ears are open, but they cannot move independently to follow the mother. These semiprecocial primate offspring must cling to the mother or, in the case of humans, be carried. It is worth noting that although humans in Western societies often place their infants in cribs (i.e., nests), as if they were altricial, ethnographic studies of human parental care stress that more continual contact between mother and baby, as seen with other primates, is the norm in most non-Western societies (Montagu 1971).

CONTINUOUS VERSUS INTERMITTENT CARE

In addition to the uniparental-biparental and the altrical-precocial dimensions, species differ in the intensity or frequency of their parental care. As we will see below, some species appear "promiscuously parental," providing nurturing behavior even towards offspring that are unrelated, whereas others avoid or attack offspring except immediately following parturition. Indeed, there are several bird species (species of cowbirds and cuckoos) that fail to show parental behavior at all. These brood parasites do not incubate their own eggs, but instead lay them in the nest of another species where they hatch and are raised as foster young. Brood parasitism introduces a number of questions about how the offspring learn species-typical behaviors (West et al. 1990) and, by comparison with closely related nesting species, provides an opportunity to identify neurobiological correlates of parental behavior (Ball 1991).

But even among mammals, the range of maternal care is profound (Rosenblatt and Snowdon 1996). At one end of the spectrum is the tree shrew, in which maternal care limited to placing the infant in a well-concealed arboreal nest and visiting it once every 48 hours to nurse. Similarly, rabbits nurse in one 3-minute bout daily, and there is neither retrieval nor contact in between. At the other end of the spectrum is the near continual contact and frequent nursing found in most primate species. These species variations in nursing behavior are matched by species differences in milk content. Rabbit milk, for instance, has nearly double the protein and fat content of monkey milk or cow milk (Rosenblatt 1993).

In summary, there is no typical mammalian or avian species for studying parental behavior. In this chapter, we will focus mostly on the Norway rat because the vast majority of the neuroendocrine research on maternal behavior has been done in this species. The rat is uniparental with altricial pups that are nursed approximately every 3 hours. Rats have been an excellent model for studying the endocrine and neural substrates of maternal care because pregnant rats avoid pups of other mothers until late in their pregnancy and then show an intense interest in nest building, retrieval, and nursing. Defining the hormonal changes necessary for the rapid onset of maternal care in this species has provided important insights into the mechanisms of maternal behavior. However, laboratory rats have been selected to breed in cages and not in a world of predation and foraging. Thus, findings in the rat may not generalize to other mammals. But then, given the diversity of parental behavior described above, no single species will suffice to fully explain all the relations among hormones and parental behavior.

Maternal Behavior in the Norway Rat

Nulliparous (literally "never parturient"—a female that has never given birth) adult rats do not display maternal behavior and will either avoid or attack pups. The gestation period for a rat is 22 days. Approximately 24 to 48 hours prior to delivery, the pregnant female shows increased interest in pups, begins to make a nest, and becomes more aggressive towards intruders, which is possibly correlated with the initiation of uterine contractions. Just prior to delivery of the first pup, the dam licks her own vaginal opening while stretching and adjusting her posture (sitting on her lower back with her legs spread) to aid in the expulsion of the fetus.

As the fetal membranes protrude through the vaginal opening, she licks and bites them, actively assisting in the delivery while covering herself in amniotic fluid. As the first pup emerges, her vigorous licking removes the fetal membranes and stimulates respiration. As with most mammals, the dam eats the placenta. Within one hour of delivery of the last pup, the first nursing bout begins. Nursing behavior involves an active crouching posture with the dam standing over the young with a pronounced dorsal arch and with her legs splayed over them. While the pups are attached to the nipples, the dam is quiescent. As with many rodents, rats exhibit postpartum estrus and usually become pregnant within 24 hours of delivery.

Newborn rats are deaf, blind, and unable to locomote or regulate their body temperature. Through the first week, rat maternal behavior involves care of the nest, retrieval and grouping of the pups, and licking the pups, typically from the head to the anogenital region (figure 9.1). Anogenital licking involves

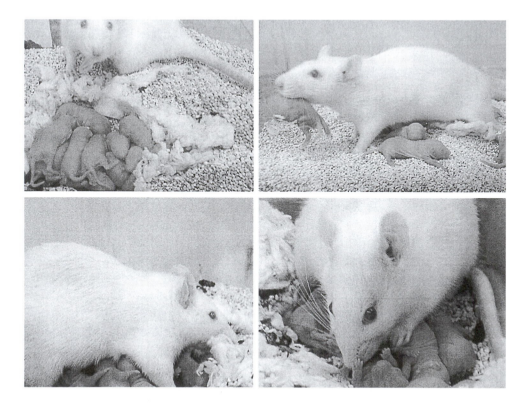

Figure 9.1 Maternal behavior in the rat consists of maintenance of the nest, retrieval and grouping of the pups into the nest, nursing with the dam situated in an arched back posture, and licking and grooming of the pups.

ingestion of a significant volume of urine from the pup, providing a recovery of fluid for the lactating dam (Gubernick and Alberts 1985). Rat dams groom their male pups more frequently than their female pups (Moore and Morelli 1979). During the first week, nursing shifts from the active crouch to a passive posture with the dam recumbent while the pups are attached to her nipples. Maternal aggression peaks in the first week.

Pups become increasingly mobile after the first week, with eyes opening on day 14. Through this period, nursing bouts begin to be initiated by the pups rather than the dam. Weaning begins around day 16 as the pups begin to eat solid food. Weaning has been reported to be completed by day 24 to 28, although because rats go into postpartum estrus, most often the dam's next litter arrives on day 22 or 23 and becomes the major focus of her maternal behavior (Stern 1996).

In summary, in the rat, pup-directed maternal behavior consists of nest building, retrieving, grouping, grooming, and nursing. While maternal behavior is often described as a composite, the various components may be dissociated under experimental conditions. Most research has focused on retrieval, as this behavior appears superficially to reflect maternal motivation. However, there is more to maternal behavior than retrieving pups. For instance, females that fail to retrieve may be able to nurse if the young are placed on the nipples. Furthermore, there are important aspects of maternal behavior that are not directed at pups. Not only are maternal rats more aggressive towards intruders, they are less fearful and markedly less responsive to stress than virgin females.

In a sense, motherhood involves a personality change for the female. How does this happen? We now understand that the onset of maternal behavior in the rat depends on specific experiential, sensory, and hormonal factors, although we still do not know how these specific factors regulate each of the components of maternal care (figure 9.2). The most salient points to remember are (1) experience appears important for both the onset and the maintenance of maternal behavior, (2) sensory inputs regulate different aspects of maternal care, and (3) hormones appear more important for the onset than the maintenance of maternal behavior.

EXPERIENTIAL FACTORS
There is some wisdom to the maxim "once a mother always a mother"—even for rats. Multiparous (many births) rats are different from primiparous (first

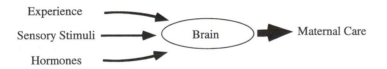

Figure 9.2 Experience, sensory stimuli, and hormonal factory interact at the level of the brain to modulate the expression of maternal care.

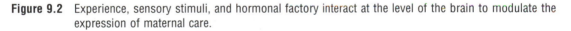

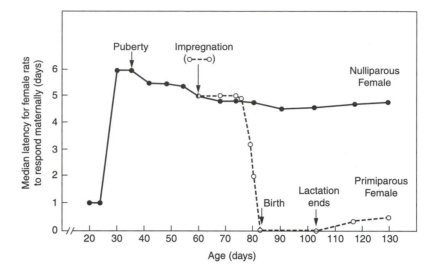

Figure 9.3 Developmental changes in maternal responsiveness in the female rat. Values represent the median number of days of pup exposure required to induce maternal behavior during a 1 hour test. The latency to respond maternally increases abruptly just prior to puberty and remains high until just before parturition. The latency remains low after the first maternal experience. (From Bridges 1990.)

birth) or nulliparous rats. This difference is most evident in their acceptance of foster pups, even when not pregnant. As noted above, nulliparous females avoid pups and fail to display maternal care. In 1933, Wiesner and Shead (Wiesner and Sheard 1933) reported that nurturing behavior can be induced by exposing virgin females to pups for several hours per day over the course of 5 or 6 days. The induction of maternal behavior by pup exposure is called "sensitization" (although the process might really be a "desensitization" to pups). As sensitization occurs in the absence of ovaries, pituitary, and adrenals, it appears to be independent of hormonal control. Even adult male rats can be stimulated to show parental behavior with repeated exposure to pups, although at a longer latency than females (Rosenblatt 1967).

The latency to express maternal behavior in nonparturient rats changes significantly over development and with maternal experience (figure 9.3). For example, juvenile male and female rats (especially at age 24 to 28 days) display maternal care within 24 hours of pup exposure without hormonal manipulation. This juvenile interest in offspring may prove adaptive in a colonial species like the Norway rat in which the dam has a new litter every 22 days. From puberty onward, 6 or more days of pup exposure are required to stimulate maternal behavior in nulliparous animals. Once a female rat has raised her first litter, she will rapidly display maternal care within 24 hours of pup exposure, regardless of her hormonal condition. Indeed, even brief experience with pups during birth promotes a long-term retention of maternal responsiveness (Morgan et al. 1992). In addition, multiparous females exhibit improved spatial learning, unlike nulliparous females, suggesting that mater-

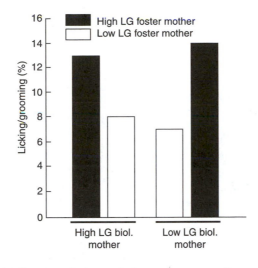

Figure 9.4 Nongenomic transmission across generations of maternal behavior patterns. Values represent the relative frequency of licking and grooming of pups for dams that were fostered as pups to either high licking-grooming (LG) or low licking-grooming mothers. Pups reared by high licking-grooming mothers exhibit high levels of licking and grooming as mothers regardless of the behavior of their biological mothers. (Data from Francis 1999.)

nal experience alters the brain not only by enhancing the acceptance of pups but more generally by facilitating learning (Kinsley et al. 1999). In this regard, it should be noted that most of the studies investigating the endocrine factors regulating the onset of maternal behavior have focused on the transition to maternal behavior in nulliparous or primiparous females, and therefore may or may not be applicable to subsequent maternal events.

Recent research has looked in great detail at the style of mothering. Michael Meaney and his co-workers have described two styles of maternal care in Long Evans rats, termed high licking-grooming and low licking-grooming (Francis et al. 1999). High licking-grooming moms spend more time grooming their pups than do low licking-grooming moms. Pups of high licking-grooming dams are less fearful and less stress-responsive in adulthood. They also show neurobiological changes, including fewer glucocorticoid receptors in the hippocampus and reduced corticotropin-releasing-hormone gene expression in the hypothalamus. It now appears, from crossfostering studies, that this style of mothering is transmitted to subsequent generations, because offspring of a low licking-grooming dam that are raised by a high licking-grooming dam will show high levels of licking and grooming towards their own pups. Thus, experiential factors that influence maternal care include not only the dam's previous experience as a mother but her own experience of being mothered as an infant (figure 9.4).

SENSORY FACTORS

What determines whether a female will approach or avoid a pup? As we have just seen, sensitization is important, but what is the dam becoming sensitized

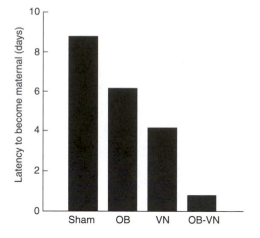

Figure 9.5 The effects of olfactory bulb (OB), vomeronasal organ (VN) or combination lesions on the latency to become maternal after daily exposure to pups. Rats with combination olfactory bulb and vomeronasal lesions show a significant reduction in the amount of pup exposure required to display maternal care relative to sham-operated animals. (Data from Fleming 1979.)

to? Given that rats are predominantly olfactory animals, it is a reasonable bet that she responds to the odor of pups. It may seem surprising, therefore, that lesions of the olfactory system actually facilitate the onset of maternal behavior in virgin female rats (figure 9.5).

In rodents, odors are processed by two olfactory systems, the main olfactory bulb and the vomeronasal organ. The main olfactory bulb can detect a broad range of odors in the environment, while the vomeronasal organ, which projects to the accessory olfactory bulb, is specialized for detecting pheromonal signals. The main olfactory system projects primarily to the piriform cortex and the cortical nucleus of the amygdala, while the accessory olfactory system projects to the cortical and medial nuclei of the amygdala. The amygdala then projects to the medial preoptic area via the bed nucleus of the stria terminalis (figure 9.6). As we will see later, the medial preoptic area plays a central role in the activation of maternal behavior. Virgin female rats with intact olfactory systems require 6 to 8 days of continuous pup exposure to show maternal care towards foster pups, whereas after complete olfactory lesions, females approached and retrieved pups after only 1 day of exposure (Fleming et al. 1979). Furthermore, lesioning the medial nucleus of the amygdala or the stria terminalis also accelerates the onset of maternal behavior in virgin females. These results suggest that pup odors normally inhibit maternal care in virgin females through an inhibitory influence of the amygdala on the medial preoptic area.

BEHAVIOR

In addition to overcoming an aversion to the smell of pups, there are specific sensory determinants for retrieval and nursing. Nearly 50 years ago, Beach

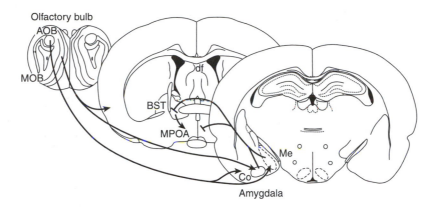

Figure 9.6   The olfactory pathway in the rodent. The main olfactory bulb (MOB) projects to the piriform cortex and the cortical (Co) amygdala. Sensory input from the vomeronasal organ projects through the accessory olfactory bulb (AOB) to the cortical and medial nuclei of the amygdala. The amygdala then projects to the medial preoptic area (MPOA) and bed nucleus of the stria terminalis.

and Jaynes (Beach and Jaynes 1956) described how retrieval depended on the dam's contact with the pup's skin. Pups with cold skin or skin covered with petroleum jelly were not retrieved. As the dam's perception of the pup's skin requires exploration with her snout and whiskers, it is not surprising that interfering with sensory processing from the perioral area reduces pup retrieval (Stern 1996). Similarly, sensory stimulation of the dam's ventrum, especially of the nipples, is essential for eliciting the nursing crouch. The arched-back nursing crouch is essentially a reflex, analogous to (although motorically the inverse of) the lordosis reflex that estrous females exhibit in response to flank stimulation (Stern 1996). After retrieval, the dam will hover over her pups, which stimulate her ventrum by rooting, pushing, and suckling. A recent study has demonstrated remarkable plasticity in the somatosensory cortex associated with lactation. Stimulation of the ventrum is so important during lactation that the receptive field for the ventrum, specifically the nipple region, within the somatosensory cortex increases by over 60%, shrinking again following the end of lactation (Xerri et al. 1994).

Hormonal Factors

HORMONAL CHANGES DURING PREGNANCY

The hormonal changes that occur from mating until parturition support pregnancy by inhibiting the normal estrus cycle, preparing the uterus for implantation, and delaying uterine contractions until term. Are these hormonal changes that prepare the uterus also priming the brain for motherhood? Terkel and Rosenblatt (Terkel and Rosenblatt 1972) provided the first clear evidence that hormonal factors associated with pregnancy were also involved in the induction of maternal behavior, since virgin rats transfused with blood from a parturient dam exhibited maternal behavior. What hormones are involved in the induction of maternal care at parturition? In the rat, the gonadal steroids, especially estrogen and progesterone, exhibit a very clear pattern across the estrus cycle and gestation. As discussed in detail in chapter 4, female rats have a 4-day cycle consisting of 2 days of diestrus followed by proestrus and estrus. During proestrus, 17β-estradiol secreted from the developing follicles stimulates physiological changes in the uterus in preparation for implantation. During the night of proestrus, ovulation occurs resulting in the release of the ovum and a surge of progesterone from the corpora lutea. Mating typically occurs in the hours following ovulation. Vaginocervical stimulation associated with mating results in a psuedopregnancy state in which the corpora lutea is stimulated by luteinizing hormone (LH) from the pituitary to secrete high levels of progesterone and relatively low levels of estrogen (figure 9.7). If fertilization occurs, around midpregnancy ovarian control is taken over by the placenta, which secretes placental lactogen to maintain the corpora lutea for the remainder of the pregnancy. Estrogen levels rise over the last half of the pregnancy. In the last days before parturition, prostaglandins and pituitary hormones end the pregnancy by terminating progesterone secretion. At the onset of parturition there is a sharp rise in prolactin, which is thought to be involved in mammary gland development. In addition, during lactation oxytocin is secreted in response to suckling to regulate milk ejection.

EXPERIMENTAL MANIPULATION DURING PREGNANCY

As noted above, the rapid initiation of maternal behavior in rats just prior to parturition provides an opportunity to ask what physiological factors are necessary for maternal care. There have been two general approaches for investigating the hormonal basis of maternal behavior. One approach has been to interrupt pregnancy at specific times to determine when females will first exhibit interest in foster pups (Rosenblatt et al. 1979). A second approach has treated virgin females with various hormonal regimens to determine which factors are sufficient to induce maternal behavior (Bridges 1996). In general, these studies have focused on inexperienced females and have measured the onset of maternal behavior over days rather than minutes.

ESTROGEN

The onset of maternal behavior in the pregnant female rat is coincident with a sharp decrease in progesterone and an increase in estrogen and prolactin. Pregnancy termination by hysterectomy (removal of the uterus and accompanying fetuses) on days 16 to 19 results in an induction of maternal behavior, but this is observed 48 hours after surgery and most animals require 1 to 2 days of pup exposure (Rosenblatt and Siegel 1975). Removal of the placenta with the uterus eliminates placental lactogen, which supports corpera leutal progesterone secretion, and stimulates estrogen secretion from the ovaries. Thus, both the induction of premature maternal behavior by pregnancy termination and the normal emergence of maternal behavior at the end of preg-

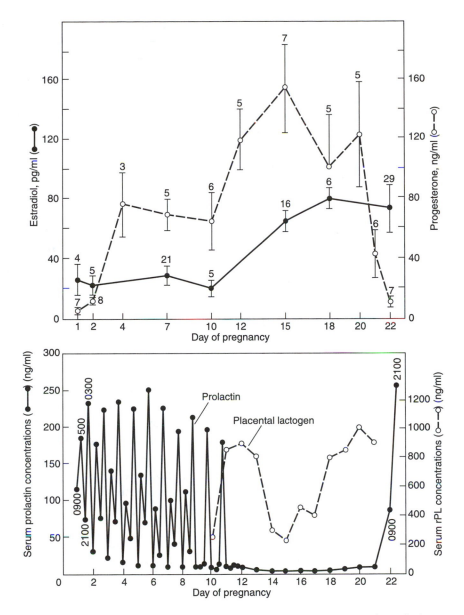

Figure 9.7 Profiles of steroid (*upper*) and lactogenic (*lower*) hormone concentrations during pregnancy in rats. (From Bridges 1990.)

nancy are associated with a fall in progesterone and an increase in estrogen levels. Combining hysterectomies with ovariectomies eliminates the increase in estrogen after pregnancy termination and delays the onset of maternal care. However, estradiol treatment reinstates maternal behavior in these females, indicating that estrogen is necessary for normal maternal behavior. Conversely, giving progesterone after pregnancy termination delays the onset of maternal behavior (Bridges et al. 1978). Thus, the combination of progesterone withdrawal in the presence of continued estrogen appears to be the optimal condition for the onset of maternal behavior.

Can similar changes in gonadal hormones induce maternal behavior in nonpregnant females? Classic studies by Moltz et al. and Bridges et al. used various steroid and prolactin treatments to simulate the physiological changes of pregnancy in ovariectomized virgin females (Moltz et al. 1970; Bridges 1984). Estrogen capsules of varying lengths were implanted on day one, and either progesterone or blank capsules were implanted on day 3. On day 13, the progesterone capsules were removed. Maternal behavior was tested beginning on day 14 of treatment. Although the low doses of estrogen alone were ineffective at inducing maternal responsiveness, the combined estrogen and progesterone treatment and withdrawal resulted in the induction of maternal care after 1 to 2 days of pup exposure. At higher doses, estrogen alone was capable of inducing similar latencies.

How does estrogen prime the brain to influence behavior? It is now clear that the effects of estradiol on behavior may be due to its actions on the estrogen receptor (ER), of which there are two subtypes, ER-α and ER-β. Estrogen receptors are abundant in specific brain regions thought to be involved in the regulation of maternal behavior, including the bed nucleus of the stria terminalis, the medial preoptic area, and the amygdala (figure 9.8).

Estrogen receptors are hormone-dependent transcription factors. That is, when they are activated by estrogen, they bind directly to regulatory sites on DNA where they alter the expression of specific genes, which in turn influence neuronal function. Thus, estrogen is best considered as an early step in a cascade of cellular events that can ultimately lead to neuronal activation, recruitment of a neural system, and ultimately behavioral change. Many of the genes regulated by estrogen receptors (e.g., oxytocin and prolactin receptors) are important for transducing the increase in estrogen concentration into changes in cellular responsiveness to other hormones associated with parturition.

What is the relative contribution of ER-α and ER-β in the induction of maternal behavior? Mice with mutated estrogen receptors provide some answers to this question. Estrogen receptor-α knockout mice are infertile; however, maternal behavior can be assessed in virgin mice since nulliparous mice display maternal behavior when exposed to pups. Estrogen receptor-α knockout mice display increased infanticide and increased latencies to retrieve pups (Ogawa et al. 1998). In contrast, estrogen receptor-β knockout mice are fertile and are capable of raising their offspring to weaning, although a detailed

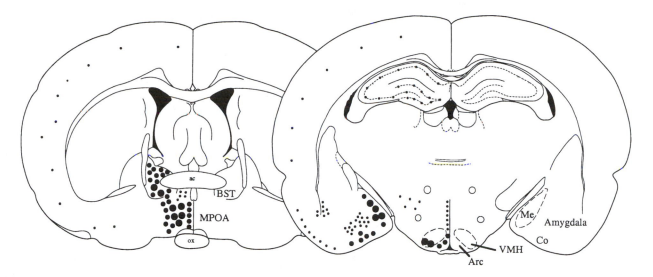

Figure 9.8 Distribution of estrogen receptor–containing cells in the rat brain. Note the abundance of estrogen receptors in the medial and cortical amygdala, the bed nucleus of the stria terminalis (BST), and the medial preoptic area (MPOA), all of which are involved in the regulation of maternal care.

analysis of their maternal behavior has not been reported. These observations suggest that estrogen receptor-α may be playing a larger role than estrogen receptor-β, but the interpretation of the behavioral deficits in the estrogen receptor-α knockout is difficult because these mice have elevated levels of estrogen and testosterone prior to gonadectomy due to a deficit in negative feedback of the HPG axis. These hormonal changes could possibly contribute to the observed effects on infanticide and retrieval behavior.

PROGESTERONE

Progesterone plays an important but complex role in the priming of neural pathways for maternal behavior. Progesterone, like estrogen, binds to specific intracellular receptors. The progesterone analogue RU 486, which blocks this intracellular receptor, antagonizes progesterone's inhibition of maternal behavior (Numan et al. 1999). Progesterone may also influence behavior via its metabolite, allopregnanolone, which modulates the activity of GABA receptors and may have diazepamlike effects. Although under most conditions, allopregnanolone may not accumulate in sufficient quantities to alter behavior physiologically, the high levels of progesterone during pregnancy may result in sufficient concentrations of this metabolite to influence GABA-ergic neurotransmission (Paul and Purdy 1992).

PROLACTIN

Plasma prolactin levels increase dramatically on the day of parturition, partially in response to the increase in estrogen (figure 9.9). There is a great deal

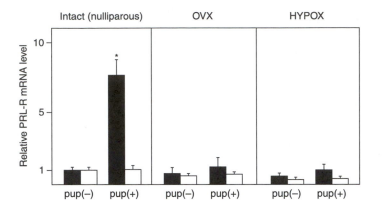

Figure 9.9 Effects of pup exposure on prolactin receptor gene expression in the brain of intact, ovariectomized (OVX) and hypophysectomized (HYPOX) female rats. The rats were exposed to pups (pups(+)) or unexposed (pups(−)) for seven days. A similar exposure paradigm had demonstrated that latency to display maternal behavior after pup exposure is significantly shorter in intact females compared to OVX and HYPOX females. Note the induction of the long form (solid bars), but not the short form (open bars) of prolactin receptor mRNA in the intact females. (From Sugiyama et al. 1996.)

of evidence suggesting that the rise in prolactin on the day of parturition is critical for the normal onset of maternal behavior. Surgical removal of the pituitary, which is the source of plasma prolactin (and many other factors), delays the onset of maternal behavior (Bridges and Ronsheim 1990). Plasma prolactin and maternal behavior can be rescued in a hypophysectomized animal by an implantation of pituitary tissue from another animal. Treating rats with bromocriptine, a substance that prevents prolactin release from the pituitary, also delays the onset of maternal behavior in estrogen-primed ovariectomized rats (Bridges et al. 1985). Finally, administering prolactin into the lateral ventricle of estrogen-progesterone-primed virgin rats induces maternal behavior (Bridges et al. 1990). However, prolactin treatment is not effective in animals that have not been primed with estrogen and progesterone. Thus, it appears that estrogen and progesterone priming are necessary for prolactin to induce maternal behavior, and, conversely, that prolactin release is necessary for the estrogen-progesterone induction of short-latency maternal behavior.

Prolactinlike hormones secreted by the placenta during pregnancy may also influence maternal behavior. Placental lactogens are released in the later stages of pregnancy in the rat and are thought to activate the prolactin receptor. Infusion of these substances into the brain also stimulates maternal behavior in steroid-primed females (Bridges et al. 1997).

The effects of rising plasma prolactin on maternal behavior raises an interesting question: How does prolactin enter the brain? The brain is surrounded by a blood-brain barrier which is impermeable to peptide hormones, although steroid hormones can pass freely from the blood to the brain. One possible explanation is the abundance of prolactin receptors in the choroid plexus, the cells lining the ventricles of the brain. These prolactin receptors may play some role in the transport of prolactin into the brain. However, prolactin mRNA can be detected in the hypothalamus, indicating that prolactin is synthesized in the brain. More importantly, prolactin receptors are present in the medial preoptic area and other regions of the hypothalamus (Chiu and Wise 1994). These receptors are candidates for mediating the induction of maternal behavior by prolactin and are regulated by estrogen and increase in density during late pregnancy and lactation (Pi and Grattan 1999).

The prolactin receptor mRNA exists in short and long forms, a result of alternate splicing of the primary RNA transcript. The significance of these two forms is not yet understood. However, the amount of the long form of the prolactin receptor in the brain is increased several fold during lactation, concommitant with the expression of maternal behavior (Sugiyama et al. 1996). Removal of the pups from a lactating female reduces the expression of the long form, and re-exposure to pups reinstates its expression. Surprisingly, the expression of the long form of the receptor also increases in virgin female rats after exposure to pups. In one study, intact, ovariectomized and hypophysectomized female rats were exposed to pups daily. Intact, but not ovariectomized and hypophysectomized females displayed maternal behavior after only a few days of pup exposure. When the brains of each of these groups were analyzed, it was found that the long form of the prolactin receptor mRNA was increased only in the intact females. Therefore, the induction of the long form of the receptor may be associated with the onset of both pup-induced and postpartum maternal behavior (Sugiyama et al. 1996).

Studies with prolactin receptor knockout mice confirm the role of prolactin in the induction of maternal care. Virgin mice of the laboratory strains used to create these knockouts exhibit maternal behavior after 1 to 2 days of exposure to pups. Virgin female mice lacking a functional prolactin receptor failed to retrieve pups even after 6 days of exposure. Females with only a single functional copy of the prolactin receptor gene exhibited a delayed onset of maternal behavior, requiring 3 to 4 days of exposure to display maternal behavior. Thus, in contrast to the hormone-independent induction of maternal behavior in rats, prolactin is involved in pup-induced maternal behavior even in nonparturient mice. Complete prolactin receptor knockout mice are infertile, but females with one copy of their prolactin receptor gene destroyed have been studied after giving birth. Whereas nontransgenic parturient mice typically retrieve all three stimulus pups into the nest immediately, mice with one mutated and one functional prolactin receptor gene only sporadically retrieve pups to the nest. Therefore, consistent with the observation discussed above in rats, the prolactin receptor appears critical for the expression of postpartum maternal care in mice.

OXYTOCIN

Oxytocin, one of the first neuropeptide hormones to be isolated and sequenced, has been studied extensively for its ability to induce uterine contractions and milk ejection. Traditionally, oxytocin has been considered a neurohypophyseal hormone: it is synthesized in the hypothalamus and then transported to the posterior pituitary (neurohypophysis) where it is stored. Vaginocervical stimulation during delivery and suckling during nursing result in the of release oxytocin from the posterior pituitary into the general circulation, leading to uterine contractions (during labor and delivery) or milk ejection (during lactation). Recently, this traditional description of oxytocin action has been revised in two key ways. First, oxytocin mRNA has been found in high concentrations in several peripheral tissues, especially the parturient uterus (Lefebvre et al. 1992). This discovery has led to a debate about the importance of pituitary versus nonpituitary sources of oxytocin in the regulation of uterine contractions. Second, there is increasing evidence that oxytocin is released within the brain where it acts on specific receptors identical to the receptors found in the uterus and mammary myoepithelium (Barberis and Tribollet 1996). Indeed, as with prolactin, changes in oxytocin receptor concentration in the brain may be as important as changes in the content of peptide for the regulation of behavior.

If oxytocin is a brain hormone or neurotransmitter, it is reasonable to hypothesize that it may serve as a trigger for parental behavior, in parallel with its peripheral role for parturition and lactation. Pederson and Prange demonstrated that in hormone-primed virgin rats, injecting oxytocin into the lateral ventricles resulted in the onset of maternal behavior within 1 hour (Pedersen and Prange 1979). Even more important, the onset of maternal behavior is delayed by reducing oxytocin neurotransmission either by injecting a specific receptor antagonist (Leengoed et al. 1987) or an anti-oxytocin antibody (Pedersen et al. 1985) into the brain, or by lesioning the paraventricular nucleus of the hypothalamus (the major source of oxytocin in the brain) (Insel and Harbaugh 1989). Remarkably, once maternal behavior has been induced, these same interventions have no effect. Thus, oxytocin has a role in the transition from pup avoidance to maternal behavior, but once established, oxytocin is not necessary for the maintenance or performance of maternal behavior.

How does oxytocin facilitate the onset of maternal behavior? As noted above, lesions of the olfactory system reduce the latency to the onset of maternal behavior. Some evidence suggests that oxytocin acting in the olfactory bulb may reduce olfactory processing, thus facilitating the approach and reducing the avoidance of pups. In one study, a low concentration of a specific oxytocin receptor antagonist infused directly into the olfactory bulb delayed the onset of maternal behavior in parturient rats; if oxytocin was infused directly into the bulb, half of the animals displayed maternal behavior within 2 hours of pup exposure (Yu et al. 1996a). In another study by the same investigators, electrophysiological stimulation of the paraventricular nucleus of the hypothalamus, the major source of forebrain oxytocin projections, inhibited the firing of olfactory bulb mitral cells (Yu 1996b). The effect was blocked by intrabulbar infusion of the oxytocin receptor antagonist, and mimicked by intrabulbar infusion with oxytocin. Thus, oxytocin in the olfactory bulb may decrease olfactory processing, potentially modulating the olfactory aversion to pup odors. As we shall see below, others have demonstrated that oxytocin influences the onset of maternal behavior by actions in the preoptic area and the ventral tegmental area. Perhaps the modulation of olfactory processing acts simultaneously with effects in other areas, such as the preoptic area, to enhance motivation or nurturing behavior.

The synthesis of and sensitivity to oxytocin in the brain changes during the course of pregnancy. Oxytocin gene expression in the hypothalamus increases during pregnancy and lactation (VanTol et al. 1988). Estrogen or progesterone alone do not increase oxytocin synthesis, but prolonged estrogen and progesterone followed by progesterone withdrawal (i.e., precisely the physiological sequence of hormonal changes that occurs during gestation) results in a marked increase in oxytocin mRNA (Amico et al. 1997). Perhaps even more important, oxytocin receptors in select brain regions increase as well. Oxytocin receptor mRNA in the preoptic area is elevated during midpregnancy and oxytocin receptor binding is elevated in the medial preoptic area, the bed nucleus of the stria terminalis, the ventromedial nucleus of the hypothalamus, and the ventral tegmental area on postpartum day 1 (Insel 1990; Pedersen et al. 1994; Young et al. 1997). Estrogen has been shown to increase both oxytocin receptor gene expression and binding in the hypothalamus (Johnson et al. 1991; Bale and Dorsa 1995). Thus, by increasing oxytocin receptors at specific brain targets, the elevations in estradiol levels during late pregnancy may serve to potentiate the actions of oxytocin released in the CNS at the onset of parturition.

Given the data suggesting a role for oxytocin in the induction of maternal behavior in rats, it is surprising that oxytocin knockout mice display apparently normal maternal care (Nishimori et al. 1996). How can this be explained? Since these mice have functional oxytocin receptors, it is possible that other peptides capable of activating the oxytocin receptor may be up-regulated to compensate for the lack of oxytocin. However, this seems unlikely since the oxytocin knockout mice continue to show normal pup retrieval and grooming behavior even when infused for several days with an oxytocin receptor blocker. A more likely explanation is that the strain of mice (SV129xC57B6J) used to create the knockout display high levels of spontaneous maternal care as virgins. In other words, they appear promiscuously parental, without the aversion to pups found in virgin rats and house mice. In this strain, oxytocin is not needed to facilitate the shift from aversion to nurturing behavior, as is the case with rats. Remember that in rats that have already developed maternal care, disruption of the oxytocin system does not significantly alter the expression of maternal behavior. Nevertheless, it is interesting to contrast these findings with those of the prolactin receptor knockout mouse described above. These results suggest that oxytocin and prolactin are playing different roles in activating behavior.

Summary

In summary, the data on the neuroendocrine factors regulating maternal behavior suggest that estrogen and progesterone serve to prime the brain in such a way that the female responds to pups by providing nurturing care. The drop in progesterone and the surge in estrogen facilitate the neuroendocrine factors that regulate this behavior. The steroid-dependent up-regulation of prolactin, prolactin receptors, oxytocin, and oxytocin receptors are likely important. Activation of prolactin receptors appears important for increasing and maintaining the motivation to provide maternal care, while the activation of oxytocin may facilitate the transition from nonmaternal to maternal care, partially by modulating the aversive quality of pup-related stimuli. Clearly other factors are involved in mediating maternal behavior. Several neuropeptides, including opiate peptides, tachykinin K, and corticotropin-releasing factor have been implicated (Numan 1994). And maternal care has been disrupted in transgenic mice deficient in epinephrine, *fosB*, and oddly enough, two paternally imprinted genes: *PEG3* and *Mest* (Brown et al. 1996; Lefebvre et al. 1998; Li et al. 1999; Thomas and Palmiter 1997). It is not clear whether the effects of these neuropeptides or these genes are specific to maternal behavior or more generally related to processes critical for maternal behavior, such as sensory processing or cognition. Again, it is important not to think one gene–one behavior, but rather to understand how these various factors fit into a cascade of cellular actions that alter neural pathways, which results in behavioral change. As we will see below, classical neurotransmitters may provide final common paths by which many of these factors modulate behavior. But first, we will examine the neural pathways by which hormones and neuropeptides may be influencing maternal behavior.

Neuroanatomy of Parental Behavior

There is not just one brain area that represents the neuroanatomical locus of maternal behavior. It is also true that much of the brain is not involved. Indeed, even large cortical lesions may have no impact on maternal care. However, a few specific regions have been implicated as important for selective aspects of maternal care, based on lesion studies. While behavioral deficits after lesions are frequently used to link a specific area to a specific behavior, there are problems with this approach. Lesions are rarely neuroanatomically specific. For instance, lesions made with electrolytic probes or suction destroy fibers of passage, such as axons from distant cells, as well as the neurons that have been targeted. Axon-sparing lesions, made with n-methyl-d-aspartate or related excitatory amino acids, destroy neuronal cell bodies and should not affect fibers of passage. But even with these more selective ablations, behavioral changes may be difficult to interpret because you are inferring the function of a nucleus from what an animal does in the absence of that nucleus.

Clearly, a behavioral change after a lesion would result if the nucleus were involved as one node in a complex circuit. It is important to remember that a decrease in maternal behavior after a lesion of area X does not mean that area

X is the neural center for maternal behavior. At most, it indicates that area X is a necessary component in a circuit that influences maternal behavior. Furthermore, the behavioral changes may be nonspecific, influencing sensory, motor, or cognitive performance, and not maternal behavior specifically. Recent studies using receptor mapping, regional gene expression, or cellular markers of activation may be more helpful for detecting the function of specific brain areas with respect to specific behaviors.

Neocortex

In spite of the role of the cortex for processing the auditory and somatosensory stimulation from pups, in general, lesions of the neocortex (i.e., excluding the limbic cortex such as the hippocampus and cingulate) do not impair maternal behavior. In rats, 40% of the cortex can be destroyed, and in hamsters, virtually the entire neocortex can be removed, with little detectable impact on maternal care (reviewed in Numan 1994). While this suggests that maternal behavior is mediated via subcortical pathways, it should be noted that females with hippocampal lesions show impairment of maternal retrieval, probably secondary to spatial deficits, and females with cingulate lesions fail to retrieve pups, as one of several deficits in goal-directed behavior. Although these interventions impair the performance of maternal care (as well as several other behaviors), there is no evidence that lesions of either the neocortex or the limbic cortex specifically decrease the female's interest in pups or her willingness to care for them. As noted earlier, olfactory pathways (olfactory bulbs and downstream targets such as medial amygdala and stria terminalis) appear important for the sensitization process.

Medial Preoptic Area

The area that has been most intensively studied for its role in maternal behavior is the medial preoptic area (MPOA), in the most anterior aspect of the hypothalamus. Both electrolytic and axon-sparing lesions of the MPOA disrupt maternal behavior (Numan 1994). These effects are seen in both pup-induced and postpartum maternal behavior. Careful behavioral observations demonstrate that the deficits are specific to nest building and retrieval, that is, those aspects of maternal care that are dependent on perioral stimulation. MPOA-lesioned females will nurse and adopt a typical crouch posture if pups are placed beneath them. Remarkably, these lesioned females show no retrieval deficits for nonpup stimuli. For instance, candy that approximates the length and weight of a pup is retrieved normally.

The MPOA is not the only region involved in maternal behavior, but it is of particular interest because of its potential role in the hormonal regulation of the onset of maternal care. The MPOA is rich in estrogen and progesterone receptors. These receptors increase in number during gestation (Giordano et al. 1990; Numan et al. 1999). Estrogen implanted directly in the MPOA facilitates the onset of pup retrieval (Fahrbach and Pfaff 1986). The MPOA also has prolactin and oxytocin receptors, both of which, like estrogen receptors, increase during pregnancy. Injections of prolactin directly into the MPOA facilitate maternal behavior in steroid-primed virgin females treated pharmacologically to inhibit endogenous prolactin release (Bridges et al. 1997). Similarly, an oxytocin antagonist injected directly into the MPOA decreases maternal behavior in postpartum females (Pedersen et al. 1994). Taken together, these results suggest that the MPOA is an important site for the actions of estrogen, prolactin, and oxytocin on maternal behavior.

Recent studies using Fos immunocytochemistry have also emphasized the importance of the MPOA for maternal behavior. Fos, the protein product of the *c-fos* immediate-early gene, is a transcription factor that influences the expression of a diverse range of genes in neurons. Fos has been used as a nonspecific marker of cellular activation. Not all neurons utilize *fos*, so negative data cannot be interpreted. But in cells that use the Fos protein as an intracellular effector, an increase in Fos staining indicates activation. If females are exposed to pups daily, regional Fos activation can be compared in those that show maternal behavior and those, given the same stimulus, that do not. Several studies have shown that Fos increases in the MPOA and the ventral bed nucleus of the stria terminalis (as well as in many other regions) of maternal females. These results are consistent with lesion and receptor mapping studies, suggesting an important role for the MPOA in nest building and maternal retrieval.

How does the MPOA work? We still do not know exactly what the MPOA does, but several approaches have given us insights into the circuit through which this region might influence maternal behavior. First, the connectivity of the MPOA includes inputs from the amygdala via the stria terminalis. Recall that the stria terminalis and amygdala appear to inhibit the onset of maternal behavior, so the MPOA may provide a gate between these limbic pathways and a variety of downstream targets. What are the projections of the MPOA? In the rat, MPOA neuron projections include the lateral septum, the lateral habenula (LH), and the ventral tegmental area (VTA) as well as several brainstem nuclei (figure 9.10). The projections from the MPOA to the VTA and brainstem pass through the lateral preoptic area (LPOA). In a series of knife cut and tract tracing experiments, Numan showed that severing the pathway from the MPOA to the LPOA could disrupt the onset of maternal behavior as much as a bilateral MPOA lesion (Numan 1994). When the MPOA to LPOA pathway was cut on one side of the brain, maternal behavior was unaffected. But if the same lesion was combined with a unilateral VTA lesion on the other side of the brain, the females showed the same deficits observed with bilateral MPOA lesions. As several additional combinations of knife cuts failed to alter the onset of maternal behavior, Numan concluded that the MPOA projection via the LPOA to the VTA (or to a site caudal to the VTA) was critical for the expression of maternal behavior (figure 9.10).

Other Brain Regions

Clearly there are other brain regions that are critical for maternal behavior, even among the projection sites of the MPOA. In addition to the VTA, lesions

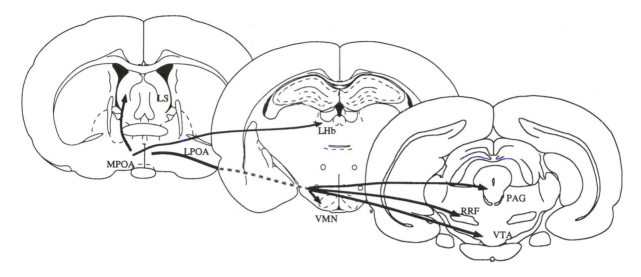

Figure 9.10 Neural projections of medial preoptic area (MPOA). Projections to the caudal areas such as the ventral tegmental area (VTA), retrorubral field (RRF) and periaqueductal gray pass through the lateral preoptic area (LPOA). LS, lateral septum; LHb, lateral habenula; VMN, ventromedial nucleus of the hypothalamus.

of the lateral habenula (LHb), the caudal periaqueductal gray (PAG), and the peripeduncular nucleus (PPN) have all been reported to disrupt maternal behavior. It is important to note that these different lesions have different effects. LHb lesions disrupt the hormonal induction of maternal behavior (Corodimas et al. 1992), PAG lesions disrupt the nursing posture (Lonstein et al. 1998), and as noted above, PPN-lesioned females fail to exhibit maternal aggression (Factor et al. 1993). In an elegant follow-up to his lesion studies, Numan used a series of retrograde tracer injections in various projection sites combined with Fos immunocytochemistry (Numan and Sheehan 1997) (figure 9.11). First, a retrograde tracer was injected into the various projection sites of the MPOA. For example, tracer injected into the VTA would be taken up by the projections and transported back to the cell bodies in the MPOA. The animals were then exposed to pups and allowed to display maternal behavior. Immunocytochemistry for both c-Fos and the tracer was then performed to determine the fraction of MPOA neurons that project to the VTA that are activated (i.e., express c-Fos) during maternal behavior. The results suggest that the MPOA cells activated when females are maternal are not a single population, but project to several targets including the VTA, the LHb, and the PAG.

In summary, there appear to be several circuits involved in maternal behavior. The MPOA is an important funnel through which olfactory and somatosensory inputs are gated and from which several midbrain and brainstem nuclei are affected. Maternal behavior is associated with activation of the MPOA and lesions of the MPOA impair nest building and retrieving, aspects of maternal care dependent on perioral stimulation. Nursing requires ventral

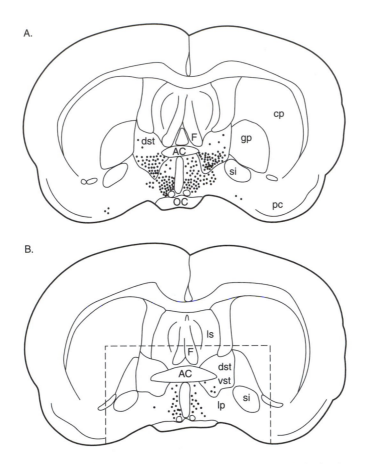

Figure 9.11 Distribution of cells labeled with Fos-like immunoreactivity in the preoptic area of a postpartum female rat that was (*a*) exposed to pups and showed maternal behavior and (*b*) exposed to candy. (From Numan and Sheehan 1997.)

stimulation, with mediation through several brainstem nulcei, including the cPAG and the PPN. Maternal aggression appears to depend on an intact PPN.

Mesolimbic Dopamine Pathway

The description of hormones and neuropeptides above stressed the role of gonadal steroids, prolactin, and oxytocin. Neuroanatomical studies have focused our attention on the MPOA and its projections to several midbrain and brainstem targets. Monoamine neurotransmitters, including dopamine, norepinephrine, and serotonin are synthesized in the midbrain and the brainstem by neurons that have diffuse terminal fields throughout the forebrain. Dopamine has been implicated in various forms of reinforcement and learning. In particular, the mesolimbic dopamine system with cell bodies in the VTA and projections to the nucleus accumbens, septum, and midline frontal cortex appears important for defining various forms of reward, from drugs like amphetamine and cocaine, to electrical self-stimulation, feeding, and even mating (Koob and Moal 1997). Pups are also believed to be rewarding, not only because rat mothers protect them from intruders, but because dams will bar-press for access to pups, just as virgin females will bar-press for amphetamine, electrical self-stimulation, and food rewards. Maternal behavior is associated with increased Fos-staining (presumably a marker of activation) in the VTA, the source of dopamine neurons that project to the nucleus accumbens and other forebrain nuclei.

Consistent with this observation, pup exposure increases the release of dopamine in the nucleus accumbens (Hansen et al. 1993). Injections of 6-hydroxydopamine, which deplete dopamine in the VTA and nucleus accumbens, abolish pup retrieval (Hanson et al. 1991). Treatment with the dopamine antagonist, haloperidol, also impairs maternal behavior (Giordano et al. 1990). Interestingly, cocaine, which transiently increases dopamine, also impairs maternal behavior in rats and possibly in humans (Johns et al. 1994). Thus, dopamine appears to be an important player in maternal behavior, potentially in the hedonic or rewarding aspects of maternal care. One model of the neurobiology of maternal behavior posits that a circuit including the MPOA projection to dopamine cells in the VTA and a projection from the VTA to the nucleus accumbens is critical for the motivation to initiate maternal care in the rat.

Other Species

Birds

Some of the earliest studies on the hormonal regulation of parental behavior were performed on birds. In fact, in 1935, Riddle identified prolactin as key factor in stimulating incubating behavior in the hen (Riddle et al. 1935). As mentioned earlier, 90% of birds exhibit biparental care. Analysis of prolactin levels in several species has demonstrated that prolactin levels increase in both males and females at the onset of incubation behavior (Buntin 1996). Interestingly, prolactin levels are also elevated in breeding cowbirds, which are brood parasites and provide no parental care at all (Dufty et al. 1987). The hormonal basis of avian parental behavior has been best studied in the ring dove. In both male and female ring doves, prolactin levels increase during incubation and peak around hatching, although prolactin levels are low at the beginning of incubation. The rise in prolactin levels parallels the development of the crop sac which produces crop milk that is regurgitated by the parents to the offspring. As in the rat, gonadal steroids also appear to play an important role in the regulation of parental behavior. Gonadectomy eliminates incubation behavior, and estrogen and progesterone replacement in females or testosterone replacement in males reinstates these behaviors (Chen and Silver 1975). Relatively little is known regarding the neural substrates underlying avian parental behavior; however, there is some evidence supporting the role of the preoptic area. For example, lesions of the preoptic area disrupt prolactin-induced feeding in the ring dove (Slawski and Buntin 1995). Thus, there appears to be a remarkable conservation in the hormonal and neural mechanisms regulating parental behavior in birds and mammals.

Sheep

Rats are useful as a model of maternal care with altricial offspring. Herd species with precocial offspring, such as sheep, face a different set of problems, including individual recognition and protection of the young while foraging. Sheep, like rats, exhibit maternal behavior for the first time at parturition. But unlike rats, the ewe develops a selective bond only to her lamb. A non-parturient virgin ewe will butt or avoid lambs, and a parturient ewe will reject a lamb that is not her own. This discriminatory care may seem nonadaptive, but it is critical for the lamb to survive. Sheep are seasonal breeders and, therefore, several lambs are born within a very short time. If the ewe were to nurse any lamb that approaches to suckle, she might not have sufficient milk to nurture her own lamb. Sheep, therefore, provide an opportunity to study not only maternal behavior, such as the nurturing behaviors observed with mothers of altricial young, but also selective bond formation, including processes of recognition and memory.

MATERNAL BEHAVIOR IN THE EWE

How does the ewe recognize her own offspring? This process is mostly olfactory (although audiovocal cues may become important in older lambs) and largely dependent on parturition (Levy et al. 1996). Ewes generally avoid amniotic fluid, but just before birth and for about 2 hours postpartum, they find the odor of amniotic fluid highly attractive. At the time of delivery, the ewe licks the amniotic fluid and placental membranes off her lamb, then eats the placenta and emits low-pitched bleats that are unique to maternal females. Within 2 hours of birth, the ewe noses the lamb towards her udder to begin suckling.

If the ewe and her lamb are separated during this period, she will not become maternal. Careful separation studies suggest that both the recognition and the bond to the lamb develop within 2 to 4 hours of parturition (Poindron et al. 1988). Approximately 50% of ewes separated for the first 4 hours and 75% separated for the first 12 hours subsequently reject their lambs. Maternal rejection includes butting of the lamb, high-pitched bleats, and udder refusal. Placing the lamb in a double-walled mesh cage so that the ewe can smell but not lick or nurse it results in only subtle disturbances of maternal responsiveness. On the other hand, housing the lamb in an airtight box to preclude smelling her lamb virtually eliminates maternal responsiveness. Lesion studies have demonstrated that maternal behavior and individual recognition in sheep is mediated by the main olfactory bulb and does not require an intact accessory olfactory bulb (Levy et al. 1996). Although the cue for selectivity has not been identified, like most ungulate offspring, lambs adopt an

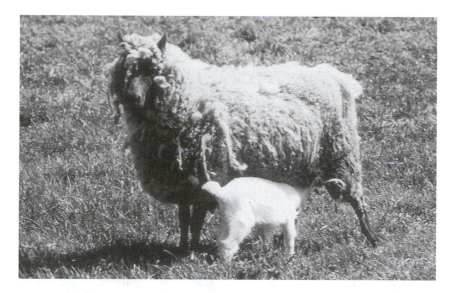

Figure 9.12 Maternal behavior in the ewe. (Photo by Keith Kendrick.)

inverse parallel position when nursing, so that the rump of the infant is close to the ewe's nose (figure 9.12). Ewes tend to focus on the anogenital region for identification at close quarters and will prefer odor cues taken from the rump of their own lamb over equivalent samples from an alien lamb. Presumably anogenital odors are requisite, although urine is a weak discriminatory stimulus and amniotic fluid will not induce acceptance of an alien lamb once a female has become bonded, even if the amniotic fluid is taken from her own lamb.

ESTROGEN AND PROGESTERONE

The changes in estrogen and progesterone during pregnancy in sheep closely resemble what has already been described in rat gestation. Gestation in sheep is 150 days. In the 2 days prior to parturition, progesterone falls while estrogen and prolactin increase. Compared to rats, there has been less success using hormones to induce maternal behavior in sheep, especially in inexperienced females (Levy et al. 1996). Priming with estrogen and progesterone in non-pregnant experienced ewes induces acceptance of alien lambs in about 50% of the subjects, but in contrast to postpartum maternal behavior, the hormonally induced maternal behavior is slow to develop and not well-organized. And, in contrast to rats, neither increasing nor decreasing prolactin appears to influence maternal behavior in sheep.

OXYTOCIN

A remarkable body of research has implicated central oxytocin pathways in the process by which the ewe bonds to her lamb (Kendrick et al. 1997). This research began with an experimental observation that in hormonally primed, nonpregnant ewes or postpartum ewes presented with alien lambs, maternal acceptance was induced within 5 minutes by vaginocervical stimulation (Keverne et al. 1983). As during parturition, vaginocervical stimulation releases oxytocin centrally. An epidural anesthetic injected to block pain fibers entering the lower part of the spinal cord also blocks the sensory signals from vaginocervical stimulation and prevents the increase in oxytocin release and inhibits maternal behavior. Administration of oxytocin directly into the brain induces maternal behavior in experienced estrogen-primed, nonparturient ewes or inexperienced ewes given an epidural anesthetic at parturition. An elegant series of in vivo microdialysis studies by Kendrick and his colleagues have demonstrated the local release of oxytocin in the paraventricular nucleus (where oxytocin is synthesized in the hypothalamus), MPOA, mediobasal hypothalamus, and olfactory bulb, concurrent with parturition (Kendrick et al. 1988).

Administration of oxytocin directly into the paraventricular nucleus by retrodialysis appears to be as potent for inducing maternal behavior as vaginocervical stimulation (DaCosta et al. 1996) (figure 9.13.) This effect may coordinate oxytocin release at several other sites shown to be sensitive for inducing maternal behavior (Kendrick et al. 1997). Oxytocin release into the olfactory bulb at parturition may facilitate lamb recognition, into the MPOA decreases aggression toward the lamb, and into the mediobasal hypothalamus inhibits sexual receptivity. It is of note that all treatments that facilitate maternal behavior, including oxytocin administration, also increase norepinephrine release in the paraventricular nucleus (DaCosta et al. 1996). It is also important to note that the oxytocin effects on maternal behavior have generally been demonstrated only in experienced, that is, multiparous, females. With the exception of the epidural anesthesia study cited above, oxytocin does not induce maternal behavior in inexperienced females, providing another example of the interplay between experience and neuroendocrine factors.

Primates

Most primates, as noted at the outset, are semiprecocial. Their infants are not capable of independent locomotion at birth, but rather than being cached in a nest, are usually carried. Human mothers can discriminate their infant from other infants within hours of birth, identifying not only visual cues but the odor, cries, and tactile features of their baby (Fleming 1990). Parental care in primates is extremely diverse, even within a species. As one example, placentophagia, which is common in virtually all primate females in the postpartum period, is practiced by only a subset of human societies. In many species, maternal behavior is mostly the passive acceptance of clinging and nursing, while in others, females actively search out nurturing behavior with young.

It is generally assumed that relative to other mammals, for primates hormonal factors will be less important than experiential factors, and that preadult alloparenting experience might be especially critical. Indeed, in marked contrast to rats and sheep, maternal behavior in primates is generally not

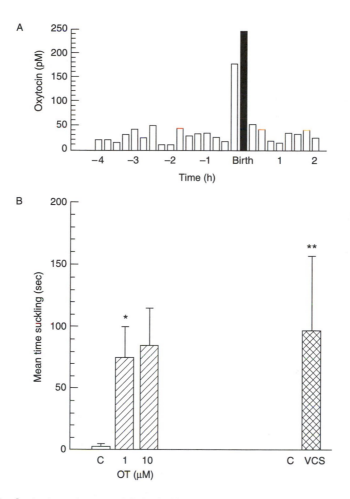

Figure 9.13 Oxytocin and maternal behavior in the sheep. (*A*) microdialysis experiments in a parturient ewe reveals a sharp increase in oxytocin release in the hypothalamus coincident with delivery of the lamb. (*B*) Infusion of oxytocin (OT) into the hypothalamus or vaginocervical stimulation (VCS) stimulates maternal behavior in multiparous, estrogen-progesterone–primed ewes. Control ewes (*C*) receiving saline did not accept the foster lamb at the udder. (Redrawn from DaCosta et al. 1996.)

restricted to the postpartum period, but can be observed in juvenile females, foster parents, grandparents—essentially in females of any endocrine status. In the same sense that other reproductive behaviors in primates (especially humans) may be uncoupled from hormonal influences, maternal behavior may be less dependent on hormonal influences and determined more by factors such as social rank or environmental stress. As pointed out by Keverne, "Any consideration of hormonal influences on behavior in our own species has to take into account the fact that behaviour has itself assumed a major controlling influence over neuroendocrine function, and, insomuch as they may be synchronised, it is now the behaviour which dictates the concordance" (Keverne 1988, p. 136).

Although there is a tendency to emphasize the role of experience, one should not assume that hormones have no influence on primate maternal behavior. This area has not received sufficient study and we remind the reader that absence of evidence is not the same as evidence of absence. Three studies are worth note.

In a particularly imaginative series of studies by Pryce, nulliparous marmosets (a New World species) with care-giving experience were treated with a regimen of estradiol and progesterone to mimic the endogenous changes of the last 15 days of pregnancy (Pryce 1996). These monkeys were tested for maternal motivation in an operant chamber where a bar-press could provide simultaneous visual exposure to an infant replica and the termination of a tape of an infant crying. In validation experiments, bar-pressing by postpartum mothers predicted the amount of time they carried their own infants. Just as with rats, the hormonal regimen of late pregnancy increased maternal interest, as measured by the frequency of bar-pressing. New World monkeys share with most nonprimate mammals a pattern of decreasing progesterone just prior to parturition. In Old World monkeys (such as macaques), apes, and humans, progesterone does not decrease at the end of pregnancy (figure 9.14).

Maestripieri and Zehr recently reported that estrogen treatment increased the interaction of ovariectomized females rhesus macaques with infants (figure 9.15) (Maestripieri and Zehr 1998). Moreover, in the last weeks of pregnancy, estrogen and progesterone concentrations in plasma correlated with an increase in the interaction with unrelated infants. Previous studies that had failed to detect an influence of estrogen on maternal interest used a caged environment, which may have obscured effects on maternal interest that could be observed in a more complex social environment with more naturalistic opportunities for interaction. In fact, a recent study in human mothers found that the changing ratio of estrogen to progesterone across gestation predicted the subsequent quality of attachment in human mothers (Fleming et al. 1997).

Fleming and her co-workers have discovered that plasma cortisol, elevated through human pregnancy, appears to be correlated with maternal feelings in first-time human mothers. Indeed, nearly half the variation in maternal attitudes among pregnant women could be accounted for by cortisol concentrations. New mothers with higher cortisol concentrations were more attracted to infant odors, were superior in identifying their infants, and were more attracted to infant cues. In the postpartum period, women with higher cortisol concentrations engaged in more physically affectionate behaviors and talked more often to their infants than mothers with lower levels (Fleming et al. 1997).

Paternal Care

Paternal care is common in birds but relatively rare in mammals. Most of the mammalian species that are biparental are monogamous (Kleiman and Malcolm 1981). Paternal behavior has been studied in California mice, prairie

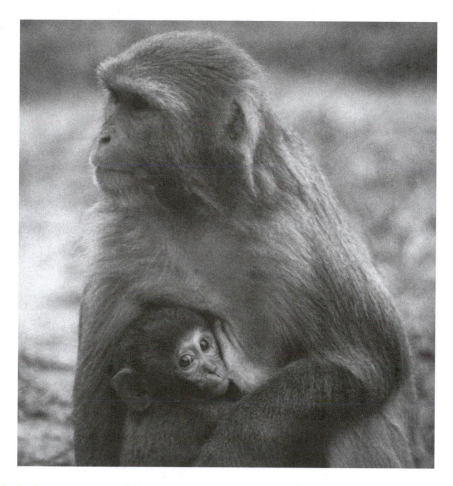

Figure 9.14 In rhesus macaques, interaction with infants increases in the later weeks of pregnancy and is correlated with levels of estrogen and progesterone. (Photo by Kim Wallen.)

voles, dwarf hamsters, gerbils, tamarins, and marmosets. Humans also exhibit paternal care, but there remains an active debate about whether our own species is monogamous.

Paternal behavior can range from passive carrying of offspring and nest defense to active caretaking of the offspring. Male dwarf hamsters have even been reported to assist in the delivery of young (Jones and Wynne-Edwards 1999). In California mice, the species most extensively studied, paternal interest increases during the mate's pregnancy and then increases again in the postpartum period. But unlike other biparental species, fatherhood in the California mouse appears to depend on the presence of the mother (Gubernick and Alberts 1989). If the female is removed, the male fails to take care of the offspring. In many species, such as marmosets, paternal care is not simply maternal care by a male: male parental care develops with a different time course and may include different behaviors (figure 9.16).

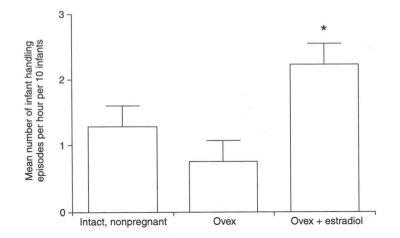

Figure 9.15 Estrogen treatment increases handling of infants in rhesus females. Shown is the mean rate of infant handling in intact, nonpregnant, untreated ovariectomized (Ovex) and estrogen-treated ovariectomized (Ovex-estradiol) females. (Redrawn from Maestripieri and Zehr 1998.)

Does paternal behavior have a hormonal basis? In gerbils, dwarf hamsters, and marmosets, paternal behavior is associated with a decrease in testosterone and a marked increase in prolactin (Dixson and George 1982; Brown et al. 1995; Reburn and Wynne-Edwards 1999). In paternal California mice, prolactin is elevated but testosterone is not depressed (Gubernick and Nelson 1989). Prolactin levels in male marmosets carrying their twin babies are elevated 5-fold (Dixson and George 1982). However, at this time, the relationship between prolactin and paternal care in mammals is only correlational: no study has demonstrated that prolactin treatment can induce paternal care or that decreasing prolactin can inhibit it. In contrast to the current lack of evidence in mammals, prolactin has been shown to induce paternal care in the ring dove (Buntin et al. 1991).

Studies in prairie voles suggest that vasopressin, a neuropeptide closely related to oxytocin, might be important for paternal behavior. Vasopressin injected into the lateral septum increased, whereas a vasopressin antagonist decreased, paternal behavior in prairie voles (figure 9.17) (Wang et al. 1994) Male prairie voles show increased paternal behavior after several days of cohabitation with a female (Bamshad et al. 1994). During this time, there is also a decrease in vasopressin immunoreactivity in the fibers of the lateral septum as well as an increase in vasopressin mRNA in the brain regions projecting to the lateral septum (Wang et al. 1994). This may indicate that during cohabitation, when paternal responsiveness increases, there is a release of vasopressin into the lateral septum (resulting in decreased fiber immunoreactivity) and a simultaneous increase in synthesis. As vasopressin in the brain is sexually dimorphic, it is intriguing to consider that just as oxytocin has been implicated in maternal care, vasopressin may have evolved to subserve male parental care.

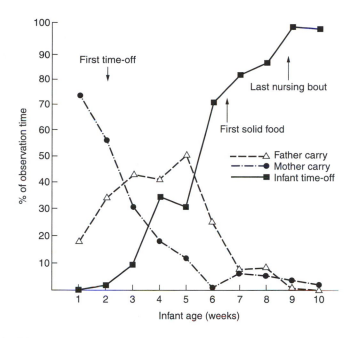

Figure 9.16 Maternal and paternal care in the pygmy marmoset develop with different time courses. Shown is the mean percent time in which infants are carried by the mother and father. During the first two weeks of life, the infant is carried mostly by the mother, after which the father plays a larger role. The mean times for three developmental milestones are noted on the graph. (From Wambolt et al. 1988.)

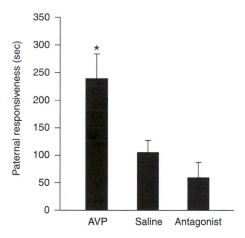

Figure 9.17 Vasopressin plays a role in modulating paternal behavior in the prairie vole. Shown is the mean paternal responsiveness in male prairie voles after receiving lateral septal injections of vasopressin (0.1 ng), saline, or vasopressin antagonist. (From Wang et al. 1998.)

General Conclusions

Roles for Hormones

We have seen that gestational steroid hormones, particularly estrogen and progesterone, play an important role in priming the brain in each of the vertebrate species studied, from birds to primates. In contrast, peptide hormones, such as prolactin and oxytocin, appear to have varying roles in different species. Prolactin facilitates maternal behavior in birds and rodents, but does not appear to be essential for sheep maternal behavior. Oxytocin, however, plays a role in the induction of maternal behavior in both sheep and rats, but not in strains of mice that display spontaneous maternal behavior. Little is known about the role of prolactin or oxytocin in primate parental behavior; however, prolactin levels are correlated with the onset of paternal care in marmosets.

Neuroanatomical Control

Neuroanatomically, the medial preoptic area appears to play a central role in regulating parental care in most species, although no data are available for primates. This region is a likely target of action of the steroid and peptide hormones controlling the behavior. In addition, olfactory-processing pathways, such as the olfactory bulbs, medial amygdala, and bed nucleus of the stria terminalis, are critical for species that use olfaction as a primary sensory modality. Very little is known about the regulation of human parental behavior, but it would not be surprising to find that similar neural mechanisms modulate parental care in our species.

Summary

1. Parental behavior is complex. It shows remarkable variation between species, between genders within a species, and within individuals over their lifespans. This variation is an opportunity for identifying the endocrine and neural mechanisms associated with parental care. Experience, sensory information, and hormones all contribute to the onset and expression of maternal behavior. These factors carry different weights in species with altricial (e.g., rat), precocial (e.g., sheep), and semiprecocial (e.g., primate) offspring.

2. In the rat, the hormones of pregnancy, particularly estrogen and progesterone, prime the brain to promote interest in and acceptance of offspring. At a cellular level, this priming involves estrogen activating one of its intracellular receptors, which in turn activates the expression of several genes at critical sites in the brain. Many of these genes have yet to be identified, but two candidate systems, prolactin and oxytocin, have been studied extensively. Estrogen influences these two systems by increasing the receptors within select brain circuits, thereby increasing cellular responsiveness to prolactin and oxytocin release.

3. One region of the rat brain that appears important for maternal retrieving and nest building is the medial preoptic area (MPOA). Neurons in the MPOA are

part of a circuit that integrates the sensory and hormonal stimuli influencing maternal behavior. As with the genes for maternal behavior, we are just beginning to identify the nodes in this circuit, but projections from the MPOA to several midbrain and brainstem nuclei appear important. Specifically, projections from the MPOA to dopamine cells in the ventral tegmental area may be critical for the motivational changes observed with the onset of rat maternal behavior.

4. Studies in sheep and primates demonstrate the problems in generalizing from results with one species. In sheep, prolactin appears less important than oxytocin, but the effects of both hormones appear less important than the role of experience. Similarly, in primates, experience may be the predominant factor. However, there are intriguing correlates of parental interest in primates, including humans.

5. Paternal care, common in birds and monogamous mammals, may also have a hormonal basis. Prolactin and vasopressin (as opposed to oxytocin) have been implicated in mammalian paternal care, but the mechanisms by which these neuropeptides influence male interest in offspring have yet to be determined.

6. Parental care provides an extraordinary opportunity to explore how genes and hormones influence the brain to modify behavior. In particular, the diversity of parental care, while discouraging simple generalizations across species, offers several remarkable experiments of nature which, properly analyzed, should yield important insights into the mechanisms by which parental care evolved.

Study Questions

1. How does parental behavior vary with the developmental stage of the young within species and across species?

2. Discuss the evidence for a hormonal basis for paternal behavior in birds and mammals.

3. Compare and contrast the roles of prolactin and oxytocin in maternal behavior in birds, rodents, and sheep.

4. Discuss the neural control of maternal behavior in rats and sheep.

5. What are the key experiments you need to do in order to determine whether hormones are involved in maternal behavior in primates? What would your hypothesis be? How would you test your hypothesis?

References

Amico, J. A., Thomas, A., and Hollingshead, D. J. (1997) The duration of estradiol and progesterone exposure prior to progesterone withdrawal regulates oxytocin mRNA levels in the paraventricular nucleus of the rat. *Endocr. Res.* 23: 141–156.

Bale, T. L., and Dorsa, D. M. (1995) Regulation of oxytocin receptor messenger ribonucleic acid in the ventromedial hypothalamus by testosterone and its metabolites. *Endocrinology* 136: 5135–5138.

Ball, G. F. (1991) Endocrine mechanisms and the evolution of avian parental care. *Acta XX Congressus Internationalis Ornithologici* 984–991.

Bamshad, M., Novak, M., and DeVries, G. J. (1994) Cohabitation alters vasopressin innervation and paternal behavior in prairie voles. *Physiol. Behav.* 56: 751–758.

Barberis, C., and Tribollet, E. (1996) Vasopressin and oxytocin receptors in the central nervous system. *Crit. Rev. Neurobiol.* 10: 119–154.

Beach, F. A. (1948) *Hormones and Behavior.* New York: Paul B. Hoeber.

Beach, F. A., and Jaynes, J. (1956) Studies on maternal retrieving in rats. III. Sensory cues involved in the lactating female's response to her young. *Behaviour* 10: 104–125.

Bridges, R. S. (1984) A quantitative analysis of the roles of dosage, sequence, and duration of estradiol and progesterone exposure in the regulation of maternal behavior in the rat. *Endocrinology* 114: 930–940.

Bridges, R. S. (1990) Biochemical bases of rat parental behavior. In N. Krasnegor and R. Bridges (Eds.), *Mammalian Parenting: Biochemical, Neurobiological, and Behavioral Determinants.* Oxford: Oxford University Press.

Bridges, R. S. (1996) Biochemical basis of parental behavior in the rat. *Adv. Stud. Behav.* 25: 215–242.

Bridges, R. S., Numan, M., Ronsheim, P. M., Mann, P. E., and Lupini, C. E. (1990) Central prolactin infusions stimulate maternal behavior in steroid-treated, nulliparous female rats. *Proc. Natl. Acad. Sci. USA* 87: 8003–8007.

Bridges, R. S., DiBiase, R., Loundes, D. D., and Doherty, P. C. (1985) Prolactin stimulation of maternal behavior in female rats. *Science* 227: 782–784.

Bridges, R. S., Robertson, M. C., Shiu, R. P. C., Sturgis, J. D., Henriquez, B. M., and Mann, P. E. (1997) Central lactogenic regulation of maternal behavior in rats: Steroid dependence, hormone specificity, and behavioral potencies of rat prolactin and rat placental lactogen I. *Endocrinology* 138: 756–763.

Bridges, R. S., Robertson, M. C., Shiu, R. P. C., Sturgis, J. J., Henriquez, B. M., and Mann, P. E. (1997) Central lactogenic regulation of maternal behavior in rats: Steroid dependence, hormone specificity, and behavioral potencies of rat prolactin and rat placental lactogen I. *Endocrinology* 138: 756–763.

Bridges, R. S., and Ronsheim, P. M. (1990) Prolactin (PRL) regulation of maternal behavior in rats: Bromocriptine treatment delays and PRL promotes the rapid onset of behavior. *Endocrinology* 126: 837–848.

Bridges, R. S., Rosenblatt, J. S., and Feder, H. H. (1978) Serum progesterone concentrations and maternal behavior in rats after pregnancy termination: Behavioral stimulation after progesterone withdrawal and inhibition by progesterone. *Endocrinology* 102: 258–267.

Brown, J. B., Ya, H., Bronson, R. T., Dikkes, P., and Greenberg, M. E. (1996) A defect in nurturing in mice lacking the immediate early gene *fosB*. *Cell* 86: 1–20.

Brown, R. E., Murdoch, T., Murphy, P. R., and Moger, W. H. (1995) Hormonal responses of male gerbils to stimuli from their mate and pups. *Horm. Behav.* 29: 474–491.

Buntin, J. D. (1996) Neural and Hormonal Control of Parental Behavior in Birds. In J. S. Rosenblatt and C. T. Snowdon (Eds.), *Parental Care: Evolution, Mechanisms, and Adaptive Significance*, vol. 25. San Diego: Academic Press, pp. 161–213.

Buntin, J. D., Becker, G. M., and Ruzycki, E. (1991) Facilitation of parental behavior in ring doves by systemic or intracranial injections of prolactin. *Horm. Behav.* 25: 424–444.

Caldwell, J. P. (1997) Pair bonding in spotted poison frogs. *Science* 385: 211.

Chen, M. F., and Silver, R. (1975) Estrogen-progesterone regulation of nest building behavior in ovariectomized ring doves. *J. Comp. Physiol. Psychol.* 88: 256–263.

Chiu, S., and Wise, P. M. (1994) Prolactin receptor mRNA localization in the hypothalamus by in situ hybridization. *J. Neuroendocrinol.* 6: 191–199.

Corodimas, K. P., Rosenblatt, J. S., and Morrell, J. I. (1992) The habenular complex mediates hormonal stimulation of maternal behavior in rats. *Behav. Neurosci.* 106: 853–865.

DaCosta, A. P. C., Guevara-Guzman, R. G., Ohkura, S., Goode, J. A., and Kendrick, K. M. (1996) The role of oxytocin release in the paraventricular nucleus in the control of maternal behaviour in the sheep. *J. Neuroendocrinol.* 8: 163–177.

Dixson, A. F., and George, L. (1982) Prolactin and parental behaviour in a male New World primate. *Nature* 299: 551–553.

Dufty, A. M., Jr., Goldsmith, A. R., and Wingfield, J. C. (1987) Prolactin secretion in a brood parasite: The brown headed cowbird, *Molothrus ater*. *J. Zool. (Lond.)* 212: 669–675.

Factor, E. M., Mayer, A. D., and Rosenblatt, J. S. (1993) Peripenducular nucleus lesions in the rat: I. Effects on maternal aggression, lactation, and maternal behavior during pre- and postpartum periods. *Behav. Neurosci.* 107: 166–185.

Fahrbach, S. E., and Pfaff, D. W. (1986) Effect of preoptic region implants of dilute estradiol on the maternal behavior of ovariectomized, nulliparous rats. *Horm. Behav.* 20: 354–363.

Fleming, A. (1990) Hormonal and experiential correlates of maternal responsiveness in human mothers. In N. A. Krasnegor and R. S. Bridges (Eds.), *Mammalian Parenting*. Oxford: Oxford Press, pp. 184–208.

Fleming, A., Vaccarino, F., Tambosso, L., and Chee, P. (1979) Vomeronasal and olfactory system modulation of maternal behavior in the rat. *Science* 203: 372–374.

Fleming, A. S., Ruble, D. N., Krieger, H., and Wong, P. (1997) Hormonal and experiential correlates of maternal responsiveness during pregnancy and the puerperium in human mothers. *Horm. Behav.* 31: 145–158.

Fleming, A. S., Steiner, M., and Corter, C. (1997) Cortisol, hedonics, and maternal responsiveness in human mothers. *Horm. Behav.* 32: 85–98.

Francis, C. M., Anthony, E. L. P., Brunton, J. A., and Kunz, T. H. (1994) Lactation in male fruit bats. *Nature* 367: 691–692.

Francis, D., Diorio, J., Liu, D., and Meaney, M. J. (1999) Nongenomic transmission across generations of maternal behavior and stress responses in the rat. *Science* 286: 1155–1158.

Gans, C. (1996) An overview of parental care among the reptilia. *Adv. Stud. Behav.* 25: 145–157.

Giordano, A., Johnson, A., and Rosenblatt, J. (1990) Haloperidol-induced disruption of retrieval behavior and reversal with apomorphine in lactating rats. *Physiol. Behav.* 48: 211–214.

Giordano, A. L., Ahdieh, H. B., Mayer, A. D., Siegel, H. I., and Rosenblatt, J. S. (1990) Cytosol and nuclear estrogen receptor binding in the preoptic area and hypothalamus of female rats during pregnancy and ovariectomized rats after steroid priming correlation with maternal behavior. *Horm. Behav.* 24: 231–255.

Gubernick, D. J., and Alberts, J. R. (1985) Maternal licking by virgin and lactating rats: Water transfer from pups. *Physiology and Behavior* 34: 501–506.

Gubernick, D. J., and Alberts, J. R. (1989) Postpartum maintenance of paternal behaviour in the biparental California mouse, *Peromyscus californicus. Anim. Behav.* 37: 656–664.

Gubernick, D. J., and Nelson, R. J. (1989) Prolactin and paternal behavior in the biparental California mouse, *Peromyscus californicus. Horm. Behav.* 23: 203–210.

Hansen, S., Bergvall, A. H., and Nyiredi, S. (1993) Interaction with pups enhances dopamine release in the ventral striatum of maternal rats: A microdialysis study. *Pharmacol. Biochem. Behav.* 45: 673–676.

Hanson, S., Harthon, C., Wallin, E., Lofberg, L., and Svensson, K. (1991) Mesotelencephalic dopamine system and reproductive behavior in the female rat: Effects of ventral tegmental 6-hydroxydopamine lesions on maternal and sexual responsiveness. *Behav. Neurosci.* 105: 588–598.

Insel, T. R. (1990) Regional changes in brain oxytocin receptor post-partum: Time-course and relationship to maternal behavior. *J. Neuroendocrinol.* 2: 539–545.

Insel, T. R., and Harbaugh, C. R. (1989) Lesions of the hypothalamic paraventricular nucleus disrupt the initiation of maternal behavior. *Physiol. Behav.* 45: 1033–1041.

Johns, J. M., Noonan, L. R., Zimmerman, L. I., Li, L., and Pedersen, C. A. (1994) Effects of chronic and acute cocaine treatment on the onset of maternal behavior and aggression in Sprague-Dawley rats. *Behav. Neurosci.* 108: 107–112.

Johnson, A. E., Coirini, H., Insel, T. R., and McEwen, B. S. (1991) The regulation of oxytocin receptor binding in the ventromedial hypothalamic nucleus by testosterone and its metabolites. *Endocrinology* 128: 891–896.

Jones, J. S., and Wynne-Edwards, K. E. (1999) Midwifery by males in a naturally biparental hamster. *Soc. Behav. Neuroendocrinol. Abst.*

Kendrick, K. M., Costa, A. P. C. D., Broad, K. D., Ohkura, S., Guevara, R., Levy, F., and Keverne, E. B. (1997) Neural control of maternal behavior and olfactory recognition of offspring. *Brain Res. Bull.* 44: 383–395.

Kendrick, K. M., Keverne, E. B., Chapman, C., and Baldwin, B. A. (1988) Microdialysis measurement of oxytocin, aspartate, gamma-aminobutyric acid and glutamate release from the olfactory bulb of the sheep during vaginocervical stimulation. *Brain Res.* 442: 171–174.

Keverne, E. B. (1988) Central mechanisms underlying the neural and neuroendocrine determinants of maternal behaviour. *Psychoneuroendocrinology* 13: 127–141.

Keverne, E. B., Levy, F., Poindron, P., and Lindsay, D. R. (1983) Vaginal stimulation: An important determinant of maternal bonding in sheep. *Science* 219: 81–83.

Kinsley, C. H., Madonia, L., et al. (1999) Motherhood improves learning and memory. *Nature* 402: 137.

Kleiman, D. G., and Malcolm, J. R. (1981) The evolution of male parental investment in mammals. In D. J. Gubernick and P. H. Klopfer (Eds.), *Parental Care in Mammals*. New York: Plenum Press, pp. 347–387.

Koob, G. F., and Moal, M. L. (1997) Drug abuse: Hedonic homeostatic dysregulation. *Science* 278: 52–58.

Leengoed, E. V., Kerker, E., and Swanson, H. H. (1987) Inhibition of postpartum maternal behaviour in the rat by injecting an oxytocin antagonist into the cerebral ventricles. *J. Endocrinol.* 112: 275–282.

Lefebvre, D. L., Giad, A., Bennet, H., Lariviere, R., and Zingg, H. H. (1992) Oxytocin gene expression in the uterus. *Science* 1553–1555.

Lefebvre, L., Viville, S., Barton, S. C., Ishino, F., Keverne, E. B., and Surani, M. A. (1998) Abnormal maternal behaviour and growth retardation associated with loss of the imprinted gene Mest. *Nature Gen.* 20: 163–169.

Lehrman, D. S. (1961) Hormonal regulation of parental behavior in birds and infrahuman mammals. In W. C. Young (Ed.), *Sex and Internal Secretions.* Baltimore: Williams and Wilkins, pp. 1268–1382.

Levy, F., Kendrick, K. M., Keverne, E. B., Porter, R. H., and Romeyer, A. (1996) Physiological, sensory, and experiential factors of parental care in sheep. In J. S. Rosenblatt and C. T. Snowdon (Eds.), *Parental Care: Evolution, Mechanisms, and Adaptive Significance.* San Diego: Academic Press, pp. 385–416.

Li, L., Keverne, E., Aparicio, S., Ishino, F., Barton, S., and Surani, M. (1999) Regulation of maternal behavior and offspring growth by paternally expressed Peg 3. *Science* 284: 330–333.

Lonstein, J. S., Simmons, D. A., and Stern, J. M. (1998) Functions of the caudal periaqueductal gray in lactating rats: Kyphosis, lordosis, maternal aggression, and fearfulness. *Behav. Neurosci.* 112: 1502–1518.

Lucas, B. K., Ormandy, C. J., Binart, N., Bridges, R. S., and Kelly, P. A. (1998) Null mutation of the prolactin receptor gene produces a defect in maternal behavior. *Endocrinology* 139: 4102–4107.

Maestripieri, D., and Zehr, J. (1998) Maternal responsiveness increases during pregnancy and after estrogen treatment in macaques. *Horm. Behav.* 34: 223–230.

Moltz, H., Lubin, M., Leon, M., and Numan, M. (1970) Hormonal induction of maternal behavior in the ovariectomized nulliparous rat. *Physiol. Behav.* 5: 1373.

Montagu, A. (1971) *Touching: The Human Significance of Skin.* New York: Columbia University Press.

Moore, C. L., and Morelli, G. A. (1979) Mother rats interact differently with male and female offspring. *J. Comp. Physiol. Psychol.* 93: 677–684.

Morgan, H. D., Fleming, A. S., and Stern, J. M. (1992) Somatosensory control of the onset and retention of maternal responsiveness inprimiparous Spague-Dawley rats. *Physiol Behav.* 251: 549–556.

Nishimori, K., Young, L., Guo, Q., Wang, Z., Insel, T., and Matzuk, M. (1996) Oxytocin is required for nursing but is not essential for parturition or reproductive behavior. *Proc. Natl. Acad. Sci. USA* 93: 777–783.

Numan, M. (1994) Maternal behavior. In E. Knobil and J. D. Neill (Eds.), *Physiology of Reproduction.* New York: Raven Press, pp. 221–302.

Numan, M., Roach, J. K., Cerro, M. C. R. D., Guillamon, A., Segovia, S., Sheehan, T. P., and Numan, M. J. (1999) Expression of intracellular progesterone receptors in rat brain during different reproductive states, and involvement in maternal behavior. *Brain Res.* 830: 358–371.

Numan, M., and Sheehan, T. P. (1997) Neuroanatomical circuitry for mammalian maternal behavior. *Ann. N.Y. Acad. Sci.* 807: 101–125.

Ogawa, S., Eng, V., Taylor, J., Lubahn, D. B., Korach, K. S., and Pfaff, D. W. (1998) Roles of estrogen receptor—a gene expression in reproduction-related behaviors in female mice. *Endocrinology* 139: 5070–5081.

Paul, S. M., and Purdy, R. H. (1992) Neuroactive steroids. *FASEB J.* 6: 2311–2322.

Pedersen, C. A., Caldwell, J. D., Fort, S. A., and Prange, A. J. (1985) Oxytocin antiserum delays onset of ovarian steroid-induced maternal behaviour. *Neuropeptides* 6: 175–182.

Pedersen, C. A., Caldwell, J. D., Walker, C., Ayers, G., and Mason, G. A. (1994) Oxytocin activates the postpartum onset of rat maternal behavior in the ventral tegmental and medial preoptic area. *Behav. Neurosci.* 108: 1163–1171.

Pedersen, C. A., and Prange, A. J. (1979) Induction of maternal behavior in virgin rats after intracerebroventricular administration of oxytocin. *Proc. Natl. Acad. Sci. USA* 76: 6661–6665.

Pi, X. J., and Grattan, D. R. (1999) Increased prolactin receptor immunoreactivity in the hypothalamus of lactating rats. *J. Neuroendocrinol.* 11: 693–705.

Poindron, P., Levy, F., and Krehbiel, D. (1988) Genital, olfacotry, and endocrine interactions in the development of maternal behaviour in the parturient ewe. *Psychoneuroendocrinology* 13: 99–125.

Pryce, C. R. (1996) Socialization, hormones, and the regulation of maternal behavior in nonhuman simian primates. In J. S. Rosenblatt and C. T. Snowdon (Eds.), *Parental Care: Evolution, Mechanisms, and Adaptive Significance.* San Diego: Academic Press, pp. 423–465.

Reburn, C. J., and Wynne-Edwards, K. E. (1999) Hormonal changes in males of a naturally biparental and a uniparental mammal. *Horm. Behav.* 35: 163–176.

Riddle, O., Bates, R. W., and Lahr, E. L. (1935) Prolactin induces induces broodiness in fowl. *Am. J. Physiol.* 111: 352–360.

Rosenblatt, J. S. (1967) Nonhormonal basis of maternal behavior in the rat. *Science* 156: 1512–1514.

Rosenblatt, J. S. (1993) Hormone-behavior relations in the regulation of parental care. In J. B. Becker, S. M. Breedlove, and D. Crews (Eds.), *Behavioral Endocrinology.* Cambridge, Mass.: MIT Press, pp. 219–260.

Rosenblatt, J. S., and Siegel, H. I. (1975) Hysterectomy-induced maternal behavior during pregnancy in the rat. *J. Comp. Physiol. Psychol.* 89: 685–700.

Rosenblatt, J. S., Siegel, H. I., and Mayer, A. D. (1979) Progress in the study of maternal behavior in the rat: Hormonal, nonhormonal, sensory and developmental aspects. *Adv. Stud. Behav.* 10: 225–311.

Rosenblatt, J. S., and Snowdon, C. T. (1996) *Parental Care: Evolution, Mechanisms, and Adaptive Significance.* San Diego: Academic Press.

Sharman, G. B. (1970) Reproductive physiology of marsupials. *Science* 167: 1221–1228.

Slawski, B. A., and Buntin, J. D. (1995) Preoptic area lesions disrupt prolactin-induced parental and feeding behavior in ring doves. *Horm. Behav.* 29: 248–266.

Stern, J. M. (1996) Somatosensation and maternal care in norway rats. *Adv. Stud. Behav.* 25: 243–294.

Sugiyama, T., Minoura, H., Toyoda, N., Sakaguchi, K., Tanaka, M., Sudo, S., and Nakashima, K. (1996) Pup contact induces the expression of long form prolactin receptor mRNA in the brain of female rats: Effects of ovariectomy and hypophysectomy on receptor gene expression. *J. Endocrinol.* 149: 335–340.

Terkel, J., and Rosenblatt, J. S. (1972) Humoral factors underlying maternal behavior at parturition: Cross transfusion between freely moving rats. *J. Comp. Physiol. Psychol.* 80: 365–371.

Thomas, S. A., and Palmiter, R. D. (1997) Impaired maternal behavior in mice lacking norepinephrine and epinephrine. *Cell* 91: 583–592.

Trumbo, S. T. (1996) Parental care in invertebrates. *Adv. Stud. Behav.* 25: 3–51.

VanTol, H. H. M., Bolwerk, E. L. M., Liu, B., and Burbach, J. P. H. (1988) Oxytocin and vasopressin gene expression in hypothalamo-neurohypophyseal system of the rat during the estrous cycle, pregnancy, and lactation. *Endocrinology* 122: 945–951.

Wambolt, M. Z., Gelhard, R., and Insel, T. R. (1988) Gender differences in caring for infant *Cebuella Pygmaea*: The role of infant age and relatedness. *Dev. Psychobiol.* 96: 87–202.

Wang, Z., Ferris, C. F., and DeVries, G. J. (1994) Role of septal vasopressin innervation in paternal behavior in prairie voles (*Microtus ochrogaster*) *Proc. Natl. Acad. Sci. USA* 91: 400–404.

Wang, Z., Smith, W., Major, D. E., and DeVries, G. J. (1994) Sex and species differences in the effects of cohabitation on vasopressin messenger RNA expression in the bed nucleus and stria terminalis in prairie voles (Microtus orchogaster) and meadow voles *(Microtus pennsylvanicus).* *Brain Res.* 650: 212–218.

Wang, Z., Young, L. J., DeVries, G., and Insel, T. R. (1998) Voles and vasopressin: A review of molecular cellular, and behavioral studies of pair bonding and paternal behaviors. *Prog. Brain Res.* 119: 483–499.

West, M. J., King, A. P., and Duff, M. A. (1990) Communicating about communicating: When innate is not enough. *Devel. Psychobiol.* 23: 585–598.

Wiesner, B. P., and Sheard, N. M. (1933) *Maternal Behavior in Rats.* London: Oliver and Boyd.

Wilson, E. O. (1971) *The Insect Societies.* Cambridge, Mass.: Harvard Univeristy Press.

Xerri, C., Stern, J. M., and Merzenich, M. M. (1994) Alterations of the cortical representation of the rat ventrum induced by nursing behavior. *J. Neurosci.* 14: 1710–1721.

Young, L. J., Muns, S., Wang, Z., and Insel, T. R. (1997) Changes in oxytocin receptor mRNA in the rat brain during pregnancy and the effects of estrogen and interleukin-6. *J. Neuroendocrinol.* 9: 859–865.

Yu, G.-Z., Kaba, H., Okutani, F., Takahashi, S., and Higuchi, T. (1996a) The olfactory bulb: A critical site of action for oxytocin in the induction of maternal behaviour in the rat. *Neuroscience* 72: 1083–1088.

Yu, G.-Z., Kaba, H., Okutani, F., Takahashi, S., Higuchi, T., and Seto, K. (1996b) The action of oxytocin originating in the hypothalamic paraventricular nucleus on the mitral and granule cells in the rat main olfactory bulb. *Neuroscience* 72: 1073–1082.

III Hormones and Regulatory Functions

We now explore how regulatory functions are affected by hormones. Some of these functions are still closely linked to reproduction, and thus perhaps the importance of gonadal, hypothalamic, and pituitary hormones in such behaviors is to be expected.

This section begins with a topic that is new to the second edition of *Behavioral Endocrinology*: psychoneuroimmunology. Chapter 10 describes research from this exciting new field of investigation. We will see that psychoneuroimmunology is important for behavioral endocrinology because the immune system can affect brain and behavior through activation of the endocrine system. Stress and the release of the stress hormones are powerful influences on the immune system, and chapter 11 continues the discussion of stress. Variables such as experience, personality, and social rank within a dominance hierarchy, however, seem to affect how an animal reacts to stressful events.

Chapter 11 also explores the beneficial short-term effects of hormones released during stress and the dire consequences caused by these same hormones when they are released chronically. The interactions among the immune system, endocrine systems, and the nervous system are explored further in this chapter. We conclude this section with an introduction to the field of biological rhythms. As you may have noticed already, when it comes to hormones and behavior, timing is everything. Without our intrinsic biological clocks to coordinate internal events with each other and with the world in which we live, we would all be in trouble.

10 Neuroendocrine and Behavioral Influences on the Immune System

Christopher L. Coe

While the first edition of Behavioral Endocrinology *did not have a chapter on immunity 10 years ago, today we are very much aware of the extensive and important interactions between neuroendocrine and immune responses. Many lines of research have converged to establish a new field known as psychoneuroimmunology, or as the study of neuroimmunomodulation. The initial goal of this field was to understand how the brain and behavior could affect immune responses and thereby influence our susceptibility to disease. But, as you will see in this chapter, many surprising and unexpected discoveries served to expand the scope of the research. Much of it is directly relevant to behavioral endocrinology because the crosstalk between the brain and the immune system is often mediated by hormones. In addition, it turns out that many of the principles that account for the relationship between behavior and hormones also apply to understanding the basis of neuroimmune interactions.*

Introduction

Asked to justify an interest in the hormonal changes induced by environmental or behavioral events, we might reply that, of course, we know that high or low hormone levels are important because they impact so many body functions, including *even* the immune system. While hormones are certainly interesting and significant in their own right, when it comes to health issues, most people are more inclined to think that a potential change in immunity is something worth worrying about. In the following pages, we review some of the new findings that indicate that immune responses are, in fact, quite malleable and responsive to hormones. These studies are part of a field called psychoneuroimmunology (PNI), which has grown up parallel to the discipline of behavioral endocrinology (Ader 1981; Schedlowski and Tewes 1999). Moreover, many of the same principles that account for the link between the brain and endocrine activity appear to also explain the associations between behavior, the brain, and the immune system. We have come to realize that the responsiveness of white blood cells to environmental events and behavioral states is almost equal to that of hormones, a realization that has modified our traditional view that these cells, or **leukocytes** as they are also known, attend only to bacterial and viral infections.

Looking back from today's vantage point, it might seem that this sensitivity of leukocytes to behavior, neuronal activation, and hormones should have been obvious all along, but to traditional immunologists it seemed that immune functions were just too important to be significantly impacted by so many other processes. After all, wouldn't it be safer for an individual if the immune system functioned independently, protecting the host at all times, irrespective of environmental insults, social disturbances, or nutritional privation? But, as we will see, the situation may be exactly the opposite. In addition to responding to pathogens, the immune system may actually be designed to act more as a sixth sense, capable of informing the rest of the body about many aspects of both the external and the internal world (Blalock 1984).

Perhaps some of the slowness in coming to this profound realization occurred because of the complex cellular makeup of the immune system. Unlike the endocrine system, where one can readily point to the major glands, or the nervous system with its obvious anatomical architecture, the primary players in the immune system are widely dispersed throughout the body. While there are several important centers of activity, including the **thymus** and **spleen**, most of the critical functions are mediated by individual cells, which are mobile and can congregate and grow in new locations as needed (figure 10.1). In fact, at any one time, only about 2% of our leukocytes are found in the bloodstream, and even these cells are often in transit to other locations in the body, such as the lymph nodes, or maybe responding to a virus in the lungs. Major breakthroughs by immunologists over the last several decades have given us much greater insight into the functioning of this amazingly intricate system, which is comprised of more than a trillion cells. These great advances in knowledge, as well as the development of new techniques and reagents for assessing immunity, allow us to tackle the question of how the immune system interacts with other physiological systems, including the endocrine and autonomic nervous systems (ANS).

Physicians and philosophers might have been more comfortable with the ideas of PNI several hundred years ago than most members of the research community were just 20 years ago.[1] The notion of **body humors**, first developed by the early Greeks, persisted well into the nineteenth century; it reflected the belief that disease was due largely to an imbalance of the body's systems. Even in the early 1800s, prominent American doctors like Benjamin Rush continued to treat infectious outbreaks of scarlet fever by blood-letting, presumably to remove the disease-causing humors. Obviously, this practice, as well as putting leeches on patients, was not particularly effective, and when more reasoned scientific approaches demonstrated later that many diseases were actually transmitted by microorganisms, the role of the host's state in accounting for disease susceptibility tended to be de-emphasized. The development of **germ theory** by Louis Pasteur and others changed the focus of scientists toward the pathogen, just as discoveries about the specific functions of immune cells may have inadvertently contributed to the view that they acted independent of the nervous and endocrine systems. During the great influenza and tuberculosis epidemics at the start of this century, it is clear that physicians continued to be quite aware that a disease course was often mediated by the nonimmune characteristics of their patients. In addition to treat-

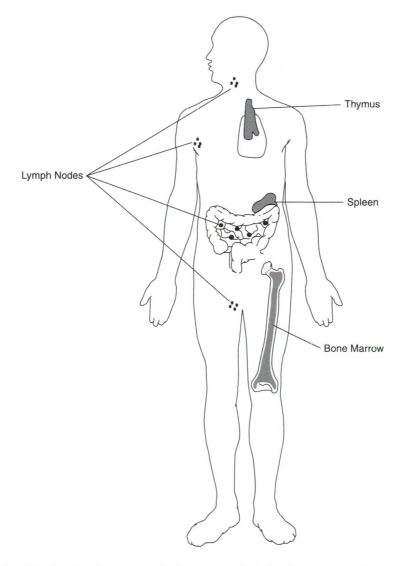

Figure 10.1 All leukocytes derive originally from stem cells in the bone marrow. Some migrate to the thymus where they become regulatory T cells. Responses to pathogens may be mounted where they are first encountered in the skin, lungs, and intestines, or in the regional lymph nodes and spleen.

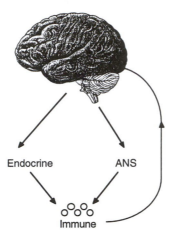

Figure 10.2 The capacity of the brain to influence the immune system via the endocrine and autonomic nervous systems (ANS) was first demonstrated in studies on stress. Later research revealed that there were also reciprocal effects of immune responses back on the central nervous system.

ing diseases and contagion through better hygiene and quarantine, these caregivers knew about the important influence of age, gender, poverty, stress, and other psychosocial factors in determining both the risk of infection and the likelihood of mortality (Dubos 1959).

Immunity and the Stress Response

But it is actually in the early writings on the topic of stress that we see the first real inklings of PNI as it is conceptualized and investigated today (figure 10.2). In a series of studies between 1900 and 1940, the American physiologist **Walter Cannon** demonstrated the important role of the sympathetic nervous system (SNS) in mediating many of the physiological changes associated with the "fight-or-flight response" (Cannon 1929). Mostly we think about this arousal response in terms of adrenaline and increased blood pressure or respiration, but there were also early reports on changes in white blood cells associated with this physiological state (Mora et al. 1926). When exposed to a fear-inducing stimulus, animals showed a transient increase in the number of leukocytes in the bloodstream, an effect we now know to be mediated primarily by one type of phagocytic cell, the **neutrophil**. Instead of remaining adhered to the walls of the blood vessels or residing in tissue, the neutrophil appears to temporarily increase in number because it becomes mobile to be better positioned to encounter and engulf an invading pathogen.

The individual who usually gets even more credit for emphasizing the significance of stress-related immune changes is **Hans Selye**. Beginning in the 1930s, this Canadian physician described the generalized physiological response commonly seen after physical trauma in both humans and animals (Selye 1936). Specifically, Selye characterized several hallmark features of the more protracted reaction to stressors, which he called the **General Adaptation Syndrome**. His three physiological criteria were: (1) endocrine activation, especially higher levels of adrenal hormones, (2) development of ulcerations in the stomach and small intestines, and (3) reduction in the size of immune glands and decreased number of immune cells. It is the latter component of the stress response that is of special interest to PNI, because Selye observed that following the initial rise in neutrophil numbers, there was a more sustained decline in other types of leukocytes in the blood, especially lower numbers of **lymphocytes** and **eosinophils**. Sophisticated assays were not available 60 years ago to test the functional consequences of this lymphocytopenia and eosinopenia, but Selye was still able to observe that the immunosuppression was so pronounced after several days that it became overtly evident by a decrease in the size of the thymus gland and lymph nodes. The technical term for this stress-related shrinkage is **thymo-lymphatic involution**. Thus, if one strictly follows the original definition of the stress response, an individual should be described as being in a stressed state only when these immune alterations occur. Following this line of reasoning, another logical prediction is that most arousing, disturbing, or traumatic events should be associated with immune changes.

With the advent of the exquisite techniques available today, that is typically what we find. The ability of cells to proliferate, to make antibody, or to attack cancerous cells is usually found to be reduced following stressful events, whether they are school- and work-related, or a consequence of negative social experiences, such as divorce (Kiecolt-Glaser et al. 1987). This may sound fairly straightforward, but understanding how and why these alterations occur requires us to delve into more complex terminology on the immune system and its functions. Moreover, to predict the magnitude of the immune changes and the possible implications for health, many subtle nuances must be considered, including the duration and intensity of the stressor.

Is Immune Suppression Adaptive?

The immune changes that occur in response to stress are actually very dynamic over time and involve many cells responding in different ways. During the immediate reaction to a stressor, it seems that immune alterations may be adaptive, such as when the neutrophils move out as a first line of defense. Accompanying this change, many lymphocytes leave the bloodstream to relocate in lymph nodes, where they could initiate the response to a foreign pathogen. Some lymphocytes also return to the bone marrow where they may stimulate the production of new cells (Cohen and Crnic 1984). However, over a period of several hours, and certainly after several days, if the stressful situation persists that long, the immune changes start to become maladaptive. The change in the number and location of one type of lymphocyte, the **natural killer cell (NK)**, nicely illustrates this bidirectional aspect of the stress response.[2] During the first 30 to 60 minutes after stress onset, we see a brief surge of NK cells into the bloodstream, but soon afterwards there is a more sustained and marked decline in the functioning of these cells, which may continue for days (Benschop et al. 1996). Because the NK cell is specialized for detecting viruses, one might hypothesize that the initial increase could be adaptive, but it is the longer-lasting decrease that is of greater concern for health. Over time the reduction in NK activity can markedly impair several important immune responses, such as the killing of virally infected and cancerous cells. Prolonged stressors also affect other immune functions, eventually reducing the ability of the neutrophil to phagocytize foreign microorganisms or the capacity of lymphocytes to make antibody against viruses.

Because this stress-induced suppression of immunity appears to increase the risk for disease, it is normally considered maladaptive, although even here one could argue that there are some overall benefits for the individual. During the sustained response to stressful and traumatic events, the body must make a cost-benefit analysis of how and where to allocate energy resources. In general, the major goal seems to be to provide more energy for brain and muscle in times of need, even at the expense of homeostatic processes, such as growth, reproduction, and immunity. Hormones, including adrenaline and cortisol, participate in effecting this shift in energy resources, and they also enable the body to make more energy available. From this metabolic point of view, the state of stress should be described as a **catabolic** one, with previously stored energy being liberated to deal with the crisis. A transient decline in immunity may be one cost of this energetic shift, because immunity normally requires protein synthesis. Later, during better times, the situation is reversed and immunity is restored, when the body is once again able to enter an energy-storing and growth mode (i.e., **anabolic state**).

For the most part, we all comfortably tolerate these transient up-and-down shifts in immunity, and that is why we typically remain healthy, despite the occurrence of many stressful events in our lives (figure 10.3). However, there are some exceptions, such as when the temporary immune suppression creates a window of opportunity for an infectious or pathogenic process to get started. One of the great challenges for PNI today is to better understand how much immune competence can decline before it really matters from a health point of view. If a certain cellular function decreases 50%, as has been found for natural killer cell activity in many studies of undergraduate and medical school students during final exam week, is there really a significant risk to health? (Kang et al. 1996) Fortunately, the research has indicated that most young adults in the prime of their lives appear to tolerate such a shift in immunity without serious concern. However, when equivalent stress-related changes occur in the elderly, who may already have weakened responses because of age-related changes in immunity, the consequences seem to be more relevant to health (Kiecolt-Glaser et al. 1995). We will return to this important point later in the chapter, when we discuss PNI within a life span perspective, but first we must review some of the fundamentals of immunology for those who have not had a class on the subject.

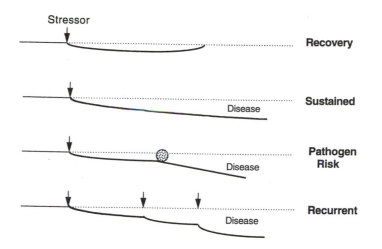

Figure 10.3 Many temporary changes in immunity can occur without disease consequence. However, sometimes a period of immune suppression creates a window of opportunity for a pathogen, especially if the immunosuppressive event is recurrent or prolonged.

What Does the Immune System Do?

We are all familiar with the symptoms of a common cold virus and the yellow pus around a cut, which provide evidence of our cellular response to a viral or bacterial infection, but there is really much more to know about the functions of the immune system. If one takes an evolutionary perspective, it is interesting to note that the precursors of immunity go all the way back to the first multicellular animals (Becker and Habicht 1996). Even in the primordial world, microorganisms needed to know when a foreign life form was invading. Thus, some of the earliest immune responses entailed making a distinction between "self" and "other," and then either engulfing the foreign invader (**phagocytosis**) or moving it to the exterior of the body cavity. A number of different types of leukocytes, including the neutrophil, the eosinophil, and the macrophage, still rely on this type of phagocytic response to protect us against bacteria and parasites (figure 10.4).

However, by the time fish appeared, over 300 million years ago, we see that more sophisticated immune cells and specialized responses had evolved, including the ability to make **antibody** (Litman 1996). In this case, one type of **lymphocyte** had acquired the ability to secrete a protein that adhered to foreign substances. Anything that elicits an antibody response is described in scientific jargon as an **antigen**, because of its *anti*body-*gen*erating capacity.[3] Antibody helps to label the antigen so that it is more readily recognized as "other" by cells of the immune system. Sometimes antibody serves to mobilize the more primitive components of the immune system (the innate immune response); alternatively, the antibody itself may directly neutralize the pathogenic capability of a virus or bacteria. In modern animals, these antibody-secreting cells are called **B lymphocytes**, because they were found to

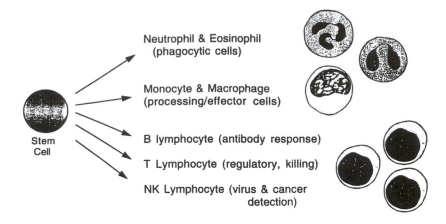

Figure 10.4   An immune response reflects the coordinated actions of many cells, including the more primitive phagocytic neutrophil and eosinophil. Lymphocytes are involved in the production of antibody and the killing of virally infected cells or cancerous tissue. Depending upon the type of pathogen or illness, different cells predominate in the mounting of the immune response.

derive from the Bursa in birds, although in mammals such cells mature in the bone marrow before moving into circulation.[4]

Cellular processes involved in other aspects of **acquired immunity** also became more refined, and this refinement included the enhanced capacity of some lymphocytes to detect if another cell was infected by a virus and, if so, to kill that transformed cell. In addition, leukocytes developed many ways to signal and recruit other cells to assist in the immune response. Such regulatory cells in modern mammals can coordinate the actions of a large number of other cells, enhancing or shutting off the response as needed. PNI researchers tend to focus on the **T lymphocytes**, which mature in the thymus, where they attain this ability to up- and down-regulate other cells (i.e., the **T helper** and **T suppressor cells**, respectively). For anyone interested in gaining a deeper understanding of PNI and immune-related disease, it is important to be conversant with this terminology and the different cell types.

Three Important Types of Immunological Disease

One other reason to know more about these various cell subsets is that each plays a different role in combating the many diseases under the jurisdiction of the immune system. An obvious first category of concern is **infectious** illness. Here the immune system serves a protective role, guarding against numerous pathogens, including viruses, bacteria, fungi, and parasitic organisms. We have recently become fully cognizant of this ongoing daily battle because of the emergence of a new disease in the 1980s that causes a profound immune suppression, making infected individuals unusually vulnerable to many pathogens simultaneously. We all know this disease as **AIDS** (acquired immunodeficiency syndrome). By now, almost everyone has become aware that this terrible disease is caused by a virus that progressively shuts down the immune system, primarily by infecting and causing the destruction of large numbers of T helper cells. AIDS has taught us one other important lesson. The increased susceptibility of immune-suppressed individuals to infections has made it clear that healthy people are also continually exposed to large numbers of pathogens. But when our immune system is functioning normally, we are assured of health, despite the presence of disease-causing microorganisms all around us. Even as you read this text, your immune system is actively at work. It is protecting you from the fungus that causes athlete's foot, the cold virus you recently inhaled into your upper respiratory tract, and also from a few old viruses that may have never actually left your body, such as the chicken pox virus that was last active when you succumbed to it as a young child.

Combating all these potential infections, as well as containing some inactive viruses in a latent state, would already seem to be a daunting task, but fortunately, many immune cells are also on duty monitoring for a second type of disease. In addition to infection, the immune system must pay attention to any cells in the body that become abnormal, especially to those that develop genetic mutations and could grow wildly into a cancerous tumor. If one thinks about **cancer** or neoplastic disease in terms of the concept of "self" and "other," then this additional surveillance role of the immune system makes sense. It can be considered one more aspect of the job of recognizing the "other" (in this case, deviant cells that should not be kept as a part of the healthy self). Here the T lymphocytes, and some other leukocytes that have cell-killing abilities, such as the NK cell and **macrophage**, play a critical role. Once a transformed cell or a small tumor is recognized, it is destroyed, often by creating a hole in the cancerous cell and causing it to burst. As one might imagine, considerable research in PNI has focused on these killer lymphocytes, because of an obvious interest in how psychological and environmental factors may affect the capacity to detect and kill cancer cells (Glaser et al. 1986). Such an influence could affect both the onset and the progression of cancer. Much excitement was generated by early PNI studies showing that the activity of the NK cell and the severity of disease in breast and skin cancer could be affected by the patient's ability to express emotions and his or her level of sociality (Levy et al. 1985; Temoshok and Fox 1984). Ongoing research today suggests that psychological interventions, including social support groups, may directly benefit certain cancer patients (Spiegel 1992).

There is a third and final category of disease that is also frequently assessed in PNI research. Although immune-related, these illnesses are quite different because they result from mistakes made by the immune system. Typically grouped together under the heading **autoimmune disease**, these conditions occur when the immune system has erroneously begun to attack healthy tissue. In some cases, these errant cells target the myelin sheath of the neuron (multiple sclerosis), the insulin-secreting cells of the pancreas (type 1 diabetes), or the tissue in the joints between bones (rheumatoid arthritis). These are a complex set of diseases but, at a general level, they too can be understood in terms of the distinction between recognizing self and other. Here the immune system appears to inappropriately designate healthy tissue as "other," and incorrectly mobilizes leukocytes to attack normal cells. These autoimmune diseases share some traits that make them of interest for PNI. For example, most seem to be extremely responsive to psychological factors, especially to stressful events, which tend to aggravate symptoms (Grant et al. 1989). Psychological effects on immunity may account for why these diseases often wane and then flare up again. In addition, many symptoms of autoimmune disorders, especially the ones involving inflammation, are also quite sensitive to hormones. As a consequence, one of the more common clinical treatments is the administration of corticosteroid drugs to inhibit the overactive and incorrect immune response. But to understand why a drug mimicking the actions of extremely high levels of cortisol could have such a beneficial and immunosuppressive effect, we need to return to the original theme of this chapter—that is, why should there be any relationship between endocrine and immune activity in the first place?

The Discovery of Neuroendocrinimmunology

At the outset, it was mentioned that the field of PNI led to some unanticipated discoveries. Although research nearly 100 years ago had indicated that certain stress-related hormones could influence immune responses, and doctors had used steroidal drugs to treat allergies and inflammation for decades, few foresaw the true extent of the interactions between the nervous, endocrine, and immune systems. To capture the excitement that ensued when these findings were first reported, we will consider them chronologically.

A number of researchers in the 1980s reported that the neural influences on immunity were much more direct than they had previously imagined. By closely analyzing the histology of the major lymphoid glands, these investigators revealed that both the thymus and the spleen were heavily innervated by the autonomic nervous system (ANS) (Bullock and Moore 1981; Felten et al. 1987). Nerves from the sympathetic and parasympathetic nervous system reached far into the tissue, where the individual neurons terminated in such close proximity to immune cells that secreted neurotransmitters could actually contact leukocytes and affect their activity. Moreover, other types of studies in animals indicated that destruction of parts of the brain or the cutting of peripheral nerves could affect immune responses, providing what appeared to be a real anatomical basis for the concept of neuroimmunity (Renoux et al. 1983).

At the same time, a growing number of reports indicated that many types of hormones were capable of influencing immune responses, other than the previously known effects of adrenaline and corticosteroid hormones. Growth hormone, thyroid hormone, and even reproductive hormones were found to be potent modulators of immune responses (Kelley ey al. 1992; Berczi 1986). These findings suggested that the brain might be able to influence immunity on a regular basis through many of the well-known neuroendocrine pathways. The hypothalamus now began to look like a common pathway through which PNI effects could be explained, especially since it is perfectly situated to regulate the release of hormones from the pituitary. In addition, via its neuronal connections to the brainstem, the hypothalamus can also affect ANS activity. With this information, it was perhaps not surprising that lesion studies in animals demonstrated that damage to the hypothalamus could affect immune responses far out in the peripheral bloodstream and spleen (Berczi and Nagy 1991).

But most of us were still unprepared for the truly seminal discoveries that revealed the extent of the overlap in the physiology of the nervous, endocrine, and immune systems. Perhaps the most provocative discoveries were the first molecular biology experiments that showed that lymphoid cells actually had the capacity to produce a number of substances previously thought to be the exclusive domain of the endocrine system (Blalock 1994). Once activated by a virus, lymphocytes were found to secrete their own hormone-like substances, including both adrenocorticotrophic hormone (ACTH) and endorphins. This secretory response proved to be due to the fact that viral infections turned on genes in lymphocytes, enabling them to make pro-opiomelanocortin (POMC), the precursor of both hormones. The story did not end there, however, and more recent studies have revealed that other endocrine products, including corticotrophin-releasing hormone (CRH), can be made by lymphocytes. Although these hormones are not produced in the same abundance as by cells found in the pituitary, it is believe that sufficient quantities are released locally in the vicinity of other nearby immune cells to affect their activity.[5] Studies of the synovial fluid in the joints of arthritic patients suggest further that this type of hormone secretion at the cellular level could aggravate the pathophysiology of the local inflammation (Chrousos 1995).

But the findings went far beyond the secretion of endocrine substances by the immune system. It appears that we may have to modify our thinking further, and maybe even our terminology, when we designate proteins as part of the immune or endocrine systems. Immune cells have long been known to release other soluble substances, including **cytokines** and **chemokines**. Typically, these were thought to be just growth factors that caused immune cells to proliferate, or specialized chemoattractants, which recruited cells to the site of an infection or inflammation. Cytokines and chemokines certainly do subserve such important functions, but they also appear to have another role that involves communication with the endocrine and nervous systems. Probably the best-studied cytokine is **interleukin-1** (IL-1), a substance secreted by both lymphocytes and macrophages, and now known to be an extremely potent stimulator of endocrine activity (Besedovsky et al. 1986). When injected into animals, small quantities of IL-1 have been found to activate hormone release maximally at all levels of the hypothalamic-pituitary-adrenal axis (HPA) (figure 10.5) (Berkenbosch et al. 1987) These observations prompted the obvious questions of why and how such stimulation could occur. Today, we know that receptors for IL-1 and many other cytokines are located on both

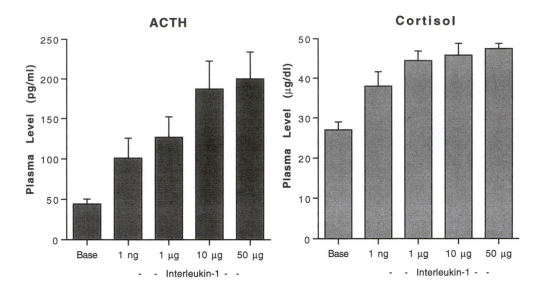

Figure 10.5 When injected into animals, proinflammatory cytokines, such as interleukin-1, cause a large increase in the release of pituitary-adrenal hormones. Here one can see increasing levels of ACTH and cortisol after different quantities of IL-1 were administered into the bloodstream of rhesus monkeys (Reyes and Coe 1996.)

neural and endocrine tissue. Moreover, the cytokines that act on these receptors do not originate only from lymphoid cells. Many of these so-called immune products are actually synthesized locally by neurons and glial cells within the nervous system, even in higher cortical regions of the brain. The field of PNI has been compelled, therefore, to broaden its scope considerably to also investigate the role of such substances in the functioning of the central nervous system (CNS). We will revisit this exciting line of inquiry later, in the discussion on **sickness behavior**, because cytokines also appear to be the critical mediators of the behavioral changes associated with illness (Dantzer et al. 1998).

Before moving on, it is probably worth pausing to summarize the discoveries made in the last two decades, which have provided us with a very different and more integrated view of the body's physiology. When discussing how environmental or psychological processes affect an immune response, we are now able to definitively trace a number of pathways from the brain to the immune system. The hypothalamus may influence immunity via changes in the secretion of pituitary hormones or through neuronal pathways to the brainstem and the nerves of the ANS. In turn, the activational state of leukocytes may be affected by hormone levels in the bloodstream or even by exposure to minute amounts of neurotransmitters, as the cells course through the major lymphoid organs. Experimental manipulation of neurotransmitter levels in the spleen has shown definitively that lymphocytes emerge in a very different state after norepinephrine has been released by the neurons of the SNS that reach into the splenic tissue.

Equally exciting findings have revealed a complementary side to the neuroimmune relationship—while the brain and the endocrine system affect immune responses, immune activation has an equivalent, reciprocal influence back on the brain. Products released by lymphocytes can alter neuronal activity, at least when leukocytes are in an activated state fighting disease. Upon reflection, such a bidirectional system of communication makes sense. If the brain is involved in the regulation and modulation of immunity, then it must also have a detection system capable of monitoring the immune system and distinguishing when such effects occur. Much of this feedback to the CNS appears to be mediated by cytokines and chemokines. It is believed that cytokines act both within the brain and indirectly by stimulating receptors along peripheral nerves. In the latter case, one of the major ways the brain monitors the immune system appears to be via the **vagus nerve**. The vagus, or 10th cranial nerve, innervates the gastrointestinal tract, lungs, and heart, and can relay information about local cytokine levels up to the brainstem, almost as if it were sending back an afferent sensory signal (Maier et al. 1998).

Examples of PNI in Everyday Life

It is one thing to demonstrate these physiological relationships in animal studies or by adding hormones to cell cultures in a test tube, but quite another to prove that they really occur in a meaningful way in humans during the course of real life events. For a variety of reasons, including the desire to show that stress could affect vulnerability to disease, the early PNI research focused largely on negative life experiences. One goal was to show that immune responses were inhibited at these times. Certainly, the most widely cited paper on this topic was the first demonstration that there is an inhibition of cellular activity during bereavement after the loss of a loved one (Bartrop et al. 1977).

Using a standard assay of the day, the investigators separated lymphocytes from the blood samples, and then stimulated them in cultures with plant proteins or **mitogens** to see how much they would proliferate. Proliferation responses were assessed by quantifying the amount of radioactive thymidine incorporated into the cells. In this pioneering study, Bastrop et al. (1977) reported that the cells from bereaved individuals were less prone to proliferate when collected during the 1 to 2 month period after the loss of a spouse. Because the diminution was found by comparing cell replication in bereaved individuals to that of hospital workers, who might not be the best control group, it was quite important for another group of investigators to repeat the study using a prospective, within-subjects design. In this case, 6 years later, men were assessed before and for 1 year after their terminally ill wives had succumbed to cancer (Schleifer et al. 1983). Again, decreases in lymphocyte proliferation were found at the 1-month time point after loss. Additional studies conducted subsequently revealed that other immune responses were also compromised. NK cell activity—measured by culturing lymphocytes in vitro in the presence of cancer cells and ascertaining the number of lysed target cells—was also reduced in bereaved individuals (Irwin et al. 1987).

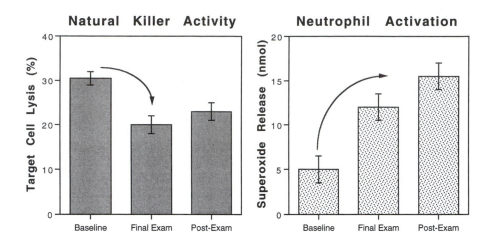

Figure 10.6 Many changes in immunity can be observed during final exam week. These graphs illustrate two of the immune changes: (1) a decrease in natural killer cell activity, as measured by the in vitro lysis of target cancer cells, and (2) an increase in the activational state of neutrophils, as revealed by the cellular release of superoxides after in vitro priming of the cells with chemical stimulators (Kang et al. 1998.)

Given that this type of personal loss is an extreme life stressor that induces both emotional sequelae and many changes in behavior, it may not be surprising that a period of immune suppression was observed. Investigators began to explore the possibility that stress-induced immune changes would also be found after other life events, and immune alterations were reported to occur after many types of negative life events, including unemployment, divorce, environmental disasters, and even in students during the weeks of school exams (Herbert et al. 1993; Ironson et al. 1997). Moreover, in addition to decreases in proliferative and killing activity, many other changes in cellular responses were demonstrated. Perhaps the most systematic studies have been conducted on students experiencing the demands of school exams because, as you know yourselves, class tests provide an easy and reliable way to induce stress at periodic intervals (figure 10.6). From this research on undergraduate, nursing school, and medical school students, we know that the responsiveness of cells to cytokine stimulation also changes during exam week and, further, that cells obtained from stressed students release different amounts and types of cytokines (Kang et al. 1997; Glaser et al. 1990). In fact, it takes about 2 weeks after final exam week for cell functions to completely return to normal.

Because the immune suppression is transient and recovery is usually assured, one obvious question is whether such alterations in students really matter. The issue of health impact requires a different approach than the measurement of cellular responses in vitro after the cells have been isolated from a blood sample. Researchers were challenged to develop creative and noninvasive strategies, because it is not ethical to purposefully infect stressed students with a virus or to implant a cancerous tumor, the way one might in an animal study. One such approach involved testing the effectiveness of a vaccine to induce protective immunity, as measured by antibody levels (Glaser et al. 1998). Medical students were vaccinated against hepatitis, which proved to be a good choice, because this vaccine must be administered repeatedly on three occasions to ensure a good antibody response in some people. It was found that emotionally distressed students required more booster shots to attain high antibody titers against hepatitis antigen, and typically needed the third rather than just the second follow-up vaccination.

This same group of investigators developed another ingenious approach for evaluating stress-induced changes in immunity in a noninvasive manner. They relied on the fact that most people have been exposed to a type of Herpes virus which permanently remains in them, even after the initial infection has resolved (Glaser et al. 1985). Their hypothesis was that stress might lead to a partial reactivation of these Herpes viruses, which are known as **latent viruses**, because they remain hidden and inactive in neurons or other cells, and reappear only periodically. One of the more common is Herpes simplex, which causes the cold sore blister when active; another is the Epstein Barr virus, which induces the disease mononucleosis when not in the latent state. During school exams and other stressful times, their studies found that there were signs of viral activation and release of viral proteins (Kiecolt-Glaser et al. 1987). This led to a renewal of the production of antibody by B cells so, paradoxically, their measure of immune suppression was an elevated titer of antibody to the specific viral proteins. Although a stress-induced *increase* in antibody may seem counter-intuitive, it is actually indicative of the failure of other cellular immune responses to maintain the virus in the latent state.

Emotions and the P in PNI

Because stressful life events are typically associated with negative emotions, there was also considerable interest in ascertaining whether anxiety and depression were involved in mediating changes in immunity. Psychiatrists, in particular, wanted to know whether similar alterations in immune status were evident in their depressed patients. Soon the literature was filled with many studies reporting that there were comparable decrements in both lymphocyte proliferation and cell-killing ability in psychiatric patients (Stein et al. 1991). Because many depressed individuals also show elevated pituitary-adrenal activity, it is tempting to speculate that the immune alterations reflect an effect of higher cortisol levels, but such a simple explanation has been difficult to prove. If anything, the evidence suggests that the immune suppression is more likely an indirect effect mediated via the SNS, or possibly by the sleep disturbances that frequently occur in depressed individuals (Irwin et al. 1992).

More progress has been made at providing mechanistic explanations within the immune system, at least with regard to attributing the functional changes to altered numbers and types of lymphocytes found in depressed patients.

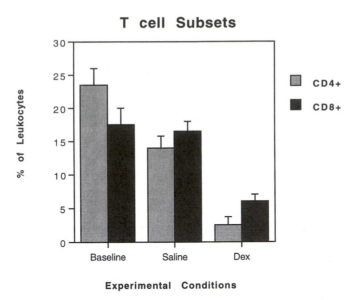

Figure 10.7 Corticosteroid drugs can suppress the immune system. Here we can see the effect on two types of T cells, CD4+ and CD8+ lymphocytes, 12 hours after an intramuscular injection of dexamethasone (Hou et al. 1996). Note that even the handling disturbance associated with injecting the control saline on a different day had some effect (compared to the number of cells found in the undisturbed baseline.)

The latter analysis usually entails marking a subject's lymphocytes with monoclonal antibodies, which adhere to proteins on the cell surface, and then counting the percentages of the labeled cell subsets on a Fluorescent Activated Cell Sorter (FACS). Typically, most PNI investigators have focused on the T helper and T suppressor cells, which are distinguished by their **CD4 and CD8** surface proteins, respectively. In a summary of the results from many studies, Herbert and Cohen (1992) concluded that the reduced proliferation responses in depressed patients appeared to be associated with a decline in the ratio of CD4 to CD8 cells. The skewed ratio is usually interpreted to mean that the inductive capacity of the T cells has been reduced relative to their suppressive activity, which is mediated by the CD8 population. Here the parallels to the effects of stress are particularly striking. As can be seen in figure 10.7, the administration of corticosteroid drugs to animals or humans can induce a decrease in lymphocyte numbers, and both cortisol and epinephrine can induce a similar shift in the ratio of CD4 to CD8 (Crary et al. 1983).

Stress Hormones and Immunity in Animal Models

For more specific information about the likely role of hormones in mediating immune changes, we need to return to animal studies, where there has been a plethora of research on the topic. Numerous experiments in rats and mice have shown that most of the traditional stress manipulations used by laboratory researchers are capable of altering immune responses. Considerable in-

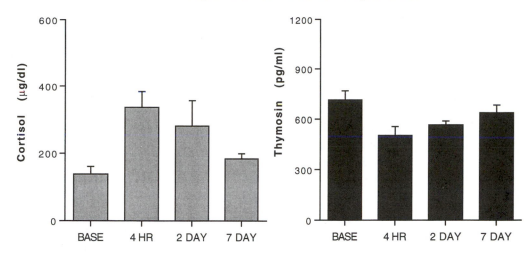

Response to Social Separation

Figure 10.8 Many stress studies in animals have indicated that immune changes coincide with the period of maximal endocrine activation. In this example, decreases in the thymic hormone, thymosin, mirrored the increases in cortisol found when juvenile monkeys were housed alone for one week away from their social group. Subsequent experiments showed, however, that the decreases in thymosin occur even if the cortisol response is blocked (Coe and Hall 1996.)

formation is available on the effects of challenges such as physical restraint and mild electric shock, as well as of social disturbances such as aggression and isolation from conspecifics (Dhabhar et al. 1995; Cunnick et al. 1990). In some cases, the role of hormones in mediating the immune alterations has been demonstrated directly by showing that the effects were ameliorated by adrenalectomy, removing the source of adrenaline or corticosterone prior to the stressor. More typically, the role of hormones has been inferred by mimicking the immune effect with an exogenous hormone treatment, or sometimes by characterizing the close association between the temporal pattern of the hormone and immune changes (figure 10.8).

For example, when mice were exposed to 3 hours of noise stress daily over a 7-week period, their lymphocyte proliferative responses were inhibited for the first 2 weeks (Monjan and Collector 1977). This reduction in cellular responses to in vitro stimulation with the mitogen concanavalin A or to lipopolysaccharide (LPS) occurred while the mice showed large corticosterone responses to the stressor. Thereafter, as they apparently adapted to the daily occurrence of noise, the elevation in adrenal activity subsided at 2 weeks and lymphocyte proliferation was no longer suppressed. In fact, by the final weeks of the study, there was actually a rebound and enhanced proliferative response.

The role of corticosterone in mediating stress-induced immunosuppression was also implicated in an experimental paradigm that assessed immunity related to cancer (Riley et al. 1981). Mice were implanted with a tumor and then stressed for 6 days by rotating their home cage on a record player turntable 10 minutes of each hour all day. While undisturbed control mice could contain the growth of the implanted lymphosarcoma over the next several weeks, the stressed mice could not. Later, in a follow-up study, other investigators showed that rotation-induced increases in corticosterone levels probably inhibited the killing ability of a T lymphocyte cell critically involved in tumor containment (Kandil and Borysenko 1988).

Not all studies have been so successful in finding the actual hormone mediator for the stress-induced immune change. While experimental stressors typically cause immune alterations in laboratory animals and most of these manipulations also affect the endocrine system, adrenal hormones are not always the exclusive or primary mediator of the immune changes. As in the example portrayed in figure 10.8, some stress-induced immune alterations cannot be prevented by inhibiting the release of adrenal hormones with drugs or blocking their actions with antagonists to the hormone receptor (Coe et al. 1996). Usually such findings are then interpreted as indicative of the multifaceted nature of the body's response, with other hormonal or immune mediators implicated in the cascading effects of stress.

Understanding the influence of hormones on immunity requires thinking about one other complex issue. Often the inhibitory effect on immune responses emerges only when the hormones reach fairly high levels. Thus, when doctors employ corticosteroid medications to reduce inflammation, they typically administer potent analogs of the natural hormone or use doses at supraphysiological levels, far above the amount that could ever be produced naturally. You can see the same effect of high doses when one adds a range of cortisol concentrations to lymphocyte cultures in vitro, the inhibition becomes most evident only when titers rise into the high stress range. For some immune responses, the levels of cortisol that occur in the undisturbed basal state may either not have an effect or may induce a moderate enhancement. We can see this type of dose-response relationship in figure 10.9, which illustrates the emergence of an inhibition of proliferation at 10^{-7} to 10^{-6} molar concentrations of cortisol, whereas normal basal levels are closer to 10^{-8} M. This perspective is important to remember when applying PNI to many topics studied by behavioral endocrinologists, where animals may be assessed in the undisturbed, not in the stressed, state.

Obviously, many hormones are secreted in unison, and thus leukocytes are bathed in a veritable soup of hormones and other substances as they circulate in the bloodstream. We are only just beginning to understand how the many different types of hormones work in concert, sometimes synergizing in their effect on an immune response, at other times antagonizing the action of another hormone.

Hormone-Immune Interactions Occur Naturally, Too

So far, our discussion has focused almost exclusively on stress-related hormones, but there are certainly other important topics to consider in a review

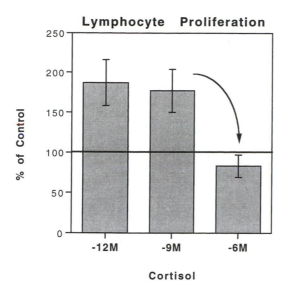

Figure 10.9 When corticosteroid hormones are added to lymphocyte cultures, there is typically an inhibition of cellular activity. However, this effect emerges primarily at doses above normal stress levels or even higher than what the body can produce naturally. In some cases, as seen in this example of proliferative responses of monkey cells to a mitogen, subphysiological levels may actually augment the immune response.

of neuroendocrine activity and PNI. Hormone influences on immunity have also been reported in animals outside the laboratory setting, where endocrine-immune interactions occur naturally without any experimental manipulations imposed by the investigators. One such example is provided by the annual variation in the physiology of seasonally breeding animals, when dramatic immune fluctuations occur in association with cyclical changes in hormones (Nelson and Demas 1996). In these species, there is often a marked shift in the size of the thymus and the spleen during the year, as well as periods of reduced cell numbers and lower lymphocyte responses. Typically, measures of immunity have been reported to be decreased during the mating season, as can be seen in figure 10.10, although the inverse pattern has sometimes been described for hibernating species, where the nadir of immune activity may be found during the dormancy stage. Understanding such seasonal changes in immunity requires an appreciation of the dual influence of both adrenal and gonadal hormones, and perhaps also the contribution of thyroid hormones.

We have not yet discussed the relationship between the pituitary-gonadal axis and the immune system. The reader is referred to review papers for more detailed information, but a few points should be highlighted here (Grossman 1985). First, the thymus gland is known to be quite responsive to gonadal hormones, and in general, thymic functions are inhibited by injections of testosterone, estrogen, and progesterone. In turn, the thymus secretes hormone-

Seasonal Changes in Antibody

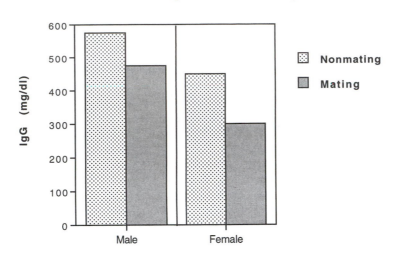

Figure 10.10   Annual changes in circulating levels of antibody (IgG) in the seasonally breeding squirrel monkey (Coe et al. 1988). Higher levels were found in the nonmating season in both males and females. In this study, the length of daylight was fairly similar. Nonmating samples were collected in November and mating season samples at the end of the breeding period in April. Males typically have higher IgG levels in this species, but that is not necessarily true for other primates.

like substances, such as **thymosin**, which have been shown to influence the release of gonadotrophins by the pituitary (Singh and Singh 1979).

Finally, we can look to variations in immune responses across the estrous and menstrual cycles in female animals to find further evidence of a relationship between reproductive physiology and immunity (Ben-Eliyahu and Shakhar 2000). It would be incorrect to say that the magnitude of the immune shift across the cycle is equivalent to that seen after stress; nevertheless, there are a few documented examples of cyclic immune changes in females that may have implications for health. For example, NK activity is known to vary across the ovarian cycle of the female rat. Thus, when cancerous cells were administered to rats at different time points, the capacity of the immune system to contain the spread of metastases was found to change in accord with the phases of the cycle (Ben-Eliyahu et al. 1996).

Anyone interested in the relationship between reproductive physiology and immunity might also want to learn more about the immune changes associated with pregnancy. Because of the placental contribution, estrogen and progesterone rise much higher than they are found in the nonpregnant state, which allows the influence of gonadal steroids on immunity to become more evident. Progesterone is known to have an inhibitory effect on certain immune responses. In fact, until it was later disproved, progesterone was once thought to be a critical mediator of several changes in immunity that were required to prevent the mother's immune system from rejecting the fetus. Other factors, including some substances produced by the fetus, have actually been shown to be more important in driving this shift in the balance of maternal immune responses during pregnancy. During the latter phase of pregnancy, some types of lymphocytes are downregulated to minimize reactions to paternal antigens on fetal cells, while a bias is simultaneously created in the mother for an enhanced humoral response, which protects her and allows beneficial antibody against viruses and bacteria to be transferred to the developing baby.[6]

Annual immune changes in seasonally breeding animals also appear to reflect a strong influence of cyclical changes in day-length. Although not easy to separate from the effects of the mating season and reproductive hormones, some immune biorhythms in animals seem to be directly driven by variation in photoperiod. Even in humans, higher numbers of cells and more robust immune responses are often found at night than during the day, when the diurnal rhythm in cortisol is tracked with a 3- to 6-hour time lag (Kronful et al. 1997). As a general conclusion, immunity in animals seems to be enhanced during the short-day/long-night season, but this depends upon whether the species is active during the diurnal or the nocturnal part of the day (e.g., humans are active during the diurnal phase, rats are active during the nocturnal phase). Within the controlled environment of the laboratory, it is relatively easy to demonstrate the potential potency of light/dark cycles by manipulating photoperiod where the standard conditions are 12h:12h, light:dark. One example dramatically illustrates this point: the size of the thymus in rats was assessed after maintaining them in either constant dark or constant light conditions for one month (Mahmoud et al. 1994). After 4 weeks in the dark, the nocturnal rat evinced over a 300% increase in thymic weight. In contrast, there was a 50% reduction in the size of the thymus during the constant light condition, as compared to standard conditions.

Although humans are not usually seen as seasonal breeders, many studies have indicated that we too exhibit annual changes in immune responses, including changes in the numbers of leukocytes circulating in the blood stream (Levi et al. 1988). You are probably very much aware of annual fluctuations in disease prevalence, especially if you happen to be reading this chapter during the flu season that occurs every winter. Some of this variation is due to climatic effects, including changes in lifestyle that affect contagion, but there are also less understood changes in our internal physiology. Even the symptoms of certain autoimmune diseases may show a seasonal pattern of exacerbation and remission. For example, epidemiological surveys indicate that autoimmune diseases like multiple sclerosis are more common in northern and southern latitude countries than in the equatorial region.

There are also some differences in immunity between the sexes. While the similarities in the immune systems of males and females are certainly much greater than the differences, it is easy to find studies reporting a wide range of subtle, and sometimes not so trivial, variations. For example, the prevalence of autoimmune diseases in humans is typically higher in women—from 3 to 8 times more frequent, depending on the disease (Solomon 1981). Often this finding is explained by suggesting that females have a more active immune system, but in truth, we really do not have a good simple explanation for this sex bias in the risk for illness. Other diseases are more common in males, including the higher prevalence of asthma in young boys, although the incidence shifts again in early adolescence, because girls are more likely stay asthmatic or to develop asthma after puberty (Mrazek et al. 1991). There is a natural temptation to explain the cause of these sex-related effects as the influence of gonadal steroids, but it is still not clear whether this action of hormones is primarily during fetal development, as the immune system is maturing, or if it reflects the ongoing influence of the hormone levels circulating in the adult. For anyone desiring to combine an interest in PNI with the field of neuroendocrinology, this is an exciting area of inquiry in need of further exploration.

PNI Is Important Across the Entire Lifespan

The preceding section raised several important points about changes in immunity over time, both with respect to the seasons and to the reproductive cycle. It alluded to the fact that different types of hormonal effects may be evident at particular stages in the lifespan. Hormones could have one influence during the maturation of the immune system in the young infant, and then another influence in the adult, which might affect the maintenance and expression of immune responses.

The study of developmental effects has been the research focus of my own group, because we have been intrigued by the possibility that PNI is especially significant at two points in the lifespan, infancy and old age. Although these two stages are obviously quite different, from an immune perspective, they have some features in common. One similarity is that immune responses are less competent in both the very young and the very old, compared to the mature adult. Moreover, in both phases, the immune system is undergoing a protracted period of developmental change. During infancy, the immune system is refining its capacity to respond to pathogens, and many cell functions are still maturing. Conversely, immune competence declines progressively in the elderly, as the body enters a normal aging process known as **immune senescence**. We have hypothesized that the immune system may be more responsive to extrinsic events during both phases, which includes being more sensitive to the actions of hormones. In the developing infant, such neuroendocrine effects could affect the set points at which certain immune responses are established. In turn, the capacity to recover from immune suppression may be impaired in the elderly, if they are already in a weaker, senescent state.

Experiments demonstrating the influence of early rearing conditions on immunity were actually among the first to stimulate an interest in PNI (Ader 1983). Separating young rats or monkeys from the mother before the normal age of weaning or altering the amount of stimulation an infant animal received was shown to influence the maturation of their immune responses and even to affect disease resistance in adulthood (figure 10.11) (Solomon et al. 1968;

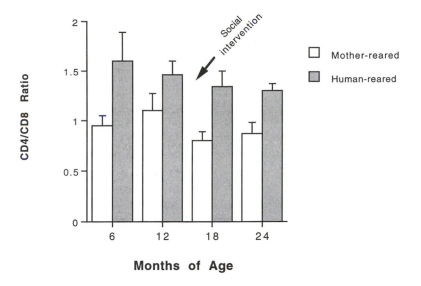

Figure 10.11   Many rearing conditions have been shown to influence the development of immunity in young animals. In this study, monkeys were raised by humans or by their biological mothers. There was a lasting effect on the ratio of CD4+ to CD8+ T lymphocytes found in circulation, even after all infants were housed with similar types of juveniles in social groups at one year of age (Lubach et al. 1995).

Coe et al. 1996). Comparable studies in children suggested that the quality and stressfulness of family life could affect the frequency and severity of bacterial and respiratory infections (Boyce et al. 1977; Meyer and Haggerty 1962). Some researchers have hypothesized further that traumatic life events in children might even influence their risk for more serious pediatric diseases, including the occurrence of leukemia or juvenile rheumatoid arthritis (Heisel 1972; Jacobs and Charles 1980).

The possibility that stress-induced immune alterations could really increase the likelihood for cancer or autoimmune disease has remained very controversial, but there is no doubt that both pregnancy and early rearing conditions can influence the development of immunity in animals (Coe 1993). While being gestated inside the gravid female, the fetus is actually quite susceptible to events experienced by the mother. In fact, the vulnerability of the immature immune system in the fetus has frequently been used as one outcome measure to show that teratogens, such as alcohol, are bad during pregnancy (Gottesfield 1990). In addition to the potential influence of nutritional factors and stressors, it is known that hormones administered to the mother can cross the placenta and affect fetal development. Because of concerns about steroidal treatments during pregnancy, many studies have examined the possible influence of dexamethasone on fetal development (Coe and Lubach 2000). At high pharmacological levels, there may be a complete regression of thymic development, but even at lower levels in the range used in obstetrical and pediatric practice, effects have been observed that may persist long after birth.

Such a sensitivity of immunity to experiential events during development makes some intuitive sense, because it has long been known that the immune system must rely on the environment for learning about pathogens. Animals raised in a germ-free condition, in the unique world of a gnotobiotic laboratory, have immune systems that appear inexperienced and understimulated compared to animals that had been exposed to pathogens in the real world. In fact, as adults they remain much more susceptible to disease. It is likely that many other factors, beyond just the level of antigenic stimulation in infancy, participate in shaping the normal development of immunity, including nutritional processes and hormone levels.

Once the set points for immune responses have become established sometime before puberty, however, we should expect to see a lessening of this sensitivity to extrinsic influence. Indeed, if we administer dexamethasone to an adult animal, the effect is transient rather than lasting: within a week or two, most immune responses have returned to normal. Similarly, if a potent immunosuppressive drug, such as cylcophosphamide, is injected in the adult rat to deplete lymphocytes, within a few weeks, the cell numbers are back to normal. This capacity to rebound to the original level has led some to hypothesize that the set point for telling the body how many cells to keep in circulation is actually determined in fetal life (Freitas and Rocha 1993). The existence of such set points would presumably help to maintain the resiliency of the adult immune system as it is buffeted by the environment and experiences the many fluctuations in physiology that we have been discussing throughout this chapter.

Nevertheless, a second period of vulnerability will inevitably reemerge later in the lifespan with the onset of the aging process (figure 10.12). In aged rodents, monkeys, and humans, there is a progressive decline in immunity associated with the process of immune senescence (Ershler et al. 1988). In elderly humans, it may be first signaled by an increased vulnerability to infectious disease, which is why many senior citizens are advised to be vaccinated against influenza. Similarly, we know that there is an increased incidence of cancer and autoimmune diseases during old age. While there are many complex processes involved in mediating these age-related changes, one of the hallmark features of old age is a decrease in the size and functioning of the thymus gland.

Some of these changes are intrinsic to the immune system, but there is also increasing evidence for a mediating role of age-related decreases in hormones. Among the obvious candidates being explored for their rejuvenating potential are growth hormone and one of the adrenal androgens, dehydroepiandrosterone (Daynes et al. 1988). Normal secretion of both hormones decreases with age, and thus investigators have been assessing whether administration of GH or DHEA to elderly individuals could mediate a partial immune restoration. The evidence is still not conclusive, but for the purposes of this chapter, such studies highlight yet another potential link between PNI and neuroendocrinology.

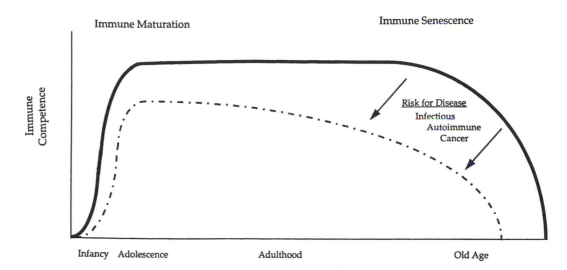

Figure 10.12 Immunity across the lifespan is characterized by a period of maturation during infancy followed by a phase of immune senescence. In old age, there is a reemergence of a vulnerability to infectious disease, and an increased risk for cancer and autoimmune disorders. However, the timing varies markedly across individuals, reflecting both intrinsic factors, such as hormones, and the extrinsic influence of environmental variables.

Here, too, the relationship between hormones and immunity will certainly prove to be reciprocal. Immunologists have long hypothesized that the thymus gland plays an important role in the aging process, and some have even speculated that it may be the site of an "aging clock." The interested reader is referred to the intriguing literature on the role of the thymus in signaling the timing of several important transitions in the lifespan, including both puberty and old age (Makindon 1978). Most of us think about puberty as an endocrine event, but immunologists have long known that the thymus changes markedly at this time, too. Removing the thymus in infancy will significantly alter the pace of aging and may even affect the age at which animals attain puberty. In a similar manner, we know that what we describe as aging at the end of the lifespan reflects the confluence of changes spanning the immune, nervous, and endocrine systems.

Can Immune Changes Occur in the Absence of Overt Hormone Changes?

Some researchers have reported evidence for behaviorally induced alterations in immunity in the absence of an overt hormonal change. Perhaps they failed to measure the right hormone, but it is also conceivable that the immune effects were driven just by the ANS or by some other neuroimmune mechanism not yet delineated. Without a doubt, in this category, the most exciting studies are concerned with the capacity to modify immunity via behavioral conditioning. Using classical or operant conditioning, it has been possible to change immune responses in both an up and a down direction, and even to modify the course of illness in animals.

Some of the most impressive conditioning results have been obtained by pairing the actions of immunosuppressive drugs with a taste or an odor (Ader and Cohen 1993). In a typical paradigm, a rat or mouse is provided with a saccharin-flavored drink, and then with an immunosuppressive drug such as cyclophosphamide. Subsequently, the animal is offered just the saccharin drink without the drug and an immune measure is assessed. In accord with the principles of classical conditioning, the previously neutral stimulus—saccharin—now induces an immunosuppressive response. While it has not yet been demonstrated that there is just one primary neural or endocrine mechanism accounting for this new learned association, the potency of the conditioned response has been definitively demonstrated in several experiments. In one of the most impressive examples, representing the saccharin-flavored drink delayed the onset of an autoimmune disease in mice genetically prone to develop such a condition at a certain age in adulthood (Ader and Cohen 1982).

Many other immune-conditioning effects have also been reported in both rodents and humans. A number were concerned with allergies, which have long been thought to be sensitive to behavioral and emotional processes. Researchers found that they could condition the release of histamine, or augment the production of inflammatory mediators, such as tryptase, by pairing allergens with a color or an odor (Russell et al. 1984; Gauci et al. 1993). The role of such relationships in normal immunity is not clear, but one can envision how these relationships could be of interest to behavioral endocrinologists studying animals. For example, rats have also been found to experience an inhibition of immune responses following re-exposure to an environment in which they had previously had negative experiences (presumably through re-eliciting the physiological correlates of the Conditioned Emotional Response) (Lysle et al. 1991). Even more relevant to events that might occur in the natural world are laboratory studies that have shown that it is possible to alter immune responses in rodents simply by exposing them to the urine of stressed animals. Presumably the fear- or anxiety-related odors in the urine elicited an arousal-related immune change in the recipient. Such studies promise many more parallels between behavioral endocrinology and PNI as these two fields continue to grow.

Induction of Hormonal Activity by Immune Responses

While it was exciting to learn that behavior and hormones can have significant influences on immunity, the extent of the reciprocal influence of immunity on neuroendocrine activity was perhaps the more unexpected finding. Physicians had long known that diseases like cancer often have secondary effects on the endocrine system. Hormones like cortisol may become quite elevated in sick patients. However, this adrenal activation was usually considered part of the nonspecific stress response first described by Selye in the 1930s. Careful scrutiny of the time course of the pituitary-adrenal response after infection in rodents has now indicated that there may be more biologic meaning to this relationship (Besedovsky et al. 1975). In fact, the pattern of the hormonal changes suggests that the endocrine activation may actually be related in a functional way to regulating the magnitude of the immune response elicited by a pathogen.

Some have hypothesized further that the increased adrenal hormones may be critically involved in containing the immune response, ensuring that it doesn't overshoot and inadvertently create its own problems for the body, such as in the out-of-control physiology of anaphylactic shock (Munck et al. 1984). Support for this viewpoint has been obtained by demonstrating enhanced immune responses in adrenalectomized animals that could not secrete corticosterone to restrain their immune responses. Although this aspect of the adrenal response seems functional and beneficial, Munck et al. (1984) have suggested that when corticosteroid levels rise too high or linger for too long, the downregulation can become excessive and result in an immunosuppression below the normal state. Here we may also find an answer to the important question of why the administration of high levels of steroidal drugs can inhibit immune responses and help in some diseases caused by inappropriate immune reactions, such as the inflammation of the airways in asthma. Physicians may be taking advantage of this normal feedback relationship between hormones and immune responses.

Some have been concerned that this explanation oversimplifies very complex hormone-immune interactions into a simple bidirectional effect, but there is no doubt about the first part of the evidence: immune activation can definitely elicit a change in the endocrine system. Research on the hormonal effects of cytokines certainly provides the strongest support. As noted earlier, one of the most potent stimulators of the HPA axis is IL-1 (Dunn 1989). Whether administered peripherally into the bloodstream or centrally within the ventricles of the brain, IL-1 can maximally drive the release of corticosteroid hormones from the adrenal gland. Not only are HPA hormones released, changes in the secretion of virtually all hormones from the anterior and posterior pituitary have been described. The pituitary-gonadal axis is also impacted, although here the actions of cytokines are typically inhibitory (Shalts et al. 1992). Not surprisingly, these pervasive neuroendocrine changes led many researchers to consider the possibility that cytokines are associated with the behavioral changes one sees during illness, perhaps explaining the fact that both animals and humans rarely show much interest in sex or in much else at this time.

Immune Stimulation of Brain and Behavioral Changes

Sick animals and humans obviously exhibit many changes in behavior beyond just a loss of libido. We all know the feeling. Even before succumbing to an illness, we experience malaise, a loss of appetite, and sleepiness. One of the more exciting areas of PNI research has been concerned with the possibility that immune activation directly causes these behavioral alterations through a coordinated effect on the CNS and endocrine activity (Hart 1988).

Such changes have been linked to the cytokines that are involved in mediating the immune response to a pathogen. One big breakthrough occurred when it was realized that cytokines involved in eliciting the fever response also had many other potent effects on the brain (Kluger 1991; Kruger and Majde 1994). Following administration of these cytokines known to have pyrogenic effects, such as IL-1 and IL-6, many brain areas became activated, in addition to the hypothalamic regions involved in temperature regulation. In the brainstem, there was a discharge from the regions involved in arousal, especially from the neurons that use norepinephrine, dopamine, and serotonin as their neurontransmitters (Dunn et al. 1989). Further up in the limbic system, especially in the hippocampus, many areas were found to have a high density of receptors for cytokines, resulting in a great sensitivity to cytokines produced locally or slowly diffusing in from peripheral circulation.

The relevance of these findings could have remained restricted to the field of neuroimmunology had it not been for the insightful realization that such an orchestrated response in the CNS probably explains the constellation of behavioral reactions in sick people. A number of researchers deserve credit for providing us with this new view of sickness behavior (Dantzer 1991; Watkins and Maier 1998; Reyes and Coe 1996). Administering pathogens or just injecting a cytokine such as IL-1 into an animal can reliably elicit this unique psychobiological state. In addition to anorexia and somnolescence, cytokine-exposed and sick animals will show a reduced interest in learning and exploration, as well as a withdrawal from social interactions. Some have suggested that this change in behavioral state is an adaptive response, which enables the organism to focus its resources on fighting the pathogen (Hart 1988). In addition, it may facilitate the re-allocation of the energy resources required to mobilize a fever response, even to the point of reducing the energy expenditure needed for obtaining food. Whether such an adaptive strategy has really been selected for in the course of evolution is still open to debate, but the syndrome of sickness behavior certainly provides one dramatic example of how a PNI discovery can be relevant to those interested in behavioral endocrinology. Here it is also interesting to note that these new observations harken all the way back to Selye's original discovery of the stress response. Some of his earliest experimental manipulations involved stimulating a stress response by causing disease—by transplanting organs and evoking an immune rejection of the tissue in the recipient—long before his ideas were applied to understanding the neuroendocrinology of psychological disturbance.

Summary

The Future of PNI and Implications for Behavioral Endocrinology

As we have seen in this chapter, the field of PNI has certainly fulfilled its initial promise to demonstrate that behavioral and neuroendocrine processes can influence immune responses. Moreover, the prodigious efforts of numerous investigators in this research area have yielded many findings with important implications for other disciplines, including behavioral endocrinology. Much of the early research in PNI was dedicated to understanding how stress-related physiology could impact the immune system. Because of this interest and a concern about the effects of negative life events, the studies naturally focused on the SNS, especially on hormones secreted by the HPA axis. Both systems were found to have potent effects on immune responses, which now makes sense because both adrenaline and corticosteroids are frequently used in clinical practice for the treatment of certain types of immunological disease. Physicians frequently take advantage of the anti-inflammatory properties of these hormones, as in the treatment of asthma. At very high doses, corticosteroids have also been routinely employed to suppress the rejection of organ transplants by inhibiting the immune cells involved in the graft-versus-host reaction. In both instances, the drugs are mimicking the normal influence of the endocrine system on immunity, but in an exaggerated manner far beyond what occurs when hormones are secreted at lower physiological levels.

Along with describing the immunomodulatory potential of stress-related hormones, we have discussed the growing literature that indicates that many other hormones can also influence immunity.

1. Growth hormone and thyroid hormone have been shown to have important immune effects (McCruden and Stimson 1991; Ansar Ahmed et al. 1985).
2. Gonadal steroids can affect immune responses. However, the actions of gonadal hormones are probably more critical at certain stages of development, for example, for establishing sex-specific biases in immunity. These developmental influences may explain the differential risk for autoimmune disease in women. While it is possible to detect the continuing influence of gonadal hormones in adulthood, such as in the cyclical variation of some immune responses across the menstrual cycle, more dramatic effects of gonadal steroids are likely to be found at other times.
3. The link between gestational endocrinology and immunity is just one of many areas that needs to be explored further. Pregnancy is the one example that we discussed.
4. Additional insights about the relationship between neuroendocrine and immune processes may also be obtained by studying animals and people at times other than in healthy adulthood. When the immune system is immature during fetal life, we know that there is an important influence of hormones on the trajectory of development. The pubertal transition is also an interesting time when significant changes in the anatomy and physiology of the thymus take place.
5. Later in the lifespan, there is the process of immune senescence, when the aged host begins to experience an increased risk for infectious diseases and an impaired ability to inhibit cancerous processes. We already have convincing evidence that age-related declines in hormone levels contribute to these immune changes in the elderly. Clinical studies also suggest that supplemen-

tation of some hormones that decline with age has some immune-enhancing benefits.

As we embark on these studies, however, we must remember that from the immunologist's perspective, the physiological system in the driver's seat may actually be the immune system (Kent 1977). The thymus undergoes many developmental changes, for instance, around the puberty. Similarly, the onset of old age is often first signaled by a decline in thymic function. On this point, there is much to be learned from further investigations of the hormone-like substances released by the thymus (Hall et al. 1991). Blood-borne, soluble secretions from the thymus have already been shown to have potent effects on the reproductive axis.

At the beginning of the 1900s, great gains in knowledge were made by dividing the body into three major systems—nervous, endocrine and immune— and then dissecting each in exquisite detail. The challenge for us now at the beginning of the twenty-first century will be to put the body back together again. It is clear that there is tremendous overlap in the structure and function of the three systems at the anatomical and physiological levels. Similarly, the new findings from molecular biology indicate that there is tremendous redundancy in the chemical signals used to regulate the activity of different cells throughout the body (Lyons and Blalock 1997; Heijnen et al. 1991). In many cases, we are being challenged to develop a new terminology that appropriately reflects this overlap in the communication signals used within and across the three systems. If hormones can be made by lymphoid cells and cytokines are produced by the brain, then the lines of demarcation between the physiological systems may have to be redrawn. At one point, some wanted the field of PNI to be called neuroendocrinoimmunology, but this name was overwhelming, and deemphasized the important contribution of psychological factors. Perhaps in another 20 years, we will have formulated a new term that adequately captures the importance of endocrinology within the field of PNI.

Study Questions

1. Why does it make sense that there is crosstalk between the brain and the endocrine and immune systems?
2. Describe some of the biological pathways involved when a stressful environmental event triggers an alteration in immunity.
3. If a syndrome of "sickness behavior" really exists, why would such a state be adaptive and what processes are involved in creating it?
4. In what ways is the organization of the immune system different from the endocrine system? In what ways are these two systems similar?
5. Try to think about some immune-related diseases that have a unique relevance for each point in the life span: (i) childhood, (ii) adolescence, (iii) adulthood, and (iv) old age.

Notes

1. The view that the mind could influence the body's physiology was espoused by the famous Spanish physician Maimonides (1135–1204) when he wrote: "The physician should make every effort that all the sick and all the healthy should be most cheerful of soul at all times, and they should be relieved of the passions of the psyche that cause anxiety."

2. Some studies on this question were quite exciting, too, especially when one investigator monitored cell changes in subjects before, during, and after skydiving out of a plane. As you might imagine, this resulted in quite a strong adrenaline response, which temporarily increased NK cells in the bloodstream by driving them out of the lungs and off the walls of the blood vessels to which they had been adhered.

3. The **acquired** immune response differs from the **innate** one; it is directed more specifically at the pathogen and involves the development of a memory for the antigen's proteins. Acquired immunity comprises two components, the **humoral response** (B cell antibody response) and the **cellular response** (primarily T cell).

4. The Bursa of Fabricus is a small gland near the cloaca in birds, and is the source of B lymphocytes. In mammals, B lymphocytes derive from the bone marrow, which is the original source of all leukocytes, even for those that migrate to the thymus and mature into T lymphocytes.

5. If a cell stimulates itself with hormones in this manner, it would be described as **autocrine**, whereas actions on adjacent cells are described as a **paracrine** effect, distinct from the more distant **endocrine** influences we typically think about.

6. This shift in the predilection of the immune system to react with a humoral response (antibody response) as opposed to a cellular response is sometimes described as a **Th2** versus a **Th1** response. The latter terminology refers to the set of cytokines released by T cells, which are predominant in driving immune responses in a certain direction (IL-2 and interferon for Th1, in contrast to IL-4, IL-5, IL-6, and IL-10 for Th2 responses). Hormones such as cortisol and DHEA are known to affect the bias of T cells to show a Th1 or Th2 pattern of cytokine release.

References

Ader, R. (1981) *Psychoneuroimmunology*. New York: Academic Press.

Ader, R. (1983) Developmental psychoneuroimmunology. *Devel. Psychobiol.* 16: 251–267.

Ader, R., and Cohen, N. (1993) Psychoneuroimmunology: Conditioning and stress. *Annu. Rev. Psychol.* 44: 53–85.

Ader, R., and Cohen, N. (1982) Behaviorally conditioned immunosuppression and murine systemic lupus erythematosus. *Science* 215: 1534–1536.

Ansar Ahmed, S., Penhale, W. J., and Tatal, N. (1985) Sex hormones, immune responses and auto-immune diseases. *Am. J. Pathol.* 121: 531–551.

Bartrop, R. W., Luckhurst, E., Lazarus, L., Kiloh, L. G., and Penny, R. (1977) Depressed lymphocyte function after bereavement. *Lancet* 1: 834–836.

Beck, G. and Habicht, G. S. (1996) Immunity and the invertebrates. *Sci. Am.* 275: 60–66.

Ben-Eliyahu, S., and Shakhar, G. (2000) The impact of stress, catecholamines, and the menstrual cycle on NK activity and tumor development. From in vitro studies to biological significance. In R. Ader, D. L. Felten, and N. Cohen (Eds.), *Psychoneuroimmunology*, 3rd edition. New York: Academic Press.

Ben-Eliyahu, S., Page, G. G., Shakhar, G., and Taylor, A. N. (1996) Increased susceptibility to metastasis during proestrus/oestrus phases in rats. Possible role of oestradiol and natural killer cells. *Br. J. Cancer* 74: 1900–1907.

Benschop, R. J., Rodriguez-Feuerhahn, M., and Schedlowski, M. (1996) Catecholamine induced leuko-cytosis: Early observations, current research and future directions. *Brain Behav. Immunity* 10: 77–91.

Berczi, I. (1986) Pituitary function and immunity. Boca Raton: CRC Press.

Berczi, I., and Nagy, E. (1991) Effects of hypophysectomy on immune function. In R. Ader, D. L. Felten, and N. Cohen (Eds.), *Psychoneuroimmunology*. San Diego: Academic Press, pp. 339–376.

Berkenbosch, F., Van Oers, J., del Rey, A., Tilders, F., and Besedovsky, H. O. (1987) Corticotropin releasing factor producing neurons in the rat are activated by interleukin-1. *Science* 238: 524–526.

Besedovsky, H. O., Del Rey, A., Sorkin, E., and Dinnarello, C. A. (1986) Immunoregulatory feedback between interleukin-1 and glucocorticoid hormones. *Science* 233: 652–654.

Besedovsky, H. O., Sorkin, E., and Mueller, J. (1975) Hormonal changes during the immune response. *Proc. Soc. Exp. Biol. Med.* 150: 466–479.

Blalock, J. E. (1984) Immune system as a sensory organ. *J. Immunol.* 132: 1067–1070.

Blalock, J. E. (1994) The syntax of immune-neuroendocrine communication. Immunol. *Today* 15: 504–511.

Boyce, W. T., Jensen, E. W., Cassel, J. C., Collier, A. M., Smith, A. N., and Ramey, C. T. (1977) Influence of life events and family routines on childhood respiratory tract illness. *Pediatrics* 60: 609–615.

Bullock, K., and Moore, R. Y. (1981) Thymus gland innervation by brain stem and spinal cord in mouse and rat. *Am. J. Anat.* 162: 157–166.

Cannon, W. B. (1929) *Bodily Changes in Pain, Hunger, Fear and Rage*, 2nd edition. New York: Appleton.

Chrousos, G. P. (1995) The hypothalamic-pituitary-adrenal axis and immune-mediated inflammation. *N. Engl. J. Med.* 332: 1351–1362.

Coe, C. L. (1993) Psychosocial factors and immunity in nonhuman primates: A review. *Psychosomat. Med.* 55: 298–308.

Coe, C. L., and Hall, N. R. (1996) Psychological disturbance alters thymic and adrenal secretion in a parallel but independent manner. *Psychoneuroendocrinology* 21: 237–247.

Coe, C. L., and Lubach, G. R. (2000) Prenatal influences on neuroimmune set points in infancy. *Ann. N.Y. Acad. Sci.* 917: 468–477.

Coe, C. L., Cassayre, P. Levine, S., and Rosenberg, L. T. (1988) Effects of age, sex, and psychological disturbance on immunoglobulin levels in the squirrel monkey. *Devel. Psychobiol.* 21: 161–175.

Coe, C. L., Lubach, G. R., Karaszewski, J., and Ershler, W. B. (1996) Prenatal endocrine activation influences the postnatal development of immunity in the infant monkey. *Brain Behav. Immun.* 10: 221–234

Cohen, J. J., and Crnic, L. S. (1984) Behavior, stress, and lymphocyte recirculation. In E. L. Cooper (Ed.), *Stress, Immunity and Aging.* New York: Marcel Dekker, pp. 73–80.

Crary, B., Borysenko, M., Sutherland, D. C., Kutz, I., Borysenko, J. Z., and Benson H. (1983) Decrease in mitogen responsiveness of mononuclear cells from peripheral blood after epinephrine administration in humans. *J. Immunol.* 130: 694–697.

Cunnick J. E., Lysle, D. T, Kucinski, B. J., and Rabin, B. S. (1990) Evidence that shock-induced immune suppression is mediated by adrenal hormones and peripheral β-adrenergic receptors. *Pharmacol. Biochem. Behav.* 36: 645–651.

Dantzer, R. (1991) Stress and disease. A psychobiological perspective. *Ann. Behav. Med.* 13: 205–210.

Dantzer, R., Bluthe, R. M., Gheusi, G., Cremona, S., Laye, S., Parnet, P., and Kelley, K. W. (1998) Molecular basis of sickness behavior. *Ann. N.Y. Acad. Sci.* 856: 132–138.

Daynes, R. A., Araneo, B. A., Ershler, W. B., Maloney, C., Li, G. Z., and Ryu, S. Y. (1993) Altered regulation of IL-6 production with normal aging. *J. Immunol.* 150: 5219–5230.

Dhabhar, F. S., Miller, A. H., McEwen, B. S., and Spencer, R. L. (1995) Effects of stress on immune cell distribution. Dynamics and hormonal mechanisms. *J. Immunol.* 154: 5511–5527.

Dubos, R. (1959) *Mirage of health.* New York: Harper and Row.

Dunn, A. J., Powell, M. L., Meitin, C., and Small, P. A. (1989) Virus infection as a stressor: Influenza virus elevates plasma concentrations of corticosterone, and brain concentrations of MHPG and tryptophan. *Physiol. Behav.* 45: 591–594.

Dunn, A. J. (1989) Psychoneuroimmunology for the psychoneuroimmunologist: A review of animal studies of nervous system-immune system interactions. *Psychoneuroendocrinology* 14: 251–274.

Ershler, W. B., Coe, C. L., Gravenstein, S., Klopp, R. G., Meyer, M., and Houser, W. D. (1988) Aging and immunity in nonhuman primates. I. Effects of age and gender on cellular immune function in rhesus monkeys (*Macaca mulatta*). *Am. J. Primatol.* 15: 181–188.

Felten, D. L., Felten, S. Y., Bellinger, D. L, Carlson, S. L., Ackerman, K. D., Madden, K. S., Olschowski, J. A., and Livant, S. (1987) Noradrenergic sympathetic neural interactions with the immune system: Structure and function. *Immunol. Rev.* 100: 225–260.

Freitas, A. A., and Rocha, B. B. (1993) Lymphocyte lifespans: Homeostasis, selection, and competition. *Immunol. Today* 14: 25–34.

Gauci, M., Husband, A. J., Saxarra, H., and King, M. G. (1993) Pavlovian conditioning of nasal tryptase release in human subjects with allergic rhinitis. *Physiol. Behav.* 55: 823–82.

Glaser, R., Kennedy, S., Lafuse, W. P, Bonneau, R. H., Speicher, C., Hillhouse, J., and Kiecolt-Glaser, J. K. (1990) Psychological stress-induced modulation of interleukin 2 receptor gene expression and interleukin 2 production in peripheral blood leukocytes. *Arch. Gen. Psychiat.* 47: 707–712.

Glaser, R., Kiecolt-Glaser, J. K., Speicher, C. E., and Holliday, J. E. (1985) Stress, loneliness and changes in Herpes virus latency. *J. Behav. Med.* 8: 249–260.

Glaser, R., Kiecolt-Glaser, J. K., Malarkey, W. B., and Sheridan, J. F. (1998) The influence of psychological stress on the immune response to vaccines. *Ann. N.Y. Acad. Sci.* 840: 649–655.

Glaser, R., Rice, J., Speicher, C. E., Stout, J. C., and Kiecolt-Glaser, J. K. (1986) Stress depresses interferon production by leukocytes concomitant with a decrease in natural killer cell activity. *Behav. Neurosci.* 100: 675–678.

Gottesfield, Z. (1990) Prenatal ethanol exposure alters immune capacity and noradrenergic synaptic transmission in lymphoid organs in the adult mouse. *Neuroscience* 35: 185–194.

Grant, I., Brown, G. W., Harris, T., McDonald, W. I., Patterson, T., and Trimble, M. (1989) Severely threatening events and marked life difficulties preceding onset or exacerbation of multiple sclerosis. *J. Neurol. Neurosurgery Psychiat.* 53: 8–13.

Grossman, C. J. (1985) Interactions between the gonadal steroids and the immune system. *Science* 227: 257–261.

Hall, N. R., O'Grady, M. P., and Farah, J. M. (1991) Thymic hormones and immune function: Mediation via neuroendocrine circuits. In R. Ader, D. Felten, and N. Cohen (Eds.), *Psychoneuroimmunology*. New York: Academic Press, pp. 515–528.

Hart, B. L. (1988) Biological basis of the behavior of sick animals. *Neurosci. Biobehav. Rev.* 12: 123–137.

Heijnen, C. J., Kavelaars, A., and Ballieux, R. E. (1991) Beta-endorphin: Cytokine and neuropeptide. *Immunol. Rev.* 119: 41–63.

Heisel, J. S. (1972) Life changes as etiologic factors in juvenile rheumatoid arthritis. *J. Psychiat. Res.* 16: 411–420.

Herbert, T. B., and Cohen, S. (1992) Depression and immunity: A meta-analytic review. *Psychol. Bull.* 113: 472–486.

Herbert, T. B., and Cohen, S. (1993) Stress and immunity in humans. A meta-analytic review. *Psychosomat. Med.* 55: 364–379.

Hou, F.-Y., Coe, C. L., and Erickson, C. (1996) Psychological disturbance differentially affects CD4+ and CD8+ leukocytes in the blood and intrathecal compartments. *J. Neuroimmunol.* 68: 13–18.

Ironson, G., Wynings, C., Schneiderman, N., Baum, A, Rodriguez, M., Breenwood, D., Benight, C., Antoni, M., LaPerriere, A., Huang, H.-S., Klimas, N., and Fletcher, M. A. (1997) Post traumatic stress symptoms, intrusive thoughts, loss, and immune function after Hurricane Andrew. *Psychosomat. Med.* 50: 128–141.

Irwin, M., Daniels, M., Smith, T. L., Bloom, E., and Weiner, H. (1987) Impaired natural killer cell activity during bereavement. *Brain Behav. Immunity* 1: 98–104.

Irwin, M., Smith, T. L., and Gillin, J. C. (1992) Electroencephalographic sleep and natural killer cell activity in depressed patients and control subjects. *Psychosomat. Med.* 54: 10–21.

Jacobs, T. J., and Charles, E. (1980) Life events and the occurrence of cancer in children. *Psychosomat. Med.* 42: 11–24.

Kandil, O., and Borysenko, M. (1988) Stress induced decline in immune responsivity in C3H/HeJ mice. Relation to endocrine alterations and tumor growth. *Brain Behav. Immun.* 2: 32–49.

Kang, D.-H., Coe, C. L., McCarthy, D. O., and Ershler, W. B. (1996) Academic exams significantly impact immune responses, but not lung function in healthy and well-managed asthmatic adolescents. *Brain Behav. Immun.* 10: 164–181.

Kang, D.-H., Coe, C. L., McCarthy, D. O., Jarjour, N. N., Kelly, E. A., Rodriguez, R. R., and Busse, W. B. (1997) Cytokine profiles of simulated blood lymphocytes in asthmatic and healthy adolescents across the school year. *J. Interferon Cytokine Res.* 17: 481–487.

Kelley, K. W., Arkins, S., and Lin, Y. M. (1992) Growth hormone, prolactin, and insulin-like growth factors: New jobs for old players. *Brain Behav. Immun.* 6: 317–326.

Kent, S. (1977) Can normal aging be explained by immunologic theory. *Geriatrics* 32: 111–121.

Kiecolt-Glaser, J. K., Fisher, L., Ogrocki, P., Stout, J. C., Speicher, C. E., and Glaser, R. (1987) Marital quality, marital disruption, and immune function. *Psychosomat. Med.* 48: 13–34.

Kiecolt-Glaser, J. K., Glaser, R., Dyer, C., Suttleworth, E., Ogrocki, P., and Speicher, C. E. (1987) Chronic stress and immunity in family caregivers of Alzheimer's disease victims. *Psychosomat. Med.* 49: 523–535.

Kiecolt-Glaser, J. K., Marucha, P. T., Malarkey, W. B., Mercado, A. M., and Glaser, R. (1995) Slowing of wound healing by psychological stress. *Lancet* 346: 1194–1196.

Kluger, M. J. (1991) Fever: Role of pyrogens and cryogens. *Physiol. Rev.* 71: 93–127.

Kronful, Z., Madhavan, N., Zhang, K., Hill, E. F., and Brown, M. B. (1997) Circadian immune measures in healthy volunteers: Relationship to hypothalamic-pituitary adrenal axis hormones and sympathetic neurotransmitters. *Psychosomat. Med.* 59: 42–50.

Kruger, J. M., and Majde, J. A. (1994) Microbial products and cytokines in sleep and fever regulation. *Critical Rev. Immunol.* 14: 355–379.

Levi, F., Canon, C., Touilou, Y. (1988) Seasonal modulation of the circadian time structure of circulating T and natural killer lymphocyte subsets from healthy subjects. *J. Clin. Invest.* 81: 407–413.

Levy, S., Herberman, R., Maluish, A., Schlien, B., and Lippman, M. (1985) Prognostic risk assessment in primary breast cancer by behavioral and immunological parameters. *Health Psychol.* 4: 99–113.

Litman, G. W. (1996) Sharks and the origins of vertebrate immunity. *Sci. Am.* 275: 67–71.

Lubach, G. R., Coe, C. L., and Ershler, W. B. (1995) Effects of early rearing on immune responses in infant rhesus monkeys. *Brain Behav. Immun.* 9: 31–46.

Lyons, P. D., and Blalock, J. E. (1997) Pro-opiomelanocortin gene expression and protein processing in rat mononuclear leukocytes. *J. Neuroimmunol.* 78: 47–62.

Lysle, D. T., Cunnick, J. E., and Maslonek, K. A. (1991) Pharmacological manipulation of immune alterations induced by an aversive conditioned stimulus. Evidence for a beta-adrenergic receptor-mediated Pavlovian conditioning process. *Behav. Neurosci.* 105: 443–449.

Mahmoud, I, Salman, S. S., Al-Kjateeb, A. (1994) Continuous darkness and continuous light induced structural changes in the rat thymus. *J. Anat.* 185: 143–149.

Maier, S. F., Glehler, L. E., Fleshner, M., and Watkins, L. R. (1998) The role of the vagus nerve in cytokine-to-brain communication. *Ann. N.Y. Acad. Sci.* 840: 289–301.

Makindon, T. (1978) Mechanism of senescence of immune response. *Proc. Fed. Am. Soc. Exp. Biol.* 37: 1239–1269.

McCruden, A. B., and Stimson, W. H. (1991) Sex hormones and immune function. In R. Ader, D. Felten, and N. Cohen (Eds.), *Psychoneuroimmunology*. New York: Academic Press, pp. 475–493.

Meyer, R. J., and Haggerty, R. J. (1962) Streptococcal infections in families. Factors altering individual susceptibility. *Pediatrics* 29: 539–549.

Monjan, A. A., and Collector, M. I. (1977) Stress-induced modulation of the immune response. *Science* 196: 307–308.

Mora, J. M., Amtmann, L. E., and Hoffman, S. J. (1926) Effect of mental and emotional states on the leukocyte count. *JAMA* 86: 945–946.

Mrazek, D. A., Klinnert, M. D., Mrazek, P., and Macey, T. (1991) Early asthma onset: Consideration of parenting issues. *J. Am. Acad. Child Adol. Psychiat.* 30: 277–282.

Munck, A., Guyre, P. M., and Holbrook, N. J. (1984) Physiological functions of glucocorticoids in stress and their relation to pharmacological actions. *Endocrinol. Rev.* 5: 25–44.

Nelson, R. J., and Demas, G. (1996) Seasonal changes in immune function. *Quart. Rev. Biol.* 71: 511–548.

Renoux, G., Biziere, K., Renoux, M., and Guillamin, J. M. (1983) The production of T cell inducing factors is controlled by the brain neocortex. *Scand J. Immunol.* 17: 45–50.

Reyes, T. M., and Coe, C. L. (1996) Interleukin-1β differentially affects interleukin-6 and soluble interleukin-6 receptor in the blood and central nervous system of the monkey. *J. Neuroimmunol.* 66: 135–141.

Riley, V., Fitzmaurice, M. A., and Spackman, D. H. (1981) Psychoneuroimmunologic factors in neoplasia: Studies in animals. In R. Ader (Ed.), *Psychoneuroimmunology*. New York: Academic Press, pp. 31–102.

Russell, M., Dark, K. A., Cummins, R. W. (1984) Learned histamine release. *Science* 225: 733–744.

Schedlowski, M., and Tewes, U. (1999) *Psychoneuroimmunology: An Interdisciplinary Introduction.* New York: Kluwer/Plenum Press.

Schleifer, S. J., Keller, S. E., Camerino, M., Thornton, J. C., and Stein, M. (1983) Suppression of lymphocyte stimulation following bereavement. *JAMA* 250: 374–377.

Selye, H. (1936) A syndrome produced by diverse nocuous agents. *Nature* 138: 32.

Shalts, E., Feng, Y.-J., Ferin, M., and Wardlaw, S. L. (1992) Alpha-melanocyte stimulating hormone antagonizes the neuroendocrine effects of corticotropin releasing factor and interleukin-1 alpha in the primate. *Endocrinology.* 131: 132–138.

Singh, J., and Singh, A. K. (1979) Age-related changes in human thymus. *Clin. Exp. Immunol.* 37: 507.

Solomon, G. F. (1981) Emotional and personality factors in the onset and course of autoimmune disease, particularly rheumatoid arthritis. In R. Ader (Ed.), *Psychoneuroimmunology*. New York: Academic Press. pp. 159–184.

Solomon, G. F., Levine, S., and Kraft, J. K. (1968) Early experience and immunity. *Nature* 220: 821–822.

Spiegel, D. (1992) Effects of psychosocial support on women with metastatic breast cancer. *J. Psychosoc. Oncol.* 10: 113–120.

Stein, M., Miller, A. H., and Trestman, R. L. (1991) Depression, the immune system, and health and illness. *Arch. Gen. Psychiat.* 48: 171–177.

Temoshok, L., and Fox, B. H. (1984) Coping styles and other psychological factors related to medical status and to prognosis in patients with cutaneous malignant melanoma. In B. H. Fox and B. H. Newberry (Eds.), *Impact of Psychoendocrine Systems in Cancer and Immunity.* Lewiston, N.Y.: C. J. Hogrefe, pp. 258–287.

Watkins, L. R., and Maier, S. F. (1999) Implications of immune-to-brain communication for sickness and pain. *Proc. Natl. Acad. Sci. USA* 96: 7710–7714.

11 Endocrinology of the Stress-Response

Robert M. Sapolsky

We all know that life can be difficult, but evolution has provided mechanisms to protect the body during crises. Such protection requires many different changes in many different parts of the body, and, as usual, hormones coordinate these widespread and diverse efforts. When the crisis is past, ebbing hormone levels signal the all-clear, and the body resumes other interests such as eating, body repair, and reproduction. But if the crisis persists, or if the individual's perception of crisis persists, hormones continue to drive the body to take desperate measures, sometimes with disastrous consequences. Stress and the interaction between stress and the immune system are the focus of this chapter.

What are the hormonal responses to stress and how do they normally provide help for the immediate future? What are the physiological consequences of long-term stress and why does stress seem to affect some individuals more than others?

Introduction

Ours is not an ideal world. If it were, nations would beat their swords into plowshares, there would always be enough parking spaces, and we'd always have exact change for pay phones. But it is not an ideal world, and our bodies are constantly challenged by this imperfection. We can get a serious illness or an injury. The rains may fail, locusts may swarm, and as a result we spend a season malnourished, walking miles daily to forage. We may be menaced by predators, or by the aggressiveness of members of our own species. Our hearts may be broken by loss. We are even smart enough to fear these things. In fact, we sometimes anxiously anticipate them before they happen.

Normally, our bodies are in a state of physiological balance, but so pervasive are the challenges and imperfections of the world that we have evolved an entire physiological system to buffer us from those perturbations. Stress physiology is the study of the response of our bodies to the perturbations that upset our physiological balance. Stress pathophysiology is the study of how, when we are knocked out of balance severely enough, disease emerges.

Some Definitions and Some History

It is an obligation of all stress physiologists to begin by reviewing some of the confusion of terms. The word stress was borrowed by biologists from engineers in a fairly imprecise way. Stress can mean the thing that creates an imbalance, or the response of your body to it, or both. Two terms have since been adopted to distinguish between the two. A **stressor** is anything that disrupts physiological balance. It can be a physical insult—famine, for example—or a psychological insult—the expectation of famine. The **stress-response** is the body's adaptations designed to reestablish the balance. Stress will be used informally to refer to the general state of stressors that provoke a stress-response (Mason 1975; Selye 1976).

While these terms are recent, the ideas underlying them go back millennia. Hippocrates, in 400 B.C., postulated that disease did not represent divine will but rather arose from logical antecedents. This rationalist view is the foundation of modern medicine. He emphasized that health consisted of a harmonious balance with the surrounding world, while disease arose from challenges to that balance. This notion of balance ran through the works of many subsequent investigators. For example, Claude Bernard coined the phrase "internal milieu." He emphasized that organisms have evolved to become more independent of the outside environment, and that a goal of physiological systems was to buffer the internal environment or milieu from environmental perturbations. By our century, this stability of the internal milieu was termed **homeostasis**.

Stress physiology emerged as a real discipline primarily owing to the work of Walter Cannon (1871–1945), who coined the term homeostasis, and Hans Selye (1907–1982). By the beginning of this century, it was clear that maintaining homeostasis was indeed a high priority of the body, but there was little understanding of how our bodies accomplished this balance.

Two endocrine systems dominate the stress-response. Both involve the **adrenal gland**. The core, or medulla, of the adrenal gland secretes the most famous hormone of the stress-response, adrenaline, also known as epinephrine. Cannon demonstrated the role of epinephrine in stress physiology. The outer layer of the adrenal, the cortex, secretes a class of hormones called **glucocorticoids**. Selye was the first to discover their role. Cannon and Selye also made critical contributions to the theoretical framework of stress physiology. They both emphasized the nonspecificity of the stress-response. In other words, the magnitude of a stress-response is determined by the magnitude of the imbalance, not by the direction of the homeostatic imbalance.

To give a concrete example, imagine a scenario from the savanna. A zebra is mauled by a lion. The lion has not hunted successfully in days and is near starvation. The zebra's stomach is ripped open, yet for the next few hours, it has just enough strength to evade the lion. The body of the lion, near starvation, and of the zebra, terrified and in pain, are having very similar stress-responses. Somewhat similar responses would be triggered whether someone is too hot, too cold, about to make a first terrifying parachute jump, or about to go to a first terrifying high school dance. Cannon termed this nonspecific reaction the flight or fight response because such very different situations trigger the same response; he found that various stressors trigger the secretion of epinephrine. Cannon thought that he was studying how the body successfully coped with a stressful situation. To some extent, he was right.

Selye noted that stressors also provoked glucocorticoid secretion, and he termed this nonspecific response the **general adaptation syndrome**. Both terms are basically synonymous with the stress-response. Selye frequently recounted the story of how he came to think about the nonspecificity of the stress-response. As a young scientist, he was investigating the physiological effects of a potential new hormone (which turned out not to really exist). Every day rats received injections of ovarian extracts containing this putative compound. He found that the rats developed peptic ulcers, enlarged adrenal glands, and shrunken tissues of the immune system.

His tremendous excitement collapsed when he found that the same symptoms were occurring in his control rats. Rats receiving extracts from other organs or with saline alone had the same symptoms. Clearly, the changes could not have been caused by his putative hormone. Selye intuited that the experience common to all the rats, experimentals and controls alike, was the unpleasantry of daily injections. Perhaps, he thought, he was observing the nonspecific response to unpleasantry itself. He tested this by subjecting rats to other unpleasantries—cold, heat, hemorrhage, illness, and so on. The rats showed the same changes. The stress-response appeared to be nonspecific; it did not matter what the emergency, only that there was an emergency.

Selye had initially thought that the stress-response was beneficial, as reflected in his use of the word "adaptive" as to describe the stress-response. Yet his rats were getting sick—they had peptic ulcers and their immune systems were collapsing. If the stress-response is adaptive, why were Seyle's rats getting sick? The answer was clear: Under some circumstances, the body's adaptations in the face of stressors are not perfect. The field of stress pathophysiology had been founded.

In the first half of this chapter, we will review the complex physiology of the stress-response. Which hormonal and neural systems are stimulated by stressors and which are inhibited? What physiological adaptations do these bring about and why do they make sense? Why do these adaptations fail at times and bring about a variety of diseases? In the second half of the chapter, we will consider why psychological stressors are stressful and why individuals differ in the quality of their stress-response and their vulnerability to stress-related disease.

The Neural and Endocrine Mediators of the Stress-Response

To understand how the body adapts to stressors, we must begin by cataloging the mediators of such adaptations. This is, in effect, an introduction to the actors (Reichlin 1998).

Systems Stimulated by Stressors

As noted, glucocorticoids and adrenaline (hereafter called epinephrine) are the two most critical hormones released during the stress-response (figure 11.1). Glucocorticoid secretion by the adrenal cortex is just the final step in a cascade of events that begin in the brain.

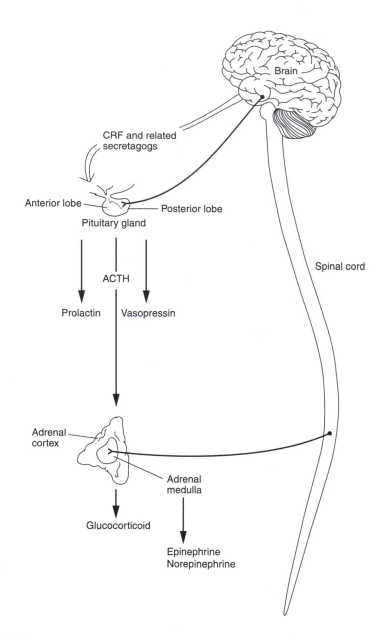

Figure 11.1 The endocrine and neural systems stimulated by stress. Stress causes the hypothalamus to release CRH and related secretagogs, which enter the hypothalamic-pituitary portal circulations. This triggers anterior pituitary release of ACTH which, in turn, stimulates glucocorticoid release from the adrenal cortex. Prolactin is also released by the anterior pituitary during stress; as with ACTH, its secretion is ultimately under complex hypothalamic control, but those hormones are deleted here for simplicity. Vasopressin is released by the posterior pituitary; in this case, hypothalamic control is neural, rather than hormonal, in that the cell bodies for the vasopressin-releasing neurons are actually located in the hypothalamus. In addition, the sympathetic nervous system is activated, releasing norepinephrine (NE) from most of its nerve endings; the sole exception is the release of epinephrine (EPI) from the sympathetic projection that terminates in the adrenal medulla. For simplicity, pancreateic release of glucagon has not been portrayed.

A stressor is perceived by the brain. The hormone corticotropin-releasing hormone (CRH) is released from the base of the brain, the hypothalamus. CRH stimulates the pituitary gland to release adrenocorticotropic hormone (ACTH), which stimulates the adrenal to release glucocorticoids. Glucocorticoids are steroid hormones, and a number of different forms occur. In humans and primates, the dominant form released is **cortisol** (also known as hydrocortisone), whereas in rodents it is **corticosterone**. During stress, there is an increase in the secretion of CRH within a few seconds, of ACTH within perhaps 15 seconds, and of glucocorticoids within a few minutes. Predictably, the picture is actually far more complicated than this. CRH, which was isolated in the 1980s after decades of work, is only one of probably a half-dozen hypothalamic hormones that modulate ACTH release from the pituitary. Recent work shows that different stressors cause different patterns of these hormones to be released by the hypothalamus.

The other main component of the stress-response is the **sympathetic nervous system**. Neural control of peripheral bodily functions is generally divided into voluntary and involuntary (or autonomic) control. The former allows you to make intentional muscle movements: You sign checks, make silly faces, tap dance, and so on. The latter mediates responses like blushing, gooseflesh, orgasms, and getting breathless. This involuntary **autonomic nervous system** has two components with opposing roles (figure 11.2). The **parasympathetic nervous system** mediates calm vegetative functions such as growth and digestion, slow heart rate, and breathing. It is typically stimulated during sleep or after a large meal. In contrast, the sympathetic nervous system is stimulated by arousal, vigilance, or an emergency. When something scares us, the sympathetic response triggers the "adrenaline" surge that we feel. Sympathetic relays originating in the spinal cord terminate in the adrenal medulla and stimulate the release of epinephrine within seconds. Other projections go to essentially every organ in the body and release the closely related hormone **norepinephrine**. Epinephrine and norepinephrine both belong to the class of compounds known as **catecholamines**. As will be seen, glucocorticoids and catecholamines together mediate most of the changes that form the stress-response.

Other hormones are typically secreted during stress as well. **Endorphin**, which is secreted by the pituitary gland, is part of a class of opiate compounds that regulate pain perception and reproductive physiology during stress. Reproductive physiology is also affected during stress by the pituitary hormone prolactin. Vasopressin (also known as antidiuretic hormone), is a posterior pituitary hormone involved in the regulation of renal function and water volume. Finally, glucagon, a pancreatic hormone, helps to regulate carbohydrate trafficking. This does not represent a complete list of the endocrine systems stimulated by stress, but these are the ones that will be referred to most frequently in this chapter. All these systems help to marshal and conserve body resources in preparation for a crisis.

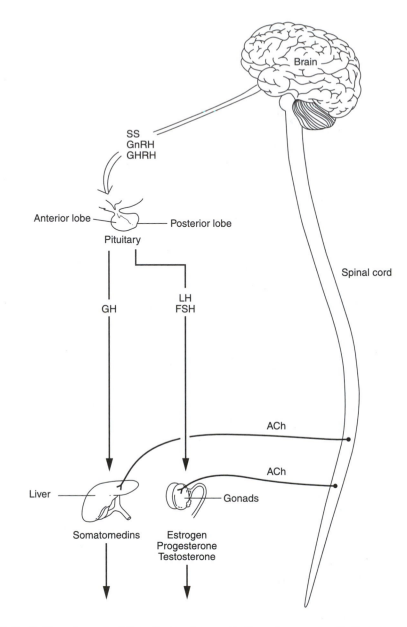

Brain

SS
GnRH
GHRH

Anterior lobe — — Posterior lobe

Pituitary

Spinal cord

GH

LH
FSH

ACh

ACh

Liver —

Gonads

Somatomedins

Estrogen
Progesterone
Testosterone

Figure 11.2 Outline of some of the effects of sympathetic and parasympathetic nervous systems on various organs and glands.

Systems Inhibited by Stressors

As noted, the sympathetic and parasympathetic branches of the autonomic nervous system usually work in opposition (figure 11.3). Thus, the parasympathetic system is inhibited promptly by stress. There is also inhibition of the numerous hormones involved in reproductive physiology and behavior. The secretion of gonadotropin-releasing hormone (GnRH), luteinizing hormone (LH), follicle-stimulating hormone (FSH), and the gonadal steroids is inhibited by stress. Finally, the secretion of insulin, the pancreatic hormone concerned with glucose storage, is typically inhibited.

A more confusing picture is seen with **growth hormone** (GH). Its secretion by the pituitary is under regulation by the brain, in that the hypothalamus secretes both **growth hormone–releasing hormone** (GHRH), which stimulates GH release, and **somatostatin**, which inhibits it. These work like an accelerator and a brake, respectively. GH, in turn, exerts many of its effects by stimulating the secretion of **somatomedins** by the liver. In rodents, the secretion of GH, and consequently of somatomedins, is promptly inhibited by stressors. In contrast, in humans, most short-term stressors stimulate GH release transiently, whereas more sustained stressors tend to inhibit release.

The Logic of the Stress-Response: What Good Is It?

It seems particularly reasonable to ask this in the context of the variety of stressors that elicit this relatively consistent set of responses. As physiologists, we are trained to understand what the body does when it is too hot and when it is too cold. Intuitively, it seems that the responses to each should be fairly different, if not opposite. Similarly, it seems that being frightened and injured (like the zebra) should be a different physiologic state from being hungry and predatory (like the lion). Why, then, should there be a whole set of physiologic changes that is elicited whether you are too hot or too cold, whether you are the zebra or the lion? Is there a logical explanation for these changes?

Much of biology has a logical structure that can be discerned. The disparate endocrine and neural changes that comprise the stress-response actually make a fair amount of sense. Such differing states as being too hot or too cold, injured or hungry, can all elicit similar responses because there is a common thread to all of them. Even though the different stressors throw the body out of homeostasis in different directions, the task of reestablishing the balance, however disrupted, is still fairly similar (Sapolsky et al. 2000; Sapolsky 1998).

First and foremost, both the zebra and the lion have an immediate need for energy. The metabolic hallmark of the stress-response is the need to mobilize energy for immediate use. Therefore energy storage is inhibited, and preexisting stores of energy are broken down into simpler, more readily utilized forms in the bloodstream. (This is the metabolic equivalent of going to the bank in a time of financial crisis and emptying your savings account in order to have cash in your pocket.) The net result is increased concentrations of

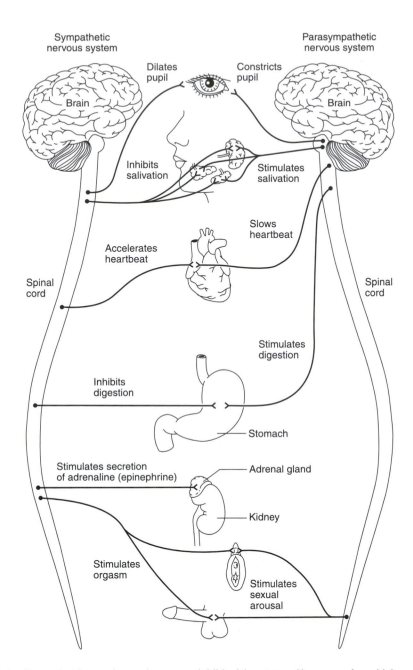

Figure 11.3 The endocrine and neural systems inhibited by stress. Hormones for which secretion is inhibited are underlined. Normally, hypothalamic GnRH stimulates the pituitary release of LH and FSH which, in turn, stimulate gonadal secretion of steroid hormones. During stress, all secretion is inhibited. Pituitary release of GH is stimulated by GHRH and inhibited by somatostatin (SS). During stress, GHRH release is inhibited, whereas there is no clear evidence that secretion of SS is changed, The result is decreased GH release and, in turn, decreased somtaomedin release. As discussed in the text, the inhibition of this growth axis is somewhat species-specific. Finally, parasympathetic nervous system activity (as represented by the release of acetylcholine [ACh]) is inhibited. For simplicity, the inhibition of pancreateic release of insulin is not included.

glucose in the bloodstream. The glucose, along with oxygen, must be delivered rapidly to the muscles that are being worked heavily in the zebra and lion. Thus, the breathing rate increases to facilitate the exchange of oxygen in the lungs. Cardiovascular tone also increases. Blood pressure and heart rate rise. Water is retained in the circulation to increase the blood volume. In addition, parts of the circulatory system are shut down to ensure that blood is preferentially shunted to the organs and muscles that need it most.

This pattern of curtailing nonessentials is seen in many other ways. If a hurricane appears to be heading for your town, this is not the afternoon to decide to paint the kitchen or to finally replant the tulip bulbs in the garden. It is an emergency, and long-term building projects can wait for tomorrow. By this logic, numerous anabolic processes are inhibited by the stress-response. For example, digestion is curtailed. While the digestive process will eventually provide the body with needed nutrients, it will not do so rapidly enough to help that lion or zebra in the coming minutes, and it is an unnecessary expense in the meantime.

By the same logic, reproductive physiology and behavior are usually inhibited by stressors. Reproduction is certainly one of the most expensive, optimistic things you can do with your body, especially if you are female, and it simply cannot be a high priority when you are sprinting for your life. Similarly, growth and tissue repair are typically inhibited. The former is dramatically the case in young, growing organisms.

Another feature of the stress-response is the suppression of inflammation and pain perception. Suppose in the initial attack on the zebra, its knee was injured. In most circumstances, the logical next step would be an inflammatory response. Capillaries dilate to allow fluid to rush into the extracellular space, leukocytes migrate into the region to scavenge damaged tissue. The knee swells and becomes painful and difficult to use. This is a way to convince the organism to rest the knee and allow it to repair. But this is a luxury that the zebra cannot afford. True, the knee joint may become even more injured if the zebra continues to use it, but the consequences will be far worse if the animal stops. Thus, inhibition of the inflammatory response makes a fair amount of sense. Pain perception can be blunted as well. For example, at the height of battle, soldiers are occasionally grievously injured and do not even notice the pain at the time. Such ''stress-induced analgesia'' has been documented in many circumstances and appears to be mediated by the release of endorphins.

Thus, when subjected to a physical stressor, it is adaptive for an organism to mobilize energy and deliver it to the parts of the body that need it, to curtail nonessential physiological processes, and to blunt pain and inflammation. As will be detailed in later sections, these are precisely the consequences of the various endocrine and neural responses.

Some investigators have begun to view these hormonal shifts not only as a way to understand how the organism initiates its response to the emergency but also how it eventually terminates the response. This could explain some puzzling features of the stress-response. For example, many metabolic consequences of the shifts in glucocorticoids, catecholamines, glucagon, growth hormone, and insulin appear to be contradictory, because opposing responses are triggered. The resolution of this puzzle is that the various hormones work at different speeds. Catecholamines, for example, produce their effects upon target tissues within seconds, whereas most of the effects of glucocorticoids or growth hormone take hours. Thus, two opposing endocrine signals may be given simultaneously, yet they may exert their effects at different times. The slower responses may not be mediators of the stress-response as much as counterregulatory signals that prepare the organism for eventually recovering from that stress-response. As we will see in some detail, considering *time course* in this way is relevant to understanding the complex effects of stress on the immune system.

The Illogic of the Stress-Response: The Emergence of Stress-Related Disease

The stress-response seems ideal for aiding the zebra or the lion in its stressful encounter. Energy is mobilized and delivered where it is needed, pain is blunted, costly anabolism is deferred until a more auspicious time. In some ways, their bodies are already gambling that the stressor will be survived and are preparing for a return to normal. From this perspective, the system seems quite adaptive. Yet, from the first day of Selye's work, it was apparent that the stress-response is not perfect; his rats had peptic ulcers and atrophied immune systems. We now know that Selye had discovered the tip of the iceberg of stress-related disease. If the stress-response is so logical and adaptive, why do such diseases emerge?

The answer lies in the sorts of disclaimers that one gets with the instructions for a new appliance: The stress-response, just like a new microwave oven, must be used properly. It is an ideal system for allowing an organism to deal with short-term physical stress, and that is exactly the sort of stressor that most organisms face most of the time. Stress-related disease appears most likely to emerge when the stress-response is activated for too long, or too frequently (i.e., chronic stressors), and when it is not activated for a physiological reason (i.e., psychological and social stressors).

Selye noted the seeming paradox that the physiological system he had discovered, so logical and adaptive under some circumstances, could cause disease. He was among the first to guess that prolonged stressors could cause disease. His explanation for the phenomenon, however, was mostly incorrect. Selye conceptualized the stress-response as coming in three stages. The first, alarm, involved noting the challenge to homeostasis, the stressor. The second, resistance, consisted of successfully dealing with the short-term physical insult. The third stage was when disease started, when the stressor went on for too long. Selye termed this stage exhaustion. In his view, at some point the capacity to mount a stress-response fails and the adrenal runs out of glucocorticoids to secrete. The sympathetic nerve endings become depleted of catecholamines, and so on. In effect, the army defending the body from the external stressor runs out of ammunition, and the stressor can now assault the body unhindered. In actuality, this scenario of exhaustion does not really occur very often. With sustained stressors, for example, the adrenal increases its capacity to secrete catecholamines by increasing the concentrations of the rate-limiting enzyme for catecholamine synthesis, **tyrosine hydroxylase**. In addition, the adrenal cortex, the zone in which glucocorticoids are synthesized, increases in size (explaining why Selye's original rats had hyperplastic—enlarged—adrenals). In some circumstances of sustained stress, the hormonal output decreases over time, but this is because the organism has become habituated to the stressor (i.e., it views the event as less stressful) rather than because it has become depleted of the hormones. This can be proved by showing that when the catecholamine response to a sustained stressor decreases, a novel stressor still elicits a large catecholamine response.

Thus, there is little evidence that sustained stressors deplete the system of the hormones it needs for the stress-response. The army does not run out of ammunition. The problem is that with sustained stress, the stress-response can eventually be as damaging as the stressor. To extend the military metaphor, if you keep spending your budget on bullets instead of on bread or education, you can ultimately destroy your country just as effectively as an invading enemy. Most features of the stress-response are damaging, inefficient, and even dangerous. Yet that zebra and that lion must activate the stress-response; it is an emergency. If the body constantly decides it is an emergency and activates the stress-response, disease eventually emerges.

It is not the stress that makes you sick. As a first qualification, stress makes you more *likely* to become sick—it is a statistical relationship, and some individuals are more prone to stress-related disease than others, a point that will be explored in detail towards the end of this chapter. As a second qualification, the statement that stress makes you more likely to become sick is more accurately stated as stress makes you more likely to get diseases that make you sick. In other words, stress interacts with the ways in which bacteria, viruses, toxins, and rogue genes make you sick—as will be seen, in many cases, what stress does is impair the body's defenses against those sources of disease.

In subsequent sections, we will review how the hormones of the stress-response bring about helpful adaptations to acute physical stressors and how the same hormones, secreted over time, endanger health.

THE METABOLIC STRESS-RESPONSE

When faced with an acute physical stressor, there are two adaptive metabolic responses. First, the body makes sure that none of the energy substrates in the bloodstream are stored away. Second, it gets access to previously stored energy and converts it back to circulating energy substrates (Goodman 1980). The first task is accomplished quite readily. In times of plenty, when there are surplus energy substrates in circulation, the body stores them in complex storage forms. Circulating fats maintained in the form of fatty acids and glycerol are stored in adipose tissue as triglycerides. Amino acids are stored throughout the body as proteins, and glucose is stored as glycogen.

The critical hormone in this storage process is insulin, which is secreted by the pancreas in response to increased circulating glucose concentrations. At fat cells, insulin promotes glucose uptake and fatty acid synthesis, and blocks the breakdown of triglycerides. All these steps promote the formation and maintenance of triglyceride stores. In muscles, insulin promotes glucose and amino acid transport and glycogen and protein synthesis, and blocks the breakdown of proteins and glycogen. Finally, in the liver, insulin promotes the formation of glycogen and blocks the breakdown of preexisting glycogen. Insulin is the prototypical hormone that signals that there is no metabolic crisis looming on the horizon.

With the onset of a stressor, insulin secretion is typically inhibited, and the storage of substrates is halted. The process of gaining access to substrates already stored is more complex, principally involving glucocorticoids, catecholamines, and glucagon. Collectively, they reverse all the effects of insulin. In fat cells, glucose uptake, protein synthesis, and fatty acid synthesis are halted. Preexisting triglycerides are broken down (lipolysis), and free fatty acids are flushed into the circulation. In muscle, the uptake of glucose and amino acids and the synthesis of glycogen and proteins are halted. Preexisting glycogen and proteins are degraded (glycogenolysis and proteolysis), and glucose and amino acids are again flushed into the circulation. This is the picture in nonexercising muscle. Things are quite different in the muscles that are working to save you from the stressor, in that all the energy substrates being mobilized are being shuttled towards such muscle. How your body differentiates between exercising and nonexercising muscle is not completely understood.

Stored energy has now been turned into cash—circulating glucose, amino acids, and fatty acids. As a final step, glucocorticoids, catecholamines, and glucagon stimulate the liver to convert fatty acids and amino acids to glucose, a process called "gluconeogensis." Thus, in the face of an acute stressor, there are increased concentrations of glucose available to whichever tissue needs it.

How do these metabolic adaptations cause disease when activated chronically? Quite simply, if you constantly mobilize energy at the cost of energy storage, it will ultimately prove disastrous. Constantly breaking down stored proteins in order to flux amino acids into the circulation produces myopathy, the wasting away of muscles, a prime storage site for protein. This causes weakness and fatigue. Fatigue will also arise from the fact that, collectively, the processes of lipolysis, proteolysis, glycogenolysis, and gluconeogenesis are inefficient. One can use a surprisingly apt metaphor from the economic world. If you open a long-term savings account in which money is put away for a stipulated period, you receive a lot of interest for keeping the money in the account and a penalty if you break the agreement and withdraw the money early. Similarly, the body is penalized for constantly mobilizing energy from storage sites and transforming it; each biochemical step is inefficient, and altogether, approximately 30% of potential energy is lost.

THE CARDIOVASCULAR STRESS-RESPONSE

In the presence of a physical stressor, it is logical to increase cardiovascular tone in order to deliver more of the mobilized glucose and oxygen to the tissues that need it. This is mostly accomplished through the sympathetic nervous system, which stimulates the heart to beat faster. Blood pressure is increased through vasoconstriction, which indirectly increases the force of cardiac contractions. Blood flow to some organs (for example, the digestive tract) is decreased; this is part of the strategy of shutting down nonessentials. Blood volume is also increased by vasopressin, which increases water resorption by the kidneys. If you are sprinting across a field with a lion on your heels and your blood pressure is 160/95, this is extremely helpful. If you have the same blood pressure whenever you have to stand in a line, you are putting yourself at risk. The danger is rarely of the "guy gets bad news, clutches his chest, and collapses dead" variety. Stress-induced sudden cardiac arrest is actually quite rare. Instead, chronic activation of the cardiovascular stress-response gradually damages heart muscle, weakens vessel walls, and promotes the deposition of cholesterol and the formation of atherosclerotic plaques.

THE GASTROINTESTINAL STRESS-RESPONSE

As discussed, it makes sense to inhibit the gastrointestinal (GI) tract during an acute physical stressor; digestion can wait for later. These changes are principally mediated by the autonomic nervous system through its shift from parasympathetic to sympathetic tone. Normally the former stimulates digestion. In the mouth, saliva is secreted, while in the stomach, acid, pepsinogen, mucus, and gastrin are secreted. In the intestines, secretion of a large array of digestive enzymes and hormones is stimulated, including lipase, trypsinogen, chymotrypsin, enterokinase, cholesystokinin (CCK), and vasoactive intestinal polypeptide (VIP). Furthermore, stomach churning and the relaxation and tightening of sphincters are all coordinated to promote digestion. With stress, all of these processes are inhibited, due both to the decreased parasympathetic tone and to the increased sympathetic outflow. We are all familiar with the first sign of the shutdown—our mouths become dry when we are nervous because we have stopped secreting saliva. In addition, the sympathetic nervous system decreases blood flow to the GI tract.

There have been major changes of opinion recently about the gastrointestinal consequences of prolonged stress. Since Selye and others in the 1930s, it was recognized that stress can cause stomach ulcers—holes in the stomach wall—and the lay public probably considers peptic ulcers to be the definitive stress-related disease. There is indeed a kind of ulcer that emerges rapidly and is tightly linked to catastrophic stress; such "stress ulcers" can develop over the course of a few days following massive stressors such as a whole body burn, and involve sufficient bleeding to be life-threatening. But most gastroenterologists now question whether the classic slowly emerging type of ulcer, the type that gives months of nonspecific gut pain until finally being diagnosed, has anything at all to do with stress. The reason for this revisionism is a revolution in the field, namely the recognition that a bacteria called *Helicobacter pylori* is implicated in the vast majority of ulcers in the Western world. No one expected this, because the dogma was that bacteria could not survive the acid bath of stomach juices; however, *H. pylori* turns out to have evolved some sophisticated defenses against the acidity. Once infecting a stomach, it causes inflammation (gastritis) which, through poorly understood mechanisms, compromises the ability of cells lining the stomach wall to defend themselves against stomach acids, and an ulcer quickly ensues. The definitive bit of evidence in favor of this *H. pylori* scenario was the enormously important clinical finding that antimicrobial drugs that kill bacteria can have miraculous effects on ulcers, far better than the traditional medications given for ulcers (such as antacids).

These findings have ushered in what has been termed the "Helicobacterization" of ulcer research. What this has meant is that most gastroenterologists reject the idea that stress is relevant to ulcers. The number of papers related to stress and ulcers has plummeted in recent years, in contrast to the increase in the number of papers related to stress and other gastrointestinal disorders. In effect, most in the field have concluded, "It's not a psychosomatic disorder after all. It's been bacterial all along."

Despite this shift, a number of stress physiologists, including myself, continue to view stress as highly relevant to understanding ulcer formation. Why should this be? For one thing, an *H. pylori* infection is neither necessary nor sufficient for a person to develop a stomach ulcer. Moreover, experimental stressors remain a very reliable means of giving a rat an ulcer, and ulcer formation is more likely to occur among people who are anxious, depressed, or undergoing severe life stressors. Careful studies have shown an interaction between stress and *H. pylori*. Specifically, ulcers are observed in individuals with mild amounts of stress yet heavy bacterial loads, or mild bacterial loads with massive amounts of stress. This is a prime example of a classic feature of stress-related disease—it is rare that stress causes you to be sick. Instead, it is more likely to worsen a preexisting disease, or to impair your defenses against some other pathogenic risk factor (Melmed and Gelpin 1996; Levenstein et al. 1995).

How might stress make the *H. pylori* more damaging? A number of possible routes exist: (1) Because blood flow to the GI tract is inhibited during stress, the delivery of oxygen and nutrients is curtailed. If this situation is prolonged, the stomach walls become weak and necrotic, making them more vulnerable to the bacteria. (2) Normally, the stomach expends considerable energy in building and thickening stomach walls and secreting mucus. Both protect the stomach walls from the potentially ulcerative effects of the powerful gastric acids. When the stress-response is prolonged (and acid secretion is inhibited chronically), the stomach curtails both of these housekeeping activities. In effect, the stomach decides that it is a waste of energy to thicken walls and make mucus if there is only minimal exposure to gastric acids anyway. Then, when the stressors abate and acid secretion resumes at its normal heavy rate, the stomach walls are vulnerable to erosions and ulcers. If that is coupled with the presence of the bacteria that impair acid defenses, the likelihood of an ulcer increases. (3) Ulcer repair is aided by a class of compounds called prostaglandins. However, glucocorticoids are powerful inhibitors of prostaglandin synthesis. The relative contributions of each of these mechanisms to ulcer formation remains controversial.

THE REPRODUCTIVE STRESS-RESPONSE
While virtually any adult organism may seek to reproduce at some point, a prolonged stressor will wreak havoc with reproductive physiology and behavior (Warren 1983; Rabin, Gold, Margioris, and Chrousos 1989). In many species, increased population density or decreased food resources are stressors that inhibit ovulation in females. This forms an elegant means by which populations self-regulate their growth rate. In some species (notably, some New World primates), reproduction is often inhibited not so much by the stressor of food shortages as by the stressor of social subordination. A high-ranking monkey ensures that she is the only member of her group to reproduce by physically harassing subordinates into anovulation. Male reproductive physiology is also vulnerable to chronic stress in varied species. Stressors such as surgical incisions, drought, sustained exercise, or defeat in social competition will suppress testosterone secretion. And among humans, there are endless psychological stressors that disrupt reproduction. To give some sense of the magnitude of our sensitivity to stress, it has been estimated that the majority of complaints of reproductive dysfunction by men in this country turn out to be psychogenic rather than organic in origin.

Much is known about how stressors disrupt reproduction in both sexes (Warren 1983; Sapolsky 1991). The summary presented here represents a consensus from studies of various mammalian species; there is, of course, phylogenetic variability. Among females, the points of inhibition are numerous. At the hypothalamus, the secretion of GnRH is inhibited by stress-induced secretion of beta-endorphin and CRH. One step below that, pituitary responsiveness to GnRH is diminished, decreasing LH and FSH secretion. This is due to the inhibitory actions of glucocorticoids or prolactin. Glucocorticoids also inhibit ovarian sensitivity to LH. The net result of these steps is to make the secretion of estrogen and progesterone and the release of a viable egg less likely.

The diminished levels of progesterone and the increased levels of prolactin, in turn, disrupt the normal maturation of the uterine wall. Thus, if an egg is fertilized against these considerable odds, it is less likely that proper implantation into the uterine wall will occur. And if that is not enough, certain stressors disrupt reproduction in another way. Females of numerous species secrete androgens (male sex hormones) from their adrenal glands. Although the amounts are small, they would normally be enough to impair reproduction. However, they are typically converted to estrogen by an enzyme (aromatase) in fat cells. When stressors involve loss of body fat in females (from famine, wasting illnesses, extreme degrees of exercise, or anorexia nervosa), this conversion step is diminished. The result is a smaller amount of circulating estrogen and a buildup of circulating androgens, which can be disruptive to reproduction.

Among males, the regulatory steps are nearly as numerous. Similarly, CRH and beta-endorphin inhibit GnRH release. As with the female, prolactin inhibits pituitary sensitivity to GnRH, and glucocorticoids inhibit testicular sensitivity to LH. The net result is decreased testosterone secretion and, under more extreme circumstances, decreased sperm production. Cell biologists have uncovered some of the ways in which beta-endorphin, prolactin, and glucocorticoids exert their inhibitory effects in both sexes. In some cases, they decrease the numbers of LH receptors; in others, they have post-receptor effects, and in still others, they sensitize the brain to the inhibitory effects of other hormones. The body is creative and varied in its means of suppressing reproduction during stress.

Another aspect of male reproduction can be maddeningly vulnerable to stressors: attaining and maintaining an erection. The initial erection requires parasympathetic tone. With continued stimulation and arousal, breathing and heart rate increase, and the physiologic profile becomes more sympathetic rather than parasympathetic in tone. Ejaculation consists of a sudden and major inhibition of the parasympathetic tone and stimulation of the sympathetic tone. With the inhibition of parasympathetic tone during stress, it becomes difficult to have an erection—resulting in impotency. And if the erection has already occurred, the tendency of a stressor to shift autonomic tone from parasympathetic to sympathetic accelerates the normal transition—resulting in premature ejaculation.

Why are there so many mechanisms by which stressors can suppress reproduction? Another way to frame this question is to ask how effective these numerous collective mechanisms are. Surprisingly, the answer is, not very. Humans continue to reproduce under dreadful circumstances; for example, in one frequently cited study, nearly 50% of the women in a Nazi concentration camp were continuing to menstruate despite starvation, slave labor, and unspeakable psychological stressors. If you are asking how readily stress causes reproductive behavior and physiology to grind to a complete halt, the answer is that it takes massive amounts of stress to do so, in virtually any mammal studied. It requires so many mechanisms to suppress reproduction during stress because reproduction is one of the strongest biological imperatives there is. But if you ask how readily stress disrupts the subtleties of sexuality—how appealing sex seems, how readily orgasms or erections occur, or how much pleasure any of this mating business brings—the answer is that it takes remarkably little. And it is this subtle realm that makes stress-induced reproductive dysfunction so common in Western life.

THE CONSEQUENCES OF A PROLONGED STRESS-RESPONSE ON GROWTH

If the stress-response involves postponing **anabolism**, then stressors should be particularly disruptive in young, growing animals, in whom anabolism is nearly continuous (Reichlin 1998). Indeed, in rats, stressors promptly inhibit circulating growth hormone (GH) concentrations, mostly due to increased somatostatin released (rather than to decreased release of growth hormone releasing hormone). If GH secretion is inhibited long enough in a young organism, growth is disrupted profoundly. For example, maternal deprivation in rat pups inhibits growth; the same thing occurs in human children living in a war zone. These examples, however, are difficult to interpret. A rat pup deprived of its mother undergoes nutritional as well as emotional deprivation. A child in a war zone is psychologically stressed but is also likely to suffer from poor nutrition and inadequate medical care. Thus, impaired growth may not be due to the nonspecific stressfulness of the situation but instead to poor nutrition or parasitic infestation.

Syndromes of growth inhibition do occur in children with no obvious organic cause (such as starvation, chronic wasting illness, and so on). Instead, in these children there is a history of major emotional disturbance and deprivation. In such cases of "psychosocial dwarfism" (also known as "stress dwarfism" or "psychogenic dwarfism"), children average half the expected height for their age and secrete little GH, even after stimuli that normally elicit GH secretion. They may even be unresponsive to exogenous GH. Typically, within a few months of being placed in a less stressful environment, GH concentrations and rates of growth become normal, and if the child has not yet reached puberty, there can be sufficient growth for the child to eventually attain normal stature. It should be emphasized that stress dwarfism is a rare disorder seen only in tragically stressful (and often psychopathologic) circumstances (Sapolsky 1998).

Adults, obviously, no longer grow. In such cases, the growth that is inhibited during stress is the repair of existing tissues. For example, calcium is normally removed from bone and replaced with new calcium. Glucocorticoids inhibit this anabolic housekeeping. Thus, with glucocorticoid overexposure, bones become decalcified, thin, and prone to fractures. It used to be thought that such glucocorticoid-induced osteoporosis required far higher glucocorticoid levels than were ever generated by stress, and were instead only seen when people were administered large amounts of synthetic glucocorticoids (to control any of a number of diseases, usually of an autoimmune nature—to be discussed below). Thus, this would be termed a "pharmacologic" effect, rather than a "physiologic" one. Recent work with captive primates indicates, however, that prolonged social stress can lead to osteoporosis in females (Shively et al. 1991). Whether the same applies to humans has yet to be determined.

The Stress-Response and Analgesia

It has long been recognized that pain perception can be blunted during extreme stress and emotional arousal (Terman et al. 1984; Olson et al. 1997). Such stress-induced **analgesia** (pain reduction) was often thought to be purely psychological. However, an understanding of the neurochemical nature of the phenomenon came from an explosion of discoveries in the early 1970s. Considerable interest had focused on opiates such as morphine, heroin, and opium, which had similar chemical structures and were analgesic. It was during that period that opiate receptors were discovered in the brain. This discovery carried a vital implication: The brain could not have evolved receptors for a plant compound. Instead, there must be "endogenous opiates" (or "opioids") somewhere in the body that normally bond to these receptors. This triggered a fevered search for opioids. Soon, three types were discovered: the endorphins, the enkephalins, and the dynorphins. They occur in the pituitary, the brain, and a number of peripheral organs and serve endocrine, paracrine, and neuromodulatory roles. Previous lesion, stimulation, and electrical recording studies had already mapped the neuroanatomy of pain pathways. These included relay sites in the dorsal horn of the spinal cord and, within the brain, the periaqueductal gray area and the raphe complex. These regions were shown to contain opiate receptors; opioids caused analgesia when microinjected at these sites, and opiate receptor antagonists blocked such analgesia.

It was soon shown that various stressors caused the secretion of beta-endorphin from the pituitary. Athletes began to call the analgesia that comes about 30 minutes into exercise the "endorphin high," and the subject appeared solved. Two complications have emerged, however. First, it is not clear whether circulating beta-endorphins, derived from the pituitary, actually cause analgesia. Variations in circulating levels of the hormone do not predict analgesia very well. Moreover, it is not clear how the peptide normally gets past the blood-brain barrier from the circulation in order to bind to these neural opiate receptors. Instead, it is probably the release of opioids from neuron terminals within the brain and spinal cord that mediates the analgesia.

As a second complexity, some aspects of stress-induced analgesia occur independently of opioids. Such analgesia shows no crosstolerance with exogenous opiates and cannot be blocked with opiate receptor blockers. Various neurotransmitters have been implicated, including serotonin and histamine. In general, early phases of stress-induced analgesia appear to be opioid-independent, while slower phases (approximately 30 minutes or more) are opioid-mediated.

Are there pathogenic consequences of analgesia following chronic stress? Seemingly not, because the analgesia wanes over the course of hours to days. This does not represent "exhaustion" of the stress-response as Selye conceptualized it (i.e., the system does not run out of opioids); rather, this represents habituation to the stressor. As proof, imposition of a novel, painful stimulus at the point where the analgesia has waned will reinstate the analgesia.

The Effects of the Stress-Response on the Brain

The hormones of the stress-response have numerous effects on the brain; they can influence learning and memory, vulnerability to depression, feeding behavior, and aggression, to name just a few of their effects. In recent years, data have emerged showing that chronic stress, acting through glucocorticoid hypersecretion, can directly damage the brain. These findings are discussed in chapter 14.

A Detailed Analysis: The Stress-Response and Immune Function

One of the most complex subjects in stress physiology is the interaction between stress and immunity, and it has fascinating potential consequences for health. Moreover, recent findings in this area have overturned some long-held beliefs on this subject, making it worth our while to review this topic in detail.

A Brief Review of the Immune System

The immune system, whose primary job is to defend the body against infectious challenges, is frighteningly complex (Dunn 1989). As discussed in chapter 10, the basic cell types that make up the circulating components of the immune system are **lymphocytes** and **monocytes**. There are two classes of lymphocytes: **T cells** and **B cells**. B cells principally produce antibodies, while there are several kinds of T cells (T helper and T suppressor cells, cytotoxic killer cells, and so on). The T and B cells mediate different forms of attack upon infectious agents. The former bring about **cell-mediated immunity** (figure 11.4). When a pathogen invades the body, it is recognized by macrophages, a type of monocyte, which present the foreign particle to a T helper cell. A metaphorical alarm is sounded, and T cells begin proliferating, ultimately producing activation and proliferation of cytotoxic killer cells, which attack and destroy the pathogen. B cells, in contrast, are central to antibody, or **humoral-mediated, immunity** (figure 11.5). Once the macrophage/ T helper cell combination has become alarmed, the latter also stimulates B-cell proliferation. In the process, the B cells generate antibodies, proteins that recognize and specifically bind to some feature of the invading pathogen. This binding immobilizes the pathogen and targets it for destruction.

A challenge for the immune system is that its cells are scattered throughout the circulation, requiring the existence of blood-borne chemical messengers that communicate between different cell types. A variety of such messengers exist, including **cytokines** (chemicals that trigger immune cell proliferation). For example, when macrophages first recognize an infectious agent, they release the cytokine interleukin-1. This triggers the T helper cell to release interleukin-2, which stimulates T-cell proliferation. On the hormonal front, T

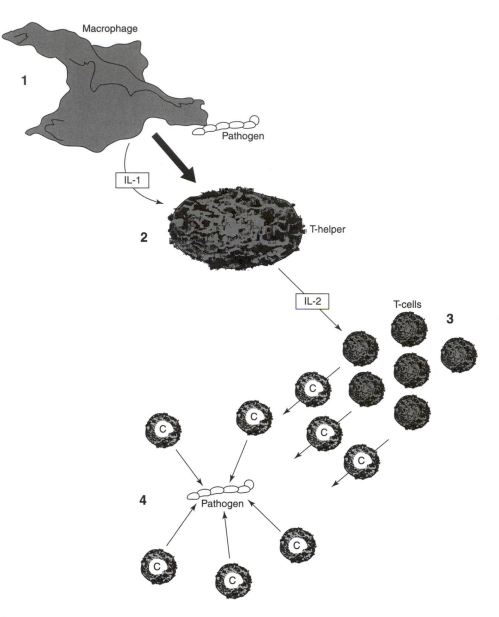

Figure 11.4 The cascade of cell-mediated immunity. (1) A pathogen is encountered by a type of monocyte called a macrophage. (2) This stimulates the macrophage to present the pathogen to a T-helper cell (a type of lymphocyte) and to release interleukin-1 (IL-1), which stimulates T-helper cell activity. (3) The T-helper cell, as a result, releases interleukin-2 (IL-2), which triggers T-cell proliferation. (4) This eventually causes another type of lymphocyte, cytotoxic killer cells, to proliferate and destroy the pathogen.

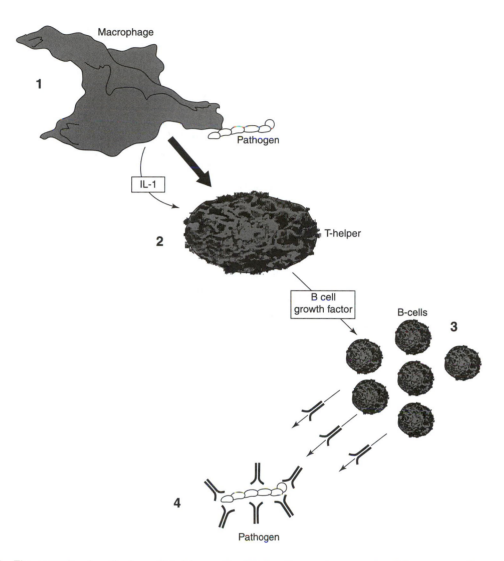

Figure 11.5 The cascade of antibody-mediated immunity. (1) A pathogen is encountered by a macrophage. (2) This stimulates it to present the pathogen to a T-helper cell, and to release interleukin-1 (IL-1), which stimulates T-helper cell activity. (3) The T-helper cell then secretes B-cell growth factor, triggering differentiation and proliferation of another lymphocyte, B-cells. (4) The B-cells make and release specific antibodies which bind to surface proteins on the pathogen, targeting it for destruction by a large group of plasma proteins known as *complement*.

cells also secrete B-cell growth factor, which stimulates B-cell differentiation and proliferation. There is also an additional class of cytokines known as the interferons. These are secreted by T cells and fibroblasts, among other cells, and have broad activating effects on lymphocytes and monocytes. The critical point in this simplistic summary is to appreciate the numerous cell types and messengers involved in immunocompetence. Numerous points in these cascades are subject to the disruptive effects of stress.

Immunosuppression During Stress

Beginning with Selye's observation that his stressed rats had atrophied immune organs, it has been known that prolonged stress can suppress immunity (Ader et al. 1991). If stress can do this, then the brain must be able to influence the immune system, since stressors are, of course, first perceived in the brain. The recognition of neural regulation of immune function arose from two types of studies. First, lesioning or stimulating different brain regions could alter immune function. Second, organisms could be conditioned to change their immune function, and conditioned learning, of course, involves the brain. These studies helped found the field of **psychoneuroimmunology** (Ader et al. 1991) and have paved the way for acceptance of the fact that neuroendocrine systems can influence immune function during stress.

While the sympathetic nervous system and opiates might play some role in suppressing the immune system during stress, the lion's share of that task goes to glucocorticoids. They were also the first hormones to be recognized (by Selye) for that function. The immunosuppressive actions of glucocorticoids are often exploited in clinical medicine. An autoimmune disease occurs when the immune system inadvertently attacks a normal part of the body, as if it is an invasive pathogen. In juvenile diabetes, for example, it is the insulin-secreting cells of the pancreas which are attacked, while multiple sclerosis involves an attack upon a part of the nervous system. Broadly, autoimmunity consists of a pathologically overactive immune system, and a standard treatment is to put the person on "steroids" (i.e., glucocorticoids, also often called "corticosteroids") in order to suppress the immunity back to normal levels (but hopefully, no further).

How do glucocorticoids suppress immunity? For starters, the hormone inhibits release of many cytokines as well as levels of their receptors. By disrupting this network of signaling, glucocorticoids inhibit proliferative responses of the immune system. Glucocorticoids also inhibit B cell-mediated immunity by inhibiting IL-1 release, and also inhibit production of certain components of **complement**, the system needed for the antibody-mediated killing of target cells.

In addition, the steroids can block the maturation of developing lymphocytes; this accounts for the involution of immune tissue first observed by Selye. The steroids also can pull lymphocytes out of the bloodstream. This effect is far more pronounced in some species (for example, humans and guinea pigs) than in others (like rats and mice). Finally, glucocorticoids can actually destroy lymphocytes, causing them to burst. This "lysis" is due to an active process of programmed cell death ("apoptosis"). Glucocorticoids induce the synthesis of a protein that is either an endonuclease (an enzyme that cleaves DNA), or which activates a preexisting endonuclease. Not surprisingly, once its DNA is fragmented into little pieces, a cell does not last long.

Why Suppress Immune Function During Stress?

Given the large number of ways that stress can suppress immunity, it is reasonable to wonder why this should have evolved. What is the physiologic advantage of suppressing immunity during stress? Investigators have offered theories for decades. A popular one fits into the framework introduced at the beginning of this chapter, namely, that unessentials are suppressed during a stressful emergency—immunity doesn't come cheap, make the antibodies tonight around the campfire, if there is a tonight, don't waste energy now on immunity while sprinting for your life.

The discovery of the glucocorticoid-induced killing of lymphocytes also killed that theory. The notion of immune suppression in order to save energy would make sense if all that happened during stress was that the immune system was stopped in its tracks (i.e., no more cell division, synthesis of cytokines, and so on). Instead, the programmed death of lymphocytes is an active process, requiring energy. The body has to *work* in order to suppress immunity.

Other, less plausible theories have been offered as well (one of which I gleefully advocated in the prior edition of this text). But the answer to this puzzle has recently become clear. This clarification is due to the increased sensitivity of a number of assays of immune function, allowing scientists for the first time to measure immune events within the first few minutes of stress, the period prior to glucocorticoids beginning to have their immunosuppressive actions. These recent studies indicate that there is actually an enhancement of immune function immediately after the onset of all sorts of stressors (Munck, Guyre, and Holbrook 1984; Sapolsky et al. 2000).

Thus, when glucocorticoids begin to have their effects some 30 to 60 minutes into a stressor, they are not suppressing immunity below a baseline. Instead, they are helping the immune system to return to baseline. If you study massive and prolonged stressors (as the stress physiologists had been doing for decades), or give an organism massive amounts of synthetic glucocorticoids, immunity is indeed suppressed far below baseline. But for the typical stressor, the immune system is first transiently activated (possibly through the sympathetic nervous system), which is followed by glucocorticoids mediating its recovery back to normal. This represents a triumph for the physiologist Allan Munck of Dartmouth, who led this revisionism (Munck, Guyre, and Holbrook 1984). His work also provides the answer to what might be the next question—why is it adaptive for the immune system to recover back to its baseline? Why not just have it work at a higher level all the time, presumably providing even better defenses against pathogens? Munck's answer was that you cannot just have immune activity climb higher and higher, because there is the danger that immunity will eventually spiral out of control into pathologic overactivation. Specifically, he predicted that if glucocorticoids did not damp the immune response back down during stress, immune activation might spill over into autoimmune disease. This turns out to be correct, and various instances of autoimmunity are now understood to involve a failure of the glucocorticoid "brake" during stressors. This also helps explain one of the persistent paradoxes in clinical medicine: synthetic versions of glucocorticoids suppress autoimmunity and help lessen the symptoms of the autoimmune disease. Yet many clinical studies and endless patient reports indicate that periods of stress *worsen* autoimmune symptoms. The resolution is now clear. If there are lots of everyday stressors, there will be bursts of transient immune activation (and thus transient worsening of symptoms in an autoimmune patient); but massive, pharmacologic doses of glucocorticoids will flatten immunity.

Recent work has added an extra subtlety to our understanding of the actions of glucocorticoids during stress. Once again, massive amounts of such steroids suppresses virtually every facet of immunity. However, as the more physiologic stress-induced levels of glucocorticoids begin to have their effects, they preferentially inhibit older constituents of the immune system. This can be seen as sculpting the immune response, bringing the newer and more helpful immune cells to the forefront (Besedovsky and Del Ray 1996). Furthermore, when glucocorticoids cause immune cells to be removed from the circulation, the classical notion was that such cells were stored, inactive, in immune tissues; recent work has shown that the early phase of glucocorticoid actions involves, instead, the diverting of immune cells to injured tissues— rather than being placed in the barracks, soldiers are being rushed to the front lines (Dharbar and McEwen 1996).

Thus, a new picture of immune function during stress has emerged. With the onset of stress, immune defenses are activated, with a number of hormones, including glucocorticoids, working to sharpen immune defenses and mobilize them to where they are needed. Shortly thereafter, glucocorticoids act to return immunity back to baseline, a critical step to avoid autoimmune overshoot. And it is only with massive and prolonged stressors that immunity is suppressed below baseline. The next section considers the controversial question of whether such immune suppression during chronic stress is enough to make you sick.

The Pathogenic Effects of Chronic Stress on the Immune System

If prolonged stress suppresses immunity, more infectious diseases should result. This seems straightforward, but is actually anything but (Booth-Kewley and Friedman 1987; Friedman and Booth-Kewley 1987; Fox 1983; House, Landis, and Umberson 1988; Sapolsky 1998; Shekelle et al. 1981, chapter 8). The stress/infection linkage is built on the following logic: during prolonged stress, there is prolonged glucocorticoid secretion; this suppresses immunity below baseline, impairing disease defenses and resulting in more illnesses. The first problem with this sequence concerns individual differences and psychological stressors (topics detailed in the next sections of this chapter). If you break someone's leg, they are going to secrete glucocorticoids, no doubt about it. But if you stick someone on a slow line at the supermarket checkout, they might fume and complain and have a robust stress-response, or they may happily daydream. When it comes to most psychological and social stressors, we differ dramatically as to what we perceive as stressful (and thus whether we mobilize glucocorticoid secretion).

Uncertainty comes with the next steps as well. We now know that, depending on the type and duration of a stressor, glucocorticoids can either stimulate or inhibit immunity, and individuals will differ as to where the transition occurs between the stimulatory and inhibitory actions. Thus, it is not even clear whether a particular stress-induced burst of glucocorticoid secretion actually inhibits immunity.

Finally, while massive suppression of immunity causes individuals to fester with infectious diseases, stress-induced immune suppression is subtler and more transient. For example, the extent of immune suppression due to a sleepless week of studying for finals doesn't remotely resemble the extent of immune suppression seen in AIDS. And it is just not clear whether the milder extent of suppression in the former case is enough to actually make a difference in defenses against disease.

When you put these various caveats together, you are left with a lot of confusion. Stress-induced immune suppression is most likely to put you more at risk for the common cold, mononucleosis, or cold-sore flare ups. But the relevance in other areas remains unclear. For example, there appears to be an increased risk of disease or mortality among individuals who are grieving for a lost loved one. Maybe this is because the stressfulness of loss leads to glucocorticoid-induced immune suppression and thus more infectious disease. However, maybe grieving, depressed people simply no longer bother taking their daily medications or eating healthy meals. In studies of such individuals, it is often quite difficult to control for some of these life-style variables. Thus, while stress-induced immune suppression almost certainly is relevant to why everyone gets colds just after finals week, it remains to be seen whether it is relevant to more serious areas of medicine.

One area in which stress-induced immune suppression plays almost no role is with respect to cancer. Many health care professionals have sensed a link between stress and cancer, as have many patients. A rather poorly controlled literature has purported to show that link as well. For example, a number of studies have reported a link between a major depression (a highly stressful state, as will be discussed below) and an increased risk of cancer, even years later. However, the effects in these studies have been tiny, and critical confounds have not been controlled for. For example, the most widely cited of these studies, carried out on a population working in an electric plant, failed to control for the fact that the depressed subpopulation also had the highest exposure to environmental carcinogens. The more careful studies have failed to show any relationship between stressors of any sort (such as depression or bereavement) and cancer incidence.

Laboratory studies have also focused on this issue. None have shown that stress can increase the rate of spontaneous tumors in a laboratory animal. A number have shown that stress can accelerate the growth of artificially induced tumors and have even uncovered likely mechanisms to explain this observation. However, the types of tumors in these studies (virally derived ones) are very rarely suffered by humans, and there is no convincing evidence that stress can accelerate the growth of the types of tumors that humans get (those that are genetic in nature or due to environmental carcinogens).

Finally, studies have shown that people who have a "fighting spirit" about their cancer (that is, those who approach the cancer as something that can be beaten) or those placed in support groups with other cancer patients are likely to survive cancer longer than cancer patients in a control group. Perhaps this is because such individuals secrete less glucocorticoids and thus have better immune defenses against the tumor. But perhaps these people are simply more compliant with treatment regimes—more likely to subject themselves to the extra chemotherapy sessions, to take their medicine although it makes them nauseous, to eat despite having no appetite, and so on.

Collectively, there is next to no scientific evidence to link stress to human cancer. It strikes me as critical to emphasize this point, given the many health care professionals and patients who believe there is a link. When you teach someone about a legitimate link between stress and disease, you are providing them with a means to improve their health. But when someone suffering from a horrible, often fatal disease is led erroneously to believe that stress had something to do with its cause or progression, you can convince them that it is their own fault that they are dying. This is not good science, good medicine, or good ethics.

Few areas of the life sciences are more exciting these days than psychoimmunology because its potential impact on health and disease is so profound. Nevertheless, it is clearly a nascent discipline, and one should be cautious about overemphasizing its findings. More research is clearly needed.

The preceding pages have reviewed the effects of stress on metabolism, cardiovascular function, and so on, detailing the adaptive features of the short-term stress-response and the pathogenic potential of chronic stress. These are summarized in table 11.1. Amid this mountain of data, two conclusions seem clear: If you are that lion or zebra and you cannot appropriately initiate a stress-response, you are in deep trouble. But just as clearly, if you are unable to terminate a stress-response appropriately, as is so often the case with modern humans, you also pay a considerable pathologic price.

How Generalized Is the Stress-Response?
Figures 11.1 and 11.3 depict the hormones and neural systems thought to be turned on by all stressors and those inhibited by all stressors, respectively

Table 11.1 The Principal Components of the Stress-Response and the Most Common Pathologic Consequences of Prolonged Exposure to Stress

THE STRESS-RESPONSE	ITS PATHOLOGIC CONSEQUENCES, WHEN PROLONGED
Mobilization of energy at the cost of energy storage	Fatigue, myopathy, steroid diabetes
Increased cardiovascular and cardiopulmonary tone	Hypertension
Suppression of digestion	Ulceration
Suppression of growth	Psychogenic dwarfism, bone decalcification
Suppression of reproduction	Anovulation, impotency, loss of libido
Suppression of immunity and the inflammatory response	Impaired disease resistance
Analgesia	
Neural responses, including altered cognition and sensory thresholds	Accelerated neural degeneration during aging

(Frakenhaeuser 1980; Mason 1968; Weiner 1992). For Selye, one of the cornerstones of the stress-response was this nonspecificity—for example, that whether you are too hot or too cold, the stress-response is essentially similar. It was no accident that Selye used the word "general" with "adaptation syndrome." He wrote:

It is difficult to see how such essentially different things as cold, heat, drugs, hormones, sorrow and joy could provoke an identical biochemical reaction in the organism. Yet this is the case; it can now be demonstrated by highly objective quantitative biochemical determinations that certain reactions of the body are totally nonspecific and common to all types of exposure.

As with many grand and sweeping statements in science, this is not entirely true; not all stressors provoke the identical package of responses. In Selye's view, any stressor would provoke norepinephrine release from all the many branches of the system. Yet there is some specificity of response. For example, hypoxia stimulates renal and gastric sympathetic activity, while hypotension stimulates only the former. Furthermore, norepinephrine and epinephrine secretion during stress can dissociate. For example, hypotension affects both renal and adrenal sympathetic activity similarly, whereas hypoglycemia does not. Thus, the entire sympathetic nervous system is not necessarily turned on in a nonspecific way in response to any stressor. This specificity of coding is also observed when comparing different endocrine systems. Some stressors provoke adrenocortical activity far more than adrenomedullary activity, while others do the opposite. Some stressors also influence glucocorticoid secretion without affecting growth hormone secretion. Broadly, you would be on safe ground if you stated that all stressors provoke some degree of catecholamine and glucocorticoid secretion. However, the exact orchestration of responses of the many hormones discussed will vary depending on the stressor, something now referred to as a "stress signature."

Psychologic Stress

We have summarized the understanding of stress that would satisfy most physiologists. Much of the remainder of this chapter examines individual differences in the stress-response. Why do two individuals differ in how often or how much they activate the stress-response? By thinking purely in terms of the physiology presented in this chapter up until now, it would be easy to approach this question. One would first point out the obvious, that the two organisms might differ in the amount of stressors they are exposed to and then move on to the next and more interesting level of analysis—two organisms that are exposed to the same stressor but differ in the resulting stress-response. We can speculate about interesting mechanisms that might explain the differences. Suppose two monkeys are both deprived of food to the point where metabolic homeostasis is disturbed and to an equal extent in both animals. Both should then secrete glucocorticoids; if there are marked differences in the amount of glucocorticoids secreted, the well-trained physiologist should immediately think of explanations such as differences in ACTH half-lives in the blood, differences in adrenal perfusion rates, numbers of glucocorticoid receptors, and so on. This would be the traditional approach of stress physiologists (Levine, Weiner, and Coe 1989; Miller 1980; Weiss 1970).

One study suffices to show how much more complex the picture really is. In the study cited above, the two monkeys differed in one critical way. While both were deprived of any nutrition, one was fed a flavored placebo. That monkey did not secrete glucocorticoids, whereas the first one had a sizable stress-response. Nothing in the world of Selye and the physiologists could have predicted this outcome because the homeostatic balance was equally disturbed in both monkeys (they were equally hypoglycemic). However, the second monkey did not *perceive* things to be as stressful as the first one did.

This study signaled a major change in the study of stress physiology. The prior view held that if you knew how physiologically disruptive the external insult was, you had a good chance of predicting the magnitude of the stress-response. Suddenly, critical intermediary—psychological factors could modulate the stressfulness of a stressor. Psychological factors could even trigger a stress-response in the absence of homeostatic disruption: Animals and humans were shown to have classic stress-responses during bereavement, difficulty in cognitive tasks, conditioned fear, and so on.

How much can psychological variables modulate the stress-response? Clearly, a great deal. Numerous physical stressors are no longer stressful when the organism is habituated to the situation and is thus accustomed to it. Yet it cannot be true that all physical stressors are stressful only to the extent that they cause emotional arousal. As evidence, an anesthetized person has a stress-response following a surgical incision.

Most scientists now accept the power of psychological variables to modulate stress physiology. The question, of course, is, what are these variables? What is stressful about psychological stress? Elegant studies have shown that the answer includes a lack of control, a lack of predictability, and a lack of outlets for frustration. Other terms and constructs have been used in the field, but these encompass the most important ideas.

Lack of control is critical. In one demonstration of this, rats were subjected to intermittent electric shocks. One rat could control the situation because it was able to press a lever to decrease the rate of shocks. The second rat received a shock whenever the first one did, but without control. The latter had far more glucocorticoid secretion and a greater chance of developing ulcers; this result occurred despite an identical extent of physical perturbation. Similar findings have emerged with dogs and humans. In a subtle elaboration, if a rat is trained to press a lever to avoid a shock and is then prevented from performing that avoidance behavior when it expects a shock, there is glucocorticoid secretion even if no shock is actually delivered. Here, loss of control is a trigger, even in the absence of a physical stressor.

Lack of predictability is also critical. If rats are given a signal indicating the impending delivery of a shock or when the shock period has ended, they have less glucocorticoid secretion than rats given identical shocks with no warning. In the former case, the signal allows the rat to predict when a shock is and is not about to occur and thus when it can relax its vigilance.

Some have noted that loss of control and of predictability share the trait of the outcome being discrepant with expectations (or, in other words, novel). Thus, the simple act of putting a rat in a novel environment—a new cage—activates the stress-response. In men learning to parachute jump, their first jump elicited a robust stress-response. With subsequent jumps, however, the response eventually habituated as the novelty of the situation lessened. Some have also emphasized that the common theme in loss of control and of predictability is the consequent arousal or vigilance, as the animal searches for the new rules of control and prediction.

A number of studies have emphasized the importance of *outlets for frustration*. For example, when rats are shocked, there is less glucocorticoid secretion and fewer ulcers if they can gnaw on a piece of wood or can attack another rat. Eating, drinking, or access to a running wheel can also serve as protective outlets.

One can ask some subtle questions. For example, does novelty stimulate the stress-response in a linear or all-or-none fashion? It appears to be linear. Thus, the more novel an environment for a rat (handled and returned to home cage, or returned to a new but similar cage, to a new type of cage, to a new type of cage illuminated with bright lights, and so on), the higher the level of glucocorticoid secretion. This demonstrates the rigor of current psychoendocrine approaches in stress research.

Thus, the extent to which a physical insult is stressful is modulated dramatically by intervening psychological variables, and psychological factors can initiate a stress-response even in the absence of a physical insult. Clearly, one vital prerequisite for responding to psychological stressors is a certain level of intelligence. One needs to have a decent memory to perceive a novelty stressor—"I know what is normal, and what's happening now is not normal, and this makes me nervous," or a conditioned stressor—"Uh oh, I remember what occurred last time this happened and it wasn't good." Thus, only the more cognitively sophisticated species can have sustained psychologic stressors (and pay the pathogenic price). And humans excel at this.

Individual Differences in Stress Physiology

Why is it interesting to study individual differences? Most physiologists hate individual variability. Just when you think you have discovered something and can announce that "X causes Y," you have to qualify your observation by saying "X causes Y most of the time, but not in a subset of animals, and don't ask me why not." Individual variability makes data messy and it's harder to know what is really going on. The emphasis in physiology on using inbred strains of animals with identical housing conditions is meant to eliminate individual variability. Why study it?

The answer must be because individual variability is a major chance to understand the prevention of stress-related disease. A mountain of data now demonstrates that stress can increase your chances of becoming sick. It sometimes seems miraculous that any of us manages to survive the lifetime of stressors that we are all subject to. Yet only some of us get stress-related diseases. To study individual differences in stress physiology is to study what some individuals are doing right and to study why some bodies and some psyches deal with stressors better than others. In the next few sections, we will review some examples of stress-responses differing systematically between individuals.

Social Rank and the Stress-Response

Among social species, dominance systems frequently emerge. Resources in the ecosystem are not infinite, competition occurs, and the resources are often divided unevenly. Every contested resource could be fought for in a bloody showdown. Instead, systems of conventionalized gestures often evolve so that individuals need not fight it out. Two animals approach a desired food item, for example, and one of them makes a facial expression, gives a certain type of growl, releases a certain pheromone, which, in that species, means dominance. And the second individual usually relinquishes the food without an overt contest. Presumably, it can remember what happened the last time conflict with this individual came to a head (Sapolsky 1990; 1993).

In some species, dominance systems are linear, in that a hierarchy of ranks emerges. Number 1 has a different quality of life from number 5, who is different from number 10. This is what is seen among chickens, for example, whose linear dominance system gave rise to the term "pecking order." In contrast, some dominance systems are nonlinear, for example, number 1 does all the mating. In this case, it is not meaningful to try to define a number 5 or a number 10. You are either a "number 1" or a "not number 1."

The quality of life of an animal depends tremendously on its social rank. Rank determines how hard it has to work for food and influences who it gets to mate with or if it gets to mate at all. Social rank determines whether it gets a safe spot during a predator attack, a warm spot in the cold, or an ideal spot to build a nest to ensure the survival of its offspring. It influences how often the individual is harassed in petty, irritating ways. Many studies have examined whether the physiology of the stress-response differs among animals of different ranks. The expectation in most studies was that subordinate animals would have chronically activated stress-responses and more stress-related disease. This was because subordinate animals are subject to the most psychological harassment, reflecting a lack of control and predictability in their lives, and because they had the fewest coping outlets available to them.

The effects of social status on the stress-response were initially difficult to discern from the large numbers of studies with conflicting results. Many findings supported the initial hypothesis—subordinate animals were reported to secrete elevated levels of glucocorticoids basally in the absence of any obvious stressor, and to have enlarged adrenal glands, elevated blood pressure, higher rates of atherosclerosis, more reproductive problems, immune suppression, and so on. In other words, for them, even everyday life was a little bit stressful. Subsequent studies showed that these physiological differences were due to being socially subordinate, rather than causing the subordinance. And some detailed neuroendocrine work uncovered the mechanisms underlying these rank differences (for example, if a subordinate primate secreted excessive glucocorticoids, was this because there was more ACTH coming out of the pituitary? More CRF coming out of the hypothalamus?). But at the same time, a substantial number of studies of other species and populations failed to find more patterns of stress and disease among subordinates. And some even found the most severe incidences of stress among dominant individuals.

Much of the confusion has now been clarified. The rank/physiology relationship appears to depend heavily on four variables (Sapolsky 1999).

1. *While rank is important, so is the species in which it occurs.* In some species (like rhesus monkeys, baboons, and rats), dominance hierarchies are typically stable. High-ranking individuals do not have to fight very often; instead, they throw their weight around merely through psychological bluff and disproportionately control access to resources. Subordinate individuals, in turn, are subjected to the highest rate of unpredictable attacks, disruptions of feeding, and so on. Not surprisingly, these are the cases where it is the subordinate individuals who show the greatest evidence of stress-related disease.

In contrast, some species exhibit "pair-bonding." This is the situation where an adult female and male pair for life, typically sharing the work of child-rearing fairly equally. Dominance hierarchies are pretty meaningless, if they even exist, in such cases. For example, among marmosets and tamarins (pair-bonding New World primates), social groups have a single breeding pair-bond. But rather than this being the dominant couple, enforcing their dominance on the subordinates through aggression and intimidation, the subordinate ranks are instead typically filled with closely affiliated younger siblings. And not surprisingly, in species such as these, there is virtually no relationship between rank and physiological profile.

Finally, in some species, dominance is something that must be reasserted constantly through physical exertion—a fight between numbers 4 and 5 in the hierarchy, for example, demands that the number 1 individual must aggress both afterward, as a reminder of the ranking. Thus, the dominant individuals have the highest rates of aggression. And in these cases (such as the one that has been reported for mongooses), it is the dominant individuals who show the markers of chronic stress-responses.

2. *While rank is important, so is the stability of the hierarchy in which the rank occurs*. As just noted, baboons are the sort of species in which the highest ranking individuals typically have all the psychological advantages, the fewest social stressors, and the healthiest profiles of stress-related physiology. That is what is seen under the typical circumstance of the hierarchy being *stable*—ranks are not particularly shifting, and the majority of interactions reinforce the status quo. In contrast, every so often, the hierarchy becomes *unstable*—a critical individual has died, some destabilizing coalition has formed, or some new aggressive individual has migrated into the troop. And for weeks to months afterward, the hierarchy fluctuates, with dramatic increases in the numbers of fights and injuries, decreased energy devoted to socially affiliative behaviors (such as grooming), and coalitions forming and disintegrating unpredictably. At the center of such unstable chaos is the top of the hierarchy, as animals battle for dominance. Not surprisingly, in such cases teetering precariously at the top of the hierarchy involves tremendous psychological stress. And in these incidences, it is dominant individuals whose physiological profiles are most prone to stress-related disease.

3. *While rank is important, so is the personal experience of rank*. Regardless of what species or type of society it lives in, a social animal's rank is not an abstraction, but a very concrete day-to-day experience. After controlling for rank, we will still find that individual animals differ as to how often and how severely they are exposed to stressors, and how readily they can make use of sources of social support. How often is your nose rubbed in your subordinance? How many friends and relatives live in your social group? In one study, the more often female baboons were subject to displacement aggression at the teeth of a particularly aggressive male, the more immunosuppressed they were. In study of female macaque monkeys, glucocorticoid levels were not just a function of rank, but of how often reconciliation behavior occurred for particular individuals after a fight.

4. *While rank is important, so is personality*. The preceding sections suggest that rank/physiology correlations must be considered in the context of the species, the society in which the rank occurs, and an individual's experi-

ence of that rank. Anyone who has ever had a pet recognizes how individualistic an animal's personality is, and careful studies have explored this more scientifically, typically with primates. A final critical variable is whether the animal has the sort of personality that sees the glass of social competition as half-empty or half-full. Consider the following example: A male baboon sits, minding his own business. A highly competitive rival of his arrives on the scene and takes a nap a dozen yards away. Does the first male continue doing whatever he was doing undisturbed, or does the mere presence of his rival napping disrupt his behavior? The more easily provoked a male is by the neutral presence of a rival, the higher the basal glucocorticoid levels after controlling for rank. After all, everyday life is filled with a lot of rivals taking naps, and if each one is considered provocative and in-your-face, stress hormone levels will reflect it. A variety of similar studies suggest that after we control for rank, we see more activated stress-responses in animals who are more reactive and readily provoked and who have fewer social outlets for support. Moreover, some of these studies have been longitudinal, following the same animals over years, and have indicated that these temperamental traits are stable over time.

Collectively, these studies do much to explain individual differences in patterns of the stress-response and of stress-related disease. Moreover, they indicate the richness of the social environment in which animals live and the subtle personality differences with which they filter the world around them.

Humans, "Rank," and Socioeconomic Status

If the rank/physiology correlates in social animals are complicated, one can imagine trying to analyze rank and physiology in a human. In general, in my view, the approach has not been successful. Some studies have found consistent differences in the physiology of humans matched in rank situations—comparing winners and losers of sporting events, for example. But we don't know whether such artificial situations (for example, a two-minute wrestling match between a pair of college-age athletes) are of any relevance to, for example, how readily someone accumulates atherosclerotic plaques in blood vessels over a lifetime.

Other studies have looked at health and rankings within large corporations. This style of study has produced some interesting findings (for example, they've shown that the notion of high-level executives having the most stress—"executive stress syndrome"—is mostly a myth (Weiss 1970)). Middle-level executives, who typically have responsibility without authority, are the ones with the greatest incidence of stress-related disease. However, a weakness there is that an individual who is low-ranking in the occupational world may, in another facet of life, be highly acclaimed—captain of the community softball team, for example—and therefore view the forty hours a week in the lowly mailroom at work as boring and irrelevant. In other words, humans are capable of being in a multitude of different hierarchies simultaneously, and it is never obvious which one they are most invested in.

Thus, I am not sure how much information this general approach has offered. There is, however, one way in which a human can be subject to the same stressors as a low-ranking animal in a tough hierarchy is, namely, being poor. When considering the range of socioeconomic status, (SES) the poor certainly have the most physical stressors—long hours of work that is often physical, the poorest diets, and the greatest likelihood of no heat in the winter. And they have the highest rates of psychological stressors as well. They lack control and predictability, often being the first to be laid off during hard times and the most likely to get the worst work hours, and so on. They also lack outlets for frustration. That relaxing vacation or weekly yoga class becomes unlikely when you're not sure where the next rent check is coming from. And they lack social support—who has time to be a shoulder to cry on when they are working two jobs?

Few studies have examined whether the poor have different stress-responses than higher SES individuals, but they certainly have a lot more disease. When comparing the poorest and wealthiest segments of our society, for example, there are up to ten-fold differences in the incidence and mortality of certain diseases (Pincus and Callahan 1995; Syme and Berkman 1976; Adler et al. 1993; Antonovsky 1968; Evans et al. 1994). A number of possible explanations for the poverty/disease link have nothing to do with stress. There are the issues of health care access—how readily you have preventive checkups and what quality doctor you see when you are sick. But it cannot all be explained by the poor having worse health care access, because the poverty/disease link exists in societies that have universal health care, and also exists for diseases whose incidences have nothing to do with health care access. The link might have something to do with the poor having more risk factors (lead paint in the crummy apartment, working in the coal mine, and so on) and fewer protective factors (lack of healthy food, lack of time for relaxing hobbies, and so on). Despite that, the link still exists after we control for many of the more obvious factors. And the link might be related to poorer education, leading to less awareness of the dangers of smoking and less ability to adhere to the details of a drug regime. But again, the link is still there for diseases that are impervious to education.

Amid those other possible explanations is stress (Pincus and Callahan 1995). This is not just because it makes sense (the poor have the most physical and psychological stressors). In addition, the diseases that show the most dramatic SES gradients are the ones that are thought to be most stress-related (heart disease and psychiatric disorders), whereas cancer shows one of the weakest gradients.

Thus, while the human picture is obviously extremely complex, there is reason to view poverty as exacting a price with respect to stress-related disease.

Psychiatric Disorders, Personality, and the Human Stress-Response

More insight into individual differences in the stress-response comes from considering a number of personality profiles and psychiatric disorders in humans. The ones I group together here are ones in which, broadly, there is a maladaptive stress-response, typically along the lines of chronic activation (Sapolsky 1998, chapter 14).

Probably the best example concerns major depression. By this, I do not mean the everyday blues that we all feel occasionally. Instead, I refer to a crippling psychiatric disorder, one in which sufferers can be incapacitated, unable to work, and unable to even get out of bed. Cognitively, major depression can best be thought of as "learned helplessness"—a state in which the individual, often because of some sort of trauma, has decided that there is no control in life, everything is hopeless, and it is not worth trying anything. On an operational level, this learned helplessness manifests itself in an individual not attempting a coping response in the face of a challenge or, if they happen to stumble on an effective coping response, not recognizing it as effective. The relevance of this to psychological stress should be obvious—the depressive feels no sense of control, predictability, and has no healthy outlets. And consonant with this, glucocorticoid levels are very significantly elevated in about half of depressives.

Anxiety disorders are also of interest. Someone suffering from such a disorder views the world as full of stressors that demand endless vigilance and endless coping, and never acknowledges the possibility that things are actually safe and they can relax. In depression, there is a mismatch between stressors and coping responses, as the individual does not bother with an attempt at coping—"What good is it, nothing matters, I have no control anyway." In the case of someone with an anxiety disorder, there is also a mismatch between stressors and coping responses. However, in this case, it is in the opposite direction, as the person assumes there are far more stressors than there actually are. And consonant with this, a number of investigators have observed an overactivation of the sympathetic nervous system during periods of anxiety. Why depression should be most interrelated with the glucocorticoid system, while anxiety is most connected to the sympathetic nervous system is a subject of ongoing research.

Another version of an overactive stress-response is seen in individuals with Type A personality disorder. As originally defined, this was a personality that was impatient and time-pressured, and had poor self-esteem and was hostile, taking pleasure only in checking things off a list of things to do. Such Type A individuals were shown to be more prone to cardiovascular disease. Subsequent refinements of the Type A concept showed that the key variable was the hostility. Type A individuals see the world as full of hostile menace that is personally directed—a slow line at the supermarket is grounds for raging about how the checkout person is doing it on purpose, just to make you late. Recent work has shown that Type A individuals, as one might expect, chronically activate the sympathetic nervous system. Again, there is a mismatch between how stressful the world actually is and what the person thinks it is like.

A final example concerns people with repressive personalities. Such individuals are not depressed, anxious, or Type A. Moreover, personality profiles show them to be fairly happy and productive. What they are, in addition, is highly regimented. These are people who like structured, predictable lives—no surprises for them. In addition, they tend not to express much emotion (hence the term "repressive") and are not good at recognizing the subtleties of emotions in others. Basically, these individuals expend enormous emotional energy making sure their worlds are under control. And recent studies have shown elevated basal glucocorticoid levels among these individuals, as well as an increased risk of cardiovascular disease. These physiological problems teach us that it can be enormously stressful to construct a world in which there are no stressors.

This section has reviewed a number of different versions in which individuals have maladaptive stress-responses. In some cases, these aberrant coping styles are explicitly linked to an increased risk of stress-related disease. Moreover, these patterns are seen in significant percentages of the population. Amid this bad news, it is important to emphasize that this need not represent biology inevitably taking its toll—various forms of psychotherapy, of stress management techniques, and so on, have been shown to have good behavioral/affective consequences (making depressed individuals feel less depressed, blunting the intensity of Type A behaviors, and so on), as well as changes in the stress physiology and the risk of stress-related disease.

Early Experience and Glucocorticoid Profiles

Two adults may also differ in their glucocorticoid profiles because of differences in early experience. In rodents, early experience can "imprint" the stress-response, in that there is a developmental critical period in which experience alters functioning of the stress-response for the rest of life (Francis et al. 1999; Liu et al. 1997; Meaney et al. 1988). Probably the best-studied of these phenomena is neonatal "handling." Removing a pup from its mother and placing it in a new cage for 15 minutes a day for the first three weeks of life induces a more efficient adrenocortical stress-response in adulthood. These rats have smaller stress-responses and return to baseline faster after the end of stress. In old age, they have lower basal glucocorticoid concentrations and less neuron loss. Handling after 3 weeks of age does not cause the effect.

Levine, in first describing this effect, called it "stress immunization," and this is an apt phrase. In medicine, infants are immunized with a mild version of a disease to stimulate the immune system into more efficient defenses against it thereafter. Similarly, handling represents stimulation of the stress-response with a mild stressor early, producing a more efficient response later.

It is reasonably well understood how handling causes these permanent changes. While the details are beyond the scope of this chapter, there is an increase in the sensitivity of the brain and the pituitary to the signal of circulating glucocorticoids, causing more efficient regulation of glucocorticoid secretion. This is accomplished by the creation of lifelong changes in the pattern of receptors for the hormones.

Rats in the real world are not normally handled by humans. Is the handling phenomenon of the laboratory relevant to the natural behavior of rats?

Recent work has shown that rat pups who are licked and groomed more than average by their mothers experience the same permanent physiological changes as seen in the handling phenomenon. Moreover, such early experience appears to make them more likely to carry out similar behaviors as mothers in adulthood, thereby passing on these endocrine traits as a case of nongenetic inheritance.

As a converse of the handling phenomenon, prenatal stress (in other words, stressing the rat during the latter stages of her pregnancy) or separating young rats from their mothers both produce elevated glucocorticoid levels in adulthood. The mechanisms underlying these lifelong changes appear to be the opposite of those that give rise to the low glucocorticoid levels in response to neonatal handling. As a final example of the importance and subtlety of these developmental effects, the deleterious consequences of prenatal stress can be reversed by increased amounts of maternal attention during the first few weeks of the rat pup's life.

Genetics and Glucocorticoid Profiles

Two individuals may also differ in glucocorticoid profiles because of genetic differences. In rats, a few strains have been shown to be congenitally less capable of dealing with mild, novelty-related stressors. They do not learn as well, are less exploratory, and defecate more (a sensitive index of anxiety in rats). They also hypersecrete ACTH and glucocorticoids at such times. Importantly, these rats are normal under basal situations or in response to major physical stressors. The genetic difference seems to be one of sensitivity to mild psychological stressors (Gentsch, Lichtesteiner, and Feer 1988; Suomi 1987).

Little is known about the causes of these strain differences. Even less is known about the genetics of the stress-response in primates and humans. In one study, emotional reactivity, glucocorticoid secretion, and styles of mothering were characterized in rhesus monkeys in which crossfostering experiments had been carried out—a child of a highly reactive high-cortisol female might be raised by an unreactive low-cortisol female, and so on. A small amount of heritability of these traits was suggested.

Some Remaining Questions About These Models and Their Interactions

These previous sections suggest that two individuals may differ in their glucocorticoid profiles because of their social rank, the stability of the society in which they live, their personality, their immediate history of frequency of exposure to stressors, their prenatal experience, or their genetics. Some critical areas of research remain in considering these individual differences and some of the questions remaining follow.

HOW DO THESE VARIOUS CAUSES OF INDIVIDUAL DIFFERENCES INTERACT?

This is an immensely complicated question. A few conclusions can be emphasized. The "good physiology" (for example, low basal glucocorticoid concentrations) does not cause the dominance rank. First, dominant males with certain personality styles are unlikely to have that physiological profile, showing that it is not a prerequisite for dominance. Second, in studies of captive primates it is generally impossible to look at adrenocortical measures in animals when they are housed alone and predict who will be dominant in a social group. Finally, artificially lowering glucocorticoid concentrations does not make someone dominant.

In contrast, personality traits involving social control and the way one deals with predictability contribute a great deal to the achievement and maintenance of high rank and to the physiology of the individual. One would then predict that males with the "low cortisol" personality had those distinctive personality traits even when they were younger and socially subordinate; this is now being studied. If it is the case, it implies that for some males the main point is that they are not in the lowest rank (whether they are number 2 or number 9 in a hierarchy of 10) whereas for others, the point is that they are still not in the highest rank (whether they are number 2 or 9). The personality differences, in turn, seem to reflect both genetic and prenatal influences.

WHERE DO THESE PERSONALITY DIFFERENCES COME FROM?
This remains an immensely complicated issue, at the center of research by large numbers of developmental psychologists.

WHAT NEUROENDOCRINE MECHANISMS UNDERLIE THESE INDIVIDUAL DIFFERENCES?
The task is to take the complex endocrine cascades encompassing the brain, pituitary, and peripheral organs and then to determine what point in the cascade works differently, depending on factors such as rank, personality, history, and genetics. Some of these complex studies have been alluded to. As a broad conclusion, these mechanisms are extremely varied. You cannot conclude that, for example, the pituitary accounts for individual differences in all of these systems or that a decreased number of receptors is the main cellular mechanism mediating these differences, and so on. For example, dominant baboons have lower basal glucocorticoid concentrations in part because their brains are more sensitive to the inhibitory effects of circulating glucocorticoids. In contrast, these same animals have higher testosterone concentrations during stress, in part because their testes are less sensitive to the inhibitory effects of circulating glucocorticoids. The individual differences occur at the brain, pituitary, or peripheral level and can involve enhanced or decreased tissue sensitivity to signals, which in turn involve probably effects on the numbers and the functioning of receptors as well as post-receptor mechanisms.

DO ANY OF THESE INDIVIDUAL DIFFERENCES MATTER?
Do organisms with the lower basal glucocorticoid concentrations live longer and have fewer heart attacks and better immune systems to combat disease?

These are difficult questions to answer. In the laboratory, animals are not exposed to the normal array of pathogens, so laboratory study requires rather artificially controlled exposure to disease. In the field, the difficulty is that the investigator must follow the same wild individuals over many decades of their lifetimes, and it is difficult to be certain what diseases they might have. Moreover, because dominance rank among male Old World monkeys tends to change over time, there is more pressure to follow the animals over their whole lifetime—a subordinate male with elevated glucocorticoid concentrations this year may be a dominant terror in a few years, with lower glucocorticoid levels. Any given year's data are like single still photographs of a very dynamic, changing scene.

Nevertheless, there is evidence that these individual differences matter. For example, in stable social groups of primates, high-ranking monkeys are less prone to atherosclerotic plaque formation in their blood vessels than are subordinates. A fair amount is known about the long-term consequences of neonatal handling in rats. Glucocorticoid exposure over the lifetime of a rat contributes to some aspects of hippocampal aging and degeneration. Thus, one might predict that handled rats, in their old age, would have less hippocampal degeneration and less of the cognitive deficits that arise from such degeneration; this is observed.

HOW READILY DO THESE FINDINGS CARRIED OUT WITH ANIMALS APPLY TO HUMANS?

This remains unclear in many cases, for a number of reasons. First, it is obviously immensely difficult to carry out studies with humans—focusing on, for example, what neonatal stress has to do with old age. Next, it is often ethically impossible to carry out well-controlled studies of stress in humans— obviously one does not want to impose serious stressors, and the spontaneously occurring stressors often come with other confounds that are difficult to control for. Finally, it is often difficult to translate findings about behavior and emotion in the animal world to that of humans.

HOW ARE THESE FINDINGS MOST RELEVANT TO US?

An inability to initiate a stress-response would obviously be catastrophic. In two human examples of this situation, Addison's disease (in which the glucocorticoid component of the stress-response is blunted because of adrenal insufficiency) and Shy-Drager syndrome (in which the sympathetic component is blunted), individuals are extremely fragile. But these are rare cases. Few of us will get sick because we have too small a stress-response. Our problem, overwhelmingly, is an overactivation.

This problem is compounded further by the circumstances under which our stress-response is overactivated. If we were to list the stressful things in our lives, the leading categories would probably be time and financial pressures, family conflicts, the tensions and disappointments of our social lives, and job dissatisfaction. Few of us are likely to list droughts, locust infestations, malaria attacks during the rainy season, or close calls with predators. In our ecologically buffered lives, we encounter few of the physical stressors that our ancestors did and that most mammals on earth still do. Instead, we have the luxury of making ourselves sick with psychological and social stressors. Given the pathogenicity of psychological stressors, we are more at risk for developing an ulcer at some point in our life than a zebra is.

Because of this, the studies concerning psychological modulation of the stress-response are profoundly important. Repeatedly, the lesson from such studies is that although external events may be stressful, the pathogenic impact of such events can be blunted considerably by psychological variables. If that is the case for a rat encountering something as unambiguously stressful as electric shocks, it should certainly be true for us and our lives, which encompass far more subtle, ambiguous stressors. We may have to rely on highly interventionist medical technology to repair us once we get sick with a stress-related disorder. But by manipulating psychological variables concerning sense of control, predictability, and so on, we have a tremendous power within ourselves to control whether we get a stress-related disorders in the first place.

Summary

1. The stress-response involves changes in a tremendous array of endocrine and neural systems. These responses are somewhat (but not entirely) nonspecific to the type of stressor that triggers them.

2. When provoked for relatively brief periods in response to physical stressors, these responses seem fairly adaptive in helping an organism survive. Thus, an inability to initiate this stress-response appropriately can be quite deleterious.

3. These same responses, when provoked chronically or repeatedly, can cause or exacerbate numerous diseases. Stress-related disease can be considered to emerge most frequently from an overactivation of the stress-response rather than from a failure of that response. Thus, an inability to terminate the stress-response appropriately can be highly pathogenic.

4. The extent to which an external stressor provokes the stress-response can be modulated by intervening psychological variables. In the right psychological setting, a stress-response can be provoked even without an external stressor. Psychological stressors appear to be stressful to the extent that they contain elements of loss of control, loss of predictability, and absence of outlets for frustration.

5. Considerable individual variation exists in the workings of the stress-response. These differences can arise from differing genetic or developmental histories and from more recent factors, such as social status and the nature of the society in which an organism lives. These differences may reflect differing psychological makeups (i.e., organisms may differ in whether they perceive the same event as stressful) and physiological makeup (i.e., once the event is perceived as stressful, organisms differ in how their various organ systems respond.

Study Questions

1. What is the logic of the stress response?
2. You are walking home late at night when all of a sudden you think you hear someone behind you. You trip and fall causing a bad gouge in your leg which starts bleeding. Whoever is behind you seems to be getting closer. You manage to get up and run down the street to your house about a mile away. Describe everything that is happening to your stress system during these events.
3. How might the events you experienced in question 2 been different if you had been with a friend? Your dog? Why?
4. What would you experience if this happened to you every night? How would your responses be different if this was a chronic stress situation?
5. How does social rank affect the stress response? Describe how this impacts your life.

References

Ader, R., Felten, D., Cohen, N. (1991) *Psychoneuroimmunology*, 2nd edition. San Diego: Academic Press.

Adler, N., Boyce, T., Chesney, M., Folkman, S., and Syme, S. (1993) Socioeconomic inequalities in health: No easy solutions. *JAMA* 269: 3140.

Antonovsky, A. (1968) Social class and the major cardiovascular diseases. *J. Chron. Dis.* 21: 65.

Besedovsky, H., and Del Ray, A. (1996) Immuno-neuro-endocrine interactions: Facts and hypotheses. *Endo. Rev.* 17: 64.

Booth-Kewley, S., and Friedman, H. (1987) Psychological predictors of heart disease: A quantitative review. *Psychol. Bull.* 101: 343–362.

Dharbhar, F., and McEwen, B. (1996) Stress-induced enhancement of antigen-specific cell-mediated immunity. *J. Immunol.* 156: 2608.

Dunn, A. (1989) Psychoneuroimmunology for the psychoneuroendocrinologist: A review of animal studies of the nervous system-immune system interactions. *Psychoneuroendocrinology* 14: 251–274.

Evans, R., Barer, M., and Marmor, T. (1994) *Why Are Some People Healthy and Others Not? The Determinants of Health of Populations.* New York: Aldine de Gruyter.

Fox, B. (1983) Current theory of psychogenic effects on cancer incidence and prognosis. *J. Psychosoc. Oncol.* 1: 17–31.

Francis, D., Diorio, J., Liu, D., and Meaney, M. J. (1999) Nongenomic transmission across generations of maternal behavior and stress responses in the rat. *Science* 286: 1155.

Frankenhaeuser, M. (1980) Psychoneuroendocrine approaches to the study of stressful person-environment interactions. In H. Selye (Ed.), *Selyes's Guide to Stress Research.* New York: Van Nostrand, pp. 46–70.

Friedman, H., and Booth-Kewley, S. (1987) The "disease prone personality": A meta-analytic view of the construct. *Am. Psychol.* 42: 539–555.

Gentsch, C., Lichtensteiner, M., and Feer, H. (1988) Genetic and environmental influences on behavioral and neurochemical aspects of emotionality in rats. *Experimentia* 44: 482–499.

Goodman, H. (1980) The pancreas and regulation of metabolism. In V. Mountcastle (Ed.), *Medical Physiology*, 14th edition. St. Louis: C. V. Mosby, pp. 1638–1676.

House, J., Landis, K., and Umberson, D. (1988) Social relationships and health. *Science* 241: 540–544.

Levenstein, S., Prantera, C., Varvo, V., Scriobano, M., Berto, E., Spinella, S., and Lanari, G. (1995) Patterns of biologic and psychologic risk factors in duodenal ulcer patients. *J. Clin. Gastroenterol.* 2: 110.

Levine, S., Weiner, S., and Coe, C. (1989) The psychoneuroendocrinology of stress: A psychobiological perspective. In F. R. Brush and S. E. Levine (Eds.), *Psychoneuroendocrinology.* New York: Academic Press.

Liu, D., Diorio, J., Tannenbaum, B., Caldji, C., Francis, D., Freedman, A., Sharma, S., Pearson, D., Plotsky, P. M., and Meaney, M. J. (1997) Maternal care, hippocampal glucocorticoid receptors, and hypothalamic-pituitary-adrenal responses to stress. *Science* 277: 1659.

Mason, J. (1968) A review of psychoendocrine research on the pituitary adrenal cortical system. *Psychosom. Med.* 30: 576–583.

Mason, J. (1975) A historical view of the stress field. *J. Hum. Stress* 1: 6–21.

Meaney, M. J., Aitken, D. H., van Berkel, C., Bhatnagar, S., and Sapolsky, R. M. (1988) Effects of neonatal handling on age-related impairments associated with the hippocampus. *Science* 766–768.

Melmed, R., and Gelpin, Y. (1996) Duodenal ulcer: The helicobacterization of a psychosomatic disease? *Israeli J. Med. Sci.* 32: 211.

Miller, N. (1980) Effects of learning on physical symptoms produced by psychological stress. In H. Selye (Ed.), *The Stress of Life*. New York: McGraw-Hill.

Munck, A., Guyre, P., and Holbrook, N. (1984) Physiological actions of glucocorticoids in stress and their relation to pharmacological actions. *Endocr. Rev.* 5: 25–48.

Olson, G. A., Olson, R. D., Vaccarino, A. L., and Kastin, A. J. (1997) Endogenous opiates. *Peptides 1998* 19: 1791–1843.

Pincus, T., and Callanhan, L. (1995) What explains the association between socioeconomic status and health: Primarily access to medical care of mind-body variables? *Advances* 11: 4.

Rabin, D., Gold, P., Margioris, A., and Chrousos, G. (1988) Stress and reproduction: Physiologic and pathophysiologic interactions between stress and reproductive axes. In G. Chrousos, D. Loriaux, and P. Gold. (Eds.), *Mechanisms of Physical and Emotional Stress*. New York: Plenum Press.

Reichlin, S. (1998) Neuroendocriology. In J. Wilson, D. Foster, W. Kronenberg, and W. Larsen (Eds.), *Williams Textbook of Endocrinology*, 9th edition. Philadelphia: Saunders.

Sapolsky, R. M. (1998) *Why Zebras Don't Get Ulcers: A Guide to Stress, Stress-Related Diseases and Coping*, 2nd edition. New York: W.H. Freeman.

Sapolsky, R. M. (1993) Endocrinology alfresco: Psychoendocrine studies of wild baboons. *Rec. Prog. Horm. Res.* 48: 437.

Sapolsky, R. M. (1991) Testicular function, social rank and personality among wild baboons. *Psychoneuroendocrinology* 16: 281.

Sapolsky, R. M. (1990) Stress in the wild. *Sci. Am.* 262: 116–123.

Sapolsky, R., Romero, M., Munck, A. (2000) How do glucocorticoids influence the stress-response? Integrating permissive, suppressive, stimulatory, and preparative actions. *Endo. Rev.* 21: 55–89.

Sapolsky, R. Hormonal correlates of personality and social contexts: From non-human to human primates. (1999) In C. Panter-Brick and C. Worthman (Eds.), *Hormones, Health and Behaviour: A Socio-Ecological and Lifespan Perspective*. Cambridge, UK: Cambridge University Press, p. 18.

Selye, H. (1976) *The Stress of Life*. New York: McGraw-Hill.

Shekelle, R., Raynor, W., Ostfeld, A., Garron, D., Bieliauskas, L., Liu, S., Maliza, C., and Paul, O. (1981) Psychological depression and 17-year risk of death from cancer. *Psychosom. Med.* 43: 117–125.

Shively, C., Jayo, M., Weaver, D., and Kaplan, J. (1991) Reduced vertebral bone mineral density in socially subordinate female cynomologus macaques. *Am. J. Primatol.* 24: 135.

Suomi, S. (1987) Genetic and maternal contributions to individual differences in rhesus monkey biobehavioral development. In N. Krasnegor, E. Blass, M. Hofer, and W. Smotherman. (Eds.), *Perinatal Development: A Psychobiological Perspective*. New York: Academic Press.

Syme, S., and Berkman, L. (1976) Social class, susceptibility and sickness. *Am. J. Epidemiol.* 104: 1.

Terman, G., Shavit, Y., Lewis, J., Cannon, J., and Liebeskind, J. (1984) Intrinsic mechanisms of pain inhibition: Activation by stress. *Science* 226: 1270.

Warren, M. (1983) Effects of undernutrition on reproductive function in the human. *Endocrinol. Rev.* 4: 363–377.

Weiner, H. (1992) *Perturbing the Organism: The Biology of Stressful Experience*. Chicago: University of Chicago Press.

Weiss, J. (1972) Psychological factors in stress and disease. *Sci. Am.* 226: 104.

Weiss, J. (1970) Somatic effects of predictable and unpredictable shock. *Psychosom. Med.* 32: 397–414.

12   Hormones and Biological Rhythms

Michael R. Gorman and Theresa M. Lee

In physiology, as in humor, timing is everything. We will find that hormones are almost always secreted in pulses and patterns across time. The timing of these pulses, both in terms of their duration and the time of day at which they occur, can have a significant impact on their effects. Animals have evolved a quite sophisticated neural clock that keeps track of the time of day and the season of the year. You will not be surprised to learn that hormones respond to this clock to help animals prepare for the future.

Why must animals keep track of the time of day and season of the year, and what neural structures provide this information? What are the various temporal patterns of hormone release and which environmental stimuli regulate the patterns? Can hormones affect the time-keeping mechanism itself?

Introduction

Unlike many of the chapters in this book, this chapter will not focus on a single class of functionally related behaviors such as feeding, mating, or parenting. Chronobiology, or the study of biological rhythms, concerns itself with the timing of events within and external to an animal. We will talk about phenomena that you will encounter in other chapters in this text, but from a different perspective. What you will learn here is that the *timing* of a performed behavior or the *timing* of a hormonal event can be as important as the behavior that is performed or the hormone that is secreted. Not surprisingly, life forms of every level of complexity, from single cells to plants to animals, have evolved timing systems that are important to virtually every type of behavior and physiology.

Almost every location on earth shows predictably recurring, or periodic, environmental fluctuations, with deep caves and the deepest oceans showing little enough variation to be considered exceptions to this rule. Most environments are alternately light and dark, hot and cold, damp and dry, food abundant and food scarce. Given the impressive evidence of natural selection generating organisms well adapted to their environments, how might animals respond to regularly *changing* environments? As discussed in chapter 7, evolution has devised multiple strategies to cope with this predictable variation. One strategy is to move from one favorable location to another and to avoid predictable extremes. Thus, many species of songbirds migrate thousands of miles from their summer territories to spend the winters at more moderate locations.

But this strategy is not a feasible response to more rapidly fluctuating conditions, such as occurs between day and night, and is not even the most predominant seasonal strategy used by mammals. Instead, most organisms remain in their local environments but alter their behavior and physiology in a way that allows them to survive changing conditions. For example, ground squirrels hibernate throughout the winter. This adaptation vastly reduces the amount of energy squirrels require when food is scarce.

A variety of environmental periodicities characterizes life on earth. The rotation of the earth on its axis generates a daily fluctuation in light (day and night) which in turn contributes to variations in temperature, humidity, and other factors. The rotation of the earth around the sun yields a yearly cycle in the earth's exposure to the warming rays of the sun. The number of hours of sunlight (referred to as day length or photoperiod) is greatest on the summer solstice and least on the winter solstice. These times of year are also characterized in temperate regions (a zone midway between the equatorial and polar regions) by warm and cold temperatures, and abundant and scare food resources, respectively.

A different, but equally important, set of periodicities characterizes life in the sea. Most marine organisms live near the shore where they are affected by tides. The rotation of the moon about the earth generates tides with periodicities of 24.8 hours (a tidal rhythm) and, superimposed upon that rhythm, approximately 29.2 days (a circalunatidal rhythm). Unfortunately, this chapter will not be able to discuss these latter fascinating rhythms except to mention that many of the general principles discussed hold true even in these seemingly quite different environments.

Not surprisingly, animals, including humans, have evolved mechanisms to alter behavior and physiology to match each of these environmental rhythms. Perhaps the most obvious biological rhythm is the daily pattern of rest and activity that characterizes most of us. But the propensity to sleep is by no means the only behavioral or physiological function to vary throughout the day. On the contrary, we are hard pressed to find more than a handful of functions that do not exhibit variation over the course of a day (figure 12.1).

One example worth remembering for future use is the daily rhythm of pain sensitivity to various dental procedures: responsiveness of teeth to cold or electrical stimulation is maximal early in the morning (when dentists seem to prefer to make appointments) and minimal in late afternoon. Moreover, the duration of effective numbing from a given dose of topical dental anesthetic is also longer in the late afternoon than at other times of day. Of greater immediate relevance to this book, the patterns of secretion of most hormones likewise vary over the course of the day. For example, the monthly surge in luteinizing hormone (LH), which induces ovulation in women, typically occurs around 4 to 6 AM, and growth hormone and melatonin are secreted predominantly, or exclusively, at night.

It is important to note that rhythmic fluctuations in physiology and behavior are not subtle: hormone concentrations commonly vary by 3 to 10-fold

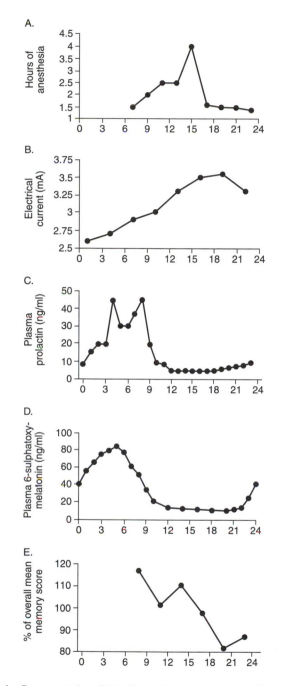

Figure 12.1   Representative 24 h fluctuations in various behavioral and physiological variables in humans. (*A*) Duration of numbness after application of local anesthetic to the jaw; (*B*) threshold values of electrical current inducing tooth pain; (*C*) plasma prolactin levels; (*D*) plasma concentrations of the major end product of melatonin, 6-sulphatoxymelatonin; and (*E*) performance on a memory task expressed as a percentage of overall mean score throughout the day. (Data redrawn from Aschoff and Wever 1981; Sassin et al. 1972; Bojkowski et al. 1987; Folkard and Monk 1980.)

over the day or across the year, and may vary by more than 100-fold. For example, the anesthetic effect of lidocaine lasts anywhere from 10 minutes at 6 AM to 30 minutes around 3 PM. Nor are the methodological, social, and medical consequences of such rhythms minor. If you are conducting an experiment involving measurement of a hormone that has a daily rhythm, any variation in collection times of your hormone sample will add unnecessary variability or "noise" to your data. Worse still, if you are comparing groups of subjects given two treatments, any difference in collection times between the two groups might look like an effect of your treatment when it may instead simply reflect the natural change in hormone levels throughout the day. Surprisingly, all scientists do not always remember this important lesson.

Outside of the scientific enterprise, daily rhythms in alertness and aspects of job performance are of critical interest for people working for the airlines, the military, nursing, or any industry in which human error can have grave consequences. Indeed, industrial accidents are most likely to occur when people are working at times of minimal alertness. In medicine, variations in physiological responses to toxic treatments (e.g., chemotherapy) are exploited to schedule therapies when their undesirable impacts are minimized and when their therapeutic effects are maximized. Lastly, a compelling rationale for studying these timed fluctuations stands apart from all of these practical implications: variation in function is one of the most basic organizational principles in biology. As you will see below, the study of biological rhythmicity represents one of the richest research opportunities to assess the intersection of behavior, hormones, brains, environments, and evolution. Additionally, few fields can rival this one for integration of, and cross-talk between, researchers in molecular biology and genetics, cellular physiology, behavior, ecology, evolution, medicine, and technology.

Circadian Clocks

Where do rhythms come from? Are they a simple byproduct of homeostatic mechanisms? In other words, do we not become sleepy at night simply because we have been awake all day and built up a "sleep debt?" And might we exhibit wakefulness the following morning because we have restored ourselves by sleeping the night before? By this view, daily rhythms might result from a chain of events, each triggering the next. Alternatively, rhythmic changes might depend on internal oscillations that *program* variation according to a strict temporal plan.

Our own experiences suggest which of these two proposed mechanisms generates some daily rhythms. Consider how alert you might feel if you deprived yourself of sleep, as most of you probably have when pulling an all-nighter—in preparation for final exams, for example. If you are typical of most people, you might report that you were quite alert until about 11 PM or 12 AM. If you failed to go to sleep, your alertness would likely decrease into the night. If you manage to remain awake throughout the night, your alertness ratings would eventually rebound, probably around 6 to 8 the following morning. Despite the fact that the number of hours since you last slept continues to grow, you become more rather than less alert at this time. If you are unfortunate enough to have to repeat your nocturnal performance the following night, this waning and waxing of alertness would continue the following night and day. There is a fluctuation, or rhythm, in your sleepiness that cannot be completely accounted for by the time elapsed since you last slept. Additionally, you probably could not sleep a full eight hours if you went to bed at noon after an all-nighter, further arguing against a "chain of events" model of rhythms.

But the persistence of varying alertness in the absence of sleep does not imply that the organism necessarily internally programs the rhythm. In the example above regarding the all-nighter, it may be the case that your alertness was simply a response to the amount of stimulation in the environment. Perhaps you get your second wind in the morning because your roommate wakes up and interacts with you. In the same way, seasonal fluctuations in allergy symptoms reflect the fact that ragweed pollens are more plentiful at certain times of year than others, and these elicit more or less severe allergy symptoms. For many years, this explanation—that rhythmic behaviors simply reflect *direct* responses to environmental fluctuations—held sway. To demonstrate that this is not the case, we need to show that the rhythm will persist when the environment is not fluctuating.

As part of this effort, humans have volunteered to live in caves away from social interactions and most environmental periodicities. Far simpler experiments, however, have been conducted on golden hamsters (also known as Syrian hamsters), which are one of chronobiologists' favorite animal subjects because of their impressive daily rhythms in their use of a running-wheel kept in their cage. If kept in a cage under otherwise natural environmental conditions, the nocturnal hamster will sleep most of the day. Shortly after dusk, the hamster will wake and begin running in its wheel (figure 12.2). This activity persists, sometimes with occasional interruptions, for most of the night. The hamster will cease running sometime before dawn.

This daily pattern repeats itself indefinitely with little variation in general form. Is this simply a response to the lights going out or the temperature dropping, or does this rhythm reflect some more complicated timing mechanism in the hamster's brain? Keeping the temperature constant does not elicit any change in the behavior, so animals are not being passively cued by temperature fluctuations. When the daily pattern of light is manipulated, some interesting results are obtained. If the lights are turned off for a few hours while the hamster sleeps in the afternoon (even if you wake the hamster), the hamster is unlikely to start running, suggesting that darkness is not a sufficient cue to elicit running. Moreover, if the lights are kept off chronically, the hamster will continue to show a rhythm of inactivity/activity indefinitely but with an important difference from that seen under natural conditions. Instead of initiating wheel-running at almost perfect 24-hour intervals, activity onset will drift to progressively later times each day. Each cycle length (i.e.,

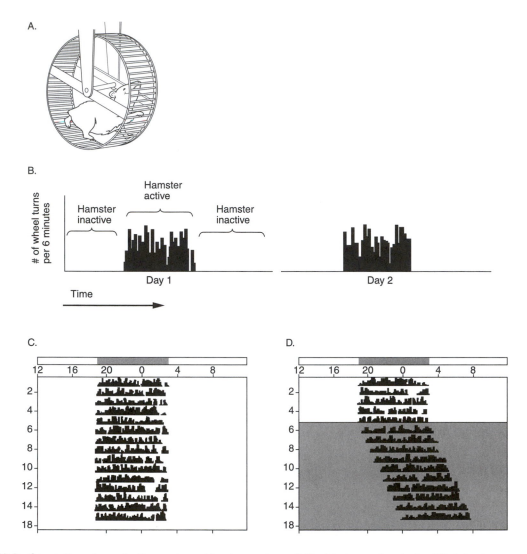

Figure 12.2 Conventions for collecting and graphing locomotor activity data in small rodents. (*A*) Animals are commonly housed in cages equipped with devices for measuring general activity around the cage or with wheels in which the animals are free to run at any time. A computer monitors the number of wheel revolutions (or alternative measures of activity) in each of many short intervals dividing the 24-hour day. (*B*) These are stored and are graphically displayed by generating a 24-hour plot of activity each day. Typically, successive days of activity are plotted below one another. (*C*) A hamster is housed in a light: dark cycle represented by the horizontal bar at the top. The shaded area of the bar indicates the hours each day that lights are off. Activity begins at approximately the same time each day. (*D*) The hamster is "free-running" in constant darkness that begins on the sixth day of the record, as indicated by the shading in the lower portion of the figure. The point at which the hamster begins running in the wheel each day (activity onset) drifts to the right as you read down graph illustrating a free-running rhythm with tau > 24 h.

period)—measured from the activity onset on one day to the activity onset the next day—would be close to, but probably not exactly, 24.0 hours.

The persistence of a daily rhythm in rest/activity in the absence of environmental fluctuation indicates that the organism is NOT being cued directly by the day/night cycle. Moreover, the fact that the length of the cycle is no longer the same as the natural day (24.0 hours) indicates that the rhythm is not being timed by any environmental fluctuation as there is no known environmental cue with such a period. In fact, a group of animals held in constant darkness will show a variety of periods (e.g., 24.10 hours, 23.92 hours, 23.95 hours), which suggests that each animal has a slightly different endogenous cycle length. Lastly, this result establishes that the daily light/dark cycle also normally serves to synchronize the endogenous rhythm to match the 24-hour period of the day.

We give the name "circadian," meaning approximately (circa) one day (dian), to describe *endogenously generated* biological rhythms. "Entrainment" is the process by which light (or other environmental cues) adjusts the endogenous circadian rhythm to 24.0 hours. The variables in the environment that entrain the rhythm are termed "zeitgebers" (meaning "time-giver" in German). Light serves this function for most organisms, although temperature, social interactions, and other environmental signals can play entraining roles in various species. Figure 12.2 illustrates an entrained rhythm and describes the conventions for graphing activity patterns.

The Freerunning Period

Studies such as these have allowed scientists to characterize the functional, or formal, properties of circadian systems—that is, without knowing anything about the physical basis of circadian clocks, we can nevertheless describe their behavior in abstract terms. The most important properties are the freerunning period in constant darkness and the response of the rhythm to light pulses which can entrain it. The freerunning period, τ (pronounced "tau"), is simply the length of the daily cycle in constant conditions such as chronic darkness or chronic light. The freerunning rhythm is measured by first identifying some characteristic portion or "phase" of the rhythm, such as the beginning or end of nocturnal wheel-running. Other common phase markers are the body temperature minimum and maximum. The length of time elapsing between the same phase markers on successive days is the period of the rhythm.

Phase-Shifting

Characterization of the response to light pulses is somewhat more complicated, but illustrates the exquisite adaptation of the circadian system. The function of light is to keep the internal rhythm synchronized with the natural day, and to re-entrain the rhythm with the natural day if it is not synchronized (for example, after a plane trip crossing several time zones). Consider the nocturnal hamster that should be limiting its time outside the burrow to the night to avoid predation. It typically leaves its burrow shortly after dusk and returns before dawn, thereby avoiding much light exposure. Suppose now that for whatever reason the hamster's rhythm runs fast so that the animal's internal clock prompts it to leave the burrow 45 to 60 minutes before dusk. In this event, the hamster will receive a substantial exposure to light from the time it emerges from the burrow until dusk. Light exposure at this time, when the animal's circadian mechanism prompts it to begin nighttime foraging (i.e., "subjective night"), causes the clock to be reset in an adaptive manner: the light pulse effectively resets the clock to an earlier time, physiologically telling the hamster "it is not 6 PM as you thought, but 5 PM." This resetting effectively adds an additional hour to the next cycle, realigning the hamster's rhythm with the natural day.

Now suppose instead that the hamster's clock runs late and therefore drifts out of synchrony in the other direction. If the hamster wakes up one hour late and leaves the burrow, it will neither "expect" light nor be exposed to any in the first half of the night. But near the end of the night the hamster's clock would expect an additional hour of foraging time in darkness when the sun comes up. Light exposure near the end of the night causes the clock to be set to a later phase—"it is not 5 AM as you think, but 6 AM." The next cycle length will thus be shortened by an hour.

Finally, consider the hamster that must leave its burrow in the middle of the day (for example, if the burrow is flooded). If the animal's time-sense tells it that it is the day, it will expect light exposure and receive it. In this event, light does not shift the rhythm at all. In summary, animals have a clock that is sensitive to resetting by light during the time that their clock tells them it is night (i.e., subjective night). Bright light falling during the subjective night tells the clock that it is improperly set (moonlight and starlight are generally not bright enough to reset animal clocks). Whether light causes the clock to be reset earlier or later depends on whether it falls early or late in the subjective night. The result is that clocks are quickly realigned with the 24-hour light:dark cycle. The use of terms such as "subjective night" notwithstanding, circadian rhythms and their resetting are not mediated at a conscious level of awareness.

Normally, clocks do not drift so far out of synchrony with the natural day as in this example. Instead, light exposures around dawn or dusk make very subtle adjustments so that the resulting phase shifts just make up for the difference between the free-running period and 24.0 hours. That is, if $\tau = 23.9$, light resets the clock to add 0.1 hour each day. If $\tau = 24.2$, light falls at a time which shortens the next cycle by 0.2 hour.

Humans, however, frequently find themselves requiring re-entrainment to the light:dark cycle. When you travel rapidly to a new time zone, your clock is initially out of phase with local time. Light and perhaps other environmental cues require several days to re-entrain the endogenous rhythm to the natural day. In the process of adjusting to local time, circadian rhythms may be temporarily disorganized and cause symptoms of jet lag. These symptoms include diminished cognitive abilities and alertness, disturbed sleep, stomach/intestinal distress, and a general feeling of malaise. The symptoms are the result of an internal desynchrony between various behavioral and physiological rhythms that occurs when readjustment to the new time zone happens at different rates for different rhythms. For example, behavioral rhythmicity (sleep onset, waking, eating) appears normal much sooner than internal rhythms such as cortisol release and core body temperature.

Phase Response Curve

A more systematic characterization of the phase-shifting light pulses at all parts of the animal's circadian cycle is called a phase-response curve or PRC and is usually derived by housing animals in constant dim light or darkness (figure 12.3). Briefly, light (or another stimulus) is presented at each phase of the daily rhythm, and the effect of each light pulse on the rhythm is measured and graphed. For example, near the beginning of the daily activity cycle, hamsters are exposed to a short light pulse. As described above, light falling at this time causes the subsequent activity onset to occur later than would be expected from the previous free-running rhythm. The size of this delay is calculated. Because our phase marker (activity onset) was shifted later, we say the rhythm was phase-shifted or phase-delayed.

Next, hamsters are exposed to similar light pulses at all phases of the endogenous rhythm (e.g., 2, 4, 6, or 8 hours after activity onset) and deflections from the free-running pattern are again calculated. The phase shift at each phase of the cycle is then plotted to yield the PRC. To adjust for the fact that τ is not exactly 24 hours in DD, the cycle is divided into 24 equivalent fractions termed circadian hours. By convention, the phase in the cycle where activity onset occurs is labeled "circadian time 12" (CT12) in nocturnal animals and CT0 in diurnal animals and other circadian times are derived in relation to these reference points. For example, CT2 occurs 2 circadian hours after CT0. PRCs differ somewhat between nocturnal and diurnal animals, between different species and even individuals, but they have more similarities than differences. Specifically, most are comprised of phase-advancing intervals that tend to fall during late subjective night (CT18–CT24), phase-delaying intervals in the early subjective night (CT12–CT18) and intervals of reduced responsiveness during the subjective day (CT0–CT12). In hamsters, light has no effect in most of the subjective day and so this interval has been called a "deadzone."

The Role of the Suprachiasmatic Nucleus (SCN)

Although circadian rhythms have been studied for decades, interest in the field exploded following the identification of a nucleus in the brain apparently responsible for generating daily rhythms. In the early 1970s it was accepted that light shifted circadian rhythms, as described above, and that the eyes were necessary for the effects of light on circadian rhythms in mammals. Moreover, anatomical studies had just identified a direct neural

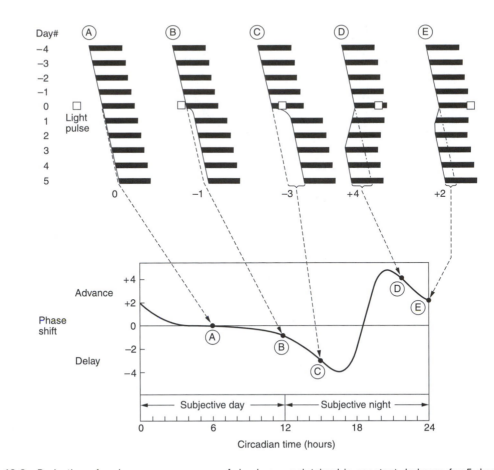

Figure 12.3 Derivation of a phase-response curve. Animals are maintained in constant darkness for 5 days before they are exposed to a brief light pulse. Darkness also persists for several days following the light pulse. In repeated experiments, the light pulse is scheduled to fall at every phase of the animal's circadian cycle. At time point *A*, in the subjective day, the free-running rhythm looks no different before and after the light pulse. Thus, there is no shift of the rhythm. At time point *B*, however, the rhythm after the light pulse is shifted by 1 hour to the right (a delay of the rhythm). Thus, in the graph below, a 1-hour phase delay is plotted for a light pulse falling at the beginning of subjective night (called circadian time 12). Similarly, large delays are seen after light pulses falling at circadian time 15 (*C*). At circadian time 22, the rhythm is seen to be shifted (after several days) to the left. This reflects a shifting earlier or phase-advance. In this fashion, a PRC for the entire circadian cycle is generated.

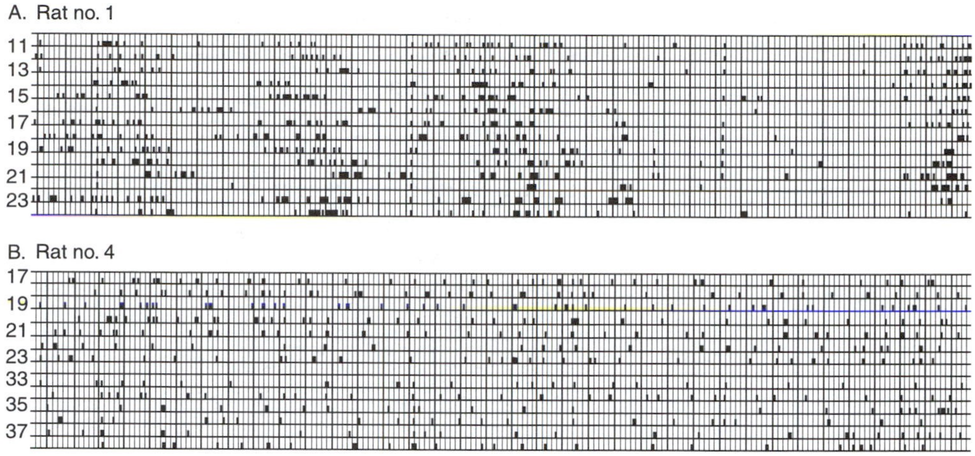

A. Rat no. 1

B. Rat no. 4

Figure 12.4 Activity records of blinded rats with intact (*top*) or lesioned (*bottom*) SCNs. *Top:* A daily rhythm is clearly present as indicated by the greater concentration of activity in the left half of the figure. *Bottom:* Activity appears to be randomly distributed throughout the 24-hour day. (Figure from Stephan and Zucker 1972.) Note that the activity rhythms collected from rats are not characterized by the clearly defined activity onset and offset collected from other species illustrated in figures 12.2, 12.7, and 12.11. The rhythms collected from different species often differ markedly, although underlying circadian principles seem to hold.

connection between the retina and the suprachiasmatic nuclei (SCN) so named because they are found just above (supra) the crossing (optic chiasm) of the optic nerves of the hypothalamus of mammals (Moore and Lenn 1972).

The SCN Is a Master Oscillator

Because the hypothalamus was additionally known to regulate multiple functions that express daily rhythms, two groups of researchers decided to lesion the target of the retinal projections, the SCN, and assess whether rhythms could still be shifted by light (Stephan and Zucker 1972; Moore et al. 1972). To their surprise, the rhythms could not be shifted because there was no rhythm left to be shifted (figure 12.4). Cortisol secretion, drinking, and activity, previously robustly rhythmic, all became arrhythmic. All of these functions continued to occur, but they showed no regular 24-hour pattern.

These results could not yet be taken to indicate that the SCN was the generator of original rhythms. For example, a circadian generator located elsewhere in the brain might send its projections through the SCN so that destruction of the SCN would disconnect the circadian pacemaker from the rest of the brain. Several other types of studies would be required to more firmly establish the SCN as the master oscillator. Briefly, investigators next demonstrated that the SCN showed daily rhythms in spontaneous neural firing rates and in metabolic activity (Schwartz and Gainer 1977). The latter was determined by injecting animals with a glucose analogue (2-DG) that accumulated in metabolically active tissues and which could be visualized in brain slices examined post mortem. Again, this evidence suggests but does not prove that there is a timing mechanism in the SCN: it could also be the case that the rhythmic function of the SCN is controlled by a timing mechanism located somewhere else.

Investigators next demonstrated that the electrical rhythms in the SCN were still present after the SCN region was disconnected from the rest of the hypothalamus by knife cuts (so-called SCN-island experiments) (Inouye and Kawamura 1979). Moreover, rhythms of neural firing outside the hypothalamus that were present prior to surgery disappeared, suggesting that the isolated SCN were their original source. Two other important methods, however, conclusively established the importance of the SCN for rhythm generation. First, thin slices of the hypothalamus containing the SCN were collected and kept alive in a petri dish, where rhythms in the rate of spontaneous neural firing could be monitored for several days (Gillette and Prosser 1988; Shibata al. 1989). The results clearly showed that SCN rhythms did not originate outside of the hypothalamic slice and also demonstrated that these electrical firing rates could be phase-shifted by pharmacological agents.

Lastly, and most definitively, investigators satisfied one of the strictest criteria for establishing a brain behavior relationship—a removal and replacement study. Adult hamsters had their SCN destroyed and, as expected, their locomotor activity rhythms were obliterated. At this point, tissue from the SCN region was collected from hamster fetuses shortly before they would have been born. When this tissue was transplanted into the third ventricle of adult hamsters lacking rhythms, the fetal SCN tissue survived and remained viable. Remarkably, the adult hamster lacking its original SCN once again began to show daily rhythms in activity (Drucker-Colin et al. 1984; Sawaki et al. 1984).

Even this incredible result, however, does not mean that the SCN is the source of the rhythm—perhaps it only produces some substance necessary to allow another clock to function. Studies with genetic mutants ruled out this possibility. Whereas most hamsters exhibit a free-running rhythm with a period very close to 24 hours, mutants were found to produce a rhythm with a 22-hour period in the heterozygous condition and 20-hour period in the homozygous state (Ralph and Menaker 1988). When fetal tissue from one of these mutants was transplanted into the ventricle of a wildtype, or normal, hamster that expressed a near 24-hour rhythm prior to ablation of its SCN, the new rhythm that emerged was characteristic of the mutant strain (Ralph et al. 1990). In other words, the donor tissue, not the host, dictated the period of the rhythm, providing the very strongest evidence that the donor SCN tissue was the source of the observed rhythmic behavior.

Despite this impressive line of evidence, the SCN cannot be considered the only oscillator in the brain capable of generating rhythmic behaviors. Studies of rats with SCN lesions illustrated that circadian activity rhythms could reappear if their drinking water was treated with methamphetamine (Honma et al. 1987). These results suggest that other, extra-SCN, oscillators are competent under certain conditions to produce circadian rhythms, although the location of these oscillators has not yet been identified.

More recently, a vast number of tissues throughout the body have been shown to be capable of transiently exhibiting circadian rhythms in the absence of control from the SCN. Rather than measuring rhythms such as activity and melatonin secretion that depend on complex physiological systems, scientists have monitored daily rhythms in cellular expression of specific genes related to circadian clocks (see below). For example, cells known as fibroblasts, derived from connective tissue of rats, can be grown on culture plates if provided with an adequate supporting solution (medium) containing all necessary nutrients. As these cells are cultured alone for many generations, there can be no ongoing influence of the SCN. While such cells were not initially rhythmic, an abrupt change in the medium (a so-called "serum shock") induced them to express a circadian rhythm in expression of many genes that lasted for several cycles (Balsalobre et al. 1998). Fresh tissue cultures of lung, liver, and skeletal muscle likewise showed circadian rhythms, at least for the first few days after dissection (Yamazaki et al. 2000).

When the whole organism is exposed to a phase-shifting light pulse, the SCN are rapidly reset (as described above), but resetting of the other rhythms requires additional time. These and other data paint a subtle but important new picture of circadian systems. Rather than thinking of the SCN as the only oscillator imparting a rhythm on nonrhythmic structures downstream, the SCN appears to be one of many oscillators and it most likely synchronizes and coordinates other very weakly rhythmic tissues. As you will see later, some of these tissues and their outputs may have reciprocal effects back on the SCN.

The SCN Generates Rhythms

The fact that the SCN can be considered a master pacemaker controlling a wide range of different behavioral and physiological rhythms does not mean that the SCN controls all these rhythms similarly. On the contrary, it appears that the connections of the SCN to other parts of the brain are extremely diverse. Here we will describe just three systems controlled by the SCN to illustrate the different output pathways used.

MELATONIN

The circadian system produces a daily rhythm in the secretion of the hormone melatonin from the pineal gland of most mammals (see figure 12.1). In most species, melatonin secretion is completely restricted to nighttime, with concentrations of the hormone in the blood increasing as much as a hundredfold each night. In many rodent species housed in a typical 14 hours of light and 10 hours of dark each day, melatonin secretion increases abruptly 1 to 2 hours after the lights go off. Secretion is high throughout most of the night and declines precipitously shortly before the lights go on in the morning (Goldman et al. 1981).

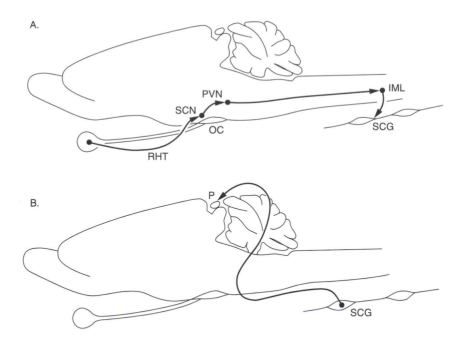

Figure 12.5 (*A*) Pathway by which the SCN controls the production and secretion of pineal melatonin. The suprachiasmatic nuclei (SCN) cells send projections to the paraventricular nucleus of the hypothalamus (PVN), which projects in turn to the intermediolateral column (IML) of the spinal cord. These neurons synapse on neurons with cell bodies in the superior cervical ganglion (SCG) in the sympathetic nervous system. (*B*) Neurons in the SCG send noradrenergic projections to the pineal gland (P). Note also that the SCN, located just dorsal to the optic chiasm (OT), receives a direct projection from the eye via the retino-hypothalamic tract.

This pattern of secretion is not a passive response to darkness but is a programmed rhythm that persists (freeruns) in constant darkness, indicating that it is controlled by the circadian system. The anatomical pathway allowing control of pineal melatonin secretion by the SCN is the best understood circadian output mechanism (Klein et al. 1983) (figure 12.5). The SCN sends efferents to the paraventricular nuclei of the hypothalamus (PVN), which in turn send projections that course through the brainstem and spinal cord where they exit and project to a group of cells (ganglion) that is part of the sympathetic nervous system. Cell bodies in the superior cervical ganglion send their projections back into the spinal cord and these travel to the pineal gland where they synapse on pinealocytes. Release of norepinephrine from the terminals of sympathetic cells onto pinealocytes triggers these latter cells to alter their production of enzymes that are necessary for making melatonin. When the levels of these enzymes are increased, melatonin production and secretion are correspondingly increased. Interruption of fibers anywhere in this convoluted trajectory, or blockade of neurotranmission at any synapse, eliminates the circadian rhythm of melatonin secretion in mammals (Klein et al. 1983).

THE OVARIAN CYCLE

The SCN uses a different set of outputs to influence LH secretion, a necessary component of the ovulatory cycle of female mammals. You may recall from an earlier chapter that the ovulatory surge in LH and the onset of behavioral estrus occur at a specific time during the light phase of female rodents. Despite the fact that the LH surge occurs only every 4th or 5th day in rats and hamsters, evidence from several sources indicates that the SCN is responsible for its precise timing. First, lesions of the SCN eliminate the ovarian cycle, although as discussed above, this cannot prove the SCN generates the ovarian cycle (Wiegand et al. 1980). More persuasively, in constant lighting the timing of the LH surge maintains its exact relationship to the locomotor activity rhythm, suggesting that it is controlled by the same circadian mechanism as the activity cycle (Fitzgerald and Zucker 1976).

Lengthening or shortening of the activity cycle by pharmacological treatments or entrainment by light is accompanied by identical lengthening or shortening of the rhythm of behavioral estrus and the LH surge (Carmichael et al. 1981). Lastly, an injection of pentobarbital on the morning of proestrus temporarily blocks the LH surge. The LH surge is not delayed merely until the pentobarbital is metabolized, nor is an entire 4- to 5-day cycle skipped. Rather, the LH surge occurs at precisely the normal time on the next day (Stetson and Watson-Whitmyre 1977).

This and other evidence suggest that there is a timed signal out of the SCN that causes the LH surge. The signal occurs daily but results in an LH surge only at the phase of the cycle supported by the appropriate milieu of gonadal hormones (see chapter 4). Because LH is secreted in a pulsatile form in direct response to its releasing hormone, GnRH, cells manufacturing the latter hormone most likely receive the circadian signal. Although GnRH is released from terminals in the median eminence, the cell bodies of GnRH neurons are found scattered throughout the rostral forebrain in the septum, diagonal band of Broca, anterior hypothalamus and preoptic area. The latter area has been particularly implicated in generating the LH surge.

How does a signal get from the SCN to GnRH cell bodies in the preoptic area? In both the hamster and the rat, the SCN makes direct projections to GnRH cells in the pre-optic area (and other areas as well) (de la Iglesia et al. 1995; van der Beek et al. 1997). Specifically, SCN cells concentrated in the ventro-lateral portion of the SCN and using vasoactive intestinal polypeptide (VIP) as a neurotransmitter are likely to project to GnRH neurons (van der Beek 1993). GnRH cells that are active around the time of the LH surge (as indicated by the presence of the marker of cell activity, c-Fos) are particularly likely to be receiving VIP inputs (van der Beek et al. 1994). Finally, because VIP is known to affect secretion of LH, this direct SCN-GnRH projection is a possible substrate for the circadian influence on the LH surge.

SCN neurons, however, project to many other nuclei besides those containing GnRH neurons. Some of these areas are just outside the SCN, and although they do not contain GnRH cell bodies themselves, they send projections in large numbers to GnRH cells in the preoptic area, raising the possibility that the SCN also indirectly innervates GnRH neurons. One of these regions, the subparaventricular hypothalamic nucleus, is a site where VIP can act to alter LH, and therefore presumably GnRH, secretion (Stobie and Weick 1990). Thus, in contrast to the straightforward series of three synapses connecting the SCN and pineal, the SCN may influence GnRH function through a more elaborate set of connections—some direct and others indirect. The specific roles of each of these pathways are still not understood.

WHEEL-RUNNING ACTIVITY

Finally, the SCN may use a completely different type of mechanism to generate daily rhythms in wheel-running activity. As indicated above, when circadian activity rhythms are eliminated following destruction of the SCN, they can be restored by implanting SCN tissue from embryonic brains into the brain of the arrhythmic animal. Notably, these transplants cannot restore circadian rhythms in melatonin secretion or several other normally rhythmic hormones known or suspected to be controlled by specific neural projections out of the SCN (Meyer-Bernstein et al. 1999). Moreover, the restoration of activity rhythms does not appear to depend on the reestablishment of neural connections between host brain tissue (the original arrhythmic hamster) and transplanted donor tissue. Fetal tissue that is encapsulated in a plastic barrier that prevents the outgrowth of axons but allows diffusion of small chemical signals is nonetheless able to restore activity rhythms (Silver et al. 1996). These results suggest that activity rhythms can be controlled humorally, by chemical signals, and that synapses of SCN neurons on tissue outside the SCN are not required. Whether the intact SCN uses exclusively humoral signals to control activity cannot be decided at this point. The identity of the chemical signal from the SCN is unknown.

Very recently it has been suggested that the chemical signal responsible for the timing of activity may derive from a small group of cells within the SCN of hamsters. In other words, these might be the specific cells that drive the circadian oscillation in activity. Original reports suggested that SCN lesions did not affect activity rhythms of hamsters as long as about 25% of the SCN was left undamaged, and that it did not matter which 25% of the SCN survived. More recent studies suggest that activity rhythms persist following SCN lesions only as long as a small group of cells expressing a calcium-binding protein, calbindin-D28K, are not lesioned (LeSauter and Silver 1999). Moreover, fetal cell transplants that restore activity rhythms in lesioned hamsters also contain calbindin-D28K cells. Transplants that lack these cells do not restore activity. In these studies, calbindin-D28K is only being used to identify a population of cells: the results do not mean that calbindin-D28K itself is the signal necessary for imparting rhythms to substrates governing locomotor activity. Indeed, some rodents show no or little calbindin-D28K but nonetheless exhibit robust circadian rhythms. Cells in the hamsters that are producing calbindin-D28K may secrete some other factor that is the critical signal.

Although all three of the rhythms described are controlled by the SCN, they illustrate the complexity and heterogeneity of the SCN and its output pathways. It is convenient to give the SCN a single label, but it is really composed of many cell populations with distinct inputs and outputs. Its mechanisms of control may include both humoral and neural actions. Understanding how other physiological and behavioral functions are controlled by the SCN will continue to be an active area of research.

SCN Function Changes with the Seasons

It may have occurred to you already that the day/night cycle is not constant throughout the year. Except at the equator, days are long in summer but short in winter and the difference between seasons becomes more extreme as you move towards the poles. If the circadian system functions to generate adaptive behaviors to match environmental variations, the system will need to be flexible to meet these seasonally fluctuating day/night conditions. Because the circadian system does indeed function very differently throughout the year, it has been considered "a clock for all seasons." We first consider how the circadian system might achieve the flexibility to program appropriate rhythms for summer and winter and then go on to consider the consequences of seasonal variation in one of the best-studied clock outputs—the pattern of daily melatonin secretion.

Evidence for seasonal variation in the circadian system can be found by looking closely at any number of rhythms that the circadian clock controls (figure 12.6). For example, locomotor activity in the cage (sometimes measured instead of wheel-running behavior) of hamsters entrained to a short night may be expressed at high levels for 4 to 6 hours, but in longer winter nights, the activity duration may be increased to 10 to 12 hours. As another example, the pattern of melatonin release during the dark period varies across the seasons and these changes also can be reproduced in the laboratory by simulating the day length of the different seasons (Bartness and Goldman 1989). Melatonin duration is short in the short nights (and long days) of summer and longer after entrainment to the long nights (and short days) of winter.

A slightly more complicated, but theoretically important, difference between circadian systems entrained to summer and winter light conditions appears in the response of the system to light pulses. Recall that the PRC was a description of how animals respond to light pulses at every phase of their near-24-hour rhythm. In the example depicted, the hamster had been entrained to a 14-hour day, 10-hour night. The PRC would look different in hamsters entrained to longer nights (e.g., 10-hour day, 14-hour night). The fraction of the PRC characterized by phase advances and phase delays would be expanded and the light-nonresponsive interval of the day would be reduced (see figure 12.6). In addition to covering a greater fraction of the cycle, the phase-shifts induced would also be larger in winter than in summer light conditions. Because we know that the SCN mediates phase-shifts, we must conclude that the SCN itself functions differently in different photoperiods.

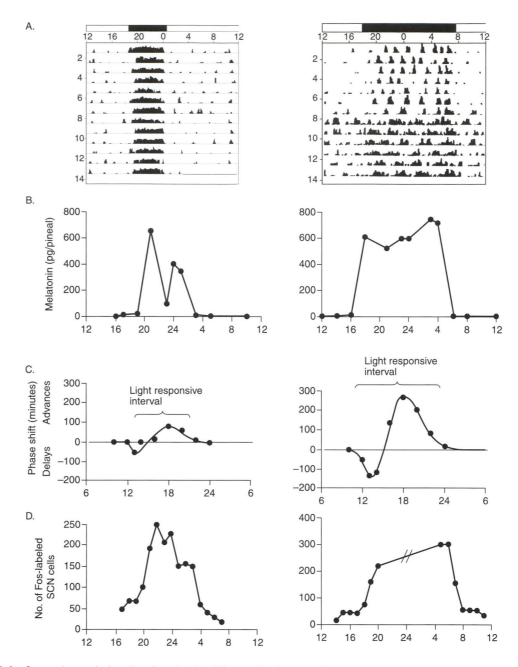

Figure 12.6 Comparison of circadian function in different day lengths. Rats or hamsters were maintained in light:dark cycles which simulated summer conditions (long days and short nights, *left column*) or winter conditions (short days and long nights, *right column*). (*A*) Hamster locomotor activity rhythms during entrainment to the light:dark conditions shown below the figure. Notice that the method of recording employed here—monitoring of general activity around the cage as recorded by infrared motion detectors above the cage—are not as noise-free as previous records of wheel-running, but a marked increase in general activity is still observed during the nighttime hours. (*B*) The concentration of melatonin present in the pineal glands of hamsters assayed at intervals throughout the day and night. (*C*) The PRCs of hamsters previously entrained to very long or short day lengths. After exposure to constant darkness for 10 days, hamsters were pulsed with light for 15 minutes throughout the circadian cycle and phase shifts were calculated and plotted. The interval of light responsiveness is marked in each plot to aid comparison. (*D*) The number of SCN cells responding to 30-minute light pulses throughout the circadian day after entrainment to long or short day lengths. (Data redrawn from Pittendrigh et al. 1984; Goldman et al. 1981; Sumova et al. 1995.)

More direct evidence comes from studies of Fos expression in the SCN after light pulses: recall that Fos immunoreactivity is a handy marker for cellular activity. At times of day where the PRC shows a phase-shift in response to a light pulse, cells in a part of the SCN that receive direct neural projections from the retina will express Fos protein after a light pulse. During the deadzone, the same light pulse causes no phase-shift and no Fos expression, presumably because those cells are unaffected by the light (see figure 12.6). In summer day lengths, Fos can be induced in the SCN for a shorter number of hours than in winter day lengths (Sumova et al. 1995).

To summarize, the circadian system generates quite different rhythms in many functions (activity, melatonin, PRC, and Fos-induction, to name just a few), depending on the "photoperiod," or number of hours of light, per day. When transferred to constant darkness, moreover, these rhythms freerun in synchrony, which implies that they are all controlled by a single mechanism (Elliott and Tamarkin 1994). Finally, the photoperiodic differences in activity duration, melatonin secretion, and so on can persist for several weeks in constant darkness.

Multiple Clocks in the SCN?

How is the SCN entrained to generate different melatonin signals in summer versus winter photoperiods? Most accounts suggest that seasonal flexibility could be achieved if the circadian pacemaker were really composed of two separate clocks linked, or coupled, together. The idea of multiple clocks was suggested by data obtained serendipitously when the light timer in an animal housing room malfunctioned causing the lights to remain on 24 hours a day. After about 6 weeks, some of the hamsters began exhibiting unusual rhythms (figure 12.7). Instead of a simple alternation between active and inactive periods summing up to slightly more than 24 hours, the rhythms split into two distinct components. Because the periods of the two components were different, it was suggested that a separate circadian oscillator controlled each component. Normally, the two oscillators were coupled and produced only a single bout of activity nightly (in nocturnal hamsters), but exposure to constant light disrupted the coupling and the oscillators drifted apart.

With two coupled oscillators, the flexible properties of the circadian oscillator can be readily modeled (figure 12.8). One oscillator, termed the evening (E) oscillator, is entrained such that it generates circadian events during the beginning of the night—melatonin secretion and activity are increased, and the SCN are responsive to light pulses. This oscillator tends to have a short period, which means that to be entrained to 24-hour light, it needs to delay slightly each day. A morning oscillator (M) programs these same functions nearer the end of night. But because its period is greater than 24 hours, it becomes phase advanced each day by morning light. The important point is that E and M can be entrained separately by evening and morning light. In short nights, E and M are pushed close together in overlapping phases so that the duration of all the nocturnal functions discussed is compressed. In longer

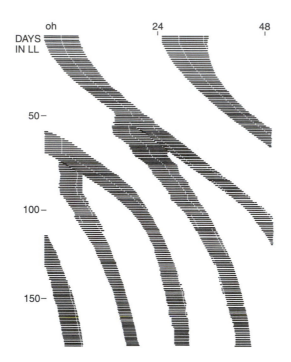

Figure 12.7 Splitting of hamster wheel-running rhythms into two components after prolonged exposure to constant light. Note that the figure is "double-plotted," meaning that each horizontal line graphs two days of data. This convention is commonly employed to aid viewing of free-running rhythms. Thus, splitting occurs midway through the figure where four activity components are observed on each horizontal line (two per day). Morning (M) and evening (E) components are identified based on the previous relationship to the unsplit rhythm. (From Earnest and Turek 1982.)

nights, the overlap is reduced as E and M drift apart so that melatonin secretion and other nocturnal functions expand to fill the available night.

Evening and morning oscillators have remained theoretical concepts—no one has been able to point to a physical part of the SCN or a particular molecular process and connect it to an evening or morning oscillator. An attractive but still speculative hypothesis is that different cell groups in the SCN correspond to the two oscillators. This hypothesis springs from exciting research threads in cellular and molecular biology that show that individual SCN cells contain all the necessary machinery to produce a circadian rhythm (this is not surprising since single-cell organisms also have daily rhythms).

As indicated earlier, fetal SCN cells could be used to restore rhythms in adult hamsters with lesioned SCN. These same fetal cells can also be cultured in vitro. Because SCN neurons are some of the smallest in the brain, it has only recently become possible to record the electrical activity of individual cells grown on specially designed tissue culture plates. Individual cells generate freerunning circadian rhythms in spontaneous neural firing for several weeks, making it clear that a single cell has the machinery to generate a circadian rhythm (Herzog et al. 1997). In dispersed cultures where cells do not

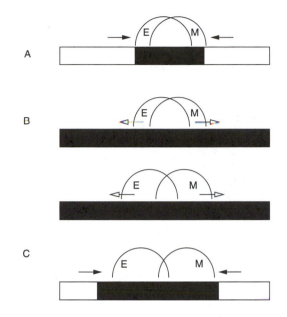

Figure 12.8 Model of evening and morning oscillators and mammalian photoperiodism. Depicted are two similar oscillators designated evening (E) and morning (M). The curves represent times of day when each oscillator programs various nighttime functions such as locomotor activity (in the nocturnal rodent), melatonin secretion, and responsiveness to shifting effects of light. In short nights (A), the two oscillators are entrained into largely overlapping phases and so the total duration of these nighttime functions is not much longer than the duration of each oscillator's individual functions. Evening light (the portion of the light:dark cycle just before night) causes daily delays in the position of E (recall that the PRC shows delays at this time) (solid arrow). Morning light causes daily advances in M (recall that the PRC shows advances at that time). In the absence of light (B), the oscillators drift apart because their free-running rhythms differ (outline arrows). E tends to drift earlier and M later. In long nights (C), the oscillators adopt an entrainment pattern where they overlap minimally. In this case, the total duration of activity, melatonin secretion, and so on will be nearly twice that of each individual oscillator.

form the same patterns of connections as they do in the mature SCN, the various cells on the culture plate will cycle out of synchrony (Liu et al. 1997; Honma et al. 1998). In contrast, cell activity is largely synchronized in hypothalamic slice preparations where the pattern of connectivity between cells is intact. These results indicate that individual cells may have individual circadian machinery and that they normally interact to regulate the activity of each other.

The Molecular Basis for Endogenous Clocks

During the last decade, molecular biologists have made tremendous strides in describing the biochemical machinery that produces approximately 24-hour fluctuations in cell function that serve as the basis of circadian rhythms. The rapid advances of the 1990s were made possible by examining the differences between normal wild type individuals and mutants of the same species that

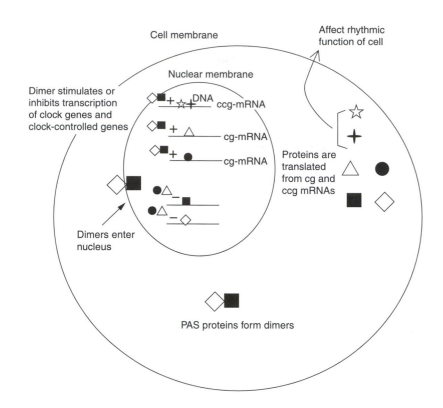

Figure 12.9 Simplified schematic representation of the molecular feedback loop principle of cellular circadian rhythms. PAS proteins transcribed from clock gene (cg) mRNA (square and diamond) form dimers, which are translocated to the cell nucleus where they stimulate (plus sign) transcription of other clock genes (triangle and circle) as well as clock-controlled genes (ccg, stars). Proteins translated from the mRNA of clock genes feed back on the elements that stimulated them by reducing the stability or production of the PAS proteins through various types of negative feedback mechanisms (minus sign). The products of clock-controlled genes are the basis for the many rhythmic functions of cells. Many fine details of their interactions among clock components are omitted here for clarity.

produced genetically inherited abnormal circadian rhythms (with particularly long or short periods) or produced no rhythms at all. Three eukaryotic organisms have been studied extensively: the fungus *Neurospora crassa*, the fruit fly *Drosophila melanogaster*, and the mouse *Mus musculus*. Surprisingly, in each species the fundamental biochemical oscillator operates under fundamentally similar principles involving negative feedback loops of molecular processes traversing the cell nucleus and the cytoplasm. In figure 12.9, we only sketch the broadest outlines of a series of feedback loops which are better understood with each passing month. (The interested reader can consult Dunlap 1999 and Shearman et al. 2000.)

In all three organisms, two proteins—each characterized by a particular molecular signature (called a PAS domain)—come together in the cytoplasm to form a "complex" or a "dimer." If both proteins are present at the same time, the resulting dimer moves into the cell nucleus where genes are transcribed into RNA. By interacting with a particular segment of DNA, this dimer stimulates the transcription of several "clock genes." These clock genes were given names such as "per1" or "per2" (for period 1 or period 2) because they were eventually shown to be genes with mutations in animals exhibiting genetically inherited abnormalities in the period of their free-running rhythms.

After these clock genes are transcribed to make RNA, the RNA moves into the cytoplasm and translation occurs, producing a protein of the same name (e.g., Per1 protein). Importantly, the clock genes have a negative feedback effect on the production or stability of the PAS domain proteins. Because the amount of PAS dimer decreases under the influence of the clock proteins, further transcription of clock genes is also diminished. In essence, the clock genes are negatively regulating their own expression. Due to the interaction of various components and time lags associated with these interactions, the negative feedback transcription/translation oscillation requires approximately 24 hours to complete a cycle of rise and fall. Some mutations stop the oscillation from occurring at all. For example, a PAS protein that is abnormal may be incapable of pairing with the other half of the dimer and therefore cannot get to the cell nucleus to drive the transcription of the clock genes. Other mutations result in the feedback cycle running faster or slower than normal because one or more steps in the chain is accelerated or slowed down.

This general scheme summarizes how a cycle lasting roughly 24 hours could exist within cells. It does not address how the cell generates circadian outputs (such as changes in spontaneous electrical firing) or how light or other zeitgebers influence the setting of the clock. Specific circadian rhythms may result because the clock proteins initiate the transcription of genes tied to various circadian outputs of cells. These latter genes are designated "clock-controlled genes" because, although they are very close to the basic molecular oscillation, they are not a necessary part of it. Rather, they are rhythmically driven by the most basic molecular mechanism.

In addition, light gains its resetting powers because it alters the levels of certain components in the feedback mechanism. Light might act directly on cells in lower organisms or indirectly via synaptic communication from the retinal projection to the SCN. In the mouse, light increases the transcription of clock genes. If light increases the levels of clock-gene products at the phase of the cycle when they are gradually rising, then they will exert their maximal negative feedback effects sooner than if no light were present. As a result, the cycle would be shifted earlier. Similarly, an increase in clock proteins at the phase of the cycle when they are gradually decreasing will prolong their negative feedback effects. As a result, they will not be turned off quite as quickly as in the absence of light and the cycle will be delayed.

How might this molecular framework be relevant for humans? The human clock appears to be quite similar to that of the mouse. In fact, all the genes identified in the mouse have also been identified in the human. This includes two genes with specific slight changes in the gene sequence that researchers suggest might be related to the differences between the nocturnality of mice and the diurnality of humans. Furthermore, within humans, a variant in one clock gene has been shown to be correlated with delayed arousal and sleep, compared to the mean population (Katzenberg et al. 1998).

To summarize, individual SCN cells produce sustained circadian rhythms in gene expression, electrical firing rates, and other functions. In the intact organism, the various cells have their rhythms influenced by the light environment and by interactions with other SCN cells. Summer and winter light conditions may entrain cells of the SCN into different phase relationships. Different cell populations may correspond to the abstract concepts of evening and morning oscillators.

The Melatonin Rhythm and Seasonality

The preceding section stressed the differences between circadian function in summer and in winter because seasonal differences in one of these circadian rhythms—the pattern of melatonin secretion—is a critical part of the mechanism by which organisms change their physiology and behavior according to the time of year. Seasonal changes that are driven by the changes in the day length (or by melatonin duration at a more physiological level of analysis) are described as photoperiodic. In such species, an annual cycle of seasonal change will not occur without exposure to alternate seasons of long and short day lengths. In other species, even annual rhythms are endogenous and do not require changing environmental conditions to drive them. These rhythms are described as circannual (by analogy with circadian). This latter category, which we will not discuss further, uses the changing day length (and melatonin duration) to synchronize, or entrain, the endogenous rhythm to match the natural year.

Different species respond to seasonal variations in the environment in different ways (Bronson 1989). Siberian hamsters, for example, decrease body weight in response to the decreased day lengths typical of autumn even if they are provided with an abundance of laboratory food. By maintaining a lower body weight and huddling together, they reduce the total number of calories they need to consume to make it through the winter. Other species, however, will increase food consumption as day lengths shorten to increase fat stores which they will expend for energy throughout the winter. In the domain of reproduction, many small rodents cease mating in autumn because winter months are challenging times to nurse a litter of pups. Sheep, on the other hand, initiate mating in the fall which, because of their long gestation period, allows them to give birth and nurse their lambs in spring when food is most plentiful. Despite these rather different adaptations, the control mechanisms are quite similar. Both depend on seasonal changes in the pattern of melatonin secretion.

The Pineal Gland

A large body of evidence indicates that melatonin is an important hormonal signal in orchestrating these seasonal transitions. Hamsters and voles have been preferred species of study because they are easily maintained in the laboratory and because they show such marked changes in reproduction and behavior across the seasons. Removal of the pineal gland, the principle source of melatonin in the blood in mammals, prevents these species from responding to winter day lengths in the typical fashion (as does interruption of any portion of the pathway between the SCN and the pineal) (Reiter 1980). In contrast to an intact animal, a pinealectomized Siberian hamster transferred to short day lengths will continue to breed, will not reduce body weight, and will not molt into a winter fur (Hoffmann 1979).

Replacement of the melatonin signal, however—a classic lesion/replacement endocrine study—restores the seasonal response. Giving injections every few hours or, more simply, implanting under the skin a permanent catheter that is attached to a pump, can restore melatonin. The pump, which can be controlled by a timer, infuses small volumes of melatonin dissolved in saline. Laboratory animals quickly adjust to the catheter and can be given months of programmed melatonin infusions while they are completely free to move about in their cages.

MELATONIN SIGNAL PARAMETERS

Using this paradigm, the critical parameters of the melatonin signal for inducing seasonal changes in physiology and behavior have been described (Goldman 1991) (figure 12.10). First and foremost, the duration (measured in hours) of exposure each day to elevated melatonin concentrations is critical. Infusions of melatonin for 4 hours a day—a condition that mimics the short nights/short melatonin pattern of summer—stimulate summer traits. Conversely, the same amount of melatonin infused over a longer interval (e.g., 12 hours), which mimics the long nights and long melatonin signal in winter, yields a winter phenotype.

Between these extreme durations, there is a critical duration of melatonin that divides the winter and summer responses: in Siberian hamsters, this critical duration is around 7 to 8 hours. Shorter infusions induce summer responses, whereas longer signals provoke winter adaptations. The critical number of hours that differentiates between long and short photoperiods varies by species and is dependent upon the prior photoperiod history of the animal (Lee and Gorman 2000). Thus, animals recently exposed to long day lengths (for example, 16 hours) require a shorter duration of daily melatonin exposure to enter a short photoperiod state than do animals that have long been exposed to an intermediate photoperiod (for example, 13 hours).

The time of day that the animal is exposed to melatonin (phase) is not critical. Although this situation would never arise in nature, pinealectomized animals will respond similarly to a 6-hour melatonin infusion delivered every afternoon or every night. Moreover, in contrast to many other hormonal systems where there is a linear or logarithmic dose-response relationship, the dosage (amplitude) of the melatonin signal is of little consequence as long as it exceeds some minimal detectable level or threshold: 10 ng of melatonin

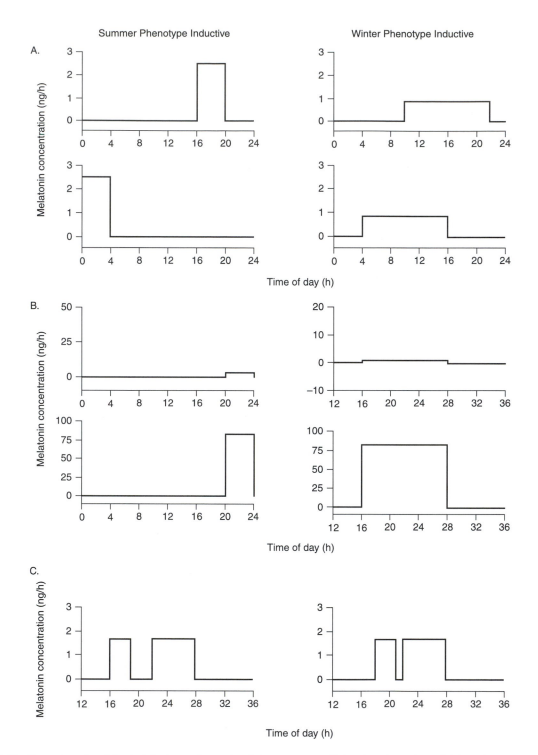

Figure 12.10 Examples of melatonin-infusion patterns that induce summer (*left column*) or winter (*right column*) phenotypes in Siberian hamsters. The summer phenotype is characterized by increased body weight, reproductive maturity, and dark fur. Under winter conditions, body weights are lower, the

infused over 4 hours induces the same response as 1,000 ng of melatonin. Of course, with extremely high dosages, the effective duration that melatonin is above the threshold will be lengthened because it will take somewhat longer to break down all the melatonin, and in that case, amplitude might be a relevant variable.

To develop a winter response, the long duration of melatonin needs to be nearly continuous. For example, if a long (12-hour) winter melatonin signal is interrupted 6 hours into it with an interval of no melatonin lasting more than an hour, the signal is no longer interpreted as a long signal. Instead, hamsters treat the signal as a stimulatory summer melatonin signal (Goldman et al. 1984). Last, melatonin conveys seasonal information only when the animal is exposed to the signal at approximately 24-hour periods (Elliott et al. 1989). Melatonin infusions at a 24-hour period caused greater gonadal regression in male Siberian hamsters than infusions every 18 hours, and infusions at 36- or 48-hour periods were not at all effective.

THE SITE OF MELATONIN ACTION

Where and how does melatonin act to induce the various seasonal changes in physiology and behavior? Specific high-density melatonin-binding sites have been localized in various structures including the SCN, pars tuberalis of the pituitary (PT), nucleus reuniens, premammillary hypothalamic area, and paraventricular nucleus of the thalamus (PVT) (de Reviers et al. 1991; Duncan et al. 1989; Malpaux et al. 1998; Reppert et al. 1988; Stankov et al. 1994; Vanacek et al. 1987; Vanacek 1988; Weaver et al. 1989; Weaver et al. 1993; Williams and Morgan 1988; Williams 1989). Different species show markedly different patterns of melatonin binding, but one substrate that binds in most, if not all, species with seasonal variations in reproduction is the PT. The PT has been particularly implicated in mediating seasonal changes in the prolactin function, which is necessary for seasonal molts in many species (Malpaux et al. 1993; Kennaway and Rowe 1995). The uniformity of PT binding between species may reflect the fact that all mammals studied increase PRL secretion in spring and summer.

The same uniformity is not observed in the secretion of gonadotropins (FSH and LH) since gonadotropins increase during the breeding season and in seasonal breeders, some animals breed in fall and others in spring and summer. Not surprisingly perhaps, seasonal regulation of reproduction probably depends on melatonin actions apart from the PT. In sheep, melatonin

Figure 12.10 (continued)

gonads regress, and the fur becomes lighter in color. (*A*) Melatonin delivered over 4 hours induces the summer phenotype but the same total amount of melatonin infused over 12 hours yields the winter condition. The time of day that melatonin is infused is without consequence. (*B*) Increasing the dosage 100-fold does not alter the response of hamsters to infusions of a given duration. (*C*) A break in the melatonin signal for 3 hours results in a summer phenotype, although a shorter 1-hour break produces the winter phenotype. For clarity, the X-axis sometimes plots the 24-hour interval beginning at midnight and sometimes at noon. (Data redrawn from Goldman 1991.)

implants (which mimic long duration infusions) in the premammillary area of the hypothalamus altered patterns of LH secretion, but not PRL. In Siberian hamsters, melatonin implants in any of three brain regions suppressed reproductive function—the SCN, PVT, and the nucleus reuniens (Badura and Goldman 1992). The necessity of the SCN for responding to melatonin, however, varies by species: Siberian hamsters but not Syrian hamsters require an intact SCN to respond to reproductively inhibitory melatonin signals (Bartness et al. 1991; Bittman et al. 1989). Thus, it is clearly a mistake to assume that photoperiodic systems are alike in all mammals. These and other results have led to the suggestion that melatonin may act on at least two distinct substrates—the PT, to regulate prolactin secretion, and the medialbasal hypothalamus (with much species variation within this area), to regulate gonadotropins (Lincoln 1999).

In summary, by using a highly reliable output of the circadian pacemaker—the nightly secretion of melatonin from the pineal gland—mammals have an internal hormonal representation of the length of the night which, of course, reflects the season of the year. The seasonally changing melatonin signal results from the circadian entrainment of two (or more) oscillators present within the SCN. By responding differently to various lengths of melatonin secretion, animals can adapt their physiology and behavior to meet seasonally changing selection pressures.

Interactions Between the SCN and Melatonin

Thus far we have focused on how a master oscillator, the SCN, generates rhythms in other behavioral and physiological functions, and the consequences of some of these outputs. Traditionally, scientists have considered the circadian system to be influenced only by the outside environment and not by the systems that it is timing. They reasoned by analogy with mechanical clocks: if your wristwatch sped up or slowed down depending on whether you were awake or asleep, you probably would not think it was a very good clock. We now know that this unidirectional view of the circadian system—from SCN to all other rhythms—is inaccurate. Several of the endocrine systems that have circadian hormonal release (these include melatonin and cortisol) as well as noncircadian gonadal steroids have effects on the function of the SCN or circadian system more generally. We will discuss two examples that involve the endocrine system: the interaction between the circadian system and pineal melatonin and the interaction between the circadian system and gonadal function.

Feedback Effects of Melatonin on Circadian Function

As described above, the mammalian circadian melatonin rhythm clearly depends upon the function of the SCN. Consistent with the idea that the information was all in one direction early studies demonstrated that surgical removal of the pineal (pinealectomy) in rats and hamsters did not affect entrained or free-running activity rhythms (Quay 1968; Aschoff et al. 1982).

More detailed assessments of circadian function in the presence or absence of the pineal gland, however, suggested that melatonin might feed back on circadian systems. For example, in rats and hamsters the rate of re-entrainment to a shift in the light:dark cycle (similar to that which you experience travelling to different time zones) was enhanced by pinealectomy (Quay 1970; Finkelstein et al. 1978).

The possibility of a dual interaction between the pineal and the SCN was not further investigated for many years, until the effect of pinealectomy was examined in rats housed in light 24 hours/day. Under such conditions activity rhythms quickly lose their circadian character and faster (i.e., ultradian) rhythms emerge with periods between 2 and 6 hours. Rats with pineal glands did not respond in this fashion (Cassone 1992). Pinealectomy also enhanced splitting of activity rhythms in hamsters in constant light (Aguilar-Roblero and Vega-Gonzalez 1993). How the pineal gland exerted its effects on the circadian system was not clear: one possibility was that that pineal melatonin influenced the animal's sensitivity to light. A heightened sensitivity in pinealectomized animals, for example, might explain why they re-entrained more readily and split in constant light.

Melatonin Entrainment of Circadian Rhythms

A very different effect of melatonin was discovered in the 1980s by Redman et al. (1983) who demonstrated that melatonin, like light, could actually entrain circadian activity rhythms. Injections of pharmacological doses of melatonin at the same time each day caused previously free-running activity rhythms of rats to become entrained to the injections. The effect was dose dependent, with minimum effective doses producing near physiological plasma levels of melatonin (Cassone et al. 1986; Warren et al. 1993) (figure 12.11) suggesting that melatonin itself, and not the act of being picked up and pricked with a needle, was responsible for the entrainment. Animals aligned their circadian activity rhythms so that the onset of their nocturnal activity occured around the time of the injection. This relationship between activity and melatonin injections mimics the relationship between activity and the nightly endogenous rise in melatonin that occurs naturally in nocturnal species. In addition to the entraining effects, rats given exogenous melatonin during a phase-shift of the light cycle accelerate re-entrainment to the new LD cycle (Redman and Armstrong 1988).

Melatonin and Treatment of Jet Lag

The potential importance of this feedback effect for dealing with human chronobiological problems due to blindness, jet lag, shift-work, or aging has been demonstrated in a growing number of studies. Retinally blind and therefore free-running, humans provided with oral melatonin at the same time each day entrain to a 24-hour schedule as measured by their activity, sleep-wake, and temperature cycles (Sack et al. 1991; Zaidan et al. 1994; Arendt et al. 1997). In contrast to the rats described above, the relationship between melatonin

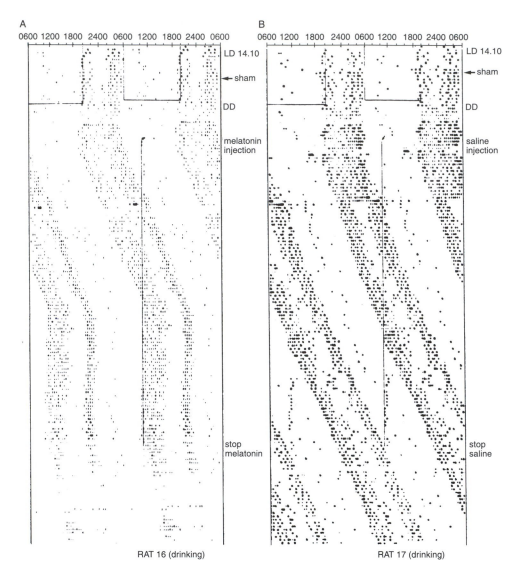

A   B

0600 1200 1800 2400 0600 1200 1800 2400 0600   0600 1200 1800 2400 0600 1200 1800 2400 0600

LD 14.10   LD 14.10

← sham   ← sham

DD   DD

melatonin   saline
injection   injection

stop   stop
melatonin   saline

RAT 16 (drinking)   RAT 17 (drinking)

Figure 12.11 Continuous records of drinking behavior of sham-lesioned rats that received (*A*) daily injection of the pineal hormone melatonin or (*B*) daily injections of ethanol:saline vehicle. (*A*) melatonin injection entrained the rats to the period of the injection regime. (*B*) Vehicle had little or no effect. Records are double-plotted to facilitate visualization of the free-running rhythm. (From Cassone et al. 1986.)

and activity peaks is reversed from that found in nocturnal animals and typical of that for diurnal animals: the active part of the cycle precedes the time of melatonin administration and rest/sleep follows it.

Melatonin administration also hastens recovery from jet lag or simulated phase-shifts in some studies (increased the rate of reentrainment to a new LD cycle) in human subjects, as it does with rats (Arendt et al. 1987; Samel et al. 1991; Deacon and Arendt 1995; Dawson et al. 1995; Arendt and Deacon 1997). These and at least ten other studies included data collection of both subjective (primarily sleep disturbance, but also cognitive function, digestive disturbance, and so on) and objective measures (body movement, body temperature, cortisol, and melatonin) of jet lag from a variety of natural and simulated protocols and compared it to similarly treated subjects given a placebo. However, not all studies reach the same conclusion about the benefits of melatonin on recovery from jet lag.

For example, a very careful double-blind study found no effect of any melatonin dosage schedule (Spitzer 1999). The subjects in this study were returning home after a 4-day period of phase-advance between Oslo and New York City. They had not fully entrained to Oslo time prior to the trip home, and therefore the timing of melatonin administration may have been inappropriate. However, this and similar study leave open the question of the effectiveness of melatonin on recovery from jet lag.

Recent work has also demonstrated improved sleep initiation and maintenance when melatonin is administered to elderly patients with typical age-associated insomnia (Haimov et al. 1995). In many elderly subjects, night time insomnia and day time sleepiness are correlated with decreased melatonin release (Haimov and Lavie 1997), and therefore replacement melatonin may be beneficial. However, many healthy, unmedicated elderly subjects demonstrate no decrease in melatonin compared to healthy young adults (Zeitzer et al. 1999), and therefore the authors suggest that individual melatonin levels should be tested before beginning nightly doses of melatonin to improve sleep. The fact that many elderly subjects are on a variety of medications that might affect circadian systems greatly complicates the assessment of melatonin effects in this population.

Site of Melatonin's Circadian Effects

Melatonin is thought to have its beneficial effects by influencing the function of the SCN directly or indirectly through other inputs to the SCN. The data from animals and from blind humans are consistent with this interpretation. The observation that the effectiveness of melatonin for jet lag depends on its time of administration suggests that it works by altering the circadian system. However, melatonin can also act independently from the circadian system inducing a noncircadian, sleep-inducing effect at higher doses (James et al. 1990). Thus, the effects on jet lag and, even more likely, the effects on insomnia in the elderly may be partly due to melatonin's soporific effects (Cassone

1998). To distinguish between these different types of actions, recent studies have been careful to use lower doses of melatonin (less than 5 mg) that minimize the noncircadian sleep-inducing effects. It is nonetheless still unclear whether all the effects of melatonin described above are due to effects on the circadian system.

As you might expect, the SCN appears to be the most important if not the only site of melatonin's circadian effects. The recent findings that the SCN of many species contains a significant number of melatonin receptors and that the numbers vary across the day suggest a possible physiological basis for the effects of melatonin on SCN function (Gauer et al. 1993; 1994a, 1994b; Weaver et al. 1993; Neu and Niles 1997). Notably, two species with reduced or undetectable numbers of melatonin receptors in the SCN (adult Syrian hamsters and mink) also do not entrain to injections of melatonin (Hastings et al. 1992; Bonneford et al. 1993). This has led to the suggestion that SCN binding sites may be necessary for the entraining effects of melatonin.

Lastly, in vitro SCN tissue studies yield results analogous to those obtained with the intact organism. For example, melatonin has its largest effects on activity rhythms when delivered around the beginning of nocturnal activity, lesser effects near the end of night, and no effect during middle of the day or night. Correspondingly, administration of melatonin to dissected SCN tissue in a dish affects both the metabolism and the neural firing rates of that tissue when added to the dish at a time that corresponds to the beginning of the night (Cassone et al. 1988; Shibata et al. 1989; Stehle et al. 1989; McArthur et al. 1991; Starkey et al. 1995).

To conclude this example of the feedback effects of melatonin on the circadian system, it is instructive to compare and contrast the mammalian pattern of circadian organization described above with that of nonmammalian vertebrates such as birds, fish, and reptiles. At first glance, circadian systems of these latter vertebrate classes differ markedly from those of mammals: in contrast to mammals where the pineal gland is the only significant source of melatonin in the blood, in some birds, the retina, Harderian glands (a structure near the eyes), and/or the gut may affect blood melatonin concentrations (Vakkuri et al. 1985; Osol et al. 1985).

The pineal gland of nonmammalian vertebrates, moreover, is not entrained to light/dark cycle by way of projections of the SCN as in mammals. Sometimes called "the third eye," the pineal gland itself contains light-sensitive cells that regulate their own secretion of melatonin in response to light penetrating the skull (Takahashi et al. 1989). Last, in contrast to the mammalian case, the pineal gland and the eyes of some birds, reptiles, and fish are circadian pacemakers that can operate independently of the SCN. In short, nonmammalian vertebrates may contain as many as three (eye, pineal, and SCN) oscillators of nearly equal influence. Because these structures are not interconnected via neural projections, melatonin may be the most important coordinating or synchronizing mechanism between them. In this light, it is not surprising that melatonin in mammals would continue to feedback on the

SCN. Although the control mechanisms of the pineal have changed over evolutionary time and the pacemaker function of the pineal and the eyes have been diminished in mammals, this evolutionarily ancient function of melatonin persists.

To summarize, the circadian system, particularly the SCN, controls the circadian pattern of melatonin release in mammals. Melatonin has multiple effects on the organism, and the SCN is a key component in those effects. The nuclei are the target of melatonin's entraining and modulating circadian effects in several species.

The Feedback Effects of Steroid Hormones

Steroid hormones from the male and female gonads influence the function of the circadian systems both during development and in adulthood. The following studies were largely conducted on mice, rats, hamsters, and a less well-known South American rodent, the degu (*Octodon degus*). Unlike the work with melatonin feedback effects on circadian function, we currently have no data on where or how these steroid-induced circadian differences occur. Nor do we have any experimentally supported theories about why the circadian system should be sexually dimorphic and/or influenced by adult hormones (i.e., why it is adaptive). Since humans also demonstrate sexual dimorphisms in circadian function, we may ultimately find it necessary to understand these differences when dealing with circadian disorders.

Circadian Systems

Adult sex differences in circadian function can be classified into three categories: (1) fundamental properties of the circadian system (tau, PRC); (2) the amplitude and timing of specific measured rhythm end points, such as peak activity, core body temperature minimum and maximum, sleep onset and pattern, and hormone release patterns; and (3) estrous effects on rhythmic expression of activity, temperature, sleep, and cognitive function.

The freerunning rhythms of male and female hamsters (Davis et al. 1983; Zucker et al. 1980), rats (Albers et al. 1981), mice (Daan et al. 1975; Daan and Pittendrigh 1976), humans (Wever 1984) and degus (Labyak and Lee 1995; Lee and Labyak 1997) differ significantly. In addition, the PRC, the stability of entrainment, and the timing of activity onset also differ between male and female hamsters (Davis et al. 1983). Few other species have been studied in as much depth as hamsters, but men and women also demonstrate differences in the timing of sleep onset and morning arousal (Wever 1984; Critchlow et al. 1963), and degus have sexually dimorphic PRCs (Lee, unpublished data). Male, but rarely female, hamsters readily demonstrate activity patterns that are split into two bouts, usually 8 to 12 hours out of phase with each other, under conditions of constant light (Daan and Pittendrigh 1976). Indeed, following phase shifts in the light:dark cycle to which animals must re-entrain or when housed in constant conditions, females maintain a more stable and coherent pattern of activity (Morin and Cummings 1982). However, male hamsters and degus recover more quickly from a phase-shift than females do (Morin and Cummings 1982; Goel and Lee 1995).

Several of these sex differences can be eliminated in adults by removing the gonads (the source of most sexually dimorphic steroid hormones) or by treatment with testosterone or estradiol, indicating an activational effect of hormones. For example, ovariectomy of female hamsters increases the incidence of splitting in constant light, but neither castration nor hormonal manipulation decreases the incidence in males (Morin and Cummings 1982).

Other sex differences appear to be unaffected by the adult hormonal state. Such a lack of an activational effect of hormones suggests a possible organizational effect of prenatal or perinatal hormones on the development of the sex difference. An interesting case study illustrating both the activational and the organization effects of gonadal hormones is the circadian system of Syrian hamsters. In adulthood, the activational effects of estrogen are readily observed in females by first ovariectomizing them and then giving them replacement implants of estradiol. The period of the free-running rhythm in darkness is shortened by exposure to estradiol in adulthood (Morin 1985; Morin et al. 1977). Concurrent exposure to progesterone blocks the effect of estradiol, indicating an interaction between these two steroids to modulate the timing and expression of circadian activity in the hamster (Takahashi and Menaker 1980). Because the period of the free-running rhythm of male hamsters was unaffected by castration and estradiol, we see that the female retains a sensitivity to hormones that is absent in males.

This sex difference in sensitivity to steroids might have an organizational basis. Indeed, a single injection of testosterone on the day of birth caused female hamsters to lose their responsiveness to estradiol in adulthood and the castration of males at birth increased adult sensitivity to estradiol (Zucker et al. 1980). Similar work has not been done yet in other species. The physiological bases of these sex differences have not been clarified, but because this first category of hormonal effects concerns the global organization of the circadian system, one would expect neuroanatomical differences in or around the SCN itself.

Activity Rhythms

The second category includes sex differences in daily amplitude of activity in rats and in the timing and amplitude of corticosterone peak (Critchlow 1963; Albers et al. 1981). Female and male humans also differ in sleep pattern, temperature rhythm, and timing of cortisol peak (Binkley 1992; Critchlow 1963; Wever 1986). These differences between males and females have been less studied than those above, but ovariectomy of female rats eliminates the sex difference in corticosterone amplitude and timing (Critchlow et al. 1963).

Temperature Rhythms

Similarly, temperature rhythms are affected by estrogen and progesterone levels in women (Short 1984) and rats (Freeman et al. 1970), but males are unaffected by changes in testosterone or other hormones (Myers et al. 1995). As with the fundamental properties of circadian rhythms, it is not clear where steroid hormones are having their impact. Earlier we saw that the SCN has many diverse outputs, which makes the number of possible sites of hormone action even greater. Steroid hormones may act on parts of the output mechanism quite close to the SCN, or they may act on the end structure, such as the adrenal gland or the neural sleep structures in the brainstem, altering the responsiveness of the structure to a steroid-independent circadian signal.

Estrous or Menstrual Cycle–Related Rhythms

The most studied effect of steroid hormones on circadian function is the impact of estrous and menstrual cycles on circadian activity and temperature rhythms. Ovarian hormones influence the timing and expression of circadian activity and core temperature rhythms in nocturnal female rodents (Albers et al. 1981; Freeman et al. 1970; Kent et al. 1991; Takahashi and Menaker 1980). During proestrus and estrus (days 3 and 4 of a 4-day estrous cycle) when estrogen levels are high, hamsters demonstrate an increase in mean daily activity (Richards 1966), an earlier activity onset (Morin et al. 1977; Refinetti and Menaker 1992), and a rise in mean core temperature (Refinetti and Menaker 1992).

WOMEN

Since species-typical patterns are evident in nocturnal species, estrous-related alterations in circadian rhythms may be distinctly different for species with longer cycles or for those that are diurnal. For example, in one case study, the circadian rhythm of a premenopausal 46-year-old woman was monitored for one year with a device that unobtrusively records movement of the wrist (from which general activity patterns can be detected). Around the time of ovulation, the subject demonstrated a significant decrease in mean activity coupled with a significant phase delay in activity onset (Binkley 1992). Although this is a case study, the findings suggest that circadian responsiveness to changing ovarian hormones may be distinctly different in diurnal humans when compared to nocturnal rats or hamsters. Wever (1986) studied changes in the freerunning core temperature rhythm across the menstrual cycle in young women, and compared them to mean temperatures in men of similar ages. While preovulatory mean temperatures in young women were similar to those of males, postovulatory mean temperatures were higher. Such postovulatory temperature changes have not been reported for hamsters and rats, and may be the result of nocturnal/diurnal differences or the difference in the length of the luteal stage (especially since progesterone can cause increased temperature in rats) (Freeman et al. 1970).

DEGUS

Several experiments examined the circadian activity and temperature rhythms of the diurnal degu, which has a 21-day estrous cycle, to determine whether a diurnal rodent with long estrous cycles would show circadian variations typical of women (28-day cycles) or of other rodents (4- to 5-day cycles). Labyak and Lee (1995) found that degus differed from both, but were more different from hamsters and rats than from humans (figure 12.12). Cyclic changes in ovarian hormones have a pronounced effect on the timing and expression of entrained circadian activity and core temperature rhythms in the diurnal degu.

However, compared with rats, hamsters, and humans, their activity/temperature relationship has several unique characteristics. First, unlike rats but similar to humans, estrous-related circadian changes in core temperature occur even in the absence of high activity (in running wheels). Second, unlike hamsters, ovariectomy reduces mean body temperature without a concomitant reduction of mean activity or change in phase for entrained animals, and without a change in tau for freerunning animals. Third, as in humans, estrogen replacement of entrained, ovariectomized degus did not significantly increase core temperature or activity as it does in hamsters and some strains of rats.

However, progesterone replacement, which has little effect on hamsters and rats, led to an immediate reduction in core temperature and mean activity in the degu. This response also differs from that of human females in whom temperature increases following progesterone treatment. Neither estrogen nor progesterone altered the timing of activity onset, in contrast to hamsters and rats. Last, unlike hamsters, in freerunning conditions (DD), estrous-related fluctuations in the timing of daily activity onset and temperature minimum were transient, and there were no significant changes in tau with the hormone treatment of ovariectomized females. Therefore, it is likely in degus that hormonal effects on circadian activity and temperature do not directly involve the central circadian neural structures. Rather, hormone-induced changes in core temperature and, perhaps, also in brain circuits controlling locomotor activity alter mean activity and activity phase in entrained, intact females during the estrous cycle.

RATS
Steroid receptors have been identified in the SCN of prenatal and early postnatal rats (Brown et al. 1989) but not in the SCN of adult rats, hamsters, mice, or degus. However, these studies only looked for the classic estrogen, progesterone, and testosterone receptors. With newer technologies, such as in situ hybridization of mRNA, it is important to look again at the SCN for steroid receptors. If they are not found, then the adult activational effects of steroid hormones must act through projections from other brain structures that are sensitive to gonadal hormones. The permanent early alterations in circadian function brought about by early hormonal exposure might occur via steroid receptors that later disappear from the structure, but leave it functionally different between the two sexes. Recent exploration of the hypothalamus of

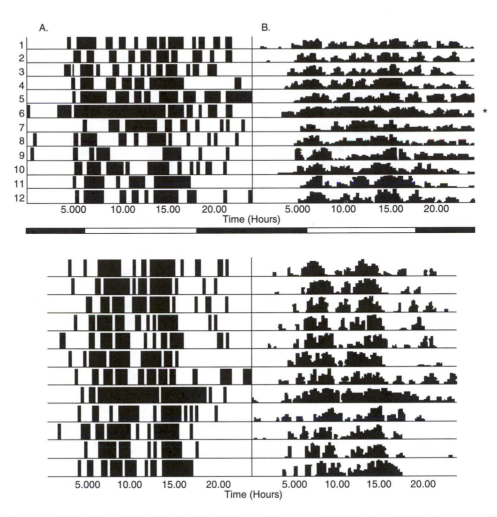

Figure 12.12 (*A*) Entrained female degu's wheel-running activity and (*B*) her core body temperature during 5 days prior to estrus, the day of estrus (asterisk on right side of figure), and several days after estrus. Body temperature is recorded continuously from transmitters implanted in the abdominal cavity and is plotted like activity data. (Bar at bottom of the top actogram denotes the light:dark schedule.) To make viewing the daily temperature elevation easier, the lowest 25% of temperature data are not displayed. Note that on the day of estrus activity and core temperature are elevated and the active period and temperature elevation are phase-advanced compared to the days before and after estrus. In the lower actogram of a degu housed in constant darkness (*C*, activity; *D*, core temperature), the elevation of activity and temperature occurs on the day of estrus, but there is no phase advance or change in tau when this occurs.

adult female rats with in situ hybridization for mRNA has revealed ERα in the area around the SCN (retrochiasmatic area) and ERβ within the SCN (Kashon et al. 1999; Shughrue et al. 1997). Much work needs to be done to determine whether cells with these receptors are involved in early organizational and/or activational effects of steroids on circadian function.

Although we still do not know the adaptive function of the differences between males and females in circadian function or why adult gonadal hormones should alter circadian function, it is clear that this is a pervasive phenomenon. The consequences of the interaction between the gonadal hormones and the circadian system are played out in human functions that should be better explored. For example, there is a strong time-of-day effect on the alertness and the cognitive performance of humans. These circadian changes are altered by the phase of the menstrual cycle and by oral contraceptives (Wright and Badia 1999). During the luteal phase or while taking oral contraceptives, the deficit in function during the early morning hours of the night is markedly less than during the follicular phase. Interestingly, men show a level of function equivalent to women during the follicular phase (Myers et al. 1995).

Summary

Environmental change is an inescapable fact of life. To the extent that this change is recurrent and predictable, like the daily alternation of light and dark or the yearly variation in temperature and food availability, organisms profit from being able to anticipate that change and modify their behavior and physiology accordingly. The neural mechanism that allows this anticipation on a daily basis is one of the best characterized brain-behavior relationships in neuroscience today. And yet, despite the recognition that the SCN comprises the dominant circadian pacemaker in mammals, close analysis reveals that the circadian system is far from simple: it reflects the interaction of multiple oscillators within the SCN, it generates outputs by multiple mechanisms, and it is influenced by myriad environmental and endogenous inputs. This system will continue to warrant significant scientific attention, and not only because of its importance to medical and social concerns but also because the evolutionarily ancient and invariant need for biological timing mechanisms makes this a tractable and profitable system in which to explore the relationship between physiology and behavior from a plethora of biological perspectives. The main points of this chapter follow.

1. Many behaviors and physiological processes exhibit regular and recurring fluctuations over time. These cycles have periods that match environmental fluctuations such as occur between day and night (daily or circadian rhythms) or between the seasons (annual rhythms), whereas other cycles are not linked to any environmental variations (e.g., estrous and menstrual rhythms).
2. The suprachiasmatic nucleus in the hypothalamus is the master pacemaker. It generates daily rhythms in physiology and behavior in mammals. The SCN

employs a variety of neural and non-neural mechanisms to impose its rhythm on other structures.

3. The circadian rhythm in the secretion of melatonin from the pineal gland changes with the seasons. Melatonin patterns characteristic of different seasons induce animals to adopt behaviors appropriate to the season—for example, the suppression of breeding in winter.

4. The circadian clock is altered by some of the hormones it helps to control. Melatonin can entrain circadian rhythms, while gonadal steroids may alter the length of the freerunning rhythms as well as the amplitude of behavioral rhythms.

5. Circadian systems of different mammalian species have much in common, such as the importance of the SCN, the entrainment to light:dark cycles, and the rhythmic production of melatonin. Species differ, however, in some of the finer details, such as the effect of gonadal hormones on body temperature rhythms and the length of the free-running rhythm.

Study Questions

1. What do we mean when we say that 24-hour rhythms in behavior are "endogenously generated"? How do we know that daily variation is not simply a direct and immediate response to variation in the environment?

2. In light of the animal studies described, what factors might influence the development of sex differences in circadian rhythms in humans? When sex differences are present in adults, where in the brain might gonadal hormones have an effect?

3. What evidence indicates that the SCN is the principal circadian pacemaker in mammals? What are the limitations associated with individual studies that contribute to this conclusion?

4. How does the pattern of melatonin secretion differ between the winter and summer solstices (December and June, respectively, in the northern hemisphere)? What are the consequences of these different secretion patterns? Which is more important—the timing of melatonin secretion or the dosage?

5. Many people develop clinical depression every fall or winter and spontaneously improve in the spring (known as seasonal affective disorder, SAD). Several scientists have suggested that the circadian system may be involved in this condition. How would you go about evaluating this claim? (Think about where dysfunction could occur along the entire circadian system: the role of the environment, the generation of rhythms, and the effects of hormones, neurotransmitters, and so on, which are controlled by the circadian system.)

References

Aguilar-Roblero, R., and Vega-Gonzalez, A. (1993) Splitting of locomotor circadian rhythmicity in hamsters is facilitated by pinealectomy. *Brain Res.* 605: 229–236.

Albers, H. E. (1981) Gonadal hormones organize and modulate the circadian system of the rat. *Am. J. Physiol.* 241: R62–R66.

Arendt, J., Aldous, M., English, J., Marks, V., and Arendt J. H. (1987) Some effects of jet-lag and their alleviation by melatonin. *Ergonomics* 30: 1379–1393.

Arendt, J., and Deacon, S. (1997) Treatment of circadian rhythm disorder: Melatonin. *Chronobiol. Int.* 14: 185–204.

Arendt, J., Skene, D. J., Middleton, B., Lockley, S. W., and Deacon, S. (1997) Efficacy of melatonin treatment in jet lag, shift work, and blindness. *J. Biol. Rhythms* 12: 604–617.

Aschoff, J., Gerecke, U. von Goetz, C., Groos, G., and Turek, F. W. (1982) Phase responses and characteristics of free-running activity rhythms in golden hamsters: independence of the pineal gland. In J. Aschoff, S. Daan, and G. Groos (Eds.), *Vertebrate Circadian Systems.* Berlin: Springer-Verlag, pp. 129–140.

Aschoff, J., and Wever, R. (1981) The circadian system of man. In J. Aschoff (Ed.), *Handbook of Behavioral Neurobiology: Biological Rhythms.* New York: Plenum Press, pp. 311–332.

Badura, L. L., and Goldman, B. D. (1992) Central sites mediating reproductive responses to melatonin in juvenile male Siberian hamsters. *Brain Res.* 598: 98–106.

Balsalobre, A., Damiola, F., and Schibler, U. (1998) A serum shock induces circadian gene expression in mammalian tissue culture cells. *Cell* 93: 929–937.

Bartness, T. J., and Goldman, B. D. (1989) Mammalian pineal melatonin: A clock for all seasons. *Experientia* 45: 939–945.

Bartness, T. J., Goldman, B. D., and Bittman, E. L. (1991) SCN lesions block responses to systemic melatonin infusions in Siberian hamsters. *Am. J. Physiol.* 260: R102–R112.

Binkley, S. (1992) Wrist activity in a woman: Daily, weekly, menstrual, lunar, annual cycles? *Physiol. Behav.* 52: 411–421.

Bittman, E. L., Crandell, R. G., and Lehman, M. N. (1989) Influences of the paraventricular and suprachiasmatic nuclei and olfactory bulbs on melatonin responses in the golden hamster. *Biol. Reprod.* 40: 118–126.

Bojkowski, C. J., Aldhous, M. E., English, J., Franey, C., Poulton, A. L., Skene, D. J., and Arendt, J. (1987) Suppression of nocturnal plasma melatonin by bright and dim light in man. *Horm. Metab. Res.* 19: 437–440.

Bonnefond, C., Monnerie, R., Richard, J. P., and Martinet, L. (1993) Melatonin and the circadian clock in mink: Effects of daily injections of melatonin on circadian rhythm of locomotor activity and autoradiographic localization of melatonin binding sites. *J. Neuroendocrinol.* 5: 241–246.

Bronson, F. H. (1989) *Mammalian Reproductive Biology.* Chicago: University of Chicago Press.

Brown, T. J., Maclusky, N. J., Toran-Allerand, C. D., Zielinski, J. E., and Hochberg, R. B. (1989) Characterization of 11-beta-methoxy-16-alpha-[I-125]iodoestradiol binding: Neuronal localization of estrogen-binding sites in the developing rat brain. *Endocrinology* 124: 2074–2088.

Carmichael, M. S., Nelson, R. J., and Zucker, I. (1981) Hamster activity and estrous cycles: Control by a single versus multiple circadian oscillator(s). *Proc. Natl. Acad. Sci. USA* 78: 7830–7834.

Cassone, V. M. (1992) The pineal gland influences rat circadian activity rhythms in constant light. *J. Biol. Rhythms* 7: 27–40.

Cassone, V. M. (1998) Melatonin's role in vertebrate circadian rhythms. *Chronobiol. Internat.* 15: 457–473.

Cassone, V. M., Chesworth, M. J., and Armstrong, S. M. (1986) Entrainment of rat circadian rhythms by daily injection of melatonin depends upon the hypothalamic suprachismatic nuclei. *Physiol. Behav.* 36: 1111–1121.

Cassone, V. M., Roberts, M. H., and Moore, R. Y. (1988) Effects of melatonin on 2-deoxy-[1-14C]glucose uptake within rat suprachiasmatic nucleus. *Am. J. Physiol.* 255: R332–R337.

Critchlow, V., Lieberit, R. A., Bar-Sela, M., Mountcastle, W., and Lipscomb, H. S. (1963) The role of light in the neuroendocrine system. *Am. J. Physiol.* 205: 807–815.

Daan, S., Damassa, D., Pittendrigh, C. S., and Smith, E. R. (1975) An effect of castration and testosterone replacement on a circadian pacemaker in mice (*Mus musculus*). *Proc. Natl. Acad. Sci. USA* 72: 3744–3747.

Daan, S., and Pittendrigh, C. S. (1976) A functional analysis of circadian pacemakers in nocturnal rodents. II. The variability of response curves. *J. Comp. Physiol.* 106: 253–266.

Davis, F. C., Darrow, J. M., and Menaker, M. (1983) Sex differences in the circadian control of hamster wheel-running activity. *Am. J. Physiol.* 244: R93–R105.

Dawson, D., Encel, N., and Lushington, K. (1995) Improving adaptation to simulated night-shift: Timed exposure to bright light versus daytime melatonin administration. *Sleep* 18: 11–21.

Deacon, S., and Arendt, J. (1995) Adapting to phase-shifts, II. Effects of melatonin and conflicting light treatment. *Physiol. Behav.* 59: 675–682.

de Reviers, M. M., Tillet, Y., and Pelletier, J. (1991) Melatonin binding sites in the brain of sheep exposed to light or pinealectomized. *Neurosci. Lett.* 121: 17–20.

de la Iglesia, H. O., Blaustein, J. D., and Bittman, E. L. (1995) The suprachiasmatic area in the female hamster projects to neurons containing estrogen receptors and GnRH. *Neuroreport* 6: 1715–1722.

Drucker-Colin, R., Aguilar-Roblero, R., Garcia-Hernandez, F., Fernandez-Cancino, F., and Bermudez Rattoni, F. (1984) Fetal suprachiasmatic nucleus transplants: Diurnal rhythm recovery of lesioned rats. *Brain Res.* 311: 353–357.

Duncan, M. J., Takahashi, J. S., and Dubocovich, M. L. (1989) Characteristics and autoradiographic localization of 2-[i-125]iodomelatonin binding-sites in Djungarian hamster brain. *Endocrinology* 125: 1011–1018.

Dunlap, J. C. (1999) Molecular bases for circadian clocks. *Cell* 96: 271–290.

Earnest, D. J., and Turek, F. W. (1982) Splitting of the circadian rhythm of activity in hamsters: Effects of exposure to constant darkness and subsequent re-exposure to constant light. *J. Comp. Physiol.* A 145: 405–411.

Elliott, J. A., and Bartness, T. J., Goldman, B. D. (1989) Effect of melatonin infusion duration and frequency on gonad, lipid, and body mass in pinealectomized male Siberian hamsters. *J. Biol. Rhythms* 4: 439–455.

Elliott, J. A., and Tamarkin, L. (1994) Complex circadian regulation of pineal melatonin and wheel-running in Syrian hamsters. *J. Comp. Physiol.* A 174: 469–484.

Finkelstein, J. S., Baum, F. R., and Campbell, C. S. (1978) Entrainment of the female hamster to reversed photoperiod: Role of the pineal gland. *Physiol. Behav.* 21: 105–111.

Folkard, S., and Monk, T. H. (1980) Circadian rhythms in human memory. *Br. J. Psychol.* 71: 295–307.

Freeman, N. E., Crissman, J. K., Jr., Louw, G. N., Butcher, R. L., and Innskeep, E. K. (1970) Thermogenic action of progesterone in the rat. *Endocrinology* 86: 717–720.

Gauer, F., Masson-Pevet, M., and Pevet, B. P. (1994a) Daily variations in melatonin receptor density of rat pars tuberalis and suprachiasmatic nuclei are distinctly regulated. *Brain Res.* 641: 92–98.

Gauer, F., Masson-Pevet, M., and Pevet, B. P. (1994b) Seasonal regulation of melatonin receptors in rodent pars tuberalis: Correlation with reproductive state. *J. Neural Transm. Gen. Sect.* 96: 187–195.

Gauer, F., Masson-Pevet, M., Skene, D. J., Vivien-Roels, B., and Pevet, B. P. (1993) Daily rhythms of melatonin binding-sites in the rat pars tuberalis and suprachiasmatic nuclei: Evidence for a regulation of melatonin receptors by melatonin itself. *Neuroendocrinology* 57: 120–126.

Gillette, M. U., and Prosser, R. A. (1988) Circadian rhythm of the rat suprachiasmatic brain slice is rapidly reset by daytime application of cAMP analogs. *Brain Res.* 474: 348–52.

Goel, N., and Lee, T. M. (1995) Sex differences and effects of social cues on daily rhythms following phase advances in *Octodon degus*. *Physiol. Behav.* 58: 205–213.

Goldman, B. D. (1991) Parameters of the circadian rhythm of pineal melatonin secretion affecting reproductive responses in Siberian hamsters. *Steroids* 56: 218–225.

Goldman B. D., Darrow, J. M., Yogev, L. (1984) Effects of timed melatonin infusions on reproductive development in the Djungarian hamster (*Phodopus sungorus*). *Endocrinology* 114: 2074–2083.

Goldman, B. D., Hall, V., Hollister, C., Reppert, S., Roychoudhury, P., Yellon, S., and Tamarkin, L. (1981) Diurnal changes in pineal melatonin content in four rodent species: Relationship to photoperiodism. *Biol. Reprod.* 24: 778–783.

Haimov, I., Lavie, P. (1997) Melatonin: A chronobiotic and soporific hormone. *Arch. Gerontol. Geriatr.* 24: 167–173.

Haimov, I., Lavie, P., Laudon, M., Herer, P., Vigder, C., and Zisapel, I. (1995) Melatonin replacement therapy of elderly insomniacs. *Sleep* 18: 598–603.

Hastings, M. H., Mead, S. M., Vindlaceravu, R. R., Ebling, F. J. P., Maywood, E. S., Grosse, J. (1992) Non-photic phase shifting of the circadian activity rhythm of Syrian hamsters: The relative potency of arousal and melatonin. *Brain Res.* 591: 20–26.

Herzog, E. D., Geusz, M. E., Khalsa, S. B. S., Straume, M., and Block, G. D. (1997) Circadian rhythms in mouse suprachiasmatic nucleus explants on multimicroelectrode plates. *Brain Res.* 757: 285–290.

Hoffmann, K. (1979) Photoperiod, pineal, melatonin and reproduction in hamsters. *Prog. Brain Res.* 52: 397–415.

Honma, K., Honma, S., and Hiroshige, T. (1987) Activity rhythms in the circadian domain appear in suprachiasmatic nuclei lesioned rats given methamphetamine. *Physiol. Behav.* 40: 767–774.

Honma, S., Shirakawa, T., Katsuno, Y., Namihira, M., and Honma, K. (1998) Circadian periods of single suprachiasmatic neurons in rats. *Neurosci. Lett.* 250: 157–160.

Hurk, R., and Wiegant, V. M. (1994) Preferential induction of c-fos immunoreactivity in vasoactive intestinal polypeptide-innervated gonadotropin-releasing hormone neurons during a steroid-induced luteinizing hormone surge in the female rat. *Endocrinology* 134: 2636–2644.

Inouye, S.-I., and Kawamura, H. (1979) Persistence of circadian rhythmicity in a mammalian hypothalamic "island" containing the suprachiasmatic nucleus. *Proc. Natl. Acad. Sci. USA* 76: 5962–5966.

James, S. P., Sack, D. A., Rosenthal, N. E., and Mendelson, W. B. (1990) Melatonin administration in insomnia. *Neuropsychopharmacology* 3: 19–23.

Kashon, M. L., Wilson, M. E., Rosewell, K. L., Shughrue, P. J., Mehta, K. D., Merchenthaler, I., and Wise, P. M. (1999) Age differentially influences estrogen receptor-β (ERβ) gene expression in specific regions of the brain. *Soc. Neurosci. Abstr.* 25: 1961.

Katzenberg, D., Young, T., Finn, L., Lin, L., King, D. P., Takahashi, J. S., and Mignot, E. (1998) A CLOCK polymorphism associated with human diurnal preference. *Sleep* 21: 569–576.

Kennaway, D. J., and Rowe, S. A. (1995) Melatonin binding-sites and their role in seasonal reproduction. *J. Reprod. Fertil. Suppl.* 49: 423–435.

Kent, S., Hurd, M., and Satinoff, E. (1991) Interactions between body temperature and wheel running over the estrous cycle in rats. *Physiol. Behav.* 49: 1079–1084.

Klein, D. C., Smoot, R., Weller, J. L., Higa, S., Markey, S. P., Creed G. J., and Jacobowitz, D. M. (1983) Lesions of the paraventricular nucleus area of the hypothalamus disrupt the suprachiasmatic spinal-cord circuit in the melatonin rhythm generating-system. *Brain Res. Bull.* 10: 647–652.

Labyak, S. E., and Lee, T. M. (1995) Estrus- and steroid-induced changes in circadian rhythms in a diurnal rodent, *Octodon degus. Physiol. Behav.* 58: 573–585.

Lee, T. M., Gorman, M. R. (2000) Timing of reproduction by the intergration of photoperiod with other seasonal signals. In K. Wallen, J. E. Schneider (Eds.), *Reproduction in Context.* Cambridge, Mass.: MIT Press, pp. 191–218.

Lee, T. M., and Labyak, S. E. (1997) Free-running rhythms and light- and dark-pulse phase response curves for diurnal *Octodon degus* (Rodentia). *Am. J. Physiol.* 273: R278–R286.

LeSauter, J., and Silver, R. (1999) Localization of a suprachiasmatic nucleus subregion regulating locomotor rhythmicity. *J. Neurosci.* 19: 5574–5585.

Lincoln, G. (1999) Melatonin modulation of prolactin and gonadotrophin secretion. Systems ancient and modern. *Adv. Exp. Med. Biol.* 460: 137–153.

Liu, C., Weaver, D. R., Strogatz, S. H., and Reppert, S. M. (1997) Cellular construction of a circadian clock: Period determination in the suprachiasmatic nuclei. *Cell* 91: 855–860.

Malpaux, B., Daveau, A., Maurice-Mandon, F., Duarte, G., and Chemineau, P. (1998) Evidence that melatonin acts in the premammillary hypothalamic area to control reproduction in the ewe: Presence of binding sites and stimulation of luteinizing hormone secretion by in situ microimplant delivery. *Endocrinology* 139: 1508–1516.

Malpaux, B., Daveau, A., Maurice, F., Gayrard, V., and Thiery, J. C. (1993) Effects of melatonin on luteinizing-hormone secretion in the ewe: Evidence for central sites of action in the mediobasal hypothalamus. *Biol. Reprod.* 48: 752–760.

McArthur, A. J., Gillette, M. U., and Prosser, R. A. (1991) Melatonin directly resets the rat suprachiasmatic circadian clock in vitro. *Brain Res.* 565: 158–161.

Meyer-Bernstein, E. L., Jetton, A. E., Matsumoto, S. I., Markuns, J. F., Lehman, M. N., and Bittman, E. L. (1999) Effects of suprachiasmatic transplants on circadian rhythms of neuroendocrine function in golden hamsters. *Endocrinology* 140: 207–218.

Moore, R. Y., and Lenn, N. J. (1972) A retinohypothalamic projection in the rat. *J. Comp. Neurol.* 146: 1–14.

Morin, L. P. (1985) Biological rhythms. In H. I. Siegel (Ed.), *The Hamster.* New York: Plenum Press, pp. 323–345.

Morin, L. P., and Cummings, L. A. (1982) Splitting of wheel running rhythms by castrated or steroid treated male and female hamsters. *Physiol. Behav.* 29: 665–675.

Morin, L. P., Fitzgerald, K. M., and Zucker, I. (1977) Estradiol shortens the period of hamster circadian rhythms. *Science* 196: 305–307.

Myers, B., Badia, P., Murphy, P., Wright, K., Jr., Hughes, R., and Hakel, M. (1995) Circadian effects of photic stimulation on the melatonin and temperature rhythms of humans. *Sleep Res.* 23: 534.

Neu, J. M., and Niles, L. P. (1997) A marked diurnal rhythms of melatonin ML1A receptor mRNA expression in the suprachiasmatic nucleus. *Mol. Brain Res.* 49: 303–306.

Osol, G., Schwartz, B., and Foss, D. C. (1985) Effects of time, photoperiod, and pinealectomy on ocular and plasma melatonin concentrations in the chick. *Gen. Comp. Endocrinol.* 58: 415–420.

Palmer, J. D. (1995) Review of the dual-clock control of tidal rhythms and the hypothesis that the same clock governs both circatidal and circadian rhythms. *Chronobiol. Internat.* 12: 299–310.

Quay, W. B. (1968) Individuation and lack of pineal effect in the rat's circadian locomotor rhythm. *Physiol. Behav.* 3: 109–118.

Quay, W. B. (1970) Precocious entrainment and associated characteristics of activity patterns following pinealectomy and reversal of photoperiod. *Physiol. Behav.* 5: 1281–1290.

Ralph, M. R., Foster, R. G., Davis, F. C., and Menaker, M. (1990) Transplanted suprachiasmatic nucleus determines circadian period. *Science* 247: 975–977.

Ralph, M. R., and Menaker, M. (1988) A mutation of the circadian system in golden hamsters. *Science* 241: 1225–1227.

Redman, J. R., and Armstrong, S. M. (1988) Reentrainment of rat circadian activity rhythms: Effects of melatonin. *J. Pineal Res.* 5: 203–215.

Redman, J. R., Armstrong, S. M., and Ng, K. T. (1983) Free-running activity rhythms in the rat: Entrainment by melatonin. *Science* 219: 1989–1091.

Refinetti, R., and Menaker, M. (1992) Evidence for separate control of estrous and circadian periodicity in the golden hamster. *Behav. Neural Biol.* 58: 27–36.

Reiter, R. J. (1980) The pineal and its hormones in the control of reproduction in mammals. *Endocrine Rev.* 1: 109–131.

Reppert, S. M., Weaver, D. R., Rivkees, S. A., and Stopa, E. G. (1988) Putative melatonin receptors in a human biological clock. *Science* 242: 78–81.

Richards, W. P. (1966) Activity measured by running wheels and observation during the oestrous cycle, pregnancy and pseudopregnancy in the golden hamster. *Anim. Behav.* 14: 450–458.

Sack, R. L., Lewy, A. J., Blood, M. L., Stevenson, J., and Keith, L. D. (1991) Melatonin administration to blind people: Phase advances and entrainment. *J. Biol. Rhythms* 6: 249–261.

Samel, A., Wegmann, H. M., Vejvoda, M., Maass, H., Gundel, A., and Schutz, M. (1991) Influence of melatonin treatment on human circadian rhythmicity before and after a simulated 9-hour time shift. *J. Biol. Rhythms* 6: 235–248.

Sassin, J. F., Grantz, A. G., Weitz, E. D., and Kapen, S. (1972) Human prolactin: 24-hour pattern with increased release during sleep. *Science* 177: 1205–1207.

Sawaki, Y., Nihonmatsu, I., and Kawamura, H. (1984) Transplantation of the neonatal suprachiasmatic nuclei into rats with complete bilateral suprachiasmatic lesions. *Neurosci. Res.* 1: 67–72.

Schwartz, W. J., and Gainer, H. (1977) Suprachiasmatic nucleus: Use of 14C-labeled deoxyglucose uptake as a functional marker. *Science* 197: 1089–1091.

Shibata, S., Cassone, V. M., Moore, R. Y. (1989) Effects of melatonin on neuronal activity in the rat suprachiasmatic nucleus in vitro. *Neuroscience* 97: 140–144.

Shibata, S., Oomura, Y., Kita, H., and Hattori, K. (1982) Circadian rhythmic changes of neuronal activity in the suprachiasmatic nucleus of the rat hypothalamic slice. *Brain Res.* 247: 154–158.

Short, R. V. (1984) Oestrous and menstrual cycles. In C. R. Austin and R. V. Short (Eds.), *Reproduction in Mammals*, vol. 3: *Hormonal Control of Reproduction,* 2nd edition. Cambridge: Cambridge University Press, pp. 115–152.

Shughrue, P. J., Lane, M. V., and Merchenthaler, I. (1997) Comparative distribution of estrogen receptor-α and -β m-RNA in the rat central nervous system. *J. Comp. Neurol.* 388: 507–525.

Silver, R., LeSauter, J., Tresco, P. A., and Lehman, M. N. (1996) A diffusible coupling signal from the transplanted suprachiasmatic nucleus controlling circadian locomotor rhythms. *Nature* 382: 810–813.

Spitzer, R. L., Terman, M. Williams, J. B. W., Terman, J. S., Malt, U. F., Singer, F., and Lewy, A. J. (1999) Jet-lag: Clinical features, validation of a new syndrome-specific scale, and lack of response to melatonin in a randomized, double-blind trial. *Am. J. Psychiatr.* 156: 1392–1396.

Stankov, B., Moller, M., Lucini, V., Capsoni, S., and Fraschini, F. (1994) A carnivore species (Canis familiaris) expresses circadian melatonin rhythm in the peripheral blood and melatonin receptors in the brain. *Eur. J. Endocrin.* 131: 191–200.

Starke, S. J., Walker, M. P., Beresford, I. J. M., and Hagan, R. M. (1995) Modulation of the rat suprachiasmatic circadian clock by melatonin in-vitro. *Neuroreport* 6: 1947–1951.

Stehle, J., Vanecek, J., and Vollrath, L. (1989) Effects of melatonin on spontaneous electrical activity of neurons in rat suprachiasmatic nuclei: An iontophoretic study. *J. Neural Transm.* 78: 173–177.

Stephan, F. K., and Zucker, I. (1972) Circadian rhythms in drinking behavior and locomotor activity are eliminated by suprachiasmatic lesions. *Proc. Natl. Acad. Sci. USA* 69: 1583–1586.

Stetson, M. H., and Watson-Whitmyre, M. (1977) The neural clock regulating estrous cyclicity in hamsters: Gonadotropin release following barbiturate blockade. *Biol. Reprod.* 16: 536–542.

Stobie, K. M., and Weick, R. F. (1990) Effects of lesions of the suprachiasmatic and paraventricular nuclei on the inhibition of pulsatile luteinizing hormone release by exogenous vasoactive intestinal peptide in the ovariectomized rat. *Neuroendocrinology* 51: 649–657.

Sumová, A., Trávníčková, Z., Peters, R., Schwartz, W. J., and Illnerová, H. (1995) The rat suprachiasmatic nucleus is a clock for all seasons. *Proc. Natl. Acad. Sci. USA* 92: 7754–7758.

Takahashi, J. S., and Menaker, M. (1980) Interaction of estradiol and progesterone: Effects on circadian locomotor rhythm of female golden hamsters. *Am. J. Physiol.* 239: R497–R504.

Takahashi, J. S., Murakami, N., Nikaido, S. S., Pratt, B. L., and Robertson, L. M. (1989) The avian pineal, a vertebrate model system of the circadian oscillator: Cellular regulation of circadian rhythms by light, second messengers, and macromolecular synthesis. *Recent Prog. Horm. Res.* 45: 279–352.

Vakkuri, O., Rintamaki, H., and Leppaluoto, J. (1985) Plasma and tissue concentrations of melatonin after midnight light exposure and pinealectomy in the pigeon. *J. Endocrinol.* 105: 263–268.

van der Beek, E. M., Wiegant, V. M., van der Donk, H. A., van den Hurk, R., and Buijs, R. M. (1993) Lesions of the suprachiasmatic nucleus indicate the presence of a direct vasoactive intestinal polypeptide-containing projection to gonadotrophin-releasing hormone neurons in the female rat. *J. Neuroendocrinol.* 5: 137–144.

Vanacek, J. (1988) Melatonin binding sites. *J. Neurochem.* 51: 1436–1440.

Vanacek, J., Pavlik, A., and Illnerova, H. (1987) Hypothalamic melatonin receptor-sites revealed by autoradiography. *Brain Res.* 435: 359–362.

Warren, W. S., Hodges, D. B., and Cassone, V. M. (1993) Pinealectomized rats entrain and phase-shift to melatonin injection in a dose-dependent manner. *J. Biol. Rhythms* 8: 233–245.

Weaver, D. R., Rivkees, S. A., Reppert, S. M. (1989) Localization and characterization of melatonin receptors in rodent brain by in vitro autoradiography. *J. Neruosci.* 9: 2581–2590.

Weaver, D. R., Stehle, J. H., Stopa, E. G., and Reppert, S. M. (1993) Melatonin receptors in human hypothalamus and pituitary: Implications for circadian and reproductive responses to melatonin. *J. Clin. Endocrinol. Metab.* 76: 295–301.

Wever, R. A. (1984) Sex-differences in human circadian rhythms—intrinsic periods and sleep fractions. *Experientia* 40: 1226–1234.

Wever, R. A. (1986) Characteristics of circadian rhythms in human functions. *J. Neur. Trans.* 21(Suppl.): 323–373.

Wiegand, S. J., Terasawa, E., Bridson, W. E., and Goy, R. W. (1980) Effects of discrete lesions of preoptic and suprachiasmatic structures in the female rat. Alterations in the feedback regulation of gonadotropin secretion. *Neuroendocrinology* 31: 147–157.

Williams, L. M. (1989) Melatonin-binding sites in the rat-brain and pituitary mapped by in vitro autoradiography. *J. Mol. Endocrinol.* 3: 71–75.

Williams, L. M., and Morgan, P. J. (1988) Demonstration of melatonin-binding sites on the pars tuberalis of the rat. *J. Endocrinol.* 119: R1–R3.

Wright, K. P., Jr., and Badia, P. (1999) Effect of menstrual cycle phase and oral contraceptives on alertness, cognitive performance, and circadian rhythms during sleep deprivation. *Behav. Brain Res.* 103: 185–194.

Yamazaki, S., Numano, R., Abe, M., Hida, A., Takahashi, R., Ueda, M., Block, G. D., Sakaki, Y., Menaker, M., and Tei, H. (2000) Resetting central and peripheral circadian oscillators in transgenic rats. *Science* 288: 682–685.

Zaidan, R., Geofriau, M., Brun, J., Taillard, J., Bureau, C., Chazot, G., and Claustrat, B. (1994) Melatonin is able to influence its secretion in humans: Description of a phase response curve. *Neuroendocrinology* 60: 105–112.

Zeitzer, J. M., Daniels, J. E., Duffy, J. F., Klerman, E. B., Shanahan, T. L., Dijk, D.-J., and Czeisler, C. A. (1999) Do plasma melatonin concentrations decline with age? *Am. J. Med.* 107: 432–436.

Zucker, I., Fitzgerald, K. M., and Morin, L. P. (1980) Sex differentiation of the circadian system in the golden hamster. *Am. J. Physiol.* 238: R97–R101.

IV Hormonal Influences on Sensorimotor Function and Cognition

This next section addresses behaviors that seem far removed from reproduction: hormonal influences and sex differences in motor patterns, responses to stimulant drugs, and learning, memory, and cognitive function. Do most boys play harder than most girls do? Are boys really better at math and girls better at language? If these things are true, is there a biological basis for these differences or are they culturally based? One way to tell whether differences in humans are biological or cultural is to study analogous behaviors in nonhuman animals. If other species exhibit the same pattern of sexual dimorphisms in certain behaviors, it might be due to biological differences.

Chapter 13 discusses the effects of gonadal hormones on nonreproductive behaviors and on neural systems that are involved in motor behavior and in "reward" systems. The fact that there are hormonal effects on these areas of the brain has implications for drug abuse, among other things. Chapter 14 will discuss the effects of pituitary, adrenal, and gonadal hormones on learning and memory in nonhuman animals. There is now substantial evidence that cognitive strategies differ between males and females of a number of species. Chapter 15 may prove especially challenging because it deals with the controversial issue of how men and women differ in cognitive abilities and whether hormones contribute to such differences.

13 Hormonal Influences on Sensorimotor Function

Jill B. Becker

In this chapter we find that hormones can affect neuronal activity in areas of the brain that are important for the complex processing of cognitive and sensorimotor information. Several interesting models have taken advantage of pharmacological methods to reveal and measure the effects of gonadal hormones on motor activity, sensory processing, and the integration of sensorimotor information. It turns out that these same neural systems are activated by drugs of abuse and are implicated in addiction. So we also will discuss the possible roles that hormones and gender may play in drug addiction.

What are the effects of gonadal steroids on neurotransmitter activity and on neural activity and structure? How can we measure the behavioral consequences of such changes? How do males and females differ in these neural systems?

Introduction

As you have learned in earlier chapters, hormones can have dramatic influences on an animal's reproductive behaviors by acting on the hypothalamus and limbic system of the brain. The behaviors that you have learned about so far—sexual behaviors, courtship behaviors, and affiliative behaviors—are just a small sample of the numerous sexually dimorphic or hormonally modulated behaviors exhibited by animals. In this chapter, we will learn about sex-related differences in, and hormonal influences on, some behaviors that are not usually considered in the context of hormonal modulation. First, we will consider sensation, activity, and the interface of these two functions—sensorimotor behavior. We ask, is an animal's ability to detect or perceive elements of the environment affected by its sex and its hormonal state? What components of how an animal moves through an environment and behaves in that environment are affected by its sex or hormonal condition? The answers to these questions have implications for a wide range of behaviors.

It is important to learn about sex-related differences in naturally occurring and spontaneous behaviors, because this gives us clues about why these behaviors are important to the animal in the wild. It is also helpful to know about sex-related differences in response to pharmacological agents or drugs, because that can help us begin to determine how the brain is sexually dimorphic. This is particularly true if we use drugs that act selectively on one neurotransmitter system. So we will also examine what happens when neurotransmitter systems are overstimulated by the administration of drugs that are typically abused by humans. For example, there are sex differences in the behavioral response to psychomotor stimulant drugs such as amphetamine or cocaine. Finally, we will examine the neural bases for sex differences in some naturally occurring and drug-induced behaviors (which turn out to be due to the same sex differences in the brain).

Sex Differences in, and Hormonal Influences on, Sensation and Activity

Sensation

If we look at the data on sex differences in, or hormonal influences on, the ability to smell, taste, and feel pain or touch, we find that in general females have lower thresholds for most sensations. This is true in rodents, women, and other species where it has been studied. For example, women tend to score better than do men on tests of odor identification and odor detection (Yousem et al. 1999). In the first demonstration of a sex difference in sensitivity to an identified mammalian pheromone, the female pig is five times more sensitive to the male pheromone, androstenone, than are intact male pigs (Dorries et al. 1995).

In rodents, odors (presumably pheromones) from conspecifics can have a profound influence on a female's neuroendocrinology. In the octodon degu, a South American rodent, a female can use the scent of another female to help entrain her biological rhythm to a new light:dark cycle, while males are not sensitive to this olfactory information (Goel et al. 1998). In mice, the scent from male mouse urine can affect a female mouse (depending on her hormonal state) by inducing estrus (Whitten effect), suppressing estrus (Lee-Boot effect), blocking pregnancy (Bruce effect), or accelerating puberty (Vandenbergh effect) (Bronson 1989; Vandenbergh 1979). These effects of odors on the female neuroendocrine system are thought to be detected by a sexually dimorphic vomeronasal system in rodents. These findings and other effects of the environment (physical and social) on hormones and behavior are discussed in more detail in chapter 18.

TASTE
Female rats exhibit a greater preference for sweet tastes (either glucose or saccharin) than males do. The ovarian hormones, estrogen and progesterone, are apparently involved in establishing taste preference in adult females. Once the sweet-taste preference has been established in the intact female rat, the preference is retained in the absence of the hormones, as ovariectomy has no effect on the behavior. Interestingly, women rate sweet tastes more intense than men do. If the taste test occurs immediately after a meal the more intense sweetness is rated unpleasant by women (Laeng et al. 1993). Adult female rats also develop a greater taste preference for salt solutions than males do. Neonatal hormone manipulations can reverse the development of salt-taste preferences in adults (Beatty 1979).

On the other hand, estrogen treatment can induce the formation of taste aversions in rats (Ganesan 1994; Merwin and Doty 1994). This suggests that estrogen may be affecting the intensity of the sensation of taste, so that either taste preferences or taste aversions are formed as a consequence of the stronger taste sensation that is produced in the presence of estrogen. Perhaps related to these hormonal influences on taste preferences is the observation that male rats, mice, and guinea pigs eat more than females of their respective species. This results in sex differences in body weight that are hormone dependent.

The effect of hormones on body weight is partly due to activational mechanisms. Estrogen will reduce body weight and testosterone will increase it in both castrated males and ovariectomized females. However, there are also organizational effects that influence the magnitude of body weight changes induced by estrogen and testosterone in guinea pigs. Male guinea pigs show greater body-weight increases in response to testosterone and less of a decrease in body weight induced by estrogen than females do (Czaja 1984). You should note that in some species (e.g., hamsters and spotted hyenas), females are bigger than males. In these species, we would not expect to find the same relations between hormones and body weight as described above for rats, mice, and guinea pigs.

TACTILE SENSATION

During the estrous cycle, estrogen has been shown to increase the size of the receptive fields for tactile stimuli delivered to the rump or perianal region of rats and hamsters. Furthermore, female rats tend to be more responsive to stimulation with electric shock to the feet than are males when they are tested in a shuttle box, where the animal moves from one side of the box to the other in response to an aversive stimulus. Female rats are found to have both lower shock thresholds and shorter escape latencies (Beatty 1979). This sensitivity to shock is modulated by perinatal androgenization and by gonadectomy in the adult, so this is thought to reflect sex differences in the neural systems mediating pain.

However, it is possible for hormonal influences on secondary sex characteristics to also change sensory sensitivity. For example, estrogen increases subcutaneous fatty deposits while testosterone increases muscle mass. Both of these hormonal effects may alter the sensitivity of an animal to tactile stimuli. By measuring both threshold and response latency (when pain thresholds are being measured, which is called nocioceptive reactivity), it is possible to determine whether secondary sex characteristics are interacting with an animal's sensitivity to stimulation. Subsequent studies of sex-related differences in response to pain and analgesia (i.e., relief from pain) have demonstrated that sex differences persist even when nocioceptive reactivity is comparable for males and females. This indicates that the sex differences reported are due to sex differences in the brain (Ryan and Maier 1988).

ANALGESIA

As discussed in chapter 11, analgesia can be induced by stress, and this is one paradigm that has been used to study sex differences in the analgesic response. In males, stress-induced analgesia is opioid-dependent and is greater in males than in females. There is also a sexual dimorphism in that females exhibit an opioid-independent response that male mice do not have. This female-specific system has been shown to be estrogen-dependent and to develop as a function of the neonatal hormone milieu (Bodnar et al. 1988; Mogil et al. 1997; Ryan and Maier 1988).

Activity and Motor Abilities

OPEN-FIELD ACTIVITY

When rats are placed in a large, open testing arena (about 90×90 cm), females tend to walk around more (ambulate) than males do. Females also rear more than males, but defecate less. The effect of gonadectomy on open-field activity is sex dependent. Castration of males has no effect, while ovariectomy causes a decrease in ambulation and rearing. The effect of ovariectomy is not consistent, however, for some authors report no effect on open-field behavior (Beatty 1979; Slob et al. 1981; Stevens and Goldstein 1981; Stewart and Cygan 1980).

The organizational effects of hormones during development on open-field behavior in the adult are quite interesting because it seems that there are two phases to the organizational process. The administration of either estrogen or testosterone to females during the perinatal period of sexual differentiation suppresses open-field behavior in the adult female rat. Therefore, the absence of androgens and estrogens during the perinatal period is necessary for feminization of this behavior. In addition, exposure of female rats to estrogen during later development appears to also be necessary for the normally high levels of activity in the adult. This additional requirement for estrogen during later postnatal development was demonstrated in experiments by Stewart and Cygan (1980) where female and male rats were gonadectomized on day 1. Animals were then treated with estrogen for 10 days, either from 10 to 20 days of age or from 30 to 40 days. Either treatment was effective at increasing ambulation and rearing in adults of both sexes. Therefore, the presence of high concentrations of testosterone or estrogen during the perinatal period suppresses open-field activity. The additional presence of estrogen later in life is necessary to complete the sexual differentiation process that results in the open-field activity seen in normal females.

Other species of rodents also show sex differences in activity, but not always under the same conditions as rats do. Mice frequently do not show sex differences in open-field activity. However, if locomotor activity is tested in the home cage, an organizational effect of perinatal hormones on general activity is reported. Intact females are more active than intact male mice are. If male mice are castrated on day 1 of life, then they are more active as adults than males that were castrated after the critical perinatal period. Conversely, if females are given androgens on day 1, they are less active than normal females (Broida and Svare 1984).

Females that are located in utero between two male fetuses (and therefore exposed in utero to the male's androgens) exhibit less locomotor activity as adults than do females located between two females in utero. Interestingly, male mice were also influenced by intrauterine position. Males located in utero between two females were more active as adults than males located between two males. Therefore, in mice there is a graded effect of perinatal hormones on adult activity (box 13.1). The hormones secreted by an individual mouse as well as those of its adjacent siblings contribute to the animal's activity as an adult, presumably through sexual differentiation of the brain. Whether there is an additional requirement for estrogen during adolescent development (as was true for rats) has not been investigated (Archer 1975; Broida and Svare 1984; Kinsley et al. 1986).

Sex differences in general activity are probably also prevalent in other species, but few have been studied as extensively as rats and mice. For example, sex differences in activity have been reported in the African clawed frog, *Xenopus laevis*. As was true in rodents, female frogs are more active than males. The organizational or activational role(s) of hormones on activity in Xenopus have not been investigated (Merkle 1989).

RUNNING-WHEEL ACTIVITY

The activity of rodents in a running wheel is a curious phenomenon. Anyone who has had a pet hamster or gerbil with an activity wheel in its cage has observed this phenomenon. During the night, hamsters, rats, or gerbils will step into the wheel and run the equivalent of miles. In female rodents, this behavior is hormonally modulated. There is a dramatic increase in running-wheel activity on the evening of behavioral estrus. This behavior has been shown to be activated by estrogen in both males and females. Since estrogen is equally effective in both sexes, hormones do not organize running-wheel activity during the perinatal period of sexual differentiation. Progesterone inhibits the effect of estrogen to activate running-wheel activity, although not completely. The *preoptic area (POA)* of the anterior hypothalamus has been implicated in the mediation of the effects of estrogen on running-wheel behavior. Implants of crystalline estradiol into the POA activates running-wheel behavior (Fahrbach et al. 1985; Wade and Zucker 1970). It is not clear that this effect is specific to the hypothalamus, however, as implants of estradiol into the striatum also activate running-wheel activity (Roy 1987).

Other hormones may also modulate running-wheel behavior in rodents. For example, in adult rats running-wheel behavior decreases when growth hormone secretion increases and vice versa (Axelson et al. 1986; Beatty 1979; Kelly 1983). However, showing that hormonal changes are correlated with a behavior does not prove causation. Further research is needed to demonstrate cause and effect relations between growth hormone and running-wheel behavior.

SOCIAL PLAY

Sex differences in social play behavior in juvenile animals has been described for a large number of species. The list includes rats, ponies, sea lions, sheep, hamsters, marmosets, squirrel monkeys, baboons, rhesus monkeys, chimpanzees, and humans. In all these species, males show both a greater incidence

Box 13.1 Intrauterine Position Affects Hormonal Exposure in Utero

Sexual differentiation of the brain of animals born in litters is more complex than of animals that have only one baby at a time. This is because the embryos all share a common blood supply. The hormones produced by neighboring embryos can affect the sexual differentiation of siblings. In order to determine intrauterine position, fetuses are delivered by cesarean section just before normal parturition. Animals are then classified by the sex of the embryos next to them. A female embryo between two other females would be called 0M (not next to a male). A female next to one female and one male would be a 1M female (next to one male). If a female is between two males she is called a 2M female. Similarly, males can be classified as 0M to 2M. The intrauterine hormones that 2M females are exposed to are not enough to completely masculinze them, but they do have significant effects on the anogenital distance and on the locomotor and aggressive behavior (vom Saal et al. 1983).

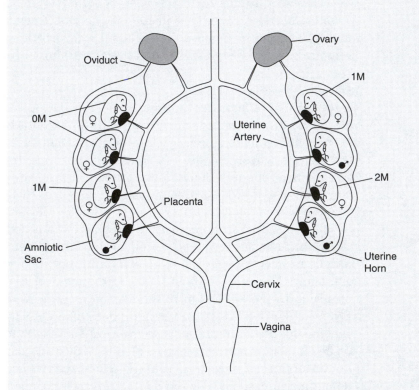

In general, male mice and rats are more aggressive than females, and this sex-related difference has been shown to be dependent on exposure to hormones during the perinatal period. In adult males, the amount of aggression is related to circulating testosterone. When aggressive behavior is assessed in female mice, however, 2M females show a greater duration of maternal aggression than 0M females postpartum. These 2M females are also more likely to be aggressive against other females in general. Males are similarly affected: 2M males are more likely to be aggressive than are 0M males.

The effects of intrauterine hormone exposure demonstrate two important points: (1) Masculine or feminine is not an all-or-none thing. Instead, there can be variations on the theme with gradations between the two extremes (2M males and 0M females being the extremes). (2) We see clear evidence that the hormone milieu that result in sexual differentiation of reproductive behaviors also affect other behaviors, including locomotor activity and aggressive behavior.

and a higher intensity of play-fighting (also referred to as rough-and-tumble play) (Meaney et al. 1985).

In rats, play-fighting is first observed shortly before weaning at about 18 days of age and reaches its peak at about 30 to 40 days of age, which is around the time of puberty. Play-fighting behavior is initiated when one rat attempts to rub its snout along the nape of another rat's neck. The recipient then uses defensive tactics to protect its nape from contact, such as rolling over in a supine position. Males tend to initiate these "nape-attacks" more frequently than females do. Furthermore, females go on the defensive earlier in the attack (when the attacker's snout is further from the nape). This may be due in part to sex differences in sensory sensitivity as discussed above. There are also sex differences in the actual defensive behaviors exhibited. Males move their bodies to block the opponent and counterattack as they are defending themselves, while females move their bodies out of harm's way. This motoric sex difference is thought to reflect sex differences in the organization of the neural systems that control motor behavior patterns (Pellis et al. 1997).

Sex differences in social play behavior have been demonstrated to be dependent on the organizational effects of early exposure to androgens. Either dihydrotestosterone or testosterone treatment of females during the critical period of sexual differentiation is sufficient to produce a masculine pattern of play-fighting in adolescent rats or rhesus monkeys. Thus, the effect of testosterone on the sexual differentiation of this behavior is due directly to testosterone and is not dependent on the conversion of testosterone to estradiol (Goy and McEwen 1980; Meaney et al. 1985). Finally, the adrenal steroids may also influence the development of play-fighting behavior, but in the opposite direction of the effect found for testosterone. Corticosterone (or the synthetic glucocorticoid dexamethasone) administered early after birth inhibited the masculinization of play-fighting in male rat pups, but had no effect in females (Meaney et al. 1985).

The effects of both androgens and glucocorticoids on the development of play-fighting are strictly organizational. The administration of either hormone during the juvenile period is without influence on this behavior. The amygdala has been implicated as the site in the brain where androgens are producing their effects. Testosterone implanted into the amygdala of 1-day-old female rats produced a masculinization of play-fighting behavior later in life. Testosterone implants in other brain regions were without effect on this behavior. Since the amygdala also has glucocorticoid receptors, it is possible that this is the site where glucocorticoids act. This possibility has not been tested experimentally yet, so it remains an open question (Meaney and McEwen 1986; Meaney et al. 1985).

Although a role for the hormonal organization of sex differences in brain function has been emphasized as an underlying mechanism mediating sex differences in play-fighting, this is not the only factor important for the development of this behavior. There is clear evidence from all species that have been examined that mothers (and fathers when they play a role in nurturing) treat male and female infants differently. The way parents treat their infants can be shown to affect the infant's behavior.

How does this occur? In the rat, mothers get 60% of their fluids from the urine of their pups, which they express by licking the anogenital region of their pups (this is necessary so that the pups can urinate). Mother rats spend more time licking the anogenital regions of their male pups than of their female pups. Handling and experience can influence the development of brain and behavior in rats. This differential treatment of males and females by the mother is quite likely, therefore, to affect their subsequent development (for additional discussion and references, see Meaney et al. 1985). In primates, including humans, mothers seem to promote independent behavior in male infants and to remain in close contact with female infants. Thus, the sex differences in juvenile behavior, while mediated in part by the organizational effects of androgens and glucocorticoids on the brain, are probably also influenced in part by the social interactions between a mother and her young (Meaney et al. 1985).

MOVEMENT PATTERNS

For most of the behaviors discussed above, the sex differences and hormonal influences have been quantitative—one sex tends to exhibit a behavior more frequently than the other does. As was the case for play-fighting, however, it turns out that there are also sex differences in the ways that male and female rats move. This can be seen when we look carefully at the way that males and females move when they exhibit species-specific behaviors.

In an elegant series of experiments, Pellis and his co-workers (Field et al. 2000; Pellis et al. 1999) have shown that there are sex differences in the movements and postural adjustments that male and female rats make. These sex differences can be seen most clearly when looking at behaviors that occur in a consistent stereotypic pattern. For example, when a rat is eating a food pellet it will pivot and move laterally to avoid another rat that attempts to take the food away. Both males and females make these evasive moves, but the exact moves are sexually dimorphic. Males pivot around a point about mid-body, moving the snout away and pushing the pelvis towards the other rat. Females pivot around a point near the pelvis, so that the snout moves away from the other rat but the pelvis stays in about the same place. This same type of sex difference in movement can be seen when an animal makes a spontaneous turn in an open field. In other words, females pivot centered on their pelvis by moving primarily their front feet, while the hind feet take small steps to stay in place. Males, on the other hand, turn around a midpoint in their body, stepping with both forelimbs and hind limbs. Finally, if one analyzes the pattern of foot placement during normal walking, one also sees a sex difference. Males tend to walk with their back feet turned in towards the midline, while female rats walk with their hind feet turned out (Field et al. 2000; Pellis et al. 1999).

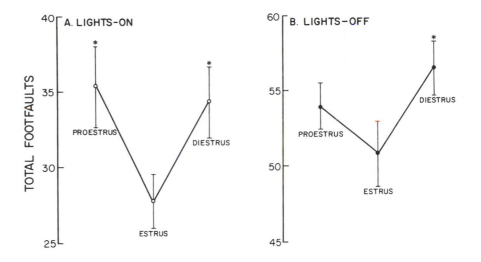

Figure 13.1 The influence of the estrous cycle and the light:dark cycle on sensorimotor performance in rats trained to walk across a narrow suspended beam. Female rats were repeatedly tested 2 hours after lights-on (*A*) or 2 hours after lights-off (*B*). The mean number of footfaults made over 3 consecutive days during the estrous cycle is depicted. Bars: SEM. Note the different ranges in the scales for A and B, suggesting that the task was more difficult when animals were tested in the dark (under red-light conditions so that the experimenter could see, but the albino rats could not). *Significantly different from estrus ($P < 0.05$). (Adapted from Becker et al. 1987.)

COORDINATED SENSORIMOTOR BEHAVIORS

It has also been shown that there are effects of the estrous cycle on behaviors that require coordination of sensory and motor information. In one study, conducted in the Becker laboratory, female rats were trained to traverse a narrow suspended beam. The rats quickly learned to walk across the beam and would do so without being food deprived. Looking at the accuracy of foot placement on the beam assessed sensorimotor function. If the foot was placed on top of the narrow beam, that was considered correct. When the foot slipped off the top, or grabbed onto the side, that was called a footfault. We found that female rats made fewer footfaults on estrus than on diestrus 1 or proestrus (figure 13.1) (Becker et al. 1987). We then wondered where in the brain ovarian hormones were acting to induce these effects.

To address this question, we trained ovariectomized female rats to walk across a suspended beam. After two or three weeks of training, their performance had stabilized. These rats then received implants of 17β-estradiol or a control substance (cholesterol or the biologically inactive estrogen 17α-estradiol). The implants were inserted bilaterally into the brain, in an area called the striatum, for 6 hours. Within 4 hours there was a dramatic improvement in sensorimotor performance: rats with cannulae that contained 17β-estradiol were making fewer footfaults. Animals continued to show improvement for 24 hours, and then behavior returned to baseline levels (figure 13.2). Importantly, control implants were ineffective, as were implants that

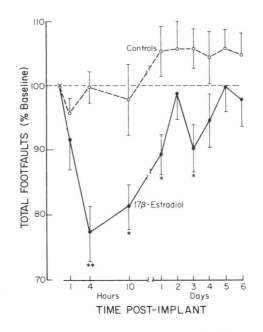

Figure 13.2 Intrastriatal cannulae containing 30% 17β-estradiol (70% cholesterol) induced a significant improvement in sensorimotor performance of ovariectomized female rats within 4 hours after implantation (closed circles). The total number of footfaults is expressed as a percentage of baseline performance (before the implants.) Control implants of 100% cholesterol or 30% 17α-estradiol: 70% cholesterol had no effect on performance (open circles). **Four hours after hormone treatment, animals that received 17β-estradiol showed a significant decrease in footfaults relative to controls ($P < 0.005$). *Significantly different from controls ($P < 0.05$). Controls did not differ from each other or from baseline at any point in time.). (Adapted from Becker et al. 1987.)

contained 17β-estradiol that missed the striatum. This suggests that estrogen can act directly on the striatum to improve sensorimotor performance. It turns out that there is considerable evidence that estrogen modulates activity of the neurotransmitter dopamine in the striatum, and that this effect of estrogen may be responsible for many of sex differences in, and hormonal influences on, the motor activity and behavior discussed above.

Gonadal Steroid Modulation of Activity in Ascending Dopamine-Mediated Behaviors

Let us consider how hormones may modulate dopamine activity in the striatum. Remember that during the estrous cycle of the rat, estrogen peaks on the afternoon of proestrus. This triggers the pre-ovulatory surge of LH, which in turn induces ovulation. The onset of behavioral receptivity (behavioral estrus) occurs 8 to 12 hours after the estrogen peak, in association with ovulation, usually after the onset of the dark phase of the light/dark cycle (see chapter 4). With each method employed, three questions should be addressed. First, does dopamine activity vary with the normal fluctuations in ovarian hormones that occur during the female rat's reproductive cycle? In other words, do ovarian hormones affect the day-to-day functions of the dopamine system in the female rat? If this proves to be the case, as discussed in chapter 1, then the question of which hormones are important comes next.

In order to determine if the gonadal steroid hormones influence the functional activity of the striatal dopamine system, a number of behavioral tests have been used. This neural system lends itself well to behavioral studies. Neurons with their cell bodies in the substantia nigra that project to striatum use the neurotransmitter dopamine. The ascending dopamine projection from the midbrain to the striatum is a massive projection, which contains over 90% of the dopamine in the brain (Lindvall and Bjorklund 1974). This means that the administration of drugs that activate or inhibit dopamine systems produces behaviors that are due primarily to activity in the ascending dopamine system. Behaviors that will be discussed have been shown through extensive experimentation to be mediated by the nigrostriatal dopamine system (Arbuthnott and Crow 1971; Costall and Naylor 1977; Fink and Smith 1980; Ungerstedt 1971; Ungerstedt 1974). Two behaviors have been used most frequently: rotational behavior and stereotyped behaviors induced by dopamine receptor agonists. Each of these behaviors has been demonstrated to depend on activation of the ascending dopamine system and to be correlated with the extent of dopamine activity in the striatum. Thus, these behaviors are used as an index, or behavioral assay, of dopamine activity in the striatum.

STEREOTYPED BEHAVIORS

When striatal dopamine activity increases, animals become hypersensitive to sensory stimuli. A rat that has received amphetamine, which induces dopamine release from dopamine terminals, becomes hypersensitive and hyperresponsive to sensory stimuli. For example, if you snap your fingers over a rat's head, normally no response is seen. If a rat has been given amphetamine, however, snapping your fingers over its head will elicit an exaggerated startle response. A similar behavioral syndrome is seen when dopamine receptor agonists are administered. In other words, the motor response to a given sensory input is greater when dopaminergic activity is increased. When high doses of dopamine mimetics such as apomorphine or amphetamine are administered to the rat, a wide variety of behaviors are induced. Shortly after drug administration the animal shows increased locomotor and exploratory behavior, and this is followed by a stereotypy phase. **Stereotyped behaviors** in the rodent are repetitive movements of the head, mouth, snout, whiskers, and forelimbs. Behaviors included are chewing movements, excessive sniffing (directed at nothing), up and down movements of the head, and jerky movements of the forelimbs. An animal will exhibit stereotyped behaviors for about an hour (depending on the dose) and then will start exhibiting locomotor activity again as the drug wears off. Experiments in the Becker laboratory have shown that female rats exhibit greater amphetamine-induced stereotypy during late proestrus/early estrus than on diestrus (Becker and Cha 1989).

A. ROTOMETER

B.

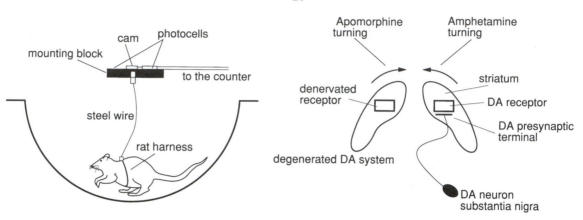

Figure 13.3 The behavioral apparatus used for assessing asymmetry in the nigrostriatal dopamine system (*A*) and a schematic model for mechanisms of dopaminergic drug-induced rotational behavior (*B*). (*A*) The behavioral apparatus employed is called a "rotometer." As is illustrated, during testing, the rat wears a nonconfining elastic harness around its chest. The harness is attached to a rigid steel wire that turns with the animal. The steel wire is attached to an assembly that can turn freely, opening and closing photocells as the animal turns. Output from the photocells is sent to a computer-controlled counter that records the number of 360° turns the animal makes during the test session. (*B*) After unilateral dopamine (DA) degeneration induced by injection of the neurotoxin 6-hydroxydopamine into the substantia nigra, rotational behavior is induced when drugs that stimulate the dopaminergic system are administered. The direction of turning is indicated by the arrows at the top of the figure. There has been considerable research to demonstrate that animals turn in circles away from the striatum that is most active. Since striatal DA receptors become supersensitive after DA denervation, administration of the DA receptor agonist apomorphine induces a greater postsynaptic response in the denervated striatum than in the intact striatum, and animals turn away from the side of the lesion. On the other hand, amphetamine induces DA release from intact DA nerve endings. Therefore, after amphetamine administration there is greater DA release in the intact striatum and animals turn away from the intact striatum.

ROTATIONAL BEHAVIOR

Another behavioral test used to assess dopamine activity in the striatum is drug-induced rotational behavior. When the nigrostriatal dopamine system is selectively damaged unilaterally (i.e., only on one side) by a neurotoxin that selectively destroys dopamine neurons (6-hydroxydopamine; 6OHDA), rats and other animals exhibit persistent circling toward the side of the lesion. A large number of studies have shown that animals typically turn in the direction that is contralateral to the nigrostriatal dopamine system that has the greatest activity (figure 13.3). Thus, after a unilateral 6OHDA lesion of the substantia nigra, the dopamine terminals in the striatum on that side degenerate and amphetamine can only release dopamine on the intact side. Activity in the intact striatum induces postural asymmetry and turning toward the damaged side. However, dopamine receptors in both striata are intact following a unilateral substantia nigra lesion. Apomorphine, acting on dopamine receptors, elicits turning in the other direction. This is thought to reflect the unilateral increase in the number of dopamine receptors on the denervated side that occurs due to process known as receptor denervation supersensitivity. Apomorphine activates more receptors on the side of the lesion, so the animal rotates away from the lesioned side toward its intact side.

As was true for stereotyped behaviors, studies examining amphetamine-induced or dopamine-induced postural asymmetries have found that female rats exhibit a greater behavioral response during late proestrus/early estrus than on diestrus (Becker and Cha 1989; Becker et al. 1987; Joyce and Van Hartesveldt 1984). Subsequent experiments demonstrated that gonadectomy resulted in a significant decrease in rotational behavior in female, but not male, rats. Furthermore, ovariectomy induced a decrease in rotational behavior on two different types of tests: amphetamine-induced rotational behavior, or rotational behavior induced by unilateral electrical stimulation of the ascending dopamine axons that project to the striatum (figure 13.4) (Camp et al. 1986; Robinson et al. 1981). This means that the effect of ovariectomy to attenuate the behavioral response induced during dopamine activation is not unique to the effect of drugs like amphetamine, but is a more general effect of stimulating the release of dopamine in the striatum.

Having found an effect of the estrous cycle on rotational behavior, and that ovariectomy attenuates this behavioral response, the next question is whether hormonal replacement could reinstate the response. So experiments tested whether estrogen treatment could enhance amphetamine-induced rotational behavior in the ovariectomized female rat. It was found that either repeated estrogen, to mimic the estrous cycle, or single dose of estrogen 30 min prior to amphetamine was sufficient to induce a significant increase in amphetamine-induced behaviors (Becker 1990b; Becker and Beer 1986). Estrogen also had a rapid effect on AMPH-induced stereotyped behaviors (figure 13.5B) (Becker and Rudick 1999). Interestingly, the results in figure 13.5 also indicate that the rapid effects of estrogen are enhanced by priming with estrogen. These findings are important for two reasons. First, they show that estrogen alone is sufficient to enhance the behavioral response to amphetamine. Second, they show that the effect of estrogen is very rapid, supporting the idea that this effect is not mediated by classical estrogen receptors (see chapter 2 for a discussion of the different types of estrogen receptors).

SEX-RELATED DIFFERENCES
The results discussed indicate that ovarian hormones are modulating behaviors mediated by the ascending dopamine system. The next question we will consider is whether there are sex differences in the behavior. In one experiment, rotational behavior was studied in male and female rats given amphetamine to induce dopamine release. In this experiment, brain and striatal concentrations of amphetamine were determined, and males received a higher dose of amphetamine than females in order to overcome sex differences in liver metabolism of amphetamine. When striatal concentrations of amphetamine were equalized during the behavioral testing period, male rats turned

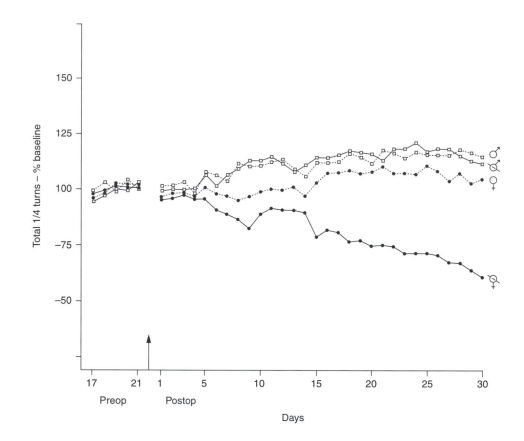

Figure 13.4 The mean total contraversive quarter turns elicited by electrical stimulation of the nigrostriatal dopamine pathway expressed as a percent change from baseline. Intact male and female rats had stimulating electrodes implanted unilaterally into the ascending nigrostriatal dopamine pathway. Animals were tested daily for 21 days and the mean number of quarter turns of the last 5 days was taken as baseline. At the arrow, half of the males and half of the females underwent gonadectomy. The other animals in each group received a sham operation. Animals were then tested daily for an additional 30 days. By day 15, post-gonadectomy, ovariectomized female rats made significantly fewer turns ($P < 0.05$) than did sham-operated females and both of the male groups. Filled circles, females; open squares, males; solid line, gonadectomized; dotted line, sham-operated ($N = 10$/group). (Adapted from Robinson et al. 1981.)

significantly less than did female rats at all stages of the estrous cycle except for diestrus 1 (figure 13.6) (Becker et al. 1982). Other studies have shown that there are sex differences in response to activation of the striatal dopamine system. Male rats exhibit lower rates of rotational behavior, locomotor activity, and stereotypy in response to amphetamine than do female rats in estrus. In addition, the behavior of female rats decreases dramatically following ovariectomy. Castration of male rats, by contrast, had no effect on rotational behavior (Becker et al. 1982; Camp et al. 1986; Robinson et al. 1981).

PACING OF SEXUAL BEHAVIOR
Demonstrating that in female rats estrogen modulates sensorimotor function and dopamine-induced behaviors through its effects on the striatum has been

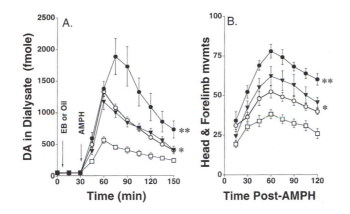

Figure 13.5 (*A*) The time line for amphetamine (AMPH)-induced (2.5 mg/kg) dopamine (DA) in dialysate from the dorsolateral striatum. DA concentration from rats undergoing in vivo microdialysis is expressed in fmole/15 min and samples were collected every 15 minutes. **Rats that received estradiol benzoate (EB; 5 µg EB in 0.1 ml peanut oil, SC) priming (72, 48, and 24 hours prior to dialysis) and then received an additional treatment of EB 30 minutes before AMPH (n = 7, closed circles) showed significantly greater AMPH-induced DA in dialysate than all other groups during the entire 2-hour period of sample collection ($P < 0.05$). *Rats that received oil priming (72, 48, and 24 hours prior to dialysis) and then received EB the day of dialysis (n = 9, open circles) showed a significant increase ($P < 0.05$) in AMPH-induced DA in dialysate over the oil primed-oil (n = 8, open squares) group. Similarly, rats that received EB priming prior to dialysis and then received oil (n = 8, closed triangles) also showed a significant increase ($P < 0.05$) in AMPH-induced DA in dialysate over the oil primed-oil group. (*B*) The average number of AMPH-induced stereotyped behaviors (head and forelimb movements) made in a 30-second sample time from rats undergoing in vivo microdialysis. **Rats that received EB priming and then EB 30 minutes before AMPH (n = 7, closed circles) exhibited significantly greater stereotyped head and forelimb movements than all other groups ($P < 0.05$). *Rats that received oil priming and then EB 30 minutes before AMPH (n = 8, open circles) also exhibited a significant increase in stereotyped head and forelimb movements than did the oil-primed oil (n = 8, open squares) group ($P < 0.05$). Similarly, rats that received EB priming and then oil 30 minutes before AMPH (n = 5, closed triangles) exhibited a significant increase in stereotyped head and forelimb movements than did the oil-primed oil group ($P < 0.05$). (Adapted from Becker and Rudick 1999.)

important for understanding how estrogen affects this neural system. However, our understanding of the role this phenomenon plays in the behavior of the rat in the wild remains relatively speculative. It may be adaptive for a female rat to be able to traverse the environment more efficiently when she is in behavioral estrus, but is this why the striatum has evolved to be sensitive to estrogen? Most evolutionary biologists believe that biological functions that vary with the reproductive cycle are likely to play a role in reproduction. Therefore, it is possible that estrogen modulation of striatal dopamine plays a role in sexual behavior.

In the male rat, the ascending dopamine system is activated during sexual behavior. Dopamine release from the nucleus accumbens is important for anticipatory or motivational components of sexual behavior, while dopamine in the striatum is important for consummatory aspects of sexual behavior (see chapter 5).

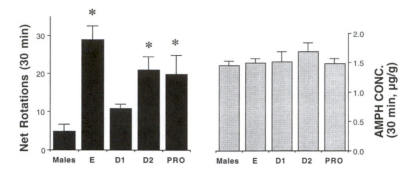

Figure 13.6 Rotational behavior and whole-brain concentrations of amphetamine (AMPH) in male and female rats at each of the four stages of the estrous cycle. Males received 1.56 mg/kg AMPH and females (E, estrus; D1, diestrus 1, D2, diestrus 2; Pro, proestrus) received 1.25 mg/kg of AMPH (i.p.). On the left are the mean (+ SEM) number of net rotations made during the first 30 min following the AMPH injection for each group (N = 16/group). On the right are the mean (+ SEM) whole-brain concentrations of AMPH (µg AMPH/g brain) 30 min after the AMPH treatment for each group (N = 8/group). (Adapted from Becker et al. 1982.)

In female rats, dopamine antagonists abolish the soliciting/proceptive behaviors of hopping and darting, while enhancing the receptive lordosis posture (Everitt et al. 1974; Everitt et al. 1975). In order to study the possible role of the ascending dopamine system in proceptive sexual behaviors of the rat, testing conditions need to be optimized for the expression of these behaviors.

As discussed in chapter 4, in seminatural conditions, the female rat will actively control the pace of copulatory behavior by exhibiting proceptive behaviors and actively withdrawing from the male (i.e., exhibit pacing behavior). The rate at which the female withdraws from the presence of the male after a copulatory contact (percent exits) and the time before she returns to the male after a contact (return latency in seconds), are used to objectively define the behavior referred to as pacing. A female that is pacing shows higher rates of percent exits and a longer return latency after an ejaculation than after an intromission or mount (Erskine 1989; McClintock 1984).

THE ROLE OF DOPAMINE IN PACING BEHAVIOR

The possible role of the ascending dopamine systems in female rodent sexual behavior has been demonstrated using a techniques called in vivo microdialysis. This is a method that lets an investigator sample the concentrations of dopamine in extracellular fluid from the brain, while simultaneously observing the behavior of the animals in vivo. With this method a small probe with a tip 250 µm in diameter and 2 to 4 mm long is placed into an area of the brain like the striatum (figure 13.7). The tip is constructed of a semipermeable membrane which allows small ions (like most neurotransmitters) to diffuse across. Pushing a physiological Ringer's solution through the probe creates a concentration gradient. This causes neurotransmitters and other small molecules in the extracellular fluid to diffuse into the probe and to be

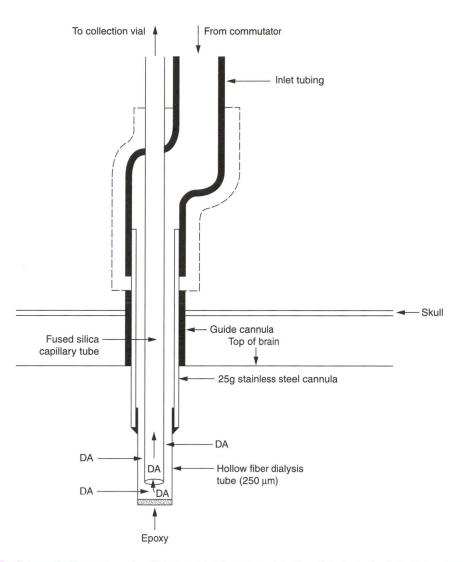

Figure 13.7 Schematic illustration of a dialysis probe (not to scale). The dialysis probe is held in place in the area of the brain of interest with a chronically implanted guide cannula. A physiological Ringer's solution flows into the probe through tubing attached to a liquid commutator to allow the animal to move about the test chamber. The Ringer's solution flows continuously through the tip of the probe and out through used silica capillary tubing into a collection vial. At the tip of the probe is a hollow fiber dialysis tube that has a low molecular weight cutoff (usually about 6000 MW). This allows small molecules to enter the probe, but keeps larger molecules out (e.g., proteins). Dopamine (DA) and other small molecules found in the extracellular fluid in the brain flow down their concentration gradient into the probe and are carried away with the Ringer's solution. The fluid is collected in a vial and analyzed chemically to determine how much DA is present in the extracellular fluid.

carried out of the brain where the investigator can collect the solution and analyze the compounds that are in the fluid.

It has been shown that there is enhanced dopamine in dialysate from striatum and nucleus accumbens during sexual behavior in female rats that are pacing sexual behavior, compared with females that are engaging in sex but not pacing. In the striatum and nucleus accumbens, the increase in dopamine concentrations in dialysate of hormone-primed ovariectomized rats pacing copulation is significantly greater than that of nonpacing animals or hormone-primed animals tested without a male rat (Becker et al. 2001; Mermelstein and Becker 1995). In female rats, dopamine in the nucleus accumbens or striatum increases in dialysate of females engaging in paced copulatory behavior (figure 13.8). In addition, female rats or hamsters tested with vaginal masks that prevent intromission by the male do not show an increase in dopamine in dialysate from nucleus accumbens or striatum (Becker et al. 2001;

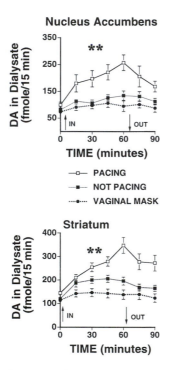

Figure 13.8 Dopamine (DA) concentrations in dialysate (fmole/15 min) obtained from nucleus accumbens (*top*) or striatum (*bottom*) of sexually receptive female rats. One group of rats was allowed to pace sexual behavior during dialysis (pacing, open squares). One group engaged in sex but could not pace sexual behavior (not pacing, solid squares). The third group was sexually receptive but could not receive intromissions due to a vaginal mask (vaginal mask, closed circles) that prevented penetration. The value obtained for time zero is the mean of two 15 min baseline samples obtained immediately prior to the introduction of the male rat into the chamber. Values indicate the mean $\pm$ SEM. **The increase in DA in dialysate during the time the male was present was significantly greater for the pacing group than for the other groups ($P < 0.003$). There were no other differences among the groups. (Adapted from Becker et al. 2001.)

Kohlert et al. 1997). These results together support the notion that dopamine in the striatum and nucleus accumbens is important for coding specific aspects of the coital stimuli received, rather than being related to specific motor behaviors.

Support for the idea that estrogen acting in the striatum and nucleus accumbens is important for pacing behavior comes from studies in which female rats were induced into behavioral estrus via hormone delivery to the ventromedial hypothalamus (VMH). Animals then received estrogen bilaterally into the striatum or nucleus accumbens (Xiao and Becker 1997). Intrastriatal estrogen was found to facilitate exits from the male after a copulatory contact (percent exits), while intranucleus accumbens implants increase the time to return to the male (return latency) (figure 13.9). Conversely, the antiestrogen ICI 182,780 applied to the striatum decreased percent exits, while in the nucleus accumbens it decreased return latency (Xiao and Becker 1997). Thus, the results together suggest that the striatum and nucleus accumbens differ-

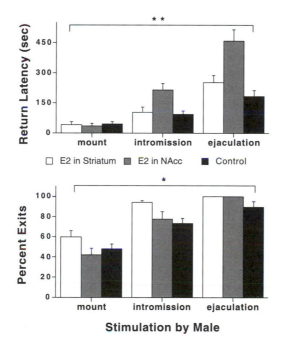

Figure 13.9 Effect of estradiol implants (E2) in the striatum and nucleus accumbens (NAcc) on pacing behavior in female rats. The mean values of return latency (top) and percent exits (bottom) following mounts, intromissions, and ejaculations recorded from 1-hr tests are plotted as a function of the intensity of mating stimuli received from the male. Sexual receptivity was induced by sequential implants of 30% E2 and then progesterone into the ventromedial nucleus. This was followed by implants of 30% E2 into either the striatum (open bars) or NAcc (shaded bars) or by cholesterol implants into either of the two areas (black bars). Vertical bars indicate the standard error of the mean. Numbers in parentheses are the sample size for each experimental group. *Significant difference between E2 in the striatum and in controls ($P < 0.05$). **Significant difference between E2 in the NAcc and in both of the other groups ($P < 0.02$). (Adapted from Xiao and Becker 1997.)

entially modulate specific components of pacing behavior, and that the effects of estrogen on dopamine in these brain areas enhances these functions.

Gonadal Hormone Influences on the Responses to Drugs of Abuse

Sensitization

So far we have dealt solely with gender differences in the acute effects of psychomotor stimulants. It is well established, however, that the effects of drugs change with repeated administration, and these changes take two general forms: tolerance or sensitization (Koob and Bloom 1988; Stewart and Badiani 1993). Tolerance is the progressive decrement in responses induced by subsequent exposures to a drug. For quite some time, the role of tolerance in the development of physical dependence has been a central focus of research on addiction (Jaffe 1990; Koob and Bloom 1988; Tiffany 1990; Watson et al. 1989; Wise and Bozarth 1987). Sensitization is the opposite of tolerance, and is sometimes called reverse tolerance for this reason. In other words, sensitization is the progressive increase in response induced by repeated treatment with the same dose of a drug. With repeated treatment with drugs like amphetamine or cocaine, one sees both sensitization and tolerance, depending on what is measured. The behavioral response to these psychomotor stimulants shows sensitization. Rats and mice exhibit more and more intense stereotyped behaviors, for example, each time they are treated with amphetamine or cocaine. On the other hand, the cardiovascular effects of these drugs show tolerance. There is increasing evidence that sensitization is playing an important role in the process of addiction (Berridge and Robinson 1995; Deminiere et al. 1989; Horger et al. 1992; Horger et al. 1990; Lett 1989; Piazza et al. 1991; Robinson 1993; Robinson and Berridge 1993; Schenk et al. 1992; Stewart and Badiani 1993).

SEX-RELATED DIFFERENCES

The literature on sex differences in sensitization of amphetamine- and cocaine-induced psychomotor behavior is quite convincing. If one looks at the increase in the behavioral response exhibited when the results of two behavioral tests are compared, female rats exhibit more robust sensitization to amphetamine or cocaine than do intact males (Camp and Robinson 1988a; Camp and Robinson 1988b; Forgie and Stewart 1994; Robinson 1984; Robinson et al. 1982; van Haaren and Meyer 1991).

The studies looking at AMPH-induced behaviors are confounded, however, by gender differences in AMPH metabolism (Becker et al. 1982). Robinson (1984) attempted to control for metabolic differences by giving females a lower dose than males (2.6 vs. 3.0 mg/kg). These doses were calculated from previous research based on brain concentration of AMPH at 30 min and 1 hour post-injection (Becker et al. 1982); however, rotational behavior was recorded for 2 hours post-AMPH. Since males exhibit more rapid AMPH metabolism, and gender differences become more pronounced with time post-injection, it is not really possible to determine from these data the magnitude of the gender difference in sensitization to AMPH. Camp and colleagues (Camp and Robinson 1988a) attempted to address this problem by giving females a substantially lower dose of AMPH on a challenge test. Females received 2.6 mg/kg AMPH during the sensitizing regimen and 1.78 mg/kg on the challenge test, while males received 3.0 mg/kg AMPH on all tests. Stereotyped behavior exhibited by females on the challenge test was significantly greater than for males on the challenge test, supporting the idea that gender differences in AMPH metabolism are not the only cause of the gender differences in reported behavior. Thus, females exhibit more robust behavioral sensitization to AMPH than do males.

Finally, it has been reported that there are gender differences in sensitization of AMPH-induced rotational behavior at a high dose of AMPH, but not at a low dose (Robinson 1984). This suggests that there may be gender differences in the dose-effect curve for sensitization. Research on gender differences in the sensitization of cocaine-induced behavioral activity is less problematic, as cocaine metabolism is the same in males and females (Bowman et al. 1999) and yet females again exhibit greater behavioral sensitization (van Haaren and Meyer 1991).

EFFECTS OF GONADECTOMY
Both ovariectomized and intact female rats show sensitization (Camp and Robinson 1988a; Camp and Robinson 1988b; Forgie and Stewart 1994; Robinson 1984; Robinson et al. 1982). In one report, however, ovariectomized females did not exhibit sensitization of cocaine-induced locomotor activity when intact females did (van Haaren and Meyer 1991). In other reports, estrogen treatments have enhanced sensitization of locomotor activity induced by AMPH or cocaine (Forgie and Stewart 1994; Peris et al. 1991).

Castration of male rats has been reported to enhance sensitization of AMPH- or cocaine-induced psychomotor behavior (see, Camp and Robinson 1988a; Camp and Robinson 1988b; Robinson 1984), although this result has not been found consistently (Forgie and Stewart 1994; van Haaren and Meyer 1991). It has been hypothesized that if castration enhances the induction and/or expression of behavioral sensitization, then testosterone treatment should reverse this effect. This is not the case, however, as testosterone treatment has not been found to affect behavioral sensitization in castrated males (Forgie and Stewart 1994). Thus, the role of testicular hormones in sensitization to psychomotor stimulants remains an open question.

Gender Differences in Humans
The gender and hormonal effects on behavioral sensitization described above have important implications for gender differences in susceptibility to cocaine addiction. According to a recent report, 9% of women age 12 and over have used cocaine. The only illicit drug used more by women is marijuana (28% have used marijuana) (Kandel et al. 1995). Among women who have used

cocaine, the prevalence of lifetime dependence for cocaine is $14.9 \pm 2.0\%$ (mean $\pm$ S.D.). This is in contrast to alcohol where 79% have used alcohol, but only $9.2 \pm 0.8\%$ have developed lifetime dependence (Kandel et al. 1995). The use of all illicit drugs has been increasing among women in the past decade, and cocaine dependence among women, in particular, is a growing public health concern (Wetherington and Roman 1995).

Neurochemical Processes Mediating the Effects of Estrogen

What are the underlying neural processes mediating the effects of estrogen on the response to amphetamine and cocaine? A number of neurochemical techniques have been used to assess the effects of ovarian hormones on striatal dopamine activity. For example, in vivo microdialysis has found that there is estrous cycle–dependent variation in the amphetamine-induced increase in dopamine in striatum. Female rats during estrus have a significantly greater amphetamine-induced increase in extracellular dopamine in striatum than do female rats during diestrus 1 (Becker and Cha 1989). As discussed above, and illustrating the power of in vivo microdialysis, data from these same animals demonstrated that females in estrus exhibit significantly more stereotyped behavior than females in diestrus 1 (Becker and Cha 1989). These results suggest that ovarian hormones modulate striatal dopamine release.

During in vivo microdialysis, a single dose of estrogen given to ovariectomized rats 30 min before amphetamine enhances the increase in extracellular striatal dopamine, coincident with enhanced rotational behavior (figure 3.5, bottom) (Becker 1990b). Treatment of ovariectomized rats with estrogen stimulates an increase in striatal dopamine turnover, as well as increasing dopamine release induced by amphetamine (Becker et al. 1986; DiPaolo et al. 1985). This is a rapid effect of acute estrogen treatment to enhance amphetamine-induced dopamine in striatum and amphetamine-induced behaviors that is seen in ovariectomized female rats, but not castrated male rats (Castner et al. 1993). Thus, there is a sex difference in the rapid effect of estrogen on the striatum.

The results of the experiments just described demonstrate that estrogen can affect both behavioral and neurochemical indices of striatal dopamine function. The question remains, however, whether the effect of estrogen on dopamine-mediated behaviors causes the effects on striatal dopamine release described above, or whether the effects of estrogen on striatal dopamine release induce the reported effects on behavior. Experiments examining dopamine release from striatal tissue slices in vitro (in glass or in the test tube) are important, therefore, to determine the causal relations between these events. In these experiments we have used an in vitro superfusion system. For this, striatal tissue slices are removed from the brain and placed into a chamber through which a Ringer's solution flows continuously. Under these conditions the brain slices retain the ability to release dopamine in response to stimulation by neurochemical or physiological stimuli that would normally induce release in the animal. Then, amphetamine, estrogen, and other compounds can be delivered directly to the pieces of brain tissue, and the effluent from the superfusion system can be sampled to measure the effect of these treatments on the release of dopamine from the striatal tissue.

Using this superfusion system, it has been shown that (1) amphetamine-induced striatal dopamine release varies with estrous cycle, so that there is greater dopamine release on behavioral estrus than on other days of the cycle (Becker 1990a), (2) ovariectomy attenuates amphetamine-induced striatal dopamine release while castration of male rats has no effect on this measure (Becker 1990a; Becker and Ramirez 1981), and (3) estrogen treatment enhances amphetamine-stimulated striatal dopamine release in striatal tissue from female but not male rats (Becker 1990a; Becker and Ramirez 1981). From the results of these experiments we conclude that the effects of estrogen on striatal dopamine release occurs in the absence of behavior. Thus, it is likely that the effects of estrogen on striatal dopamine release mediate the changes in behavior that occur.

Mechanisms Mediating the Effects of Estrogen on the Striatum

The superfusion system is a particularly powerful tool, because it is possible to use this method to determine where estrogen is acting in order to produce its effects on the striatum. The previous experiments described have used systemic estrogen treatments to manipulate striatal dopamine activity, so the results discussed could be due the effects of estrogen almost anywhere in the brain or body. With the superfusion system, estrogen can be delivered directly to the striatum, so it is possible to determined whether the effects described above are due to direct effects on the striatum. Thus, we have used the superfusion to show that estrogen in physiological concentrations (100 pg/ml) acts directly on the striatum of OVX female rats to enhance amphetamine- or K^+-stimulated dopamine release (Becker 1990a). Furthermore, we have found that the pulsatile administration of estrogen directly stimulates dopamine release in striatal tissue from female rats, but not male rats (Becker 1990a). We believe, therefore, that the acute effects of estrogen that we are investigating are due to the direct effects of estrogen on the striatum.

How does estrogen induce effects on the striatum? Autoradiography is usually used to identify neurons with estrogen receptors. Studies of this type have suggested that the striatum contains very few neurons, if any, that concentrate estrogen in their nucleus. With the discovery of a second estrogen receptor (ERβ; see chapter 2), the possibility that there might be other receptors for estrogen in the brain became a more likely possibility. Nevertheless, neither ERα or ERβ are found in the striatum.

However, as the discussion above indicates, there is both behavioral and neurochemical evidence that estrogen can act directly on the striatum to modulate neuronal activity. As discussed in chapter 2, it is now clear that estrogen and other steroid hormones can have rapid effects on cellular activity by binding to receptors located on or in the exterior cell membrane. These rapid membrane effects of steroids are usually associated activation of intracellular signaling systems, such as those associated with metabotropic receptors for neurotransmitters and protein hormones. Experiments from the Becker laboratory have shown that 17β-estradiol bound to BSA (a large protein), which prevents estrogen from getting into the cell, is just as effective as 17β-estradiol at enhancing amphetamine-induced striatal dopamine release (Xiao and Becker 1998). These results further support the idea that estrogen is acting in the striatum at membrane-associated estrogen receptors.

Membrane-Associated Estrogen Receptors

For the striatum, electrophysiological studies indicate that the rapid effects of estrogen are mediated by a second messenger-coupled membrane receptor. In these experiments, estrogen has been found to inhibit voltage-activated calcium channels in striatal neurons that use the neurotransmitter GABA. Remember that when the action potential arrives at a synapse, the change in membrane voltage opens calcium channels, allowing calcium influx, which triggers the exocytotic release of neurotransmitter. So a decrease in calcium current would result in decreased GABA release. The effects of estrogen on calcium current in striatal neurons occur within seconds, reverse as soon as estrogen delivery ceases, and are seen at physiological concentrations of estrogen.

There is also strong electrophysiological evidence that estrogen is acting at the membrane on the outside of the cell in the striatum. As was true in the superfusion system, estrogen attached to BSA is effective at blocking calcium current, indicating that estrogen does not need to get inside of the cells in order to produce an effect. Interestingly, when estrogen is applied internally to striatal neurons through the recording electrode it does not reduce calcium current, nor does it block the effect of a very low dose of estrogen applied externally. Collectively, these results indicate that the effect of estrogen occurs externally at the membrane surface.

In the presence of GTP-gamma-S (which prevents inactivation of G-protein-mediated second messenger events), the effect of 17β-estradiol does not reverse when hormone delivery ceases. These results indicate that the effect of estrogen on striatal neurons is dependent upon a G-protein-coupled, metabotropic receptor. Finally, the effect of 17β-estradiol is stereospecific as 17α-estradiol does not mimic the modulation, and steroid-specific as estrone and 3-methoxyestriol were ineffective while estriol or 4-hydroxy-estradiol mimic the effect of 17β-estradiol. It is concluded, therefore, that estrogen has rapid stereospecific effects on striatal neurons that alter signaling pathways independent of the classical estrogen receptor (Mermelstein et al. 1996).

How does inhibition of the activity of striatal GABA neurons by estrogen affect the release of dopamine from terminals in the striatum? While this question is still under investigation, the current hypothesis is that normally GABA inhibits the release of dopamine and estrogen acts to remove this inhibition (see Becker 1999 for a discussion).

Summary

1. The gonadal hormones have a wide range of influences on behavior, suggesting that many different brain regions in addition to the hypothalamus are either organized or activated (or both) by the secretion of gonadal hormones. In general, adult female rodents tend to be more active and have lower thresholds to sensory stimuli than males do. These sex differences in motor and sensory systems are mediated in part by the organizational effects of developmental hormones and in part by activational hormone effects.
2. The evidence discussed here indicates that estrogen has rapid, direct effects on the striatum that act to enhance sensorimotor function and specific components of sexual behavior in the female rat. Estrogen also enhances striatal dopamine release.
3. It is suggested that hormonal modulation of the striatum and the consequences for enhanced sensorimotor function may have evolved to facilitate reproductive success in female rats by enhancing pacing behavior.
4. Electrophysiological studies suggest that the effects of estrogen on the striatum are indirectly mediated by novel membrane receptors for estradiol.
5. These findings have important implications for our understanding of how gonadal hormones act in the brain to alter neuronal function. They also have implications for the mechanisms mediating gender differences in abuse of the psychomotor stimulant drugs.

Study Questions

1. If you are a world-famous psychologist and you want to show that male and female rats are different behaviorally, what test would you do to illustrate the differences? What results would you expect to find?
2. Why do rats turn in circles when there is unilateral stimulation of the ascending dopamine pathway?
3. How do male and female rats differ in their responses to psychomotor stimulant drugs?
4. Why do female rats pace sexual behavior?
5. How does the author suggest that estrogen produces its effects on the striatum?

Acknowledgements

Supported by the National Science Foundation (IBN 9816673) and the National Institute on Drug Abuse (RO1 DA 12677). My thanks to Robert Meisel for comments on an earlier version of this manuscript.

References

Arbuthnott, G. W., and Crow, T. J. (1971) Relation of contraversive turning to unilateral release of dopamine from the nigrostriatal pathway in rats. *Exp. Neurol.* 30: 484–491.

Archer, J. (1975) Rodent sex differences in emotional and related behavior. *Behav. Biol.* 14: 451–479.

Axelson, J. F., Zoller, L. C., Tomassone, J. E., and Collins, D. C. (1986) Effects of silastic progesterone implants on activity cycles and steroid levels in ovariectomized and intact females rats. *Physiol. Behav.* 38: 879–85.

Beatty, W. W. (1979) Gonadal hormones and sex differences in nonreproductive behaviors in rodents: Organizational and activational influences. *Horm. Behav.* 12: 112–163.

Becker, J. B. (1990a) Direct effect of 17β-estradiol on striatum: Sex differences in dopamine release. *Synapse* 5: 157–164.

Becker, J. B. (1990b) Estrogen rapidly potentiates amphetamine-induced striatal dopamine release and rotational behavior during microdialysis. *Neurosci. Lett.* 118: 169–171.

Becker. J. B. (1999) Gender differences in dopaminergic function in striatum and nucleus accumbens. *Pharmacol. Biochem. Behav.* 64: 803–812.

Becker, J. B., and Beer, M. E. (1986) The influence of estrogen on nigrostriatal dopamine activity: Behavioral and neurochemical evidence for both pre- and postsynaptic components. *Behav. Brain Res.* 19: 27–33.

Becker, J. B., and Cha, J. (1989) Estrous cycle-dependent variation in amphetamine-induced behaviors and striatal dopamine release assessed with microdialysis. *Behav. Brain Res.* 35: 117–125.

Becker, J. B., and Ramirez, V. D. (1981) Sex differences in the amphetamine stimulated release of catecholamines from rat striatal tissue in vitro. *Brain Res.* 204: 361–372.

Becker, J. B., Robinson, T. E., and Lorenz, K. A. (1982) Sex differences and estrous cycle variations in amphetamine-elicited rotational behavior. *Eur. J. Pharmacol.* 80: 65–72.

Becker, J. B., and Rudick, C. N. (1999) Rapid effects of estrogen or progesterone on the amphetamine-induced increase in striatal dopamine are enhanced by estrogen priming: A microdialysis study. *Pharmacol. Biochem. Behav.*

Becker, J. B., Rudick, C. N., and Jenkins, W. J. (2001) The role of dopamine in the nucleus accumbens and striatum during sexual behavior in the female rat. *J. Neurosci.* 21: 3236–3241.

Becker, J. B., Snyder, P. J., Miller, M. M., Westgate, S. A., and Jenuwine, M. J. (1987) The influence of estrous cycle and intrastriatal estradiol on sensorimotor performance in the female rat. *Pharmacol. Biochem. Behav.* 27: 53–59.

Berridge, K. C., and Robinson, T. E. (1995) The mind of an addicted brain: Neural sensitization of wanting versus liking. *Curr Direct. Psychol. Sci.* 4: 71–76.

Bodnar, R. J., Romero, M.-T., and Kramer, E. (1988) Organismic variables and pain inhibition: Roles of gender and aging. *Brain Res. Bull.* 21: 947–953.

Bowman, B., Vaughan, S., Walker, Q., Davis, S., Little, P., Scheffler, N., Thomas, B., and Kuhn, C. (1999) Effects of gender and gonadectomy on cocaine metabolism in the rat. *J. Pharm. Exp. Therapeut.* 290: 1316–23.

Broida, J., and Svare, B. (1984) Sex differences in the activity of mice: Modulation by postnatal gonadal hormones. *Horm. Behav.* 18: 65–78.

Bronson, F. H. (1979) The reproductive ecology of the house mouse. *Quart. Rev. Biol.* 54: 265–299.

Camp, D. M., Becker, J. B., and Robinson, T. E. (1986) Sex differences in the effects of gonadectomy on amphetamine-induced rotational behavior in rats. *Behav. Neural. Biol.* 46: 491–495.

Camp, D. M., and Robinson, T. E. (1988a) Susceptibility to sensitization. I. Sex differences in the enduring effects of chronic D-amphetamine treatment on locomotion, stereotyped behavior and brain monoamines. *Behav. Brain. Res.* 30: 55–68.

Camp, D. M., and Robinson, T. E. (1988b) Susceptibility to sensitization. II. The influence of gonadal hormones on enduring changes in brain monoamines and behavior produced by the repeated administration of D-amphetamine or restraint stress. *Behav. Brain Res.* 30: 69–88.

Castner, S. A., Xiao, L., and Becker, J. B. (1993) Sex differences in striatal dopamine: In vivo microdialysis and behavioral studies. *Brain Res.* 610: 127–134.

Costall, B., and Naylor, R. J. (1977) Mesolimbic and extrapyramidal sites for the mediation of stereotyped behavior patterns and hyperactivity by amphetamine and apomorphine in the rat. In E. H. Ellinwood and M. M. Kilbey (Eds.), *Cocaine and Other Stimulants*. New York: Plenum Press, pp. 47–76.

Czaja, J. A. (1984) Sex differences in the activational effects of gonadal hormones on food intake and body weight. *Physiol. Behav.* 33: 553–558.

Deminiere, J. M., Piazza, P. V., Le Moal, M., and Simon, H. (1989) Experimental approach to individual vulnerability to psychostimulant addiction. *Neurosci. Biobehav. Rev.* 13: 141–147.

Di Paolo, T., Rouillard, C., and Bedard, P. J. (1985) 17 beta-Estradiol at a physiological dose acutely increases dopamine turnover in rat brain. *Eur. J. Pharmacol.* 117: 197–203.

Dorries, K. M., Adkins-Regan E., and Halpern, B. P. (1995) Olfactory sensitivity to the pheromone, androstenone, is sexually dimorphic in the pig. *Physiol. Behav.* 57: 255–259.

Everitt, B. J., Fuxe, K., and Hokfelt, T. (1974) Inhibitory role for dopamine and 5-hydroxytryptamine in the sexual behavior of the female rat. *Eur J. Pharmacol.* 29: 187–191.

Everitt, B. J., Fuxe, K., Hokfelt, T., and Jonsson, G. (1975) Role of monoamines in the control of hormones of sexual receptivity in the female rat. *J. Comp. Physiol. Psychol.* 89: 556–572.

Field, E. F., Whishaw, I. Q., and Pellis, S. M. (2000) Sex differences in catalepsy: Evidence for hormone-dependent postural mechanisms in haloperidol-treated rats. *Behav. Brain Res.* 109: 207–212.

Fink, J. S., and Smith, G. P. (1980) Relationships between selective denervation of dopamine terminal fields in the naterior forebrain and behavioral responses to amphetamine and apomorphine. *Brian Res.* 201: 107–127.

Forgie, M. L., and Stewart, J. (1994) Sex difference in amphetamine-induced locomotor activity in adult rats: Role of tetosterone exposure in the neonatal period. *Pharmacol. Biochem. Behav.* 46.

Fahrbach, S. E., Meisel, R. L., and Pfaff, D. W. (1985) Preoptic implants of estradiol increase wheel running but not the open field activity of female rats. *Physiol. Behav.* 35: 985–992.

Ganesan, R. (1994) The aversive and hypophagic effects of estradiol. *Physiol. Behav.* 55: 279–85.

Goel, N., Lee, T. M., and Pieper, D. R. (1998) Removal of the olfactory bulbs delays photic reentrainment of circadian activity rhythms and modifies the reproductive axis in male *Octodon degus.* *Brain Res.* 792: 229–236.

Goy, R. W., and McEwen, B. S. (1980) *Sexual Differentiation of the Brain.* Cambridge, Mass.: MIT Press.

Horger, B. A., Giles, M. K., and Schenk, S. (1992) Preexposure to amphetamine and nicotine predisposes rats to self-administer a low dose of cocaine. *Psychopharmacology* 107: 271–276.

Horger, B. A., Shelton, K., and Schenk, S. (1990) Preexposure sensitizes rats to the rewarding effects of cocaine. *Pharmacol. Biochem. Behav.* 37: 707–711.

Joyce, J. N., and Van Hartesveldt, C. (1984) Behaviors induced by intrastriatal dopamine vary independently across the estrous cycle. *Pharmacol. Biochem. Behav.* 20: 551–557.

Kandel, D. B., Warner, M. P. P., and Kessler, R. C. (1995) The epidemiology of substance abuse and dependence among women. In C. L. Wetherington and A. R. Roman (Eds.), *Drug Addiction Research and the Health of Women.* Rockville, Md.: U. S. Department of Health and Human Services, pp. 105–130.

Kelly, P. H. (1983) Inhibition of voluntary activity by growth hormone. *Horm. Behav.* 17: 163–168.

Kinsley, C., Miele, J., Konen, C., Ghiraldi, L., and Svare, B. (1986) Intrauterine contiguity influences regulatory activity in adult female and male mice. *Horm. Behav.* 20: 7–12.

Kohlert, J., Rowe, R., and Meisel, R. (1997) Intromissive stimuli from the male increases extracellular dopamine from fluoro-gold-identified neurons within the midbrain of female hamsters. *Horm. Behav.* 32: 143–154.

Koob, G. F., and Bloom, F. E. (1988) Cellular and molecular mechanisms of drug dependence. *Science* 242: 715–723.

Laeng, B., Berridge, K. C., and Butter, C. M. (1993) Pleasantness of a sweet taste during hunger and satiety: Effects of gender and "sweet tooth." *Appetite* 21: 247–254.

Lett, B. T. (1989) Repeated exposures intensify rather than diminish the rewarding effects of amphetamine, morphine, and cocaine. *Psychopharmacology (Berlin)* 98: 357–362.

Lindvall, O., and Bjorklund, A. (1974) The organization of the ascending catecholamine neuron systems in the rat brain as revealed by the glyoxylic acid fluorescence method. *Acta Physiol. Scand. [Suppl.]* 1974, 1–48.

McClintock, M. K. (1984) Group mating in the domestic rat as context for sexual selection: Consequences for the analysis of sexual behavior and neuroendocrine responses. *Adv. Study Behav.* 14: 1–50.

Meaney, M. J., and McEwen, B. S. (1986) Testosterone implants into the amygdala during the neonatal period masculinize the social play of juvenile female rats. *Brain Res.* 398: 324–328.

Meaney, M. J., Stewart, J., and Beatty, W. W. (1985) Sex differences in social play: The socialization of sex roles. *Adv. Study Behav.* 15: 1–58.

Merkle, S. (1989) Sexual differences as adaptation to the different gender roles in the frog *Xenopus laevis Daudin. J. Comp Physiol [B]* 159: 473–480.

Mermelstein, P. G., and Becker, J. B. (1995) Increased extracellular dopamine in the nucleus accumbens and striatum of the female rat during paced copulatory behavior. *Behav. Neurosci.* 109: 354–365.

Mermelstein, P. G., Becker, J. B., and Surmeier, D. J. (1996) Estradiol reduces calcium currents in rat neostriatal neurons through a membrane receptor. *J. Neurosci.* 16: 595–604.

Merwin, A., and Doty, R. L. (1994) Early exposure to low levels of estradiol (E2) mitigates E2-induced conditioned taste aversions in prepubertally ovariectomized female rats. *Physiol. Behav.* 55: 185–187.

Mogil, J. S., and Belknap, J. K. (1997) Sex and genotype determine the selective activation of neuro-chemically-distinct mechanisms of swim stress-induced analgesia. *Pharmacol. Biochem. Behav.* 56: 61–66.

Palanza, P., Parmigiani, S., and vom Saal, F. S. (1995) Urine marking and maternal aggression of wild female mice in relation to anogenital distance at birth. *Physiol. Behav.* 58: 827–835.

Pellis, S. M., Field, E. F., Smith, L. K., and Pellis, V. C. (1997) Multiple differences in the play fighting of male and female rats. Implications for the causes and functions of play. *Neurosci. Biobehav. Rev.* 21: 105–120.

Pellis, S. M., Field, E. F., and Whishaw, I. Q. (1999) The development of a sex-differentiated defensive motor pattern in rats: A possible role for juvenile experience. *Devel. Psychobiol.* 35: 156–164.

Peris, J., Decambre, N., Coleman-Hardee, M., and Simpkins, J. (1991) Estradiol enhances behavioral sensitization to cocaine and amphetamine-stimulated [^{3}H] dopamine release. *Brain Res.* 566: 255–264.

Piazza, P. V., Deminière, J.-M., Maccari, S., Le Moal, M., Mormède, P., and Simon, H. (1991) Individual vulnerability to drug self-administration: Action of corticosterone on dopaminergic systems as a possible pathophysiological mechanism. In P. Willner and J. Scheel-Krüger (Eds.), *The Mesolimbic Dopamine System: From Motivation to Action.* New York: Wiley, pp. 473–495.

Robinson, T. E. (1984) Behavioral sensitization: Characterization of enduring changes in rotational behavior produced by intermittent injections of amphetamine in male and female rats. *Psychopharmacology (Berlin)* 84: 466–475.

Robinson, T. E. (1993) Persistent sensitizing effects of drugs on brain dopamine systems and behavior: Implications for addiction and relapse. In S. G. Korenman and J. D. Barchas (Eds.), *Biological Basis of Substance Abuse.* New York: Oxford University Press, pp. 373–402.

Robinson, T. E., Becker, J. B., and Presty, S. K. (1982) Long-term facilitation of amphetamine-induced rotational behavior and striatal dopamine release produced by a single exposure to amphetamine: Sex differences. *Brain Res.* 253: 231–241.

Robinson, T. E., and Berridge, K. C. (1993) The neural basis of drug craving: An incentirve-sensitization theory of addiction. *Brain Res. Rev.* 18: 247–291.

Robinson, T. E., Camp, D. M., and Becker, J. B. (1981) Gonadectomy attenuates turning behavior produced by electrical stimulation of the nigrostriatal dopamine system in female but not male rats. *Neurosci. Lett.* 23: 203–208.

Roy, E. J. (1987) Estradiol implants in the rat striatum stimulate locomotor activity in running wheels. *Soc. Neurosci. Abstr.* 13: 224.

Ryan, S. M., and Maier, S. F. (1988) The estrous cycle and estrogen modulate stress-induced analgesia. *Behav. Neurosci.* 102: 371–380.

Schenk, S., Valadez, A., McNamara, C., and Horger, B. A. (1992) Blockade of sensitizing effects of amphetamine preexposure on cocaine self-administration by the NMDA antagonist MK-801. *Soc. Neurosci. Abstr.* 18: 1237.

Stevens, R., and Goldstein, R. (1981) Effects of neonatal testosterone and estrogen on open-field behaviour in rats. *Physiol. Behav.* 26: 551–553.

Stewart, J., and Badiani, A. (1993) Tolerance and sensitization to the behavioral effects of drugs. *Behav. Pharmacol.* 4: 289–312.

Stewart, J., and Cygan, D. (1980) Ovarian hormones act early in development to feminize adult open-field behavior in the rat. *Horm. Behav.* 14: 20–32.

Tiffany, S. T. (1990) A cognitive model of drug urges and drug-use behavior: Role of automatic and nonautomatic processes. *Psychol. Rev.* 97: 147–168.

Ungerstedt, U. (1971) Striatal dopamine release after amphetamine or nerve degeneration revealed by rotational behavior. *Acta. Physiol. Scand.* 82(Suppl. 367): 49–68.

Ungerstedt, U. (1974) Functional dynamics of central monamine pathways. In F. O. Schmitt and F. G. Worden (Eds.), *The Neurosciences: Third Study Program.* Cambridge, Mass.: MIT Press, pp. 979–988.

Vandenbergh, J. G. (1989) Coordination of social signals and ovarian function during sexual development. *J. Anim. Sci.* 67: 1841–1847.

van Haaren, F., and Meyer, M. (1991) Sex differences in the locomotor activity after acute and chronic cocaine administration. *Pharmacol. Biochem. Behav.* 39: 923–927.

vom Saal, F. S., Grant, W. M., McMullen, C. W., and Laves, K. S. (1983) High fetal estrogen concentrations: Correlation with increased adult sexual activity and decreased aggression in male mice. *Science* 220: 1306–1309.

Wade, G. N., and Zucker, I. (1970) Modulation of food intake and locomotor activity in female rats by diencephalic hormone implants. *J. Comp Physiol Psychol.* 72: 328–36.

Watson, S. J., Trujillo, K. A., Herman, J. P., and Akil, H. (1989) Neuroanatomical and neurochemical substrates of drug-seeking behavior: Overview and future directions. In A. Goldstein (Ed.), *Molecular and Cellular Aspects of the Drug Addictions.* New York: Springer-Verlag, pp. 29–91.

Wetherington, C. L., and Roman, A. R. (Eds.). (1995) *Drug Addiction Research and the Health of Women.* Rockville, Md.: U. S. Department of Health and Human Services.

Wise, R. A., and Bozarth, M. A. (1987) A psychomotor stimulant theory of addiction. *Psychol. Rev.* 94: 469–92.

Yousem, D. M., Maldjian, J. A., Siddiqi, F., Hummel, T., Alsop, D. C., Geckle, R. J., Bilker, W. B., and Doty, R. L. (1999) Gender effects on odor-stimulated functional magnetic resonance imaging. *Brain Res.* 818: 480–487.

Xiao, L., and Becker, J. B. (1997) Hormonal activation of the striatum and the nucleus accumbens modulates paced mating behavior in the female rat. *Hormones and Behavior* 32: 114–124.

Xiao, L., and Becker, J. B. (1998) Effects of estrogen agonists on amphetamine-stimulated striatal dopamine release. *Synapse* 29: 379–391.

14 Hormones and Cognition in Nonhuman Animals

Christina L. Williams

Hormones from the adrenal gland, the pituitary gland, and the gonadal hormones can affect cognitive functioning. How does this happen? Some hormones affect neuronal development and morphology in the hippocampus. Sometimes this is a beneficial effect. But, as we saw in chapter 11, release of glucocorticoids during prolonged stress can kill neurons and impair memory. How does long-term hormone exposure affect the neural substrates of these behaviors?

How do males and females differ? Do they use different cognitive strategies? For some time it was argued that there were no differences between males and females in learning or memory. While the differences are small, they are clearly present and provide important information about how cognitive strategy may be affected by hormones during development and in adults.

Introduction

Learning and memory endow us with the flexibility to adapt to an ever-changing environment. However, we don't learn about our environment indiscriminately. Some individuals, events, and places have greater importance than others and these are often learned more easily and retained for longer periods of time. Infants need to learn quickly to identify their mothers, and mothers need to attach securely to their infants. Feeding sites and territorial boundaries need to be identified, learned, and held in memory. However, this knowledge must be flexible so that it can be updated daily or seasonally. Mates need to recognize each other and to bond in such a way that they cooperate to raise their offspring. Emotionally charged events need to be recalled vividly and without much rehearsal, so that similarly stressful and potentially dangerous situations can be avoided in the future. These are all examples of social situations in which specific hormonal systems are activated. The same hormones that function to coordinate mating, parental care, lactation, and feeding are also activated in times of stress and may have evolved to modulate learning and memory systems, which are important for allowing adaptation to novel and important environmental events.

Hormones also play a special role in modifying the brain systems involved in cognitive processes during early development and in old age. You have learned that gonadal hormones released early in development have organizational effects on the brain mechanisms involved in sexual behavior (see chapter 3). In a similar fashion, gonadal hormones have organizational effects on brain regions important for cognition (e.g., the neocortex and the hippocampus), and there is increasing evidence that these hormonally organized differences in brain morphology lead to sex differences in cognition. In addition, exposure to certain stressors during early development may imprint a developmental pattern that is useful in coping with stress throughout our lifespans. In old age, as secretion of reproductive hormones decline and adrenal hormones increase, there appears to be an accompanying decline in cognitive function that can be partially ameliorated by manipulation of hormone systems. In fact, age-related decline in gonadal hormone secretion and age-related increases in adrenal activation may contribute to a decline in the brain plasticity that is necessary for normal cognitive function.

Given the variety of roles hormones play throughout our lifespans, how do we study their effects on learning and memory? Which hormones modulate cognitive processing? Where and by what mechanisms are hormones acting in the brain? Under what naturally occurring conditions may these hormonal changes in learning and memory be adaptive? Might hormonal therapy be used to improve memory or alleviate deficits in memory? These are the issues that we will address in this chapter.

Performance versus Learning and Memory

Before we examine what researchers have discovered about the effects of hormones on cognition, let me caution you that it is not always easy to determine if a hormone has direct effects on learning and memory. Take this simple experiment. Two groups of male college students are selected such that one group has a high level of a circulating hormone (let's call it "hormone X") and one group has very low levels of hormone X. The students are asked to study a 20-word list for one minute and then to recall the words immediately. This procedure is repeated until the students recall all the items. Errors are scored for both omissions and incorrect words. If the students with high hormone X levels make fewer errors during the task than those with low levels, can you conclude that the hormone enhanced memory? If you answered yes, you are not considering a number of alternate interpretations.

Learning versus Memory

Learning and memory are two distinct, yet intimately associated, processes. Quite simply, without memory, there is no learning. However, it is possible to determine if a hormone is altering one process or the other. Studies that focus on learning tend to examine the formation of a memory, while studies of memory tend to examine the permanence of that learning. In our example, we tallied the number of errors students made while they were learning a 20-word list. Their memory of those words was not examined. To do so, we could have brought them back after delays of increasing duration and determined how many items they could remember at each time point. This would have allowed us to assess memory decay or interference with memory over time. Or we could have used multiple groups of subjects and varied the memory load (e.g., the number of words on the list). If high levels of hormone X had decreased errors made after a long but not a short delay or only when the memory load was large, then X might be a hormone that improves memory. In the following section, we will consider some of the many types of learning and memory tasks that have commonly been used in the laboratory. Hormones may alter how easily something is learned, the strategy that is used to learn a new skill, the retention, accuracy, or clarity of memory, and even the type of information that is placed in memory.

Nonmnemonic Factors

As you all know, performance on an exam is not just influenced by how well you learned or how well you can remember the test material. You might be less motivated to do well because you recently got admitted to medical school and your course grade this semester no longer seems important. You might perform poorly because you are really excited that your basketball team is playing for the national championship, or you are groggy after having taken cold medication, or you are having difficulty writing with a newly broken finger. These examples demonstrate that measures of performance do not necessarily tell us about how well information was learned and can be remembered. Because hormones orchestrate changes in many physiological systems, it is especially important to consider whether hormonal effects on cognition are occurring directly via actions on the neural substrates of learning or memory, or whether hormones are influencing cognition indirectly via effects on **nonmnemonic factors** (e.g., attention, motivation, sensory responsivity, and motor capabilities). For example, we know that estradiol influences sexual receptivity (see chapter 4), feeding (see chapters 13 and 16), motor systems (see chapter 13), and the **receptive fields** of somatosensory cells (see chapter 4 and 13). Thus, hormones may indirectly influence learning and memory by altering attention to the task, the reward properties of food, the response to sensory input, or the ability to perform the correct motor output.

How can we determine if hormones alter performance through their effects on nonmnemonic factors? One method is to examine hormonal effects using several different tasks that rely on different sensory and motor systems and different forms of motivation. Another method is to apply the hormone directly to a brain region that may be modulating a learning or memory effect (e.g., the neocortex or the hippocampus) and compare the results with the effects of the hormone administered **systemically**, or the effects the hormone applied to brain regions that might be responsible for its sensory or motor effects. Alternately, if we find that a hormone improves test performance, we can investigate the behavioral mechanisms underlying the difference in performance. But it is often very difficult to tease apart the direct and the indirect effects of hormones on cognition, and in many studies these effects have not been dissociated. For this reason, we often know that a hormone improves or interferes with test performance, but we cannot yet explain how and in what way a hormone contributes to this change.

Memory Has Stages

To determine the underlying neural mechanisms upon which a hormone might be acting to influence test performance, we can administer the hormone during a particular stage of memory formation, during the period when associations are rehearsed and stored, or during test performance rather than during learning. When a subject studies a list of words, time is spent reading and rehearsing the information so that it is encoded in memory. Rehearsal of new information (e.g., word lists) or associations between events (e.g., a red light signals that a shock will be administered unless a lever is pressed) continue even after the learning period. That is, we replay new associations while we are resting and even while we are dreaming (Maquet et al. 2000; Sutherland and McNaugton 2000). The new associations are very labile and interference from nonmnemonic factors can disrupt the rehearsal process. Over time, with continued reactivation and analysis of new memory traces, the associations are incorporated into the brain's long-term memory base, which is probably represented in the brain by a relatively durable form of synaptic alteration. Information is maintained for varying lengths of time: until later in the day, later in the semester, and perhaps, even for a lifetime. At the time of the test, the list of words must be retrieved from memory storage.

Because learning and memory processes occur in stages, researchers interested in hormones and cognition often try to determine where and in what way a hormone might influence encoding, rehearsal, consolidation, storage, or retrieval of information by administering the hormone so that it is present or absent during only one stage of the process. If hormone X were administered to half of our subjects only during recall and test performance was enhanced, we might conclude that hormone X did not improve test performance by altering the brain mechanisms involved with learning, rehearsal, or consolidation. It is more likely that the hormone increased attention or arousal factors in a way that improved the retrieval of information from memory.

Now that you have learned a bit more about some of the factors to consider when studying hormonal effects on cognition, let's return to our study of male college students with high and low levels of hormone X. Because the experimental group of students had high levels of X throughout all stages of learning and memory, it is difficult to determine how hormone X might be influencing performance. It is also impossible to assess the effects of X on nonmnemonic factors that might influence performance. Even if we did another experiment in which we could manipulate X levels directly and we could have levels high only during a particular stage of learning and not during test performance, we would still know little about where and how the hormone was acting to improve cognition. So what is a poor neuroendocrinologist to do? One good strategy is to select a learning and memory task for which the neural architecture is reasonably well understood. Then we have a good starting point from which to look for the site of hormone action. Some well-known tasks and their neural underpinnings are described in the next section.

Methods of Assessment

Hormonal effects on cognition can be examined by observing the effects of naturally occurring or manipulated hormonal states. That is, it is possible to take advantage of variations in hormone levels that occur daily or seasonally or in response to an environmental event. For example, we can test the learning abilities of human females at different stages of the menstrual cycle or of rodents at different stages of the estrous cycle. Or we can examine memory after a stressor (e.g., a mild electrical shock or the approach of a predator) has occurred. The stressor, whether it is naturally occurring or artificially induced, will alter the release of a number of neurochemicals, including hormones (see chapter 11). Alternately, we can manipulate the hormonal state of the subject in a controlled fashion. This might be done by removing the hormone-producing gland, pharmacologically altering hormone synthesis, blocking receptors, or using a genetically altered animal that has no receptors for a particular hormone or no ability to produce that specific hormone. These methods are particularly valuable if they are used in combination to provide converging evidence for hormonal modulation of learning and memory under both natural and experimental conditions.

Regardless of the method used to vary exposure to hormones, neuroendocrinologists have relied heavily on research on the neurobiology of learning and memory to choose cognitive tasks. The most common research strategy has been to utilize tasks for which the underlying neural circuitry has been partially or fully elucidated. The advantage of this approach is that if hormones do modify performance on the task, then the likely hormonal site of action can be identified and examined. Below, I will introduce you to a few tasks that are commonly used to examine learning and memory in animals and humans and tell you briefly about the neural circuitry underlying these tasks.

Spatial Tasks

Migrating birds and food-storing animals need prodigious memory abilities to survive (see Sherry and Schacter 1987). Black-capped chickadees hide seeds, nuts, and invertebrate prey in hundreds of cache sites each day and find these food stores after a few days by remembering their exact location. Homing pigeons find their way to their home loft from distant sites using a variety of navigational techniques. Other species need to be able to learn and recall spatial information to defend their territories and to forage efficiently. Because these amazing feats of spatial memory are performed to improve reproductive success, it seems quite possible that the hormones of reproduction might modulate spatial skills or memory. Although it is possible to study these abilities in the field, most researchers, even those who study wild-trapped animals, often bring subjects back to the laboratory to examine their

A. Eight-Arm Radial Maze

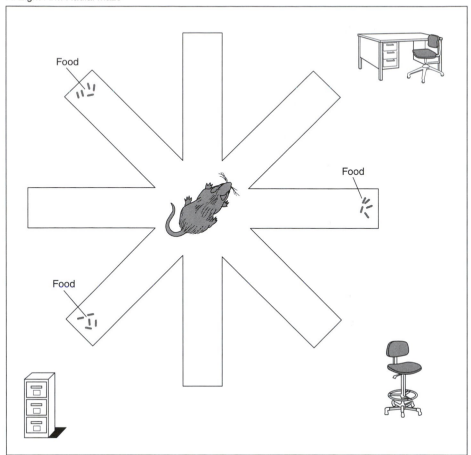

B. Morris Water Maze

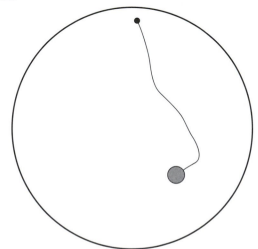

spatial abilities. To do so, researchers have developed laboratory-based tests that allow them to tap into the natural spatial abilities of many species.

One standard maze used to study spatial memory is called the **radial-arm maze** (figure 14.1A). It consists of 8 or 12 alleyways radiating from a central platform. Other mazes that have fewer choices, such as T-mazes or Y-mazes, are really just radial arm mazes with two possible food sites. Food rewards are placed in a well at the end of each arm or subset of arms. The subject is then placed on the central platform and allowed to wander freely until all the food sites have been found. Over days of training, subjects make fewer and fewer errors, learning to avoid arms that never have food and to avoid revisiting arms that have been previously visited on that day. Rat subjects, for example, learn this task easily over 7 to 14 days of training, though it often takes weeks of daily training for rats to reach steady-state performance on this task. Rats locate the food sites by remembering the location of the sites within the room, not by following scent trails or using a response algorithm (e.g., one simple algorithm is to take a sharp left each time you exit an arm). We know this because when a rat is removed from the maze in the middle of the trial and returned after the maze is rotated 180°, the rat will go to the correct room locations, which are now incorrect maze-arm choices (Olton and Samuelson 1976).

It is easy to study learning with this task because it takes many days of training for rats (and mice) to perform with few errors. It is also easy to vary the memory load by varying the number of food sites or interposing delays between choices. We can also monitor memory retention or strategies for solving the task. There are, however, several disadvantages for researchers interested in hormonal effects on cognition. Many training trials are required for rats to reach steady-state performance on this task, so hormonal effects must be assessed over a period of days, and sometimes weeks, which results in increased difficulty in isolating the effects of hormones to one particular stage of learning or memory.

For this reason, researchers often use another spatial maze task that is quickly and easily learned in just a few trials. The **water maze** (Morris 1981) takes advantage of a rodent's natural tendency to escape to dry land if it is placed in water (see figure 14.1B). In the standard water-maze task, subjects are placed in a round swimming pool and required to navigate using spatial cues to find an escape platform that is just beneath the surface of the water.

Figure 14.1 (*A*) Eight-arm radial maze. The object of this spatial maze task is to visit all the food sites (pellets placed at ends of some arms). The animal must remember which arms are baited and which arms it has already visited. When an animal returns to an arm it has previously visited, that is a working memory error. (*B*) Morris water maze. The object of this spatial task is to find the submerged platform that is hidden under opaque liquid. The animal is placed into the water at different locations around the perimeter of the pool and must swim to locate the platform. Swim time, path length, and the initial direction that the animal swims in are used to determine if the rat remembers where the platform is located.

The water is made opaque with water-soluble paint or powdered milk so that the platform is not visible. The standard procedure is to place the subject at the edge of the pool and record the time and swim path until the platform is located. The subject is allowed to remain on the platform for 20 to 30 seconds, and then after a delay, is returned to the pool at a randomly chosen location from which it must find the platform again. With a short delay between trials, rats (and some other rodent species as well) learn this task within 10 trials, so it is very easy to assess the effect of a hormone within a few hours.

It is also possible to examine memory of the platform location by seeing how well the subject recalls the platform location after a long delay, say 24 hours following the last training trial. On this trial, often called a "probe trial," no platform is available. A rat with an accurate memory of the platform location will swim to the place where the platform should be, and then swim around that region to try to find it. Time spent searching in the correct location can be used as a measure of the rat's memory. An obvious disadvantage to this and other aversively motivated tasks is that the stress of training and testing may activate other hormonal systems not under study. Another disadvantage is that this task is extremely easy to learn because only a single place must be committed to memory; therefore, hormonally induced improvements in memory may not be detectable unless task difficulty is increased, by lengthening the delay prior to a probe or by varying the platform location each day.

Social Recognition

Rats and mice along with many other social rodents are especially adept at recalling the smell of another **conspecific** that they met several hours or days ago. This type of **social recognition memory** has been studied extensively in the laboratory by arranging a meeting between two conspecifics and allowing them to smell one another for several minutes. After a delay in which they are separated from one another, they are returned for a second meeting. If recognition occurs, then the subject spends less time actively investigating the familiar stimulus animal during this encounter. If no memory is present, the subject investigates the stimulus animal for a long time, as if it were a novel stimulus. It is likely that the type of learning that is being examined in this paradigm is **habituation**, a diminution of response after repeated stimuli lacking reinforcement (Thor and Holloway 1982). In social recognition, rodents habituate to the smell of a novel conspecific over several minutes of contact, and this memory can last many days. As with the water maze task, social recognition is learned rapidly, can be tested immediately after learning, or delays of various lengths can be imposed prior to testing to increase the memory demands of the task. All these characteristics make this an excellent task to use in studies of hormonal modulation of cognition. One disadvantage is that many hormones alter olfactory processing, so it is necessary to be careful that hormonal effects are altering cognitive and not just sensory mechanisms.

Avoidance Tasks and Fear Conditioning

Other common tasks used to assess learning and memory in the laboratory are avoidance tasks and conditioned fear-response tasks. Avoidance tasks rely on an animal's species-specific tendencies to avoid certain stimuli. Rats and mice are nocturnal animals that avoid brightly lit areas, presumably because in daylight they would be easy targets for predators. Animals also have species-specific responses to threat and startle responses that are almost automatic. Some animals freeze in place to avoid being seen; others try to run away and find cover as quickly as possible.

Active avoidance studies are usually conducted by giving an animal a signal, such as a light or tone, that an aversive event like a shock is going to occur. The animal then learns to move to a safe area of the cage or to press a lever to avoid the shock. **Passive avoidance** simply requires the animal to learn to stay put—for example, on a small wooden platform over a wire grid floor—in order to avoid a shock delivered to the wire grid. In **fear conditioning**, a conditioned stimulus (e.g., a light, tone, or the context of the training cage itself) is paired with an unconditioned stimulus like a shock. When the shock is first given, the autonomic nervous system is activated, heart rate and blood pressure increase, and stress hormones are released. The animal might also leap into the air to try to avoid the shock. If learning occurs, then the presentation of the conditioned stimulus results in a conditioned response. That is, the tone or light comes to elicit the activation of the autonomic nervous system and a behavioral fear response, such as a startle response or a freezing response. When animals learn the association between the tone or light and the shock, they respond to the cue as if they were expecting to receive a shock. Since conditioned responses are acquired after just a few pairings and retained for many days, they have been used extensively to examine the stage of memory when hormones may be acting. As with the aversively motivated water maze, the stress of the task itself activates many hormonal systems and this may confound an interpretation of test performance.

The Neural Basis of Learning and Memory

Many of the tasks and procedures that have been selected for use in studies of hormones and cognition depend upon neural pathways involving the **hippocampal formation**, **amygdala**, and various **neocortical regions**. These brain regions are critically important for memory, learning, and emotion; they contain receptors for several different hormones, and they receive input from other brain regions that express hormone receptors. Although these brain regions are all interconnected, it is possible to directly examine their role in various stages and types of cognitive processes. It is beyond the scope of this chapter to explain all that is known about the neural basis of learning and

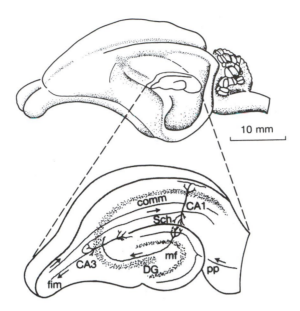

Figure 14.2 The hippocampus in the rat brain. The top illustration shows the position of the C-shaped hippocampus in the rat brain. A cross-section of the hippocampus is enlarged to illustrate the cell fields of the hippocampus known as CA1 and CA3, and the dentate gyrus (DG). Field CA2 is located between CA1 and CA3, CA4 is found between CA3 and the DG. The perforant pathway (pp) arrives from the overlying region of cortex referred to as the entorhinal cortex and perforates the DG. Axons arriving from the contralateral hemisphere, referred to as the commisural projection (comm), and collaterals from neurons within the hippocampus (Schaffer collaterals, Sch) sprout in response to perforant pathway deafferentation. Fim, fimbria; mf, mossy fibers. (Reprinted from Dudai (1989) with permission.)

memory (see Gallistel 1999; Martinez and Kesner 1998; and Gazzanaga, Ivry, and Mangun 2002). However, you need to know about several major structures and systems that provide the neural architecture for spatial navigation, social recognition, avoidance, and fear-learning, and how these may function in human cognition.

Hippocampus and Associated Input Pathways

The hippocampal region (figure 14.2) consists of a group of structures located deep within the medial **temporal lobe** of the brain. The hippocampal formation has two interlocking C-shaped structures, the hippocampus and the **dentate gyrus**. The dentate gyrus receives information via the surrounding **entorhinal cortex**, which has inputs from a wide spectrum of sensory modalities and from cortical association areas. Information flows from the entorhinal cortex to granule cells in the dentate gyrus. These cells send projections to pyramidal cells in the CA3 region of the hippocampus, which send projections to the CA1 region. Axons then exit the hippocampus in a region called the **subiculum**.

The subiculum sends information back to the entorhinal cortex before sending that processed information back to the same cortical regions from which it came. The hippocampal region also receives modulatory inputs via the **fimbria-fornix** from both **GABAergic** and **cholinergic** neurons that originate in the **basal forebrain** (structures such as the medial septum, diagonal band of Broca, and nucleus basalis magnocellularis). In humans, damage to the hippocampus produces **anterograde amnesia**, an impairment in the ability to learn new information (Squire 1987), and a temporally graded **retrograde amnesia** (where more recent memories appear to be more seriously disrupted than older ones).

This suggests that the hippocampus is necessary for the initial acquisition of certain memories and also may be needed for rehearsal and eventual consolidation of memory traces over time. The amnesia is specific for **declarative memory**, which is defined as the memory for events and experiences that are accessible to conscious control. For example, you use declarative memory to recall material for an exam and to remember the lyrics to your favorite songs. Hippocampal damage does not disrupt **procedural memory**, which is defined as the memory for the rules and motor procedures necessary to perform new behaviors. You use procedural memory to play the piano, shoot a free throw, and recall the rules of chess. In addition, there are other types of memory for which the hippocampus is not required: perceptual recognition, face recognition, simple stimulus-response associations, and emotional memories. For example, when I recall the 2001 National Championship basketball game, I feel the happiness I experienced when Duke beat Arizona. This emotional memory does not require the hippocampus.

Using animal models of hippocampal damage, experimenters have difficulty determining the loss of declarative memory because animals do not have the ability to report what they remember. Talking to animals is something Dr. Dolittle could accomplish but most of us must access an animal's knowledge in an indirect fashion. Rodents with hippocampal lesions or with lesions to cholinergic neurons in the basal forebrain that project to the hippocampus are disrupted in their **working memory** (for review, see Wenk 1997). They cannot remember the location of the food sites they just visited on the radial-arm maze (Olton, Walker, and Gage 1978) or the location of the escape platform in the water maze (Morris et al. 1982). However, the lesion does not interfere with procedural memories of how to perform the task (i.e., avoid arms that never contain any food), and does not interfere with navigation if the goal is marked directly with a beacon or a flag, or if the task can be solved using a simple stimulus-response rule (i.e., keep taking a left turn each time you have a choice). The hippocampus is not just specialized for spatial tasks; social-recognition memory also appears to be dependent upon an intact hippocampal complex (Kogan, Frankland, and Silva 2000).

One important characteristic of the hippocampus is that it develops **long-term potentiation (LTP)**, an enduring increase in postsynaptic responsivity

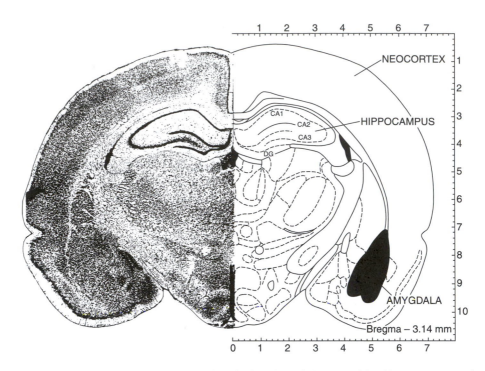

Figure 14.3 Coronal section of the rat brain showing the location of the amygdala, hippocampus, and neocortex. (Redrawn from Paxinos and Watson 1998.)

following a period of stimulation (Bliss and Lømo 1973). In other words, for several weeks following repeated electrical stimulation of cell groups in the hippocampal region, the postsynaptic cells show an increase in the magnitude of excitatory postsynaptic potentials. This physiological change in synaptic strength may be similar to the type of change that accompanies memory formation after repeated rehearsal of new associations.

Amygdala

The amygdala (figure 14.3) is located at the anterior medial portion of each of the temporal lobes, near the hippocampus. It is made up of many distinct neural groups, called **nuclei**, each with a distinct set of connections to other brain regions. The major regions of the amygdala are the medial nucleus, the basolateral nuclei, the central nucleus, and the basal nucleus. The medial nucleus receives projections from a host of sensory systems and sends information to the hypothalamus and basal forebrain. The basolateral region receives sensory information from cortical areas and also has reciprocal connections to the hippocampus. Output from the amygdala, especially from the central nucleus, projects to regions of the hypothalamus, midbrain, and pons, and produces emotional behavior as well as various **autonomic responses** (e.g., sweating and alterations in heart rate and blood pressure). Lesions to this region reduce or eliminate a wide range of emotional behaviors and accompanying autonomic responses. For example, amygdalar lesions abolish or diminish fear conditioning as well as the acquisition of aversively motivated tasks (Davis 1992), presumably because the information about the conditioned stimulus (e.g., that a tone is always followed by shock) is integrated within the nuclei of the amygdala to cause the emotional response (e.g., freezing or running). Without the amygdala, this association does not occur. Note that if the tone is present when the shock is administered, the hippocampus is not needed for the simple association to be learned. However, if a delay is interposed between the presentation of the tone and the aversive stimulus (e.g., the shock), the hippocampus is required to bridge the delay (McEchron et al. 1998). This is called **trace conditioning**.

The amygdala also appears to modulate rehearsal and retrieval processes, probably through its interactions with the hippocampus. The human amygdala also appears to participate in conditioned emotional responses. For example, the amygdalar region of human subjects was examined using functional magnetic resonance imaging (fMRI) during conditioned fear acquisition and extinction. The activity of the amygdala during acquisition was significantly correlated with autonomic indices of conditioning (e.g., heart rate or blood pressure) in individual subjects. These results provide further evidence for the conservation of amygdala function across species and implicates an amygdalar contribution to associative emotional learning tasks (LaBar et al. 1998).

Neocortex

The neocortex (figures 14.2 and 14.3) has two symmetrical hemispheres that consist of large sheets of layered neurons connected by a band of axons called the corpus callosum. Both the hippocampus and the amygdala have reciprocal connections with the neocortex and work with it to process information and lay down memories. The neocortex has four functional divisions: temporal lobes for audition, parietal lobes for somatosensation, occipital lobes for vision, and frontal lobes for motor control. However, each region also has specialized modules for specific types of learning or memory. For example, regions of the temporal lobe appear to be critical for recognizing and perceiving faces. Specialized regions of the parietal lobe are critical in identifying where an object is located, whereas regions of the temporal lobe are important for discriminating between two objects. There are also specialized modules in temporal, frontal, and parietal lobes for acquiring, understanding, and expressing language. Regions of the frontal cortex are critical for maintaining information and selecting an action, as well as for organizing and planning actions. And in many organisms, but especially in humans, functions of the neocortex and associated structures are lateralized, that is, one hemisphere of the brain is the dominant one for certain processes. This is especially true for language (mainly a left hemisphere function) and for spatial functions (mainly a right hemisphere function). With the increasing resolution of functional imaging techniques that allow the examination of brain structures and function in awake human subjects, we are just beginning to examine how hormones might modulate perceptual and memory functions of neocortical regions in humans.

Stress and Arousal Hormones

I can vividly recall the day when John F. Kennedy was assassinated. I fell hard on the playground that day and the gravel gashed my knees. I heard the first news report on the car radio as my mother rushed me to the hospital. I can also recall the details of my brief encounter with a mugger in New York City on a warm, sunny late-August afternoon. He was dressed in immaculately clean white pants and he carried a shiny, thick-handled knife. These events happened a long, long time ago, but I still remember them as if they had occurred recently. We all have experienced emotionally charged events and have found them to be easily and vividly remembered. These types of experiences provide anecdotal evidence to suggest that the hormonal systems activated by arousing experiences may directly or indirectly aid learning and long-term memory. (Note that it is also likely that continued rehearsal of these emotionally charged events throughout my lifetime has aided my memory for these particularly salient experiences.)

Why, then, do we often feel that stress or arousal blocks memory? On the first day of my Hormones and Behavior seminar each year, I have all the students introduce themselves. I'm sure it's my anxiety about making a good first impression (and not my aging brain) that prevents me from storing this information clearly because I always have difficulty recalling students' names at the very next class meeting. You can probably think of your own examples of both the performance-enhancing and blocking effects of stress and arousal. These seemingly paradoxical findings were documented almost a century ago and form the foundation of the Yerkes-Dodson law (Yerkes and Dodson 1908). Robert Yerkes and John Dodson found that mice quickly learned to avoid a chamber in which they had received a moderate shock intensity; however, learning was much slower at lower or higher shock intensities (figure 14.4). We now know that the duration of stress and not just the stress level is an important determinant as to whether stress aids performance or causes forgetfulness. Stressors that last minutes to hours (moderate arousal) tend to sharpen performance, although under certain circumstances even moderate arousal can interfere with learning or rehearsal and disrupt performance. If the stressor persists (high arousal), the enhancement is replaced by forgetfulness.

During and immediately after emotionally charged or stressful events, a number of physiological systems are activated, and as you read in chapter 11, several different hormones are released. Many of these hormones, including those released from the adrenal medulla (epinephrine), the adrenal cortex (glucocorticoids), and others, such as adrenocorticoptropin (ACTH), vasopressin, and oxytocin, are known to modulate learning and retrieval. It is likely that the amygdala is the site of the short-term modulating effects of arousal-induced hormone secretions. Under conditions of long-term or re-

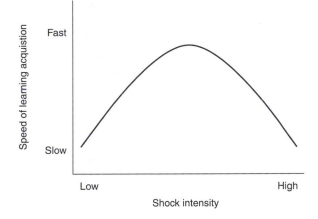

Figure 14.4 Relationship between shock intensity and speed of acquisition of an active avoidance response. Rats learned the task best at an intermediate shock intensity. Too little shock or too much shock was less effective, which indicates that there is an optimal arousal level that facilitates learning this response. (Adapted from Yerkes and Dodson 1908.)

peated stress, adrenal hormones alter memory by altering synapse formation and dendritic structure, as well as cell birth and death within regions of the hippocampal formation.

Activation of the Sympathetic Nervous System

Activation of the sympathetic nervous system and the consequent release of epinephrine (adrenaline) and norepinephrine mediate some of the performance-altering effects of emotionally charged events. Removal of the adrenal glands results in poorer performance on aversively motivated tasks, and replacement with epinephrine, either during or immediately following training, appears to restore performance to levels seen in intact animals. Research by Paul Gold and colleagues (Gold and van Buskirk 1975) was the first to show that post-training injections of epinephrine enhance the performance of a passive avoidance task. The effects of epinephrine are both dose- and time-dependent (Gold 1987). As would be predicted by the Yerkes-Dodson law, moderate doses were more effective than high or low doses. The greatest degree of enhancement was observed when epinephrine was administered immediately following training rather than before, during, or long afterwards. One interpretation of this finding is that epinephrine is acting on the process of memory consolidation directly (Gold 1987); however, we know that rats and humans continue to mentally rehearse new associations following training. Thus, epinephrine may be acting indirectly to alter attention to the rehearsal process rather than on the initial encoding process or retrieval during task performance. This performance-enhancing effect of epinephrine has been seen with a variety of learning and memory tasks, including those that are **appetitively motivated** (e.g., tasks where rats work for a reward), suggesting that the effect is generalizable across many different types of learning.

So where does epinephrine act to cause these effects? We might expect that epinephrine acts directly on the cortical regions important for cognition; however, we have known for many years that epinephrine does not cross the **blood-brain barrier** (Weil-Malharbe, Axelrod, and Tomchick 1959). If epinephrine does not have direct **central actions**, it must stimulate peripheral receptors that, in turn, activate the brain. Epinephrine released from the adrenal medulla binds to several classes of peripheral receptors, called **α-** and **β-adrenergic receptors**, which are located on the plasma membrane of neuroeffector cells that transduce epinephrine interactions with the cell into a physiological response. Blockade of peripheral α-adrenergic receptors prevents the performance-enhancing effects of arousal-induced epinephrine release in rats (Introini-Collison et al. 1992).

To determine whether β-adrenergic receptor activation is also critical for arousal-induced improvements in performance in humans, Cahill and his colleagues designed a clever experiment (Cahill et al. 1994). First they read a group of control subjects a fairly unexciting story—a boy and his mother walk through town, pass several stores, cross the street, enter a hospital where the boy's father works, and while they are in the hospital, they see an X-ray machine. Then they read a group of experimental subjects a similar story that varied only in the final details. When the boy crosses the street, he is hit by a car and taken to the hospital where his father works and is brought to the X-ray room. After a delay, the experimental subjects recall the story better than the control subjects, but just the final stressful part, not the whole story. To show that activation of β-adrenergic receptors is critical for the performance-enhancing effects of arousal, half of the subjects in a second study were given **propanolol**, a drug that specifically blocks β-adrenergic receptors. The group who received this drug and were read the arousing version of the story had a poorer recall for the story details than did subjects receiving a saline injection.

When their recall for the story details was examined closely, it was discovered that both groups were just as accurate on details occurring at the beginning and middle parts of the story, but the drug-treated group showed poorer recall of the arousing events in the story. This demonstrates that propranolol's blockade of β-adrenergic receptors prevented arousal-enhanced performance but did not interfere with performance more generally. So how does activation of peripheral β-adrenergic receptors lead to alteration in performance? Two mechanisms that are not mutually exclusive have been described.

Arousal and epinephrine activate central noradrenergic mechanisms by stimulating the release of the neurotransmitter norepinephrine in the brain (Gold and Van Buskirk 1978). The key neural site of action for norepinephrine is probably in the amygdala because the improvement in performance produced by systemic injections of epinephrine post-training can be blocked by infusing propranolol directly into the amygdala (Liang et al. 1986). These findings provide a second mechanism by which arousal-induced epinephrine release can alter the rehearsal process. However, two critical pieces of information are needed to complete the story. Does peripheral epinephrine alter norepinephrine release in the amygdala and what is the pathway by which epinephrine exerts this effect?

Cedric Williams and his colleagues (Williams et al. 1998) recently measured the change in extracellular concentrations of norepinephrine in the amygdala of rats after they had been injected with epinephrine or given an arousing footshock. They assessed norepinephrine release using a technique called microdialysis (see chapters 5 and 13) which allows the collection of extracellular fluid in particular brain regions. They found that both a mild shock to the feet and epinephrine administration caused an elevation in norepinephrine in the amygdala that persisted for up to 60 min (figure 14.5).

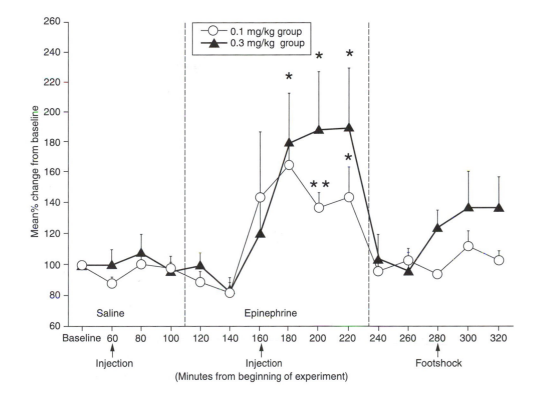

Figure 14.5 Norepinephrine concentrations in dialysis samples obtained from the amygdala of rats, expressed as a percentage of baseline values. Arrows indicate where animals received an injection or footshock. At the first arrow, all animals received saline and there was no change in norepinephrine. At the second arrow, animals received epinephrine (open circles, 0.1 mg/kg; closed triangles, 0.3 mg/kg) and both groups had a significant increase in norepinephrine in the amygdala. At the third arrow, animals received escapable footshock. While there is a trend for an increase in norephinphrine after footshock, this was not statistically different from baseline. Treatment with inescapable footshock does result in an increase over baseline, however. (*$P < 0.05$ relative to baseline at these time points; **$P < 0.01$ relative to baseline at these time points.) (Redrawn from Williams et al. 1998.)

They also found that this increase in norepinephrine could be attenuated if a brainstem region called the **nucleus of the solitary tract** (NST) was anesthetized prior to epinephrine administration. This brainstem region is activated by the **vagus nerve**, and norepinephrine is the major neurotransmitter in the projection of neurons from the NST to the amygdala. These findings suggest that epinephrine's effect on performance may be mediated by actions of vagal afferents on the noradrenergic NST neurons that send axons to the amygdala; however, there is an alternate explanation.

One well-known effect of epinephrine is to increase glucose levels in the blood, which increases glucose availability to the brain. If glucose levels are increased in humans (Parsons and Gold 1992) or in laboratory animals (Gold et al. 1986) by ingestion of a sweetened drink immediately following learning, performance on a variety of tasks is potentiated in an inverted-U shape dose-response manner. Because infusion of glucose directly to the brain also augments performance, the effects of epinephrine-stimulated glucose release are likely to be central and not peripheral. One effect of increased glucose availability is to increase delivery of glucose to neurons, particularly neurons that are active and in need of energy. Just after learning, the active cells are likely to be the ones involved in the rehearsal of previously learned information. Another consequence of increased glucose levels is to increase the synthesis and release of the neurotransmitter acetylcholine (Raggozino et al. 1996). Recall that acetylcholine is a critical modulator of hippocampus-dependent memory. During behavioral testing, both acetylcholine (Ragozzino et al. 1998) and norepinephrine (Men et al. 1999) levels increase in the hippocampus, but only acetylcholine release is augmented by **systemic** or central injections of glucose at doses that enhance performance. These data suggest that there may be two independent mechanisms by which arousal-induced epinephrine release modulates cognitive performance. So moderate arousal following studying may aid your test performance, though consuming a sugar-laden drink might work just as well.

Glucocorticoids

As you read in chapter 11, stressful emotional events not only cause the release of epinephrine from the adrenal medulla but also stimulate glucocorticoid release from the adrenal cortex. The first experiments to suggest that hormones of the hypothalamic-pituitary-adrenal axis might influence performance on learning tasks were done in the 1950s using adrenocorticotropic hormone (ACTH), a hormone released from the pituitary to stimulate the adrenal gland (Mirshky et al. 1953). Other studies (DeWied 1966) confirmed that ACTH could ameliorate the impairment in avoidance learning caused by removal of the pituitary gland. Was ACTH acting on the brain to alter learning or was ACTH causing the release of adrenal glucocorticoids and in that fashion altering cognition? Both actions appear likely. **Neuropeptides** derived from the amino-terminal end of ACTH, which do not stimulate the adrenal, enhance performance (Greven and De Wied 1973), though it is not clear that these effects occur under natural conditions. In contrast, it has been shown that glucocorticoids have multiple effects on memory function throughout an individual's lifetime. Short-term effects of glucocorticoids on performance are dependent upon the dose (i.e., much like the effects of epinephrine) and the time of administration during training. In contrast, long-term or repeated exposure causes a reversible **atrophy** of **dendrites** and an inhibition of **neurogenesis** in various cells populations of the hippocampus, resulting in an impairment of cognitive function. And exposure to high and low levels of glucocorticoids during early development also appears to program the hypothalamic-pituitary-adrenal axis' response to stress during adulthood.

SHORT-TERM EFFECTS

Single injections of a moderate dose of **dexamethasone** (a synthetic steroid that mimics corticosterone, the major glucocorticoid in rodents, and **cortisol**, the major glucocorticoid in primates) enhances performance of inhibitory avoidance learning when administered immediately following training (Roozendaal 2000). However, low and high levels of glucocorticoids appear to interfere with performance. For example, **adrenalectomy** impairs performance of a spatial water maze task, and post-training injections of moderate doses of dexamethasone can reverse this impairment. If this same dose of dexamethasone is given to control rats, however, their performance is impaired. Presumably, in control rats the stress of training causes endogenous cortisol release that sums with the injected dexamethasone, causing a high level of total glucocorticoid (**endogenous** plus synthetic) that is detrimental to performance. If training is made less stressful by increasing the water temperature, post-training injections of the same dose of dexamethasone to control rats can actually improve their performance.

Glucocorticoid effects on performance occur partly via activation of the same β-adrenergic receptors in the amygdala that are involved in the effects of epinephrine. We know this because lesions of the basolateral region of the amygdala (BLA), but not the central region, block the performance-enhancing effects of a systemic injection of a glucocorticoid receptor **agonist** (Roozendaal and McGaugh 1996a). Furthermore, infusions of a specific glucocorticoid receptor stimulant directly into the BLA also enhance performance (Roozendaal and McGaugh 1997). However, if propranolol is infused into the BLA, it blocks post-training glucocorticoid-induced enhancement of performance (Quirarte et al. 1997). These results strongly suggest that β-adrenergic activation is a critical step in mediating glucocorticoid effects on performance, and that the BLA is the site of interaction between these systems. However, circulating glucocorticoids not only occupy receptors in the amygdala, but they also bind to glucocorticoid receptors throughout the brain, including the hippocampal formation, which has an especially high density of glucocorticoid receptors. Administration of corticosterone directly into the hippocampus has also been shown to enhance performance in a dose-dependent fashion (Roozendaal and McGaugh 1997).

Glucocorticoids interact with both the amygdala and the hippocampus via two types of receptors. Type I receptors have a high affinity for corticosterone and cortisol and are located mainly in the limbic system of the brain (structures including but not limited to the hippocampal region, amygdala and **septal region**, and hypothalamus). Type II receptors have a lower affinity for endogenous glucocorticoids than type I but have a higher affinity for the synthetic glucocorticoid, dexamethasone, and are distributed quite widely throughout the brain (Reul and De Kloet 1985). At moderate glucocorticoid levels like those seen during our normal daily diurnal variation in glucocorticoid secretion (blood levels of glucocorticoids are highest right before we wake up in the morning), the high affinity type I receptors are heavily occupied (McEwen, De Kloet, and Rostene 1986). After stress-induced increases in glucocorticoid secretion, the low affinity type II receptors also bind glucocorticoids. Does this mean that the performance-enhancing effects of glucocorticoids are modulated by the type II receptors? The answer is that both types of receptors probably play different roles in the modulatory effects of glucocorticoids on cognitive processes.

Oitzl and De Kloet (1992) were the first to examine the roles of type I and type II receptors on spatial memory performance. They used **antagonists** that were specific to each type of receptor and treated **intact** rats with these drugs either before training on the water maze, after training, or right before a probe recall test. They found that the type II antagonist administered either before training or just after training impaired spatial memory in a water maze. In contrast, blockade of the type I receptor did not disrupt the ability of mice to find the escape platform; however, it did modify the swimming strategy used by the mice on their training and test trials. These data suggested that while type II receptors appear important for glucocorticoid enhancement of performance, type I receptors may be involved in sensory integration or environmental exploration (Lupien and McEwen 1997). However, another study suggests that at moderate hormone levels, type I receptors are also needed for accurate performance. When type I and type II receptor agonists were given to adrenalectomized rats (remember that in the previous study, rats were intact and had circulating adrenal hormones), either 2 hours before training on a maze task, immediately after training, or 2 hours after training, treatment with a type I receptor agonist restored the performance of the adrenalectomized rats to a level comparable to control rats if given before or immediately after training. Treatment with type II agonists did not improve the performance of the adrenalectomized rats (Conrad et al. 1997). Together these studies suggest that type I and type II receptors form a two-tier response system to modulate performance.

Further support for this idea comes from research on the effects of receptor agonists on hippocampal LTP. Administration of a type I agonist to intact rats produced an enhancement in LTP compared to either adrenalectomized or intact rats not treated with the agonist. In contrast, treatment with a specific type II agonist markedly decreased the induction of dentate gyrus LTP (Pav-

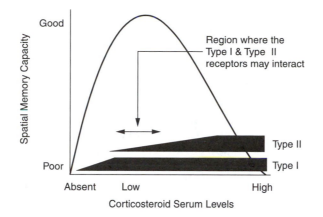

Figure 14.6 Model illustrating how the activation of hippocampal corticosteroid receptors could affect spatial memory (Conrad, Lupien, and McEwen 1999). As serum concentrations of corticosterone increase, type I hippocampal receptors become nearly completely occupied whereas type II hippocampal receptors are occupied at low levels leading to normal (or enhanced) spatial memory. As serum corticosterone levels increase further (e.g., during severe stress), more hippocampal type II receptors become activated. This results in impaired spatial memory. The double-headed arrow indicates the range at which the type I and type II hippocampal receptors could interact with each other to affect spatial memory. When serum corticosterone levels are elevated beyond the range indicated by the double-headed arrow, the interplay between the two receptor subtypes becomes insignificant as the impairing effects of the type II receptors become dominant. (Redrawn from Conrad et al. 1999.)

lides et al. 1995). A recent study suggests that the inverted U-shaped curve seen in many studies of glucocorticoid effects on performance and LTP may be related only to type II receptor activation (Conrad et al. 1999). As you can see in figure 14.6, the level of occupancy of the hippocampal type II receptor, as measured by a binding assay, was significantly correlated with spatial memory performance following an inverted U-shaped curve, whereas the level of type I receptor occupancy was not.

Taken together, these results suggest that both glucocorticoid activation of type I and type II receptors in amygdala and hippocampus contribute to the process of learning and memory in a time-dependent fashion and may play different roles in glucocorticoid modulation of behavior. Type II receptors that are occupied at the time of high-circulating glucocorticoids appear to be more important for the performance enhancement.

Have you been wondering whether anyone has treated human subjects with the synthetic corticosterone, dexamethasone, or used natural variations in glucocorticoid levels to examine their effects on memory? A number of investigators have done these experiments and they have revealed a pattern of results that is similar to that of animal studies. For example, there is some indication that the inverted U-shaped dose-response function between cortisol levels and cognitive performance is seen in humans (Fehm-Wolfsdorf et al. 1993). On a free recall task, subjects were found to make the fewest errors in the morning, when endogenous cortisol levels are highest, than in the late afternoon. If 50 mg of **hydrocortisone** is given to subjects in the morning, it increases errors compared to untreated controls, but if this same dose is given in the afternoon, it does not impair performance. Thus, the added glucocorticoids appeared to shift the dose-response function, as we have seen it do in animal studies.

Other studies indicate that exposure to high levels of glucocorticoids for several days impairs the type of memory that requires hippocampal function, that is, declarative memory. A 4-day treatment of human subjects with dexamethasone impaired performance on both immediate and delayed recall of verbal information, whereas there was no disruption of more procedural tasks (e.g., line orientation tasks, serial addition tasks) that do not require intact hippocampal function (Newcomer et al. 1994). These data suggest that there may be direct effects of glucocorticoids on the hippocampus in humans.

To date, it is not clear whether the performance-modulating effects of glucocorticoids and epinephrine actually influence memory directly, or whether the U-shaped dose-response function on performance is due to indirect effects on attention or arousal. The fact that short-term effects of adrenal hormones on performance are most effective if administered just before or just after training suggests that effects may alter nonmnemonic factors like attention or arousal that may alter the salience of the associations to be remembered or modulate interference with rehearsal processes. A moderate level of arousal during or immediately after learning could enhance attention to the task, while high levels of arousal could interfere with rehearsal processes. Because we know that glucocorticoids influence both hippocampal function and amygdalar function, it may be that there are two mechanisms underlying their effects on performance: (1) a direct hippocampal contribution to memory and (2) an indirect amygdala effect on attention and arousal.

LONG-TERM EFFECTS
Although the consequences of stress-activated epinephrine and glucocorticoid release may be beneficial in the short-run because arousing and potentially dangerous events are remembered and avoided in the future, studies of rodents, monkeys and humans suggest that long-term or repeated exposure to high levels of glucocorticoids cause cognitive impairments that result from neuronal atrophy and impaired **neurogenesis**. Free-ranging animals are unlikely to experience long term stressors. The antelope either eludes the hungry lion that has chased it across the savanna or it is caught and eaten. When a monkey falls from an unstable tree branch into the high waters of a raging river, it either swims to safety and remembers to avoid this site in the future or it drowns. However, in our modern world it is possible for psychological stressors (e.g., the pressure to get good grades or commuting to work every day in heavy traffic) to be repeated many times each day and to continue for months or years.

In the laboratory, the consequences of daily elevations in glucocorticoids have been evaluated using animal models. For example, a 21-day exposure to elevated glucocorticoids induced by a daily injection of corticosterone or 6 hours/day of restraint stress caused atrophy of the apical dendritic branches of hippocampal pyramidal cells (McEwen et al. 1995). The significance of this change in dendritic morphology is that these atrophied cells make fewer synaptic connections, which leads to poorer memory performance in spatial and other short-term memory tasks (Luine et al. 1994). Unlike the rapid effects on performance of glucocorticoids present during or immediately following training, these brain and cognitive impairments are relatively slow to develop, taking at least 3 weeks under daily stressful laboratory conditions. However, if stress is alleviated, both the changes to hippocampal dendrites and the impairments in cognition can be reversed in about a week or so.

The mechanisms underlying this reversible atrophy of dendrites are complex; however, we know that the first step is via glucocorticoid activation of type II receptors (Eldridge et al. 1989). Both stress and corticosterone-induced atrophy are prevented by **Dilantin**, an anti-**epileptic** drug, and by blocking **NMDA receptors**, which interact with the excitatory amino acid **glutamate**. Therefore, the release and actions of **excitatory amino acids** are another step in the process of dendritic atrophy (see McEwen (1999) for review). In a simple way, you can liken the actions of chronic glucocorticoids on the hippocampus to the effects of repeated and prolonged **seizures**. At this time, we do not know the mechanism by which the hippocampal dendrites undergo repair and elongation following the removal of stress, although we do know that stress alters the expression of various **growth factors** (e.g., Ueyama et al. 1997). One possible model for how these processes are acting in the hippocampus has been suggested by McEwen and is illustrated in figure 14.7.

Other cell populations in the hippocampus are also sensitive to glucocorticoid exposure. Elizabeth Gould and her colleagues have demonstrated that adrenalectomy increases the birth of new **granule cells** in the dentate gyrus in adult rats (Cameron and Gould 1994), and this increase in neurogenesis is accompanied by an increase in a form of programmed cell death called **apotosis** (Sloviter et al. 1989). This may come as quite a surprise to you because some textbooks still report the "no new neuron doctrine"—a strongly held belief that during early development we acquire all the neurons we are to have throughout life, that no new neurons are born in the brain of mammals in adult life. In fact, it was discovered in the mid 1960s that granule cells in the dentate gyrus of rats are continuously born throughout life (Altman and Das 1965). Gould and her colleagues have provided convincing new evidence that thousands of new hippocampal granule cells are produced daily in adult rodents (Gould and Tanapat 1999), and that this phenomenon also occurs in primates (Gould et al. 1999), including humans (Eriksson et al. 1998).

Both adrenal steroids and stressful experiences inhibit granule cell proliferation in rats (Tanapat et al. 1998). In an attempt to demonstrate that cell proliferation in the hippocampal region of primates can be modified by a

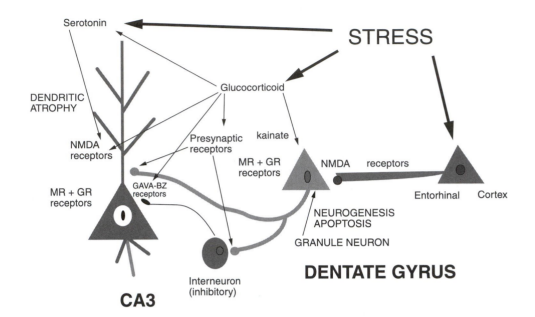

Figure 14.7 Schematic diagram of the postulated role of neurotransmitters and glucocorticoids in regulating neurogenesis and dendritic atrophy in the dendate gyrus-CA3 system of the hippocampal formation. MR, mineralocorticoid or type I adrenal steroid receptor; GR, glucocorticoid or type II adrenal steroid receptor. Granule neurons are replaced in adult life, and neurogenesis and apoptotic neuronal death are regulated by stress and by enriched environments, as well as by seizurelike activity. The balance between the excitatory input and the inhibitory tone from the interneurons is presumed to be important to the excitability of CA3 neurons. Excitatory amino acid release during stress, aided by circulating glucocorticoids, leads to a reversible atrophy of apical dendrites over 3 to 4 weeks in rats and tree shrews. Serotonin also participates and may exacerbate the atrophy induced by stress. Excitatory input to the dentate granule neurons from entorhinal cortex acts via glutamate/NMDA receptors in concert with circulating adrenal steroids to regulate the rate of neurogenesis and apoptotic cell death. Both acute and chronic stress seem to be able to inhibit neurogenesis in the dentate gyrus. (Adapted from McEwen 1999.)

natural stressor, Gould and colleagues (Gould et al. 1998) placed individual marmoset monkeys into the home territories of another group of marmosets. Although the intruders were safely enclosed in cages, they could interact with the residents. After just one hour of exposure to social stress, the intruder monkeys showed a decrease in the number of proliferating cells in the dentate gyrus compared with that of unstressed controls (figure 14.8). In real life, the intruder monkey would probably be chased out of the resident's territory or the intruder would fight with the resident and win a place in the territory, so it is unlikely that an hour of social stress would occur. However, this test situation might be comparable to an hour or more of stress during an especially difficult exam or an hour spent in an overheated car in heavy traffic.

If severe traumatic stress is prolonged for several months or years, hippocampal cells die (Sapolsky et al. 1985), and in general, repeated glucocorticoid elevation or treatment in humans is accompanied by cognitive decline.

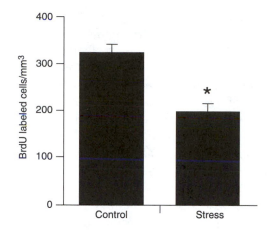

Figure 14.8 A single exposure to a resident results in a significant decrease in the number of BrdU-labeled cells in the dentate gyrus of the intruder marmoset monkey. Adult monkeys were placed individually in the home cage of a conspecific for 1 hour. After this time, the monkeys were removed and injected with BrdU, a marker for proliferating cells and their progeny. BrdU labels neurons that are being born in the same way that thymidine labels neurons (see chapter 3). Two hours later, the brains were taken for analysis. Bars: mean + SEM. *different from control $P < 0.05$. (From Gould et al. 1998.)

One clinical population that has been studied extensively is patients with **Cushing's syndrome**, who suffer from an overproduction of adrenal glucocorticoids. Using **brain imaging technologies** (**PET** or **fMRI**), it has been revealed that these patients have decreased hippocampal volumes and lower scores on verbal recall tests (Starkman 1992). However, in this case, as in other studies of patient populations, it is difficult to determine whether the cognitive deficits are due to increases in adrenal output or to the underlying illness itself.

AGING

This finding led researchers to explore the consequences of reduced glucocorticoid exposure during normal aging in humans. Most individuals show a slow increase in glucocorticoid levels as they age, and individual differences in stress reactivity and lifestyle may determine the lifetime pattern of glucocorticoid exposure. Using animal models, it has been possible to demonstrate that a lifelong reduction of exposure to glucocorticoids slows the normal age-related decline in cell death in the hippocampus and the normal age-related decline in spatial memory (see Sapolsky (1992) for review).

A study by Lupien and colleagues (Lupien et al. 1994) has examined the relationship between cortisol levels and cognitive function in an aging human population. They tracked the cortisol levels of 19 healthy elderly subjects (60 to 80 years old), and at the end of this period administered a neuropsychological test battery that assessed memory, attention, and language. Correlational analyses showed that the slope of the cortisol levels over the 4 years prior to the cognitive assessment was an accurate predictor of cognitive function. The performance of men and women with rising basal cortisol was poorer on tasks measuring declarative memory and selective attention than that of subjects with lower basal levels or declining or stable levels. These data strongly suggest that cognitive deficits in the elderly are associated with individual differences in adrenal output. Further support for this hypothesis comes from studies of aged rats (Issa et al. 1990). As is typical in all aged populations, most individuals were memory-impaired compared to young adult control rats, but a subset of rats was spared. These memory-intact aged rats also had the least hippocampal cell loss and the lowest glucocorticoid levels. These data suggest that for whatever reason (a less reactive adrenal gland, a calmer life, or less sensitive glucocorticoid receptors), some rats and people are spared the toxic effects of lifelong glucocorticoid exposure.

What is the source of these individual differences? Variation in adrenal output and differences in sensitivity of glucocorticoid receptors may be regulated by developmental differences in maternal care (Francis and Meaney 1999). One important model for the environmental regulation of the development of physiological responses to stress is research investigating the effects of postnatal handling in rodents on the stress response. "**Handling**" is a 3- to 15-minute daily separation of mother and pups, followed by a reunion. Upon reunion, mothers of handled pups spend significantly more time licking and grooming their infants than do mothers of unhandled pups. Postnatal handling of this sort makes the offspring less sensitive to stress throughout its life. That is, it does not respond as quickly or release as much glucocorticoid when arousal occurs. It appears that the type of maternal care received by pups following a handling episode is responsible for mediating these long-term changes in hypothalamic-pituitary-adrenal responsivity.

When a population of mother rats is examined, some mothers naturally lick and groom their infants more than other mothers. Pups of mothers that lick and groom extensively show a lower plasma-glucocorticoid response to restraint-stress compared to offspring of mothers that are less attentive. This is true for both biological offspring of highly attentive mothers and for pups that have been adopted into a litter with a highly attentive mother. These data are exciting because they suggest that individual differences in stress reactivity occur in part because of differences in maternal care. This may explain why some individuals may show greater age-related glucocorticoid secretion and more age-related memory loss. Together these data suggest that you should try to avoid long-term or repeated stressor in your daily life. This may be a good reason to find a job that you enjoy, avoid "road rage," and engage in regular relaxation. At this time, we do not know how to translate the early experience of being licked and groomed more as an infant rat to human mother-child interactions. However, it seems likely that variations in early social experiences can serve as the basis for programming individual differences in stress reactivity that have consequences for how glucocorticoids alter your brain and your memory.

Posterior Pituitary Hormones

The posterior pituitary gland contains two main hormones: **oxytocin** and **vasopressin** (also called argnine vasopression or AVP); both have been implicated in cognitive processes. At first, this seems quite surprising. Nerve impulses in the hypothalamus travel down axons in the stalk of the pituitary to cause the release of these hormones into the general circulation. Secretion of vasopressin increases blood pressure and inhibits the formation of urine (this is why it is sometimes called antidiuretic hormone). Oxytocin stimulates contractions of uterine muscles for childbirth. **Pitocin**, a synthetic oxytocin, is sometimes administered to accelerate the birth process in humans. Oxytocin also stimulates milk release during nursing. These actions are due to the effects of these hormones on peripheral receptors in the breast, uterus, and muscle, but there are also receptors for these hormones in the brain, which appear to be involved in cognition.

Vasopressin

The neuropeptide arginine vasopressin was one of the first hormones discovered to have a role in learning and memory. In the mid 1960s, DeWied and his colleagues in the Netherlands showed that retention of an active avoidance task was impaired in rats with pituitary ablations and that an extract of the pituitary containing vasopressin reversed this effect (DeWied 1971). A physiological role for endogenous vasopressin was later discovered using a strain of rats that was genetically deficient in vasopressin. Systemic administration of vasopressin into the **lateral ventricles** of the brain of these rats improved performance on avoidance tasks (VanWimersma Greidanus et al. 1986). Later studies showed that vasopressin facilitated passive avoidance behavior when it was administered immediately following learning or right before recall, suggesting that vasopressin may act on the neural processes involved in rehearsal and recall.

Interestingly, the behavioral effects of vasopressin were known many years before the brain systems underlying these effects were discovered. We now know that vasopressin receptors are located in both the dorsal and the ventral hippocampus, the dentate gyrus, and in neurons in the basal forebrain, including the medial septal region and diagonal band. Central target sites for the performance-enhancing effects of vasopressin appear to be the hippocampus and the medial septal region of the basal forebrain. Lesions to these areas prevent vasopressin's performance-enhancing effects, while microinjection of vasopressin into these regions produces improved performance. Fibers (axons of neurons) coming from the amygdala are a source of hippocampal vasopressin (DeVries et al. 1985). Thus, it is likely that one mechanism for elevating vasopressin in the brain is via activation of the amygdala by emotionally charged events. Vasopressin, therefore, may act in concert with the adrenal hormones to improve memory for events occurring right after arousal.

Under what naturally occurring situations may vasopressin be involved in cognition? Two lines of work suggest important adaptive functions for this peptide. Vasopressin appears to play an important role in modulating social recognition. A rat treated with vasopressin immediately after the first presentation of a another novel conspecific spends less time investigating the same individual when it is presented again 2 hours later, a time after which there is usually no recognition (Dantzer et al. 1987). Administration of a vasopressin agonist either peripherally or centrally into the lateral ventricles or into the medial **septum** (a region of the basal forebrain that sends projections to the hippocampus) greatly enhances social-recognition memory, whereas administration of a vasopressin antagonist immediately following an encounter disrupts social memory. The latter finding is particularly important because it suggests that endogenous vasopressin in normal rats may contribute to their ability to form social memory (Bluthe and Danzer 1993).

A specialized form of social recognition occurs in **monogamous species**. To be monogamous, individuals must recognize and stay bonded to one another after mating. In fact, 24 hours after mating, monogamous male and female prairie voles exhibit affiliative behavior only toward their mates; males immediately attack conspecific strangers (Shapiro and Dewsbury 1990). This change in behavior from "investigation and affiliation" to "attack" is dependent upon the act of copulation; simple exposure to a female for 24 hours will not alter a male's behavior towards novel individuals. Mating also induces increases in the release of vasopressin into the medial septum. This effect is not observed in females or in males from polygynous vole species. (**Polygynous species** have sex with many mates, and do not stay attached to a single individual.) It is therefore not surprising that administration of a vasopressin antagonist following mating interferes with pair bonding in normally monogamous male prairie voles (for review, see Wang et al. 1998).

Two recent findings suggest that vasopressin may have a very specialized role in affiliation in general and social recognition more specifically. The neuroanatomical distribution of vasopressin receptors varies greatly between vole species with different social structures. Montane voles, a polygynous species, have a high level of binding in the lateral septum, while prairie voles, a monogamous species, have high levels of binding in the diagonal band. These differences may contribute to the relative importance of this hormone for pair bonding in these species.

The techniques of molecular biology have been used to produce mice with prairie vole vasopressin receptor genes. To do this, mice were genetically manipulated so that their own vasopressin receptor gene was **knocked out**. Then the prairie vole vasopressin receptor gene was inserted. These mice showed a pattern of vasopressin receptor distribution similar to prairie voles and not mice, and exhibited more affiliative behavior after injection with vasopressin than control mice (Young et al. 1999). As yet, we do not know whether vasopressin will improve social memory in a controlled test more effectively in these **transgenic mice** than in control mice, but this might be a useful way to test the prediction.

Oxytocin

Another hormone of the posterior pituitary, oxytocin, has effects on social recognition memory that are usually opposite to that of vasopressin. That is, oxytocin appears to interfere with performance on social recognition tasks. In the brain, oxytocin receptors are present in only a few discrete forebrain locations, including a region of the anterior olfactory nucleus, the rostral area of the hippocampus, a region of the **bed nucleus of the stria terminalis**, the dosal medial region of the **caudate**, and the central nucleus of the amygdala (Insel 1992). The distribution of receptors is quite similar in males and females (Tribollet et al. 1990). Central administration of oxytocin antisera blocks the formation of avoidance responding, and at physiological doses, oxytocin decreases social recognition memory when administered after the first social encounter (Insel 1992). One way to interpret these findings is to suggest that oxytocin may work with vasopressin to enhance social affiliation. Oxytocin's role may be to inhibit normal avoidance behaviors, a first step in the initiation of new social bonds. Vasopressin may then aid memory for the new social partner. For example, female rats normally avoid infant rats; however, just after parturition when oxytocin levels are high, or after exogenous administration of oxytocin, mother rats inhibit their normal avoidance responses and become maternal towards pups (Pedersen et al. 1994). Although this is probably an indirect effect on cognitive performance, oxytocin does appear to work in concert with vasopressin to enhance social affiliation.

Gonadal Hormones

Gonadal hormones not only influence reproductive behavior and behaviors related to reproduction (see chapters 4, 5, and 6), but they also influence cognitive processes by acting on receptors in regions of the basal forebrain, hippocampus, and neocortex. At first glance, this seems rather surprising. Why should hormones that orchestrate the complex behavioral and physiological mechanisms that lead to finding a mate, producing sperm and eggs, mating, maintaining a pregnancy, and taking care of offspring also modulate learning and memory? One possibility is that hormonal modulation of learning and memory provides some benefit that enhances reproduction. For example, males of some species acquire and defend a large territory in order to attract a mate while females stay closer to home. One might predict that males of these species need a better spatial memory to help them accurately recall territorial boundaries and food sites than the females do. An alternate hypothesis is that the memory changes that accompany natural fluctuations in levels of reproductive hormones may just be a positive side effect of gonadal steroid effects on cell growth and plasticity. Gonadal hormones promote cell growth (Torand-Allerand 1996), modulate neuron birth and death (Gould 1999), and increase synapse formation (Woolley and McEwen 1993). Because learning and memory require the strengthening of synaptic connections, these forms of plasticity, when they occur in brain regions utilized for specific types of learning and memory functions, may modulate these processes.

Only in the last 10 to 15 years has it been clearly established that gonadal hormones influence learning and memory throughout the lifespan. Early in development, gonadal hormones organize neural circuits in cortical regions, which leads to sex differences in cognitive function. After puberty, circulating hormone levels fluctuate across the reproductive life of an individual, and these transient hormonal changes modulate learning and memory processing. Age-related decreases in gonadal hormone production, which is especially pronounced in females at reproductive senescence, probably contribute to age-related memory decline and may prove to be a risk factor for Alzheimer's disease. The major findings that lead to these conclusions are explored next. Whether hormone replacement can slow or prevent cognitive changes in both healthy and diseased individuals remains to be determined.

Organizational Effects

As you will learn about in greater detail in the next chapter, on average, men and women differ in performance on a number of cognitive tasks. Females outperform males on tasks of perceptual speed and verbal fluency, as well as memory for verbal material and the location of objects. Males are better than females at a variety of spatial skills, especially tasks that require mental rotation and navigation (see Kimura (1999) for an extensive review of the human research demonstrating sex differences in a variety of cognitive skills). As in humans, male rodents, both laboratory and wild-born, learn spatial tasks like a radial-arm maze or water maze more quickly and with fewer errors than females (Williams and Meck 1991). However, with practice, males and females perform equally well. Chapter 15 will discuss evidence for sex-related differences of cognitive tasks in humans.

Because males and females can both learn spatial memory tasks and differences in performance between the sexes are most apparent during learning, some researchers are of the opinion that sex differences in cognitive function are small and transient, and therefore, relatively unimportant. Maybe the differences in task performance are due to sex differences in motivation, motor ability, or sensory responsivity, rather than differences in the neural substrates for learning or memory? One way to evaluate these alternatives is to determine the underlying behavioral difference between the sexes that causes one sex to be better at a particular task than another. This type of analysis has been done in an attempt to understand why males tend to outperform females on spatial navigation tasks.

In any navigation task, the location of food sites or places to be visited needs to be practiced and learned. This information must also be stored accurately and then retrieved during the navigation task. Using the animal model of rats solving a radial-arm maze, we have determined that males and females have the same memory capacity (i.e., the number of items that can be held in short-term memory). You would predict that a rat with a larger memory capacity could hold more arm choices in memory before it began to make errors. However, research reveals no sex difference in this measure. After rats learn to find food sites without errors, males and females are equally good at remembering this information during a delay; thus, storage and retrieval mechanisms do not seem to be sexually dimorphic. Another possible explanation for sex differences during acquisition but not at steady-state performance is that males and females solve the task using different strategies, with males using a more efficient method. In fact, this is exactly what has been discovered (Williams et al. 1990).

First, male and female rats were trained on a radial-arm maze task until no sex differences in performance were apparent. Then cues in the test room were altered or removed to determine what information the rats might be using to solve the task. Male performance was found to be disrupted only when the shape of the room (e.g., the angles and distances in the room) was altered, but not when large salient landmarks (e.g., tables, computer desk, researchers, or cart with rat cages) were removed or rearranged in the room. In contrast, female rats were disrupted only when the landmarks were rearranged within the room. They were able to solve the task with either landmarks alone or room shape alone. These results reveal that male and female rats rely on different cues or cue combinations to solve a spatial task, suggesting the following interpretation of sex differences in performance during acquisition. Males may be better initially during training because they have a brain in which the shape of the room is easily processed and room shape overshadows other cues. Females have a brain that processes all available cues, and this increase in memory load may require more practice to learn all the spatial locations.

This sex difference in the use of landmarks and geometric information is also apparent in human males and females, and can be easily demonstrated by asking males and females to give directions: men generally use distances and cardinal directions (N, S, E, and W), while females will use landmarks and some distance and direction information (Ward, Newcombe, and Overton 1986; Galea and Kimura 1993). The rat experiment described above has also been modified to allow human subjects to navigate on a water maze in a virtual room on the computer, in which the room shape and local landmarks can be easily altered. Male and female college students both learned the task readily, but when the landmarks were removed after the maze was learned, males easily relearned the task with room shape only, whereas female subjects had difficulty finding the platform when accurate navigating required reliance on the room geometry only (Sandstrom et al. 1998). Like rats, male and female college students differ in the ease with which they use landmark and geometry cues to navigate. These studies indicate that males and females differ on the strategy they use to solve a spatial task and in the contents of their memory stores, but they do not differ in learning ability, ease, or strength of consolidation or retrieval. To date, this type of analysis has not been done to examine the female's advantage in perceptual speed or verbal fluency tasks.

Obviously the demonstration of a sex difference in adult cognition is not proof that differential exposure to gonadal hormones, either early in development or after puberty, are the cause of this difference. However, there is considerable evidence that treatment with estrogens or androgens around the time of birth will masculinize the spatial abilities of female mice and rats, whereas early castration (removal of the testes) of males will feminize their spatial abilities. This is similar to the process by which gonadal hormones organize neural circuits for sexual behavior (see chapter 3). For example, if males rats are castrated within 24 hours of birth and as adults are trained on a radial-arm maze, they use both landmarks and geometry to navigate, just like female rats. If female rats are treated with estradiol for the first 10 days after birth, they show faster acquisition on a radial-arm maze task and they use only room shape and angles to navigate, just like adult male rats.

It has also been shown that testosterone treatment to females just before or after birth makes their adult performance on a water-maze task more malelike (Isgor and Sengelaub 1998). Treatment of newborn males with an **aromatase** inhibitor that prevents the enzymatic conversion of testosterone into estradiol also produces males that learn a radial-arm maze task more slowly than untreated males and use both landmark and geometry cues. This suggests that for testosterone to masculinize spatial abilities, it must first be converted to estradiol. Again, this is much like the process by which sexual behavior becomes sexually dimorphic in rats (chapter 3). The site of action for these effects may well be the hippocampus. If estradiol is administered directly to the hippocampus of newborn male rats after their testes are surgically removed, they show male-type spatial abilities as adults. If the hormone is implanted in the hypothalamus, however, the neonatally castrated males show femalelike spatial abilities as adults (Williams and Meck 1991). The exact **sensitive period** for these hormonal effects on spatial abilities in the rat is unknown. Females may also require some low-level estradiol exposure prepubertally in order to develop normal female spatial abilities (Fitch and Denneberg 1998).

By what mechanism does estrogen cause sexual dimorphisms in the brain that might lead to differences in cognitive ability? At this time, the answer to this question is not known. There are, however, a number of important clues. The hippocampus as well as the neocortex, brain regions known to be involved in learning and memory, transiently express high levels of estrogen receptors during the first week of life in the rat (Clark et al. 1988; O'Keefe et al. 1990). In the hippocampus the α-estrogen receptor (ERα) is expressed in a few interneurons while the β-estrogen receptor (ERβ) is expressed in pyramidal cells (Handa et al. 2000). The distribution of these two receptor types has not yet been examined in the developing neocortex. The aromatase enzyme that converts testosterone to estradiol has also been detected perinatally in the hippocampus and in a region of the neocortex (Mac-Closky et al. 1987). The **basal forebrain**, which contains cholinergic neurons that project to the hippocampus and the neocortex, also contains estrogen receptors. Cholinergic cells in this brain region express ERα. Therefore, we know that androgens secreted by the developing testes can be converted to estradiol and can act on local estrogen receptors, potentially leading to the sexually dimorphic development of cortical morphology, neurochemistry, and neurophysiology.

If estrogens modify sexually dimorphic cognitive ability by altering the structural development of brain regions involved in cognitive processes, then we would predict that these structures would be sexually dimorphic. In many species, hippocampal volume is larger in males than in females. In rats, the CA1 pyramidal cell field is 16% larger in males than in females, and this difference is modifiable by perinatal androgen exposure (Isgor and Sengalaub 1998). The basal forebrain is also sexually dimorphic. Females have more cholinergic cells than males, and they are smaller and more densely packed (Gibbs 1996). Sex differences have also been reported in hippocampal physiology. Both castrated and intact males show greater hippocampal LTP than females (Anagnostaras et al. 1998). The differences in hippocampal LTP are probably established early in development by the organizational effects of gonadal hormones.

Other **telencephalic** areas are also sexually dimorphic. Juraska and colleagues (1988) have painstakingly examined the **corpus callosum** and visual regions of the neocortex and have carefully documented sex differences as well as interactions between experience and sex in cell type and number in these structures. In males, the **splenium**, a region in the corpus callosum, has more myelinated axons, yet the total number of axons remains the same (Juraska and Kopcik 1988). Male rats have 18% more cells and more **glia** in most regions of visual cortex than females (Reid and Juraska 1992). Recent findings show that human males and females may utilize different brain regions when they are performing a navigational task (Gron et al. 2000). When males and females were asked to search for a way out of a complex, 3-dimentional virtual-reality maze, functional magnetic resonance imaging (fMRI) of their brains revealed that navigation activated a variety of brain regions. A sex-specific group analysis revealed distinct activation of the left hippocampus in males, while females consistently recruited the right parietal and the right pre-frontal cortex. Together, these and other findings support the hypothesis that exposure to steroid hormones early in development leads to the formation of sexually dimorphic substrates for learning and memory.

It is not immediately obvious how sexual dimorphisms in cognitive abilities might be adaptive. Gaulin and FitzGerald (1986) suggest that sexually dimorphic spatial ability should only be present in polygynous species in which females and males exploit home ranges of different sizes (e.g., humans, rats, and meadow voles). Monogamous species that do not have sexually dimorphic ranging patterns (e.g., pine and prairie voles) should not be sexually dimorphic in spatial ability. They also predict that spatial ability should be positively correlated with both the size of the home range and the size of the hippocampus. These relationships are supported by data on range size, laboratory tests of spatial ability, and hippocampal volume from several related species of voles (Jacobs et al. 1990). Male prairie voles have large home ranges and large hippocampi and perform better on laboratory-based spatial tasks than female prairie voles. In contrast, meadow vole males and females have similar sized ranges and hippocampi, and perform equally well on spatial tasks. Importantly, these differences can be observed in both wild and laboratory-raised voles, despite their rearing in drastically different environments, suggesting that differences in hippocampal size and spatial ability are not driven by experience with home ranges of different sizes. So although the processing of spatial information need not be utilized in the context of reproduction, it may have evolved in a sexually dimorphic fashion in species that developed sexually dimorphic range patterns associated with reproductive fitness.

There are a few issues worth highlighting. First, unlike sexual behavior, these sex differences in spatial ability do not require the activational effects of androgens or estrogens to be expressed (Williams et al. 1990). However, as we will see next, the circulating hormones in adulthood may actually exaggerate these sexually dimorphic abilities. Second, the fact that early hormone exposure organizes brain mechanisms for spatial abilities does not mean that experience and training, either directly or indirectly, cannot modify sexually dimorphic brain regions and alter spatial abilities. For example, if female rats are raised in an enriched environment with new objects placed in their large cage each day, the granule cells in the dentate gyrus of their hippocampal complex are more branched than they are in females reared in standard laboratory cages. The same environmental enrichment of male rats increases branching of neurons in the occipital region of their cortex but not their hippocampal neurons (Juraska 1984). Third, we still do not know how and in what fashion early hormone exposure may modify verbal abilities, at which females excel. One study has shown that CAH females, who are exposed to androgens in utero because of an error in steroid metabolism, show slightly depressed verbal abilities compared to normal females, suggesting that early exposure to androgens may also modify this sexually dimorphic ability (Helleday 1994).

Cognitive Effects in Adults

As we've mentioned above, sexual dimorphisms in cognition do not require **activational** hormones to be expressed, but there is increasing evidence that variations in the levels of circulating gonadal hormones can modify, in a transient fashion, learning and memory as well as the structure and function of the basal forebrain, hippocampus, and regions of neocortex. Although there is still considerable disagreement as to the magnitude of these effects in real-life learning situations, and to whether alterations in memory can be tied to specific alterations in brain morphology and physiology, it is clear that variations in estrogens and androgens in the adult modify performance on a variety of learning and memory tasks. After evaluating the evidence presented below and the information in chapter 15, you will have to decide whether you should time your studying with your menstrual cycle variations in estrogens and progestins or your circadian and seasonal variations in androgens.

To determine how and in what fashion circulating gonadal steroids of the adult organism influence cognition, researchers have used rodent models to examine the effects of both natural and manipulated variations in hormone levels on a variety of tasks. At first glance, the findings appear to be consistent with the data on estrogen effects on human performance described above. That is, on some spatial tasks, high estrogen levels interfere with performance. For example, during proestrus, when estrogen levels are high, female rats and mice usually exhibit slower acquisition of the standard version of the water-maze escape task (Warren and Juraska 1997) compared to females tested at diestrus, when estrogen levels are low. This effect appears to be due to estrogen activation of ERα. Ovariectomized mice that have been genetically modified so that they cannot express ERα do not show a decrement in performance on a water-maze task when estrogen replacement is given, while control mice with ERα expression show slower learning (Fugger et al. 1998). Because the water-maze task requires spatial abilities, some researchers have interpreted these findings as being remarkably consistent with human studies that show the deleterious effects of estrogen on spatial tasks. However, there are several reasons to be cautious before accepting this conclusion. First, mental rotation tasks on which activational hormonal effects on human performance measure inherent abilities; no practice is required of the subjects.

In contrast, the water-maze task is designed to examine both speed of acquisition and memory after a delay. Perhaps more striking is the fact that a host of other studies have shown that performance on a variety of tasks that examine memory directly is worse in rodents and humans that have been depleted of estrogen by ovariectomy and much improved if estrogen is replaced. For example, Barbara Sherwin (Sherwin 1994) has examined 30 to 40 year old women who have had a loss of estrogen output due to ovariectomy. Following surgery, these ovariectomized women do less well on verbal memory tasks (i.e., learning and remembering word lists) than women who begin hormone replacement therapy at the time of surgery. And chronic administration of estrogen to ovariectomized rats and mice appears to enhance performance on both spatial and nonspatial tasks, including the radial-arm maze, passive avoidance, fear conditioning, and social recognition when memory is the variable being examined (see Packard 1998 for review, and Hlinak 1993). So why do some studies show negative effects of low estrogen and others show beneficial effects of estrogen replacement? We do not know for sure, but it is likely that because estrogen has multiple effects on the brain, it may also have multiple effects on cognition under a variety of different test conditions. It may interfere with water-maze acquisition via its effects on nonmnemonic factors. It may activate brain mechanisms designed for fine-motor abilities in females and this may, in some way, interfere with the fast processing of spatial information. And it may improve memory function by enhancing the plasticity of the hippocampal neurons needed for the laying down of new memories.

Neural Systems Activated by Gonadal Hormones

What neural systems are activated by estrogen in the adult rat that might account for its effects on cognition? Estrogen has been shown to exert effects on the structure and function of the neocortex, hippocampus, basal forebrain, and amygdala, all regions essential for cognitive function. ERα is the predominant receptor subtype in cholinergic neurons of the basal forebrain, in some interneurons in the CA1 region of the hippocampus, as well as regions of the ventral hippocampus. ERβ is expressed in layers of the neocortex and in pyramidal cells of the hippocampus. Both receptor subtypes are found in subregions of the amygdala (Shughrue et al. 1997). Because of these differences in receptor location, estrogen can have diverse actions. Acting at ERβ estradiol can directly modulate specific oxytocin and vasopressin systems (Alves et al. 1998). Through ERα, estradiol can stimulate the anterolateral amygdala, a major route through which the amygdala communicates with the hippocampus.

In the last decade, Catherine Woolley, Elizabeth Gould, and Bruce McEwen (see Woolley 1998 for review) discovered that variations in estrogen exposure cause transient alterations in the morphology of some hippocampal neurons. When they administered two small doses of estrogen to ovariectomized rats, they found that within 48 hours there was a 20 to 30% increase in spines on the apical dendrites of pyramidal cells in the CA1 region of the hippocampus. Spines are small protrusions from the dendrite that make synapses with nearby neurons. No changes in spine density were observed in pyramidal neurons in CA3 or in the granule cells of the dentate gyrus in young adult rats. Moreover, spine density changed cyclically during the rat estrous cycle, with the highest spine density occurring at proestrus, when estrogen levels are at their peak. The significance of these changes in dendritic spines is that they represent increases in synapses induced by estrogen (Woolley et al. 1996). These morphological studies indicate that synapses within identified regions of the hippocampus are formed and broken down rapidly during natural cyclical variations in estrogen and progesterone in the female rat (figure 14.9).

How does estrogen cause these alterations in spine density? At doses that interfere with cognition, blockers of cholinergic receptors do not stop the formation of estrogen-induced spines, suggesting that inputs from basal forebrain cholinergic neurons are not critical for this morphological change. In

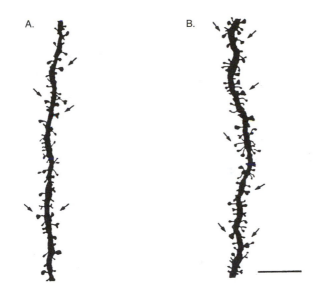

Figure 14.9 Drawings based on photomicrographs of dendrite segments in the apical trees of CA1 pyramidal cells from (*A*), an ovariectomized rate treated with sesame-oil vehicle alone and (*B*), an ovariectomized rat treated with estradiol. Some of the dendritic spines are indicated with arrows. The density of spines is greater on the dendrite from the estradiol-treated animal. Bar: 10 µm. (Redrawn from Woolley 1998.)

contrast, drugs that block NMDA receptors that are located in the hippocampus block estrogen-induced spines. The NMDA receptor is one of two main kinds of receptors (the other is the AMPA receptor) activated by glutamate, the major excitatory synaptic transmitter found throughout the nervous system. The name "NMDA receptor" is given because this receptor is especially sensitive to one particular glutamate mimic, *N*-methyl-D-aspartate. The current view (Woolley 1998) is that the majority of spine synapses on hippocampal pyramidal cells use the neurotransmitter glutamate. Estradiol appears to increase binding only to the NMDA glutamate receptors in CA1, and has no effect on non-NMDA receptors. These data are important because NMDA receptor activation is essential to learning. If a drug is used that blocks NMDA receptors in the hippocampus of an adult rat, it blocks the rat's ability to remember the location of a platform in a water-maze task, and it interferes with hippocampal LTP. Thus, these changes in spine density induced by estrogen may enhance hippocampal neural plasticity that aids the rapid strengthening of memory traces.

Do these changes in spine density in the hippocampus and the accompanying alterations in hippocampal LTP reflect the neural underpinning of estrogen modulation of memory? As a first step in answering this question, Noah Sandstrom and I examined whether hormone-induced alterations in spine density occur in parallel with alterations in memory function (Sandstrom and Williams 2001). We made use of Woolley's finding that progesterone appears to have a biphasic effect on spine density after estradiol priming.

Within a few hours of progesterone treatment, spine density continues to increase rapidly, but then falls within 8 to 10 hours (Woolley and McEwen 1993). With estradiol priming only, spines remain high for at least a week after treatment.

To examine memory at various times after estrogen and progesterone administration, we used a version of the water-maze task in which rats were asked to remember a platform location for 10, 30, or 100 minutes. Rats were tested on all 3 durations within a single day, and for each memory duration the platform was placed in a new location. We tested every rat in each hormone treatment condition. We found that memory retention of a platform location and spine density were enhanced for 4 days after two small injections of estradiol (figure 14.10). However, if progesterone was administered 2 days after estradiol priming, memory was enhanced for only 2 to 4 hours, but then returned to baseline within 24 hours. These data show a remarkable time-course parallel with the changes in hippocampal spines, and suggest that these morphological changes may underlie the memory-enhancing effects of estradiol. Further proof would require that estrogen be administered only to the hippocampus, or only to the CA1 pyramidal cell region, and that similar alterations in spines and memory would be seen.

Estradiol not only effects hippocampal morphology directly though interactions with NMDA receptors, but also acts on basal forebrain cholinergic neurons to modulate their interactions with the hippocampus. Victoria Luine (1977) was the first to show that chronic estradiol replacement to ovariectomized rats increases the activity of the enzyme choline acetyltransferase (ChAT), which converts choline to acetylcholine for packaging in vesicles in the basal forebrain, hippocampus, and frontal cortex (Luine and McEwen 1977). Robert Gibbs has shown that following an acute injection of estradiol, ChAT mRNA is increased after 24 to 48 hours. He has also found that when progesterone is administered following estradiol priming, it enhances the effect of estrogen by accelerating and prolonging its effects on cholinergic activity (Gibbs 2000). Therefore, the effects of estradiol and progesterone on memory function may also occur because estrogen stimulates cholinergic neurons of the basal forebrain to modulate hippocampal activity. To test this hypothesis, Gary Dohanich (Dohanich et al. 1994) examined the interactions between estradiol and the activation of cholinergic neurons on the performance of a maze task. He knew that the administration of **scopolamine**, a cholinergic receptor blocker, given during or immediately following a learning task (e.g., avoidance training or water-maze training) disrupts performance (Introini-Collison and Baratti 1992). If rats are treated with estradiol prior to training and then treated with scopolamine at the time of training, Dohanich found that the pre-training estradiol treatment blocked the memory impairment normally caused by scopolamine. These data strongly suggest that at least part of the memory-enhancing effect of estradiol may be mediated via estradiol activation of the cholinergic system. Increased ac-

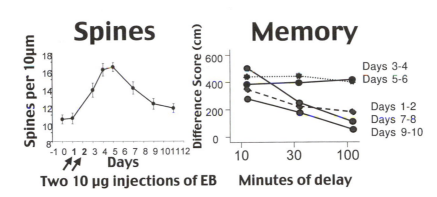

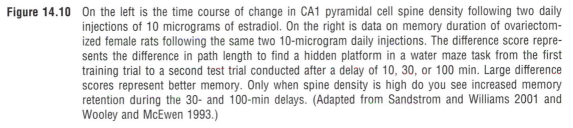

Figure 14.10 On the left is the time course of change in CA1 pyramidal cell spine density following two daily injections of 10 micrograms of estradiol. On the right is data on memory duration of ovariectomized female rats following the same two 10-microgram daily injections. The difference score represents the difference in path length to find a hidden platform in a water maze task from the first training trial to a second test trial conducted after a delay of 10, 30, or 100 min. Large difference scores represent better memory. Only when spine density is high do you see increased memory retention during the 30- and 100-min delays. (Adapted from Sandstrom and Williams 2001 and Wooley and McEwen 1993.)

tivity of basal forebrain cholinergic neurons may activate neurons in the hippocampus indirectly and in this fashion enhance the laying down of new memories.

Why should estrogen modulate memory functions in female mammals? Is there a benefit to having a better memory at times of higher estrogen? Although individually housed laboratory animals and human females living in modern cultures go though many cycles of estrogen and progesterone throughout their lifetimes, pregnancy and motherhood may be the more typical life-state of our female ancestors. That is, alterations in estrogen and progesterone levels during pregnancy and/or lactation and their effect on hippocampal function and behavior may have been selected for because nest building and locating, pup recognition and retrieval, and foraging for food during pregnancy and lactation may rely on good hippocampal functioning. A recent report (Kinsley et al. 1999) has shown that maternal rats are quicker at learning the location of food wells in a circular arena than rats that had never given birth or cared for pups. Possibly the hormones produced by rats during pregnancy, combined with the stimulation gained from caring for offspring, improved the animals' performance. Unfortunately, in this study, no attempt was made to assess memory directly. Whether it is the sensory stimulation that parenting provides, or the accompanying hormones of maternity, or both, that improves performance on this task has not yet been determined. Ultimately, it may be discovered that variations in hippocampal function are extremely adaptive in this context.

Aging and Gonadal Hormones

As we age, the gonads slow or stop their production of steroid hormones. In men, testosterone declines gradually over several decades, with free testosterone decreasing by as much as 40% between the age of 40 and 70 (Davidson et al. 1983). In women, following menopause around age 50 to 55, estrogen and progesterone levels plummet, and cycles cease. Although reproductive senescence in many animals, including early humans, occurred at about the end of their lifespan, woman now regularly live 30 or more years after menopause, and men live though years of declining testosterone production. What are the consequences on brain and cognition of a decrement or loss of gonadal hormones? You just read about studies showing that young female rats that are deprived of estrogen for a short period of time lose synapses in the hippocampus. Is it possible that the loss or decline of gonadal steroid secretion as we age contributes to the changes in brain morphology and cognitive function that are seen in an aging population?

We all know that our elderly parents or grandparents seem to lose their keys more often and repeat stories they have told just a few hours or days before. As we age, some brain region decrease in synaptic and spine density, and in dendritic arbor and width, and our neurons have more difficulty sprouting and growing new connections after damage. In studies of aging rats, induction and maintenance of hippocampal LTP are also compromised, and there is also a decline in memory in all animal populations that have been studied (see Barnes 1998). In the last 10 years, many studies have examined aging humans and other animals to investigate whether replacement estrogens and androgens slow or prevent cognitive aging. At this time, the general consensus is that there are beneficial effects of both estrogen and testosterone replacement therapies on certain components of cognitive function. However, we do not know the best method (cyclic or chronic) in which to administer replacement hormone, nor the dose or duration of treatment. We have also found that under some conditions, estrogens can protect the brain against damage caused by stroke (oxygen loss to tissue) and decrease the risk of Alzheimer's disease.

REPLACEMENT HORMONES DURING NORMAL AGING

Many studies examining aging populations have reported a beneficial effect of estrogen on cognition. Postmenopausal women who were using **estrogen hormone replacement therapy (HRT)** performed significantly better on proper name recall, on immediate and delayed paragraph recall, and on visual design recall than age-matched nonusers. The beneficial effects of postmenopausal estrogen use may also be enduring. Women who used HRT around perimenopause but were no longer using HRT also showed better performance on a word recall task than women who had never used HRT (Sherwin 2000). The major limitation of these types of observational studies is that there is no random assignment to treatment condition. Although researchers try to match subjects for age, socioeconomic class, and years of education, there may be a variety of other factors that contribute to cognition (see also chapter 15).

In the few studies that have actually used randomized controlled trials in which women were assigned to treatment conditions, the results were often equivocal, in part because of methodological problems (Yaffe et al. 1998). Nevertheless, a few studies have evaluated the role of estrogen in newly postmenopausal women with subjects serving as their own controls. Pre-menopausal women were tested before total **hysterectomy** and **oophorectomy** (removal of uterus and ovaries) and again some time after surgery and treatment with either estrogen or a placebo. Following cognitive testing, subjects were crossed over to the other treatment. A group of women who underwent a hysterectomy but did not have their ovaries removed also served as a control. Women who received HRT performed significantly better on a variety of cognitive tests (e.g., digit span, paragraph recall, and abstract reasoning) than the placebo group (Sherwin 1988). Another recent study investigated the effects of a 2-week estradiol treatment on the memory of healthy elderly women (with a mean age of 70) (Wolf et al. 1999). All women in this study had been menopausal for an average of 17 years prior to entering the study. Women were randomly assigned to either estrogen or placebo treatment groups and testing occurred 2 weeks after a daily administration of estrogen. When estradiol levels were higher, performance on a verbal memory task (delayed recall of words) was better than when estradiol levels were low. These data suggest that even after years of estrogen deprivation, the brain is still sensitive to fairly rapid effects of estrogen on cognition.

Relatively few animal studies have been done to examine how estrogen replacement during aging may influence cognition. One reason for this may be that female rats and mice, unlike human females, do not undergo a complete loss of estrogen at a point comparable to human menopause. Instead, their estrus cycles become longer and more erratic and they maintain constant, moderate estrogen levels until they reach very old age, at which point estrogen levels become very low and constant (Lefevre and McClintock 1988). One recent study using rats examined the effect of different regimens of estrogen or estrogen plus progesterone replacement beginning either immediately, or at 3 months or 10 months after ovariectomy at 13 months of age (Gibbs 2000). Eight to 12 months after ovariectomy (i.e., at 21 to 24 months of age), rats were tested on a spatial memory task in which rats were required to recall which one of two food locations recently contained food. The results showed that long-term replacement of estrogen or estrogen plus progesterone given continuously or via weekly injections improved performance relative to untreated controls and rats that had not received replacement until 10 months following ovariectomy. In contrast to the human study described above, these data suggest that estrogen may not be able to rescue performance unless treatment begins soon after estrogen loss. Whether these effects are due to a specific memory-enhancing effect of estrogen replacement or whether estrogen is working indirectly by aiding some nonmnemonic contributor to performance remains to be determined (see also Maki and Resnick 2001).

Because estrogen appears to have enhanced cognition in elderly rats and humans, we might predict that estrogen replacement to aged rats would increase spine density, as it does in young female rats. Gillian Einstein, Phillippa Miranda, and I tried to answer this question (Miranda et al. 1998). We examined the morphology of neurons in the hippocampus of aged rats that had been subjected to long-term deprivation of gonadal steroids, and we found that the spine density of the granule cells of the dentate gyrus was lower in aged females than in young females, but that no change in spines in this cell population occurred in males. Note that all the rats, both old and young, were gonadectomized, so that this is an effect of aging, not of loss of estrogen per se. When we replaced estrogen chronically for many months we found that we could not save dendritic spines; they declined in females. However, if we gave aged females two short pulses of estrogen, spine density increased to the level normally seen in young females (figure 14.11). The functional significance of increased or decreased spine density in these granule cells is still an open question, but we know that spine density and the number of excitatory synapses correlate with the efficiency of learning spatial tasks (Moser et al. 1994). Exacerbation of spine loss by estrogen deprivation in normal aging suggests that the estrogen-deficient state after human menopause my be one of decreased excitatory input, and this may contribute to cognitive decline.

NEUROPROTECTIVE EFFECTS OF ESTROGEN

Animal studies have shown that as male and female rats age, there is a pronounced sex difference in the rate of development of and the magnitude of cognitive decline. The mnemonic ability of female rats declines more rapidly than that of males, and in spatial-memory tasks, the magnitude of the impairment is greater in females than in males (Markowska 1999). In human populations, one of the most common forms of dementia, Alzheimer's disease, affects 1.5 to 3 times more women than men. This sex difference in the occurrence of Alzheimer's disease may, in part, reflect the fact that women, on average, live longer than men. However, the prevalence of Alzheimer's disease among women is higher than men even after adjusting for the effects of age (Henderson 1997). Does lack of estrogen after menopause increase the risk of Alzheimer's disease? Does estrogen replacement decrease the risk of Alzheimer's and can it be used to slow or reverse the dementia associated with Alzheimer's disease once it has been diagnosed? These types of clinical studies are now being done and the results suggest that estrogen under some conditions may serve a neuroprotective function.

Retrospective studies of women who have been diagnosed with **Alzheimer's disease** show that they are less likely to have ever used HRT than age-matched controls (Henderson 2000). These studies suffer from the same

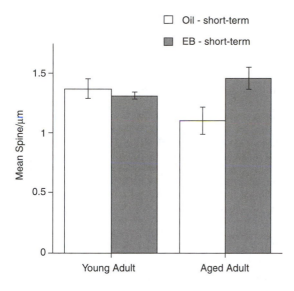

Figure 14.11 Young adult female rats ovariectomized at 4.5 months of age have high spine density on their hippocampal dentate gyrus granule cells, and spines do not appear to increase in number after short-term estrogen (EB) replacement. By 16–20 months of age, spine density of these neurons declines and short-term EB replacement can return spines to the high density seen in younger females. (Redrawn from Miranda et al. 1999.)

problems as other nonrandomized designs. Some other variable that is not matched between groups may be the important factor. A recent prospective study from the Baltimore Longitudinal Study on Aging found that the incidence of Alzheimer's disease was about 45% lower in women with a history of HRT use than in women who never used HRT (Kawas et al. 1997). And, since 1986, a handful of intervention trials have used estrogen to treat women with Alzheimer's disease (Henderson 2000). Although not all studies have used a **placebo** control and most have used brief cognitive screening tests, and a short duration of estrogen treatment, the results suggest that estrogen may have beneficial effects for verbal memory and for attention. Recently, it has been suggested that not all women may respond to HRT with improvements in cognitive function—that is, there may be a gene-environment interaction. One gene that appears to be a risk factor for Alzheimer's disease is the E4 **allele** of the **apolipoprotein** gene. Estrogen use was associated with less cognitive decline among E4-negative women but not E4-positive women (Yaffe et al. 2000).

A number of neural mechanisms have been proposed to explain the neuroprotective or cognitive-enhancing effects of estrogen. We have already discussed findings that indicate that in both young and older female rats, estrogen increases synapse formation in the hippocampus and this may strengthen neural connections. Another potential mechanism is via estrogen stimulation of the basal forebrain cholinergic neurons. This enhanced excitatory input to hippocampus and frontal cortex may also strengthen neural connections and help protect against Alzheimer's disease. This excitatory input is also known to increase the expression of a variety of neuronal growth factors that may allow for neuronal plasticity and repair (Singh et al. 1995).

It is also increasingly likely that there may be specific neuroprotective effects of estrogen that prevent cell death under conditions of excitation, injury, or oxygen deprivation. Investigators now know that estrogen exerts profound protective effects against neuronal cell death in a variety of in vivo and in vitro models of injury. Phyllis Wise (Dubal et al. 1998) has shown that physiological levels of estrogen just prior to an ischemic injury (occlusion of the middle cerebral artery preventing oxygen flow to the rat's brain) protects against the neuronal cell death that usually follows oxygen deprivation. Work from her laboratory suggests that this effect occurs via estrogen-receptor-mediated genomic events. Other laboratories (Green et al. 1997) have also shown that 17-α–estradiol, an estrogen that does not activate receptor-mediated genomic events, is also neuroprotective to cells in vitro. In sum, a number of cellular and molecular mechanisms may explain estrogen's neuroprotective actions and may provide the mechanisms underlying estrogen's ability to decrease the incidence and the rate of neurodegeneration associated with Alzheimer's disease.

Summary

As you have now seen, hormones have a variety of effects on cognition. We have focussed this chapter on the effects of several types of hormones in non-human animals: neuropeptides like oxytocin and vasopressin, steroid hormones like the glucocorticoids, estrogens, and androgens, as well as amines such as epinephrine and norepinephrine. Each works through separate receptor systems in brain regions important for cognition: the hippocampus, the amygdala, and the regions of the neocortex. Effects of some hormones occur throughout the lifespan.

1. You have learned that that glucocorticoids and gonadal steroids act during early development to blueprint brain mechanisms that will be used for cognitive function in adult life. These same hormones activate these neuronal blueprints in adult life, often via a U-shaped dose-response function. That is, there is often an optimal range of hormone; too little or too much appears to impair performance. And for some hormones, like the glucocorticoids, timing is everything. Short-term exposure is beneficial for cognition, but long-term chronic exposure causes a loss of synapses and severe memory decay.

2. You have learned that it is easy to see that hormones influence performance on a variety of cognitive tasks, but it is often difficult to assess whether this is by a direct effect on the learning and memory mechanisms or by indirect effects on attention, motivation, and sensory or motor systems. In fact, in many cases, hormones like estrogen may have a variety of effects, both direct and indirect, all of which influence performance. Clearly there are many naturally occurring variations in the adrenal, posterior pituitary, and gonadal secretion of hormones during your lifetime that will probably impact your

cognitive skills, your speed of learning, and aspects of your memory formation and decay. Some of these effects may be quantitative in nature. Estrogen may protect against memory decay. Glucocorticoids may impair, though not prevent, rehearsal processes that are critical for memory consolidation. On the other hand, in some cases hormonal effects on cognition may be qualitative. Hormonally induced sex differences in spatial navigation are probably due to qualitative differences in the use of the visual spatial cues that guide navigation.

3. As the use of hormones as clinical agents for the treatment of a variety of ailments (e.g., cortisol for inflammation, estrogen to treat osteoporosis, or androgens for building muscle) increases, we must remember that the brain, especially the brain regions involved in thinking, learning, and remembering, are targets for hormones. One of the challenges for future research will be to understand under what circumstances hormonal treatments trigger cognitive enhancement and under what circumstances they lead to transient impairment in cognitive function or permanent damage.

Study Questions

1. Describe some of the effects of posterior pituitary versus gonadal hormones on cognitive abilities in nonhuman animals.
2. If you were testing a newly discovered species of rodent and wanted to find out if males and females differed on cognitive tasks, what tests would you use to assess these differences? What would your results tell you about how the brains of males and females of your species might be different?
3. One of the things that doctors sometimes give patients with acute head injuries is prednasone (a glucocorticoid) to reduce the swelling. If you had a traumatic head injury, would you want them to give you prednasone? Why or why not? Discuss the short-term and the long-term consequences.
4. Discuss what we know about the organizational effects versus activational effects of gonadal hormones on cognitive strategies.

References

Altman, J., and Das, G. D. (1965) Autoradiographic and histological evidence of postnatal hippocampal neurogenesis in rats. *J. Comp. Neurol.* 124: 319–335.

Alves, S. E., Lopez, V., McEwen, B. S., and Weiland, N. G. (1998) Differential colocalization of estrogen receptor beta (ER beta) with oxytocin and vasopressin in the paraventricular and supraoptic nuclei of the female rat brain: An immunocytochemical study. *Proc. Natl. Acad. Sci. USA* 95: 3281–3286.

Anagnostaras, S. G., Maren, S., DeCola, J. P., Lane, N. I., Gale, G. D., Schlinger, B. A., and Fanselow, M. S. (1998) Testicular hormones do not regulate sexually dimorphic Pavlovian fear conditioning or perforant-path long-term potentiation in adult male rats. *Behav. Brain Res.* 92: 1–9.

Barnes, C. A. (1998) Memory changes during normal aging: Neurobiological correlates, In J. Martinez and R. Kesner (Eds.), *Neurobiology of Learning and Memory*. San Diego: Academic Press, pp. 247–288.

Bliss, T. V. P., and Lømo, T. (1973) Long-lasting potentiation of synaptic transmission in the dentate gyrus of the anaesthetized rabbit following stimulation of the perforant path. *J. Physiol.* 232: 331–356.

Bluthe, R. M., and Dantzer, R. (1993) Vasopressinergic modulation of social recognition in rats. *Brain Res.* 604: 205–210.

Cahill, L., Prins, B., Weber, M., and McGaugh, J. L. (1994) Beta-adrenergic activation and memory for emotional events. *Nature* 371: 702–704.

Cameron, H. A., and Gould, E. (1994) Adult neurogenesis is regulated by adrenal steroids in the dentate gyrus. *Neuroscience* 61: 203–209.

Clark, A. S., MacLusky, N. J., and Goldman-Rakic, P. S. (1988) Androgen binding and metabolism in cerbral cortex of the developing rhesus monkey. *Endocrinology* 123: 932–940.

Conrad, C. D., Lupien, S. J., and McEwen, B. S. (1999) Support for a bimodal role for type II adrenal steroid receptors in spatial memory. *Neurobiol. Learn. Mem.* 72: 39–46.

Conrad, C. D., Lupien, S. J., Thanasoulis, L., and McEwen, B. S. (1998) The effects of Type I and Type II corticosteroid receptor agonists on exploratory behavior and spatial memory in the Y maze. *Brain Res.* 759: 76–83.

Dantzer, R., Bluthe, R. M., Koob, G. F., and Le Moal, M. (1987) Modulation of social memory in male rats by neurohypophyseal peptides. *Psychopharmacology* 91: 363–368.

Davis, M. (1992) The role of the amygdala in fear and anxiety. *Annu. Rev. Neurosci.* 15: 353–375.

DeWied, D. (1971) Long-term maintenance effect of vasopressin on the maintenance of a conditioned avoidance response in rats. *Nature* 232: 58–60.

DeWied, D. (1966) Inhibitory effect of ACTH and related peptides on extinction of conditioned avoidance behavior in rats. *Proc. Soc. Exp. Biol.* 122: 28–32.

DeVries, G. J., Buijs, R. M., van Leeuwen, F. W., Caffe, A. R., and Swaab, D. F. (1985) The vsopressingergic innervation of the brain in normal and castrated rats. *J. Comp. Neurol.* 233: 236–254.

Dohanich, G. P., Fader, A. J., and Javorsky, D. J. (1994) Estrogen and estrogen-progesterone treatments counteract the effect of scopolamine on reinforced T-maze alternation in female rats. *Behav. Neurosci.* 108: 988–992.

Dubal, D. B., Kashon, M. L., Pettigrew, L. C., Ren, J. M., Finklestein, S. P., Rau, S. W., and Wise, P. M. (1998) Estradiol protects against ischemic injury. *J. Cereb. Blood Flow Metab.* 18: 1253–1258.

Eldridge, J. C., Brodish, A., Kute, T. E., and Landfield, P. W. (1989) Apparent age-related resistance of type II hippocampal corticosteroid receptors to down-regulation during chronic escape training. *J. Neurosci.* 9: 3237–3242.

Eriksson, P. S., Perfilieva, E., Bjork-Eriksson, T., Alborn, A. M., Nordborg, C., Peterson, D. A., and Gage, F. H. (1998) Neurogenesis in the adult human hippocampus. *Nature Med.* 4: 1313–1317.

Fehm-Wolfsdorf, G., Reutter, D., Zenz, H., Born, J., and Lorenz-Fehm (1993) Are circadian variations in taste thresholds cortisol-dependent? *J. Psychophysiol.* 7: 65–72.

Fitch, R. H., and Denenberg, V. H. (1998) A role for ovarian hormones in sexual differentiation of the brain. *Behav. Brain Sci.* 21: 3113–27.

Francis, D. D., and Meaney, M. J. (1999) Maternal care and the development of stress responses. *Curr. Opin. Neurobiol.* 9: 128–134.

Fugger, H. N., Cunningham, S. G., Rissman, E. F., and Foster, T. C. (1998) Sex differences in the activational effect of ERα on spatial learning. *Horm. Behav.* 34: 163–170.

Galea, L. A., and Kimura, D. (1993) Sex differences in route-learning. *Pers. Indiv. Diff.* 14: 53–65.

Gallistel, C. R. (1999) The replacement of general-purpose learning models with adaptively specialized learning modules. In M. S. Gazzaniga (Ed.), *The Cognitive Neurosciences*, 2nd edition. Cambridge, Mass.: MIT Press, pp. 1179–1191.

Gaulin, S. J. C., and FitzGerald, R. W. (1986) Sex differences in spatial ability: An evolutionary hypothesis and test. *Am. Nat.* 127: 74–88.

Gazzanaga, M. S., Ivry, R. B., and Mangun, G. R. (2002) *Cognitive Neuroscience: The Biology of Mind*, 2nd Ed. New York: Norton.

Gibbs, R. B. (1996) Fluctuations in relative levels of choline acetyltransferase mRNA in different regions of the rat basal forebrain across the estrous cycle: Effects of estrogen and progesterone. *J. Neurosci.* 16: 1049–1055.

Gibbs, R. B. (2000) Long-term treatment with estrogen and progesterone enhances acquisition of a spatial memory task by ovariectomized aged rats. *Neurobiol. Aging* 21: 107–116.

Gold, P. E. (1987) Sweet memories. *Sci. Am.* 75: 151–155.

Gold, P. E., and van Buskirk, R. (1975) Facilitation of time-dependent memory processes with posttrial amygdala stimulation: Effect on memory varies with foodshock level. *Brain Res.* 89: 509–513.

Gold, P. E., Vogt, J., and Hall, J. L. (1986) Glucose effects on memory: Behavioral and pharmacological characteristics. *Behav. Neural Biol.* 46: 145–155.

Gouchi, C., and Kimura, D. (1991) The relationship between testosterone levels and cognitive ability patterns. *Psychoneuroendocrinology* 16: 323–334.

Gould, E., Reeves, A. J., Fallah, M., Tanapat, P., Gross, C. G., and Fuchs, E. (1999) Hippocampal neurogenesis in adult Old World primates. *Proc. Natl. Acad. Sci. USA* 96: 5263–5267.

Gould, E., and Tanapat, P. (1999) Stress and hippocampal neurogenesis. *Biol. Psychiat.* 46: 1472–1479.

Gould, E., Tanapat, P., McEwen, B. S., Flugge, G., and Fuchs, E. (1998) Proliferation of granule cell precursors in the dentate gyrus of adult monkeys is diminished by stress. *Proc. Natl. Acad. Sci. USA* 95: 3168–3171.

Green, P. S., Bishop, J., and Simpkins, J. W. (1997) 17 alpha-estradiol exerts neuroprotective effects on SK-N-SH cells. *J. Neurosci.* 17: 511–515.

Greven, H. M., and De Wied, D. A. (1973) The influence of peptides derived from corticotrophin (ACTH) on performance: Structure-activity studies. *Prog. Brain Res.* 39: 429–442.

Gron, G., Wunderlich, A. P., Spitzer, M., Tomczak, R., and Riepe, M. W. (2000) Brain activation during human navigation: Gender-different neural networks as substrate of performance. *Nature Neurosci.* 3: 404–408.

Handa, R. J., Price, R. H., Solum, D. T., and Suzuki, S. (2000) Any way you splice it: Diversity of estrogen action in the developing brain. Neuroendocrine Workshop. *Neuroendocrinol. Soc. Abst.* 22.

Hampson, E. (1990) Variations in sex-related cognitive abilities across the menstrual cycle. *Brain Cog.* 14: 26–43.

Hampson, E., Rovet, J. F., and Altmann, D. (1998) Spatial reasoning in children with congenital adrenal hyperplasia due to 21-hydorxylase deficiency. *Devel. Neuropsychol.* 14: 299–320.

Helleday, J., Bartfai, A., Ritzen, E. M., and Forsman, M. (1994) General intelligence and cognitive profile in women with congenital adrenal hyperplasia (CAH). *Psychoneuroendocrinology* 19: 343–356.

Henderson, V. W., Paganini-Hill, A., Emanuel, C. K., Dunn, M. E. E., and Buckwalter, J. G. (1994) Estrogen replacement therapy in older women: Comparison between Alzheimer's disease cases and nondemented control subjects. *Arch. Neurol.* 51: 896–900.

Henderson, V. W. (1997) Estrogen, cognition, and a woman's risk of Alzheimer's disease. *Am. J. Med.* 103: 11S–18S.

Hlinak, Z. (1993) Social recognition in ovariectomized and estradiol-treated female rats. *Horm. Behav.* 27: 159–166.

Insel, T. R. (1992) Oxytocin—A neuropeptide for affiliation: Evidence from behavioral, receptor, autoradiographic, and comparative studies. *Psychoneuroendocrinology* 17: 3–35.

Introini-Collison, I. B., Saghafi, D., Novack, G., and McGaugh, J. L. (1992) Memory enhancing effects of posttraining dipivefrin and epinephrine: Involvement of peripheral and central adrenergic receptors. *Brain Res.* 572: 81–86.

Introini-Collison, I. B., and Baratti, C. M. (1992) Memory-modulating effects of centrally acting noradrenergic drugs: Possible involvement of brain cholinergic systems. *Behav. Neural Biol.* 57: 248–255.

Isgor, C., and Sengelaub, D. R. (1998) Prenatal gonadal steroids affect adult spatial behavior, CA1 and CA3 pyramidal cell morphology in rats. *Horm. Behav.* 34: 183–198.

Issa, A. M., Rowe, W., Gauthier, S., and Meaney, M. J. (1990) Hypothalamic-pituitary-adrenal activity in aged, cognitively impaired and cognitively unimpaired rats. *J. Neurosci.* 10: 3247–3254.

Jacobs, L. F., Gaulin, S. J., Sherry, D. F., and Hoffman, G. E. (1990) Evolution of spatial cognition: Sex-specific patterns of spatial behavior predict hippocampal size. *Proc. Natl. Acad. Sci. USA* 87: 6349–6352.

Janowsky, J. S., Oviatt, S. K., and Orwoll, E. S. (1994) Testosterone influences spatial cognition in older men. *Behav. Neurosci.* 108: 325–332.

Juraska, J. M. (1984) Sex differences in developmental plasticity in the visual cortex and hippocampal dentate gyrus. *Prog. Brain Res.* 61: 205–214.

Juraska, J. M., and Kopcik, J. R. (1988) Sex and environmental influences on the size and ultrastructure of the rat corpus callosum. *Brain Res.* 450: 1–8.

Kawas, C., Resnick, S., Morrison, Brookmeyer, R., Corrada, M., Zonderman, A., Bacal, C., Lingle, D. D., and Metter, E. (1997) A prospective study of estrogen replacement therapy and the risk of developing Alzheimer's disease: The Baltimore Longitudinal Study of Aging. *Neurology* 48: 1517–1521.

Kinsley, C. H., Madonia, L., Gifford, G. W., Tureski, K., Griffin, G. R., Lowry, C., Williams, J., Collins, J., McLearie, H., and Lambert, K. G. (1999) Motherhood improves learning and memory. *Nature* 402: 137–138.

Kimura, D. (1999) *Sex and Cognition.* Cambridge, Mass.: MIT Press.

Kogan, J. H., Frankland, P. W., and Silva, A. J. (2000) Long-term memory underlying hippocampus-dependent social recognition in mice. *Hippocampus* 10: 47–56.

LaBar, K. S., Gatenby, J. C., Gore, J. C., LeDoux, J. E., and Phelps, E. A. (1998) Human amygdala activation during conditioned fear acquisition and extinction: A mixed-trial fMRI study. *Neuron* 20: 937–945.

Le Doux, J. E. (1995) Emotion: Clues from the brain. *Annu. Rev. Psychol.* 46: 209–235.

Lefevre, J., and McClintock, M. K. (1988) Reproductive senescence in female rats: A longitudinal study of individual differences in estrous cycles and behavior. *Biol. Reprod.* 38: 780–789.

Liang, K. D., Juler, R., and McGaugh, J. L. (1998) Modulating effects of posttraining epinephrine on memory: Involvement of the amygdala noradrenergic system. *Brain Res.* 368: 125–133.

Luine, V. N., and McEwen, B. S. (1983) Sex differences in cholinergic enzymes of diagonal band nuclei in the rat preoptic area. *Neuroendocrinology* 36: 475–482.

Luine, V., Villegas, M., Martinez, C., and McEwen, B. S. (1994) Stress-dependent impairments of spatial memory. Role of 5-HT. *Ann. New York Acad. Sci.* 746: 403–404.

Lupien, S., Lecours, A. R., Lussier, I., Schwartz, G., Nair, N. P. V., and Meaney, M. J. (1994) Basal cortisol levels and cognitive deficits in human aging. *J. Neurosci.* 14: 2893–2903.

Lupien, S., and McEwen, B. S. (1997) The acute effects of corticosteroids on cognition: Integration of animal and human model studies. *Brain Res. Rev.* 24: 1–27.

MacClosky, N. J., Clark, A. S., Naftonlin, F., and Goldman-Rakic, P. S. (1987) Estrogen formation in the mammalian brain: Possible role of aromatase in sexual differentiation of the hippocampus and neocortex. *Steroids* 50: 459–463.

Maquet, P., Laureys, S., Peigneux, P., Fuchs, S., Petiau, C., Phillips, C., Aerts, J., Del Fiore, G., Degueldre, C., Meulemans, T., Luxen, A., Franck, G., Van Der Linden, M., Smith, C., and Cleeremans, A. (2000) Experience-dependent changes in cerebral activation during human REM sleep. *Nature* 3: 831–836.

Maki, P. M., and Resnick, S. M. (2001) Effects of estrogen of patterns of brain activity at rest and during cognitive activity. A review of neuroimaging studies. *Neuroimage* 14: 789–801.

Markowska, A. L. (1999) Sex dimorphisms in the rate of age-related decline in spatial memory: Relevance to alterations in the estrous cycle. *J. Neurosci.* 19: 8122–8133.

Martinez, J., and Kesner, R., eds. (1998) *Neurobiology of Learning and Memory.* San Diego: Academic Press.

McEchron, M. D., Bouwmeester, H., Tseng, W., Weiss, C., and Disterhoft, J. F. (1998) Hippocampectomy disrupts auditory trace fear conditioning and contextual fear conditioning in the rat. *Hippocampus* 8: 638–646.

McEwen, B. S. (1999) Stress and hippocampal plasticity. *Annu. Rev. Neurosci.* 22: 105–122.

McEwen, B. S., Albeck, D., Cameron, H., Chao, H. M., and Gould, E., et al. (1995) Stress and the brain: A paradoxical role for adrenal steroids. In G. D. Litwack (Ed.), *Vitamins and Hormones.* New York: Academic Press, pp. 371–402.

McEwen, B. S., Dekloet, E. R., and Rostene, W. H. (1986) Adrenal steroid receptors and actions in the nervous system. *Physiol. Rev.* 66: 1121–1188.

Men, D., McCarty, R., and Gold, P. E. (1999) Enhanced release of norepinephrine in rat hippocampus during spontaneous alteration tests. *Neurobiol. Learn. Mem.* 71: 289–300.

Miranda, P., Williams, C. L., and Einstein, G (1999) Granule cells are sexually dimorphic in their response to estradiol. *J. Neurosci.* 19: 3316–3325.

Mirsky, L., Miller, R., and Stein, M. (1953) Relation of adrenocortical activity and adaptive behavior. *Psychosom. Med.* 106: 39–46.

Moffat, S. D., Hampson, E., and Hatzipantelis, M. (1998) Navigation in a "virtual" maze: Sex differences and correlations with psychometric measures of ability in humans. *Evol. Human Behav.* 19: 73–87.

Moser, M. B., Trommald, M., and Andersen, P. (1994) An increase in dendritic spine density on hippocampal CA1 pyramidal cells following spatial learning in adult rats suggest the formation of new synapses. *Proc. Natl. Acad. Sci.* 91: 12673–12675.

Morris, R. G. M. (1981) Spatial localization does not require the presence of local cues. *Learn. Motiv.* 12: 239–261.

Morris, R. G. M., Garrud, P., Rawlins, J. N. P., and O'Keefe, J. (1982) Place navigation is impaired in rats with hippocampal lesions. *Nature* 297: 681–683.

Newcomer, J. W., Craft, S., Hershey, T., Askins, K., and Bardgett, M. E. (1994) Glucocorticoid-induced impairment in declarative memory performance in adult humans. *J. Neurosci.* 14: 2047–2053.

Oitzl, M. S., and de Kloet, E. R. (1992) Selective corticosteroid antagonists modulate specific aspects of spatial orientation learning. *Behav. Neurosci.* 108: 62–71.

Oitzl, M. S., de Kloet, E. R., Joëls, M., and Cole, T. J. (1998) Spatial learning deficits in mice with a targeted glucocorticoid receptor gene disruption. *Eur. J. Neurosci.* 9: 2284–2296.

O'Keefe, J. A., and Handa, R. J. (1990) Transient elevation of estrogen receptors in the neonatal rat hippocampus. *Devel. Brain Res.* 57: 119–127.

Olton, D. S., and Samuelson, R. J. (1976) Rememberance of places passed: Spatial memory in rats. *J. Exp. Psychol. Anim. Behav. Process.* 2: 97–116.

Olton, D. S., Walker, J. A., and Gage, F. H. (1978) Hippocampal connections and spatial discrimination. *Brain Res.* 139: 295–308.

Packard, M. G. (1998) Posttraining estrogen and memory modulation. *Horm. Behav.* 34: 126–139.

Parsons, M. W., and Gold, P. E. (1992) Glucose enhancement of memory in elderly humans: An inverted-U dose-response curve. *Neurobiol. Aging* 13: 401–404.

Pavlides, C., Watanabe, Y., Margarinos, A. M., and McEwen, B. S. (1995) Opposing role of adrenal steroid type I and type II receptors in hippocampal long-term potentiation. *Neuroscience* 68: 387–94.

Paxinos, G., and Watson, C. (1998) *The Rat Brain in Stereotaxic Coordinates.* San Diego: Academic Press.

Pedersen C. A., Caldwell, J. D., Walker, C., Ayers, G., and Mason, G. A. (1994) Oxytocin activates the postpartum onset of rat maternal behavior in the ventral tegmental and medial preoptic areas. *Behav. Neurosci.* 108: 1163–1171.

Quirarte, G. L., Roozendaal, B., and McGaugh, J. L. (1997) Glucocorticoid enhancement of memory storage involves noradrenergic activation in the basolateral amygdala. *Proc. Natl. Acad. Sci. USA* 94: 14048–14053.

Raggozzino, M. E., Pal, S. N., Unick, K. E., Stefani, M. R., and Gold, P. E. (1998) Modulation of hippocampal acetylcholine release and of memory by intrahipocampal glucose injections. *J. Neurosci.* 18: 1595–1560.

Raggozzino, M. E., Unick, K. E., and Gold, P. E. (1996) Hippocampal acetylcholine release during memory testing in rats: Augmentation by glucose. *Proc. Natl. Acad. Sci. USA* 93: 4693–4698.

Reid, S. N., and Juraska, J. M. (1992) Sex differences in the gross size of the rat neocortex. *J. Comp. Neurol.* 321: 442–447.

Resnick, S. M., Berenbaum, S. A., Gottesmann, I. I., and Bouchard, T. J. (1986) Early hormonal influences on cognitive functioning in congenital adrenal hyperplasia. *Devel. Psychobiol.* 22: 191–198.

Reul, J. M. H. M., and De Kloet, E. R. (1985) Two receptor systems for corticosterone in rat brain: Microdistribution and differential occupation. *Endocrinology* 117: 2505–2512.

Roozendaal, B. (2000) Glucocorticoids and regulation of memory consolodation. *Psychoneuroendocrinology* 25: 213–238.

Roozendaal, B., and McGaugh, J. L. (1996a) Amygdaloid nuclei lesions differentially affect glucocorticoid-induced memory enhancement in an inhibitory avoidance task. *Neurobiol. Learn. Mem.* 65: 1–8.

Roozendaal, B., and McGaugh, J. L. (1997) Glucocorticoid receptor agonist and antagonist administration into the basolateral but not central amygdala modulates memory storage. *Neurobiol. Learn. Mem.* 67: 176–179.

Sandstrom, N. J., Kaufman, J., and Huettel, S. A. (1998) Males and females use different distal cues in a virtual environment navigation task. *Cog. Brain Res.* 6: 351–360.

Sandstrom, N. J., and Williams, C. L. (2001) Memory retention is modulated by acute estradiol and progesterone replacement. *Behav. Neurosci.* 115: 384–393.

Sapolsky, R., Krey, L., and McEwen, B. S. (1986) The neuroendocrinology of stress and aging: The glucocorticoid cascade hypothesis. *Endocr. Rev.* 7: 284–301.

Sapolsky, R., Krey, L., and McEwen, B. S. (1985) Prolonged glucocorticoid exposure reduces hippocampal neuron number: Implications for aging. *J. Neurosci.* 5: 1222–1227.

Shapiro, L. E., and Dewsbury, D. A. (1990) Differences in affiliative behavior, pair bonding, and vaginal cytology in two species of voles (*Microtus ochrogaster*, and *M. montanus*). *J. Comp. Psychol.* 104: 268–274.

Sherry, D. F., and Schacter D. L. (1987) The evolution of multiple memory systems. *Psychol. Rev.* 94: 439–454.

Sherwin, B. B. (1988) Estrogen and/or androgen replacement therapy and cognitive functioning in surgically menopausal women. *Psychoneuroendocrinology* 13: 345–357.

Sherwin, B. B. (1994) Estrogenic effects on memory in women. *Ann. NY Acad. Sci.* 743: 213–231.

Sherwin, B. B. (2000) Mild cognitive impairment: Potential pharmacological treatment options. *J. Am. Geriat. Soc.* 48: 431–441.

Shrugrue, P. J., Lane, M. V., and Merchenthaler, I. (1997) The comparative distribution of estrogen receptor-α and β in the rat central nervous system. *J. Comp. Neurol.* 388: 507–525.

Singh, M., Meyer, E. M., and Simpkins, J. W. (1995) The effect of ovariectomy and estradiol replacement on brain-derived neurotrophic factor messenger ribonucleic acid expression in cortical and hippocampal brain regions of female Sprague-Dawley rats. *Endocrinology* 136: 2320–2324.

Sloviter, R., Valiquette, G., Abrams, G., Ronk, E., Sollas, A., Paul, L. A., and Neubort, S. (1989) Selective loss of hippocampal granule cells in the mature rat brain after adrenalectomy. *Science* 243: 535–538.

Squire, L. (1987) *Memory and Brain.* New York: Oxford University Press.

Starkman, M., Gebarski, S., Berent, S., and Schteingart, D. (1992) Hippocampal formation volume, memory dysfunction, and cortisol levels in patients with Cushing's syndrome. *Biol. Psychiat.* 32: 756–765.

Sutherland, G. R., and McNaughton, B. (2000) Memory trace reactivation in hippocampal and neocortical neuronal ensembles. *Curr. Opin. Neurobiol.* 10: 180–186.

Tanapat, P., Galea, L. A., and Gould, E. (1998) Stress inhibits the proliferation of granule cell precursors in the developing dentate gyrus. *Int. J. Devel. Neurosci.* 16: 235–9.

Tanapat, P., Hastings, N. B., Reeves, A. J., and Gould, E. (1999) Estrogen stimulates a transient increase in the number of new neurons in the dentate gyrus of the adult female rat. *J. Neurosci.* 19: 5792–5801.

Thor, D. H., and Holloway, W. R. (1982) Social memory of the male laboratory rat. *J. Comp. Physiol. Psychol.* 96: 1000–1006.

Torand-Allerand, C. D. (1996) The estrogen/neurotrophin connection during neural development: Is co-localization of estrogen receptors with the neurotrophins and their receptors biologically relevant? *Devel. Neurosci.* 18: 36–48.

Tribollet, E., Audigier, S., Dubois-Dauphin, M., and Dreifuss, J. J. (1990) Gonadal steroids regulate oxytocin receptors but not vasopressin receptors in the brain of male and female rats: An autoradiographic study. *Brain Res.* 511: 129–140.

Ueyama, T., Kawai, Y., Nemoto, K., Sekimoto, M., Tone, S., and Senba, E. (1997) Immobilization stress reduced the expression of neurotrophins and their receptors in the rat brain. *Neurosci. Res.* 28: 103–110.

Vandenberg, S. G., and Kuse, A. R. (1978) Mental rotations, a group test of three-dimensional spatial visualization. *Percep. Motor Skills* 47: 599–604.

Van Wimersma Greidanus, T. B., Burbach, J. P. H., and Veldhuis, H. D. (1986) Vasopressin and oxytocin: Their presence in the central nervous system and their functional significance in brain processes related to behavior and memory. *Acta Endocrinol.* 112(Suppl. 276): 85–103.

Warren, S. G., and Juraska, J. M. (1997) Spatial and nonspatial learning across the rat estrous cycle. *Behav. Neurosci.* 111: 259–266.

Wang, Z., Zhou, L., Hulihan, T. J., and Insel, T. R. (1996) Immunoreactivity of central vasopressin and oxytocin pathways in microtine rodents: A quantitative comparative study. *J. Comp. Neurol.* 266: 726–737.

Ward, S. L., Newcombe, N., and Overton, W. F. (1986) Turn left at the church, or three miles north: A study of direction giving and sex differences. *Envir. Behav.* 18: 192–213.

Weil-Malharbe, H., Axelrod, H., and Tomchick, R. (1959) Blood-brain barrier for adrenaline. *Science* 129: 1226–1228.

Wenk, G. L. (1997) The nucleus basalis magnocellularis cholinergic system: One hundred years of progress. *Neurobiol. Learn. Mem.* 6: 85–95.

Williams, C. L., Men, D., Clayton, E. C., and Gold, P. E. (1998) Norepinephrine release in the amygdala following systemic injection of epinephrine or escapable footshock: Contribution of the nucleus of the solitary tract. *Behav. Neurosci.* 112: 1414–1422.

Williams, C. L., and Meck, W. H. (1991) The organizational effects of gonadal steroids on sexually dimorphic spatial ability. *Psychoneuroendocrinology* 16: 155–176.

Williams, C. L., Barnett, A. M., and Meck, W. H. (1990) Organizational effects of early gonadal secretions on sexual differentiation in spatial memory. Behav. Neurosci. 104: 84–97.

Wolf, O. T., Kudielka, B. M., Hellhammer, D. H., Torber, S., McEwen, B. S., and Kirschbaum, C. (1999) Two weeks of transdermal estradiol treatment in postmenopausal elderly women and its effect on memory and mood: Verbal memory changes are associated with the treatment induced estradiol levels. *Psychoneuroendocrinology* 24: 727–741.

Woolley, C. S. (1998) Estrogen-mediated structural and functional synaptic plasticity in the female rat hippocampus. *Horm. Behav.* 34: 140–148.

Woolley, C. S., and McEwen, B. S. (1990) Roles of estradiol and progesterone in regulation of hippocampal dendritic spine density during the estrous cycle in the rat. *J. Comp. Neurol.* 336: 293–306.

Woolley, C. S., and McEwen, B. S. (1993) Roles of estradiol and progesterone in regulation of hippocampal dendritic spine density during the estrous cycle of the rat. *J. Comp. Neurol.* 336: 293–306.

Woolley, C. S., Wenzel, H. J., and Schwartzkroin, P. A. (1996) Estradiol increases the frequency of multiple synapse boutons in the hippocampal CA1 region of the adult female rat. *J. Comp. Neurol.* 373: 108–117.

Yaffe, K., Sawaya, G., Lieberburg, I., and Grady, D. (1998) Estrogen therapy in postmenopausal women: Effects on cognitive function and dementia. *JAMA* 279: 688–695.

Yerkes, R. M., and Dodson, J. D. (1908) The relation of strength of stimulus to rapidity of habit-formation. *J. Comp. Neurol. Psychol.* 18: 459–482.

Young, L. J., Nilsen, R., Waymire, K. G., MacGregor, G. R., and Insel, T. R. (1999) Increased affiliative response to vasopressin in mice expressing the V1a receptor from a monogamous vole. *Nature* 400: 766–768.

15 Sex Differences in Human Brain and Cognition: The Influence of Sex Steroids in Early and Adult Life

Elizabeth Hampson

This may be one of the more controversial and challenging chapters in this book. There is one species that, because it has an excellent brain and will attempt even very difficult tasks, allows us to examine higher cognitive function. That species is Homo sapiens, *of course. But humans are very complicated creatures. It is not too surprising, therefore, that there are great individual differences in cognitive function that make it difficult to detect differences between populations (say, men versus women, or women during the luteal phase versus those during the follicular phase of the ovulatory cycle). As you will see, there are small but reliable sex differences in cognitive function. There is even evidence that adult hormones contribute to these subtle differences in humans. Furthermore, contrary to popular notions, one sex does not have superiority in all cognitive functions in which there are sex differences. Sometimes males are better; sometimes females are better.*

How do we measure cognitive function in humans, and which of these measures reveal sex differences? Are such differences the result of hormonal or experiential differences? How do changes in gonadal hormone levels affect cognition and the lateralization of function?

Introduction

As you have already learned in previous chapters, the gonadal steroid hormones are involved in sexual differentiation of the vertebrate brain during early development. We have also seen how these hormones can influence the expression of sexually dimorphic behaviors throughout life. In this chapter, we will examine evidence that *human* brain function may be influenced by reproductive hormones. This should come as no surprise given the evolutionary continuity between *Homo sapiens* and other mammals. Still, progress in describing hormone-brain relationships in humans has been slow. This is partly because of methodological constraints in doing human research (e.g., we cannot manipulate hormones for experimental purposes). There has also been resistance to the idea that we, as a species, are still influenced by our evolutionary past. As a result, we are just beginning to understand how hormones, in conjunction with cultural and psychosocial factors, are able to influence human behavior and cognition.

In this chapter, we will discuss hormonal regulation of cognitive and motor functions. These effects are important because they show that sex steroids can affect human brain function in neural regions outside the hypothalamus and pituitary, and may help to establish other behavioral markers of sex.

Table 15.1 Abilities That Are Sexually Differentiated in Humans

MALES BETTER	FEMALES BETTER
Spatial abilities including mental rotations, route learning, and visualization of spatial relationships	Verbal skills, including fluency, rate of speech acquisition, spelling, and grammar
Mathematical reasoning and problem solving	Computational accuracy and procedural knowledge of arithmetic and mathematics
Gross motor skills that involve strength	Fine motor skills and finger dexterity
	Short-term memory including memory for object locations

Sex Differences in Cognitive Abilities

In humans, sex differences in cognitive abilities have been studied since the early part of the twentieth century. Reliable differences in a number of cognitive functions have been discovered (for reviews, see Halpern 1992; Jarvik 1975; Maccoby and Jacklin 1974; Tyler 1965; Voyer, Voyer, and Bryden 1995). Several of these are listed in table 15.1. In humans, unlike most species, it is usually assumed that all behavioral sex differences are the products of learning. Some differences, such as sex differences in how men and women dress, are clearly controlled by the cultural environment. But when it comes to intellectual abilities, the relative roles of nature and nurture are far less clearly defined. The challenge facing researchers is to figure out whether hormones, either acting alone or interactively with environmental experiences, are responsible for any portion of the cognitive differences between individuals. Researchers have only recently begun to consider whether cognitive differences might have a hormonal basis. It is this highly specific class of abilities—**sexually differentiated abilities**—that have been the focus of recent neuroendocrine studies.

Before we begin, there are several facts you should keep in mind. First, there are no sex differences in overall IQ. The abilities we will be discussing are quite specific. Second, the direction of the sex difference is not the same for all abilities. For some, the difference favors females, and for others, the difference favors males. Finally, sex differences in human cognitive or motor functions are small in relation to the striking sex differences in behavior often studied in other species. Figure 15.1 shows a typical sex difference. Because there is so much overlap in the scores of the two sexes, it is not possible to predict, merely on the basis of sex, whether an individual male or female will be good or poor at a particular ability. With a few exceptions, it is only in the group averages that we see the sex differences emerge.

Now let us consider some of the cognitive functions that exhibit sex differences.

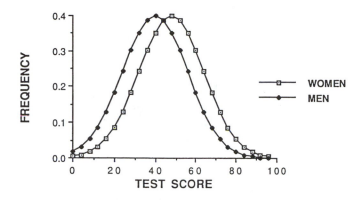

Figure 15.1 Sex differences in cognitive abilities are typically modest in size. Here, the frequency distribution of scores on a hypothetical cognitive test has been plotted separately for males and females. We see a systematic difference between the means, but there is also large overlap in the scores obtained by men and women. A consequence of the offset in the means is that the number of individuals scoring above a given point will differ in the two sexes. In our example, the mean for women is higher than the mean for men such that only 25–30% of males score above the female mean. Actual sex differences may favor either sex, but several cognitive abilities do show sex differences of approximately this size.

Spatial Abilities

Spatial abilities are a diverse range of functions that enable us to perceive or reason about the positions of objects or their movements in space. Box 15.1 shows example items from three tests that can be used to measure spatial abilities in the lab. Many spatial abilities exhibit a male advantage. This sex difference is found in both Western and non-Western cultures. It occurs in other species, too, insofar as comparable tasks can be devised (Gaulin and Fitzgerald 1986; Williams et al. 1990). Even though sex differences in spatial abilities can be observed in children (Kerns and Berenbaum 1991; McGuinness and Morley 1991; Voyer et al. 1995), the sex difference does not appear in full force until puberty. This raises the possibility that the organizational and activational effects of sex steroids might conceivably be involved in its expression. The largest sex differences occur on tests that require the imagination of three-dimensional rotations in space (e.g., box 15.1, top) or on tests where the observer or the external stimuli are in motion. Here, sex differences may be large. On the test shown in box 15.1, for example, men's average scores are often 35 to 40% higher than women's average scores (e.g., Sanders, Soares, and d'Aquila 1982). On simpler spatial tests, males typically outscore females by 10 to 25%.

Verbal Abilities

Sex differences that favor females have been reported in a variety of verbal skills, including spelling, grammar, rate of acquisition of speech in childhood, and the ability to comprehend or decode language. Boys more often

Box 15.1 Tests of Spatial Abilities

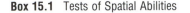

Spatial abilities are often assessed using paper-and-pencil tests. These may ask a person to imagine the rotation of a depicted object, or what an object would look like if folded together or seen from a different perspective. Other tests ask a person to recognize designated shapes that are embedded in a complex visual pattern. In this chapter, we refer to these collectively as tests of spatial abilities. As far back as the 1940s, factor analytic studies identified at least three subtypes of spatial ability, all showing a sex difference in favor of males. These are called *spatial orientation*, *spatial visualization*, and *flexibility of closure*. Sample items from tests that assess each of the three spatial factors are shown here. In the top item, you are asked to view the figure on the left and then identify which two figures on the right are rotated depictions of that same figure (1 and 3 are correct). In the middle item, you must imagine the flattened pattern folded along the dotted lines into a 3-dimensional object. Which parts of the folded figure will now correspond to each of the numbered edges? (B = 2). In the bottom item, you must identify which of the five simple figures is embedded within the more complex design (A is correct) (reprinted with permission from S. G. Vandenberg's *Mental Rotations Test*, © 1971 and from the *Manual for the Kit of Factor-Referenced Cognitive Tests* (pp. 177, 21) by R. B. Ekstrom, J. W. French, and H. H. Harman. Copyright © 1976 by Educational Testing Service).

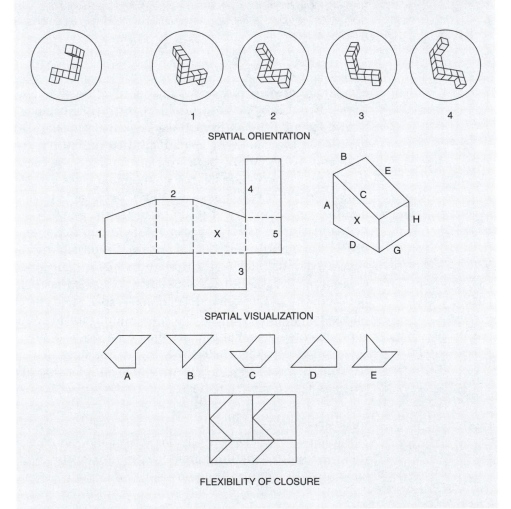

than girls show language impairments such as stuttering or dyslexia (a learning disorder characterized by the inability to recognize and comprehend the written word). One aspect of language production that shows sex differences is verbal fluency, defined as facility in thinking rapidly of appropriate words, phrases, or sentences. In the lab, fluency can be assessed by having subjects write down or orally report, within a specified time limit, as many words as possible that meet a particular phonetic or semantic criterion. For example, subjects may be asked to report all the words they can think of beginning with the letter "J" within one minute, or all the words they can think of that belong to some category, such as birds.

Sex differences in verbal abilities are usually smaller than differences in spatial abilities, but vary tremendously depending on the exact verbal function being measured. For example, Hines (1990) reported a very large sex difference in favor of females on a difficult associational fluency task (a task where people must generate many words similar in meaning to a given word). Less than 16% of men exceeded the average score for women. At the other extreme, sex differences in vocabulary are virtually nonexistent. (Vocabulary can be assessed by tests sampling knowledge of word meanings.) In a recent review, Hyde and Linn (1988) speculated that sex differences in verbal skills might be decreasing in size over time. But their review emphasized abilities such as vocabulary and reading comprehension, which are known not to show reliable sex differences in adults. It should also be noted that many current verbal tests have been standardized over time to help eliminate the sex differences favoring females that appeared on earlier versions of the tests (e.g., SAT-V).

Memory

Women often perform slightly better than men on tests of short-term memory. Many studies have found a modest female advantage on tasks that require learning lists of words or recalling the details of a short story (e.g., Kramer et al. 1988; Mann et al. 1990). There are indications that the sex difference might extend to memory tests that appear, on the surface at least, to be nonverbal. For example, Galea and Kimura (1993) gave men and women 1 minute to view a display consisting of 40 pictures of animals and common objects, randomly arranged. Twenty minutes later, women were able to recall significantly more of the items than men. This was true even though there was no sex difference in their immediate recall right after the stimuli were presented. A similar sex difference was found by Wilson and Vandenberg (1978) in a large-scale study of cognitive abilities conducted in Hawaii. This female advantage in remembering items might seem paradoxical in light of the male advantage in spatial ability. But it is important to realize that the key requirements of the tasks are different. No dynamic transformations are required in memorizing designs or other figural material. It is only important to remember the exact objects seen. Also, in many cases, memory tests are open to the use of verbal strategies as an aid to recall, even when the items to be remembered don't consist explicitly of words. We know that "dual-encoded" material is better retained (Paivio 1971). If women tend more than men to utilize verbal encoding as an aid to recall, even on pictorial tasks, it might give them an additional edge.

Recently it has been suggested that women may have an advantage in remembering the spatial *locations* of objects. Again, no dynamic changes in either the objects themselves or their positions need to be visualized. In a series of studies, Silverman and Eals (1992) gave males and females equal opportunities to learn the positions of objects in an array (figure 15.2). Women were more accurate than men at detecting if switches had been made in the positions of the objects when they were reshown later on. A female advantage in remembering object locations has now been found in other studies, too (Eals and Silverman 1994; James and Kimura 1997; McBurney et al. 1997), but the basis for this sex difference is not well understood. One view is that object-location memory is a special form of spatial ability that evolved in a sexually differentiated manner in response to selection pressures associated with foraging (Silverman and Eals 1992). Another view is that the female memory system is adept at tightly integrating object identity and location information (James and Kimura 1997). This is a general adaptation that would be useful not just in foraging but also in navigating in familiar terrain where local landmarks can be used effectively as navigational cues. This theory meshes nicely with recent studies suggesting that females do rely more heavily than males on landmarks for spatial navigation (Choi and Silverman 1997; Galea and Kimura 1993; Sandstrom, Kaufman, and Huettel 1998; Williams et al. 1990).

Perceptual Speed and Accuracy

Women also exhibit better performance than men on tests of perceptual speed and accuracy (box 15.2). This is defined as the ability to quickly and accurately perceive fine details of visual stimuli. The sex difference in this ability favors women regardless of whether the visual material is verbal or pictorial. The sex difference is comparable in size to the sex difference in spatial ability, but in favor of women instead of men (Tyler 1965). It is logical to wonder whether the newly found female advantage in object-location memory that we just described could be the result of the female advantage in perceptual speed. This has not been put to an adequate test. The two abilities could be sexually differentiated yet still be separate phenomena.

Motor Skills

Sex differences in motor skills are widely recognized. Males dramatically excel in strength, especially after the early teenage years (Jones 1947), while women show greater speed and agility in a number of fine motor skills, both manual and articulatory. The sex differences are evident in tasks such as speeded syllable repetition, grip strength, or tests of manual dexterity. For example, a person may be asked to quickly place pegs into holes or to assemble metal components in a specified order under tight time constraints.

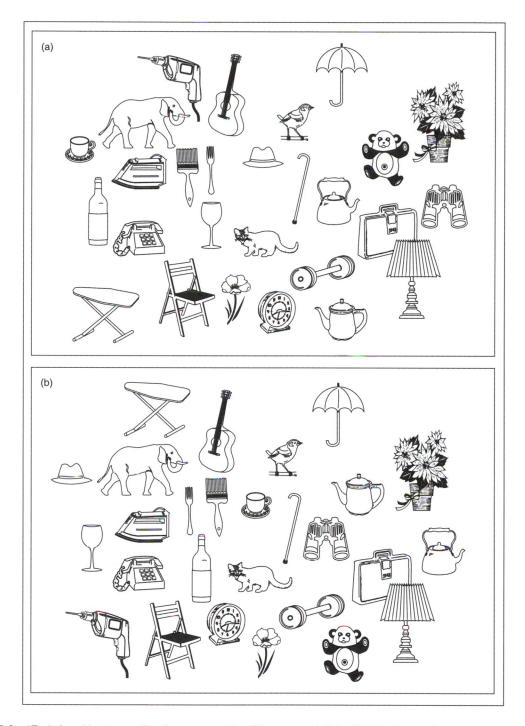

Figure 15.2 (*Top*) An object array like the one used by Silverman and Eals (1992). Men and women were allowed to study the array and then it was removed. (*Bottom*) A short time later, a second array was exposed. Note that some of the items have switched places, relative to the original arrangement. Participants were asked to indicate which objects had moved. (Redrawn from Silverman and Eals 1992.)

Box 15.2   Tests of Perceptual Speed and Accuracy

Two items from a test used to assess perceptual speed and accuracy in children. Tests of perceptual speed usually require rapid comparisons of figures or symbols or else require rapid visual scanning with the eyes to find a target having a designated visual configuration. In these examples, the child is asked to mark the 2 patterns on each line that are identical in all respects (redrawn from *Primary Mental Abilities* by L. L. Thurstone and T. G. Thurstone. Chicago: Science Research Associates 1963).

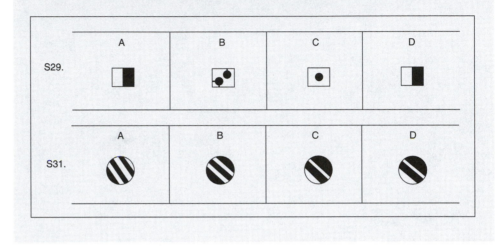

On many tests, sex differences are large enough to warrant separate norms for men and women. The female advantage on fine motor tasks may be at least partly related to smaller finger size, but CNS factors are believed to contribute, too. A study by Nicholson and Kimura (1996) suggested that females may be able to program a sequence of movements more efficiently than males. This points to a sex difference in the central processing of motor commands.

We know from studies of patients with localized brain damage that there is a motor system in the left hemisphere that is invoked when certain types of manual and articulatory movements must be programmed (Kimura 1982). If this system is destroyed by a stroke or other sudden brain event, then patients will show a fascinating phenomenon. They are able to move their limbs freely, but have great difficulty in organizing sequences of movements, so make errors in movement selection and ordering. This is called **manual apraxia**. The same patients have similar difficulty in controlling movements of the mouth region (**oral apraxia**). When they speak, they display a speech disturbance called **aphasia**, in which syllables or even larger parts of speech are omitted, misarranged, or substituted. Analysis of the speech errors made in aphasia suggests that the same motor-programming problem is at least partly responsible for the disturbances in overt speech as well.

Neuropsychological tests are a special class of tests that can be used to assess the integrity of sensory, perceptual, cognitive, or motor functions that

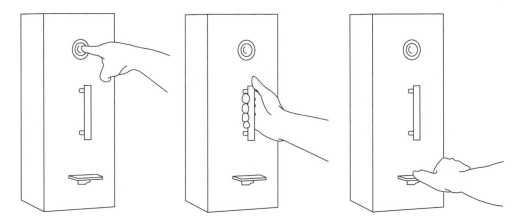

Figure 15.3 The Manual Sequence Box. If patients have brain damage that intrudes on the manual praxis system in the left hemisphere, they have great difficulty in mastering the simple sequence of three movements shown here. Even though there is adequate limb strength and mobility, motor sequences cannot be programmed accurately.

are linked to identifiable regions or pathways in the brain. Figure 15.3 shows a neuropsychological test that can tap the kinds of movements programmed by the motor system we've been discussing, the manual **praxis system.** We shall return to this test again later in the chapter. The fact that a common motor system in the left cerebral hemisphere contributes to high-level programming of both the mouth and upper limbs may be important to understanding the basis for sex differences in manual and articulatory speed and accuracy. As we shall see, a sex difference already has been discovered in the cortical localization of the praxis system.

Sex Differences in the Functional Organization of the Cortex

Why do sex differences in cognitive abilities exist? The underlying reasons are hotly debated. Some people believe that sex differences in upbringing or experience can provide a complete account of any sex differences in cognitive abilities. Others point to recent evidence of sexual dimorphism in the human brain to argue that we shouldn't be too hasty to rule out biological explanations. Structural differences could lead to cognitive differences by altering processing efficiency, capacity, or the preferred strategies used to tackle cognitive problems. In other species, we know brain dimorphisms are often caused by the actions of sex steroids. The presence of sex differences in the human brain raises the possibility that our brains, too, may be subject to modification by sex steroids.

Sex Differences in Interhemispheric Organization

You know from chapter 3 that sex differences have been discovered in the anatomy of the human hypothalamus and, possibly, the cerebral commissures. While it is not possible to see them with a microscope, it is suspected that sex differences also exist in the functional organization of the cortex. These may include sex differences in patterns of lateralization.

It is well established that the two hemispheres in humans are not equally adept at all functions. For example, in most people the left side of the brain is the one responsible for controlling speech and programming sequences of manual and oral movements, as described earlier. This is an example of lateralization of function. Since the 1970s, researchers have been hypothesizing that sex differences might exist in the *degree* to which linguistic and non-verbal functions are lateralized to the two hemispheres. Typically, it is argued that the two sides of the brain are more fully differentiated or specialized in men than in women, whereas women have a more bilateral representation of function in which the two hemispheres share certain processing capabilities (e.g., Bryden 1979; Harshman and Remington 1976; McGlone 1980).

Two types of evidence support this position. The first source of evidence comes from people with brain injuries. A number of studies have indicated that damage restricted to one side of the brain, that is, unilateral damage, has less devastating consequences in women than in men. For example, McGlone (1977) investigated the effects of unilateral brain damage on intelligence quotients (IQ). She found that left hemisphere damage impaired verbally weighted aspects of IQ more than right hemisphere damage, as we would expect if the left hemisphere is the one primarily responsible for language. But this was true only in men. One interpretation is that females with left-sided damage were able to rely on residual language capabilities in their intact right hemisphere in order to perform the verbal tasks. In another study, Lansdell (1961) gave a proverb comprehension test to 55 patients having brain surgery. Left temporal lobe lesions disrupted the ability to do the proverbs task in males but not in females. Again, this is consistent with a greater degree of right hemisphere participation in complex verbal functions in females.

The second source of evidence for sex differences in lateralization comes from the perceptual asymmetries that appear in normal adults if they are tested using **dichotic** listening or **divided visual field** tests. In these tests, simple auditory or visual stimuli are presented in a special lateralized fashion at extremely short durations. If the stimuli are verbal (e.g., words or syllables), a typical person is able to accurately report more of the stimuli presented to the right ear or right visual field. Because of the way the visual and auditory pathways project to the brain, the right-sided superiority is a marker of left hemisphere lateralization of language. Conversely, a left ear or left visual field superiority typically is seen when stimuli are briefly presented that tap the specialized processing capacities of the right hemisphere (e.g., melodies or dot arrays). Using such tests, many investigators have found that the size of the resulting perceptual asymmetries is smaller in women than in men. The fact that women tend to perform more equivalently in the two ears or visual fields is thought to be a reflection of reduced lateralization of function (see McGlone 1980 for a review).

Recently, new imaging techniques have become available that enable researchers to see relative levels of activity in different brain regions when people are actively engaged in cognitive processing. These techniques capitalize on the fact that more active brain areas use proportionately more glucose and oxygen and exhibit changes in blood flow relative to less active brain areas. The metabolic differences can either be mapped using radioisotopes, in a technique called *positron emission tomography* (PET), or by measuring changes in the oxygen content of blood in the presence of a strong magnetic field (*functional magnetic resonance imaging,* fMRI). So far, these techniques have seldom been used to study sex differences. But sex differences periodically pop up anyway. For example, using fMRI, Shaywitz and colleagues (1995) discovered a prominent sex difference in the functional activity of the frontal cortex when male and female volunteers performed an experimental task that required phonological processing, that is, decoding sound from printed words. The task involved detecting rhyme. Males showed activity only in the left inferior frontal gyrus (IFG), but many females showed both left- and right-sided activity in the IFG during the rhyme-judgment task (figure 15.4). This is a particularly compelling demonstration of a sex difference in lateralized brain function.

Sex Differences in Intrahemispheric Organization

The evidence we have been describing is fairly straightforward. Recent evidence, though, paints a more complex picture of sexual dimorphism in the human cerebral cortex. First, not *all* functions are less lateralized in females, and some may even be more lateralized (Desmond et al. 1994). When sex dif-

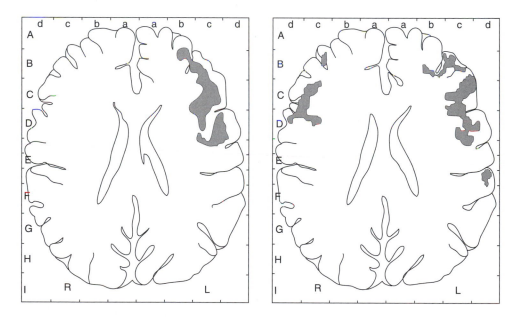

Figure 15.4 A sketch taken from the fMRI study by Shaywitz et al. (1995) showing brain regions activated during phonological processing. (*Left*) Brain regions activated in men; (*right*) brain regions activated in women. Activation was exclusively left-sided in males, but bilateral in females. Activated areas were in the inferior frontal gyrus (IFG).

ferences do occur, they are not always differences in the degree of reliance on one hemisphere versus the other. Sex differences might also exist in the anterior-posterior arrangement of certain functions.

The first indication that there might be sex differences in cortical organization *within* the two hemispheres came from a study by Kimura (1983). The study was a detailed analysis of speech disturbances in 81 patients with brain damage restricted to the anterior or posterior left hemisphere. Kimura (1983) found that in women, aphasia and apraxia almost always resulted from damage to the anterior left hemisphere, not the posterior left hemisphere. The pattern reversed in men, who most often developed aphasia after posterior damage. Of 169 patients with right hemisphere lesions, only a tiny fraction were aphasic. These were no more likely to be women than men. This is contrary to what we would expect if basic speech capacities are more dependent on the right hemisphere in females. Kimura concluded that the anterior left hemisphere is more critical in women than in men for the production and comprehension of speech. This has now been replicated in other studies of patients with aphasia (Cappa and Vignolo 1988; Hier et al. 1994; Vignolo, Boccardi, and Caverni 1986).

The possibility of anterior-posterior differences in the localization of speech within the left hemisphere is supported by cortical mapping studies (Mateer, Polen, and Ojemann 1982). Cortical mapping is a procedure used to determine safe boundaries for resection in patients about to undergo neurosurgery so they will not be left with a lasting speech deficit. The left cortex is exposed and stimulated with a mild electrical current in order to map out areas of the cortex that are involved in the control of speech. Mateer discovered that stimulation evoked naming deficits from more sites throughout the left cortex in males than in females. In the posterior parietal cortex, stimulation evoked naming errors in almost 60% of men but 0% of women.

Thus, sex differences in at least two planes have been identified in the human brain. The secret to reconciling the results may lie in the fact that different researchers have focused on very different verbal functions. Basic motor or acoustic functions related to speaking seem to show sex differences in intra- but not inter-hemispheric organization, while higher-order, abstract, or more complex verbal functions seem, if anything, to show inter-hemispheric differences. A lesson to be learned from all this is that sex differences in cortical organization are function-specific. In retrospect, early researchers overstepped the limits of their data by drawing conclusions about the lateralization of "verbal function" as a whole.

New Approaches

There is increasing acceptance of the idea that the human brain is sexually dimorphic. Recently a few studies have started to take a strategic approach—they have begun to search for structural dimorphism in brain regions we know to be involved in dimorphic cognitive functions. Language regions of the cortex have received special attention because the regions involved in language are more thoroughly mapped out than for most cognitive functions and because the female advantage in fluency and other verbal abilities is well-established. Initial results are promising. Using neuron cell counts, Witelson, Glezer, and Kigar (1995) discovered that the number of neurons per unit volume was about 11% greater in women than in men in the planum temporale. The planum temporale is involved in auditory speech processing. Schlaepfer and colleagues (1995) found that women had a 23% larger gray matter volume than men in a region of the frontal cortex having to do with language and a 13% larger gray matter volume in the superior temporal gyrus, once corrected for overall brain size. This dimorphism was not seen in a non-language region of the cortex examined for comparison.

There is no reason to think that cortical differences will be restricted to the language zones. It is likely that other sexual dimorphisms will be discovered. We are only beginning to map out sex differences in the human brain. While progress has been slow, it represents a significant departure from the old view, held until recently, that human brains do not exhibit any sexual dimorphism. So far, researchers have not attempted to relate the dimorphisms to hormonal events. Whether hormones are involved in their genesis is a matter of speculation only.

Organizational Effects of Early Hormones on Cognition

Dramatic evidence of organizational effects in other species leads us to wonder if the early hormone environment also shapes human behavior. Do cognitive differences between the sexes have their roots in the hormones we're exposed to? Do our experiences build upon a path toward sexual differentiation that is already set in motion by exposure to hormones in the womb? In this section, we consider this important question.

Techniques for Studying Organizational Effects

Testing the organizational hypothesis in humans is slow and difficult. For ethical reasons, we can't manipulate hormones in the human fetus or infant. We are also restricted in our ability to study organizational effects at the neural level, because we do not yet have technology that permits the microscopic analysis of neural organization in living people. Most of the current evidence in favor of organizing effects of sex steroids comes from people exposed to atypical hormone environments, either before birth or in infancy. Such exposure may result from genetic errors which lead to abnormalities in the synthesis, metabolism, or sensitivity to, specific hormones. Another cause is the ingestion of synthetic hormones by the mother during pregnancy. In the past, synthetic estrogens and progestins were prescribed to prevent miscarriage in at-risk pregnancies.

We hope that studying such "experiments of nature" will inform us about the role of hormones in normal behavioral development. But clinical studies are subject to limitations: (1) double-blind studies are often impossible because affected individuals and their parents are aware of the condition, (2) many of these conditions are extremely rare, making it hard to obtain large enough sample sizes to adequately test hypotheses, and (3) the childhood upbringing may be atypical—for example, aside from needing medication or other medical interventions, either the parents or the child may have difficulty in coming to terms with the psychological dimensions of these conditions. Individuals exposed to exogenous hormones provide a research population with its own difficulties: (1) the timing and type of hormone exposure varies markedly from case to case, and the potencies of different synthetic steroids can vary enormously, (2) the medical conditions that necessitated hormonal intervention in the first place might have their own effects on CNS development, and (3) families that choose to receive prenatal therapy may not be representative of the population at large. Higher socioeconomic or educational levels may be over-represented among families who chose treatment, or they might differ in other personal characteristics, making generalizations difficult.

However imperfect clinical data may be, they provide most of our current information about the role of early hormones in human development. Recently two new paradigms have emerged that provide new avenues for testing the organizational hypothesis:

1. Since organization of the human brain by sex steroids is believed to be a prenatal or early postnatal event, researchers have begun to measure T or other hormones during the hypothetical critical periods to determine if hormone concentrations at those times do correlate with behavioral or cognitive measures obtained in the same individuals later in development or at maturity (Finegan et al. 1992; Jacklin et al. 1988; Udry, Morris and Kovenock 1995). So far, hormones have been measured in umbilical cord blood at the time of birth (e.g., Jacklin et al. 1988) or in second trimester amniotic fluid (Finegan et al. 1992). Sampling amniotic fluid is only permissible in at-risk pregnancies. Such studies are valuable but extremely rare. The need to track children longitudinally over many years to monitor behavioral development makes this kind of study impossible in most research settings.

2. The newest technique for investigating organizational effects involves studying female members of opposite-sex twin pairs. This technique is based on the assumption that the uterine environment allows minute amounts of T to diffuse from the male to the female fetus. While diffusion effects do occur in litter-bearing species such as rats or gerbils, it is uncertain whether such fetal exchanges can occur in human multiple births. Nevertheless, a few researchers have already begun to use the twin method.

In the past few years, evidence from all these techniques has combined to suggest that organizational effects do occur in some realms of human development. Exposure to steroids during critical periods can influence our future behavioral tendencies in a manner similar to other species, though to a more modest degree.

Table 15.2   Examples of Sexually Differentiated Childhood Gender Role Behaviors

Patterns of childhood toy preferences

Sex of preferred playmates during childhood

Rehearsal through play of adult roles as spouse or caregiver

Interest in infants and infant care

Preference for rough-and-tumble play

Physical aggressiveness

Gender Role Behaviors

Early hormones *might* exert predisposing effects on a number of social behaviors that exhibit sex differences (table 15.2). Even though cultural or social factors play an undeniable role in promoting these differences, they may not be the only factors involved. Evidence favoring a biological contribution comes from clinical studies.

CONGENITAL ADRENAL HYPERPLASIA

Congenital adrenal hyperplasia (CAH) is an inherited condition in which an enzyme deficiency in the cortex of the adrenal glands causes massive overproduction of androgens. Overproduction begins prenatally and continues until a diagnosis is made, usually at birth or shortly afterward. Females with CAH are therefore exposed to malelike hormones throughout the gestational period when the organization of CNS function hypothetically occurs. Once identified, androgen overproduction can be normalized with medication. Any visible genital anomalies can be corrected in infancy with surgery. Typically, females with CAH are raised as females and develop a female gender identity.

Most of the evidence favoring an effect of early androgens on sexually differentiated gender role behaviors comes from studies of girls with CAH. They exhibit more masculine patterns of toy preferences than their unaffected sisters (Berenbaum and Hines 1992; Ehrhardt and Baker 1974), greater preference for male playmates, greater tomboyism, reduced rehearsal in childhood play of adult female roles as wife and mother, reduced interest in infants, reduced interest in physical appearance and attractiveness, and possibly greater aggression than control females (Berenbaum and Resnick 1997; Ehrhardt and Baker 1974; Ehrhardt, Epstein, and Money 1968; Hines and Kaufman 1994; Leveroni and Berenbaum 1998). These behavioral changes are assumed to arise from the malelike gestational environment since the genotype, postnatal phenotype, and environmental upbringing of girls with CAH are all distinctively female. Unfortunately, most CAH studies have relied exclusively on self-reports or parental reports rather than on direct behavioral observations. This weakens the evidence by leaving open the possibility of bias in reporting. Only recently have a few studies, such as the one by

Hines and Kaufman (1994), begun to use objective quantification of behavior. These researchers studied rough-and-tumble behaviors in children with CAH by videotaping play interactions in a controlled laboratory setting. Further use of objective methods will help to solidify the quality of the research coming from CAH studies.

EXPOSURE TO EXOGENOUS HORMONES

Support for organizational effects on gender role behavior comes from children whose mothers took masculinizing progestins during pregnancy to prevent miscarriage (Ehrhardt and Money 1967). These hormones are no longer prescribed. In some cases, the female offspring of these pregnancies were born with partly masculinized genitals, which had to be surgically corrected. Using semistructured interviews, Ehrhardt and Money (1967) reported that such girls showed high levels of energetic play in childhood, which is more typical of boys. They also had a strong interest in traditional boys' toys, such as guns and trucks, rather than in dolls and other toys traditionally preferred by girls. They were described as "tomboys" by their parents and themselves. Reinisch (1981) found that progestin-exposed individuals also had a heightened potential for physical aggression. This was true even though none of Reinisch's females were genitally masculinized. Gender identity and sex of rearing in the progestin-exposed women were female.

TWIN STUDIES

Recently the opposite-sex twin method has been applied to the study of gender role behaviors. Results have been mixed. Resnick and colleagues (1993) found increased sensation-seeking behavior in female members of opposite-sex twin pairs. This is consistent with the male preponderance usually seen on this personality trait. But Henderson and Berenbaum (1997) failed to find any alterations in sex-typed play in a well-controlled study of opposite-sex twins. In theory, any behavioral masculinization reported in twin studies could alternatively be caused by the social effects of having a brother the same age. To rule out social learning effects, twin studies must include appropriate control groups. So far, few studies have done this. As we noted earlier, the twin technique is yet to be validated. A finding by McFadden (1993), though, suggests that environmental factors are not the only mechanisms at work. McFadden found that females with male co-twins exhibited defeminization in the incidence of **spontaneous otoacoustic emissions**, weak tonal sounds emitted by the cochlea. Because cochlear emissions are strictly a physical characteristic, it is hard to imagine how social factors could account for this.

To summarize, data from females with CAH and females exposed to masculinizing progestins suggest that hormones in the uterine environment may be capable of exerting a lasting influence on certain gender role behaviors. The evidence, however, is weakened by small sample sizes, over-reliance on subjective reports, and the limited control groups used. Therefore, while promising, most of the findings can only be considered preliminary and are in need of rigorous substantiation.

Cognitive Abilities

The effects of early hormones on cognitive functions have been assessed by studying general intelligence and, more recently, sexually differentiated abilities.

Available evidence does not support an effect of prenatal androgens on intelligence. This makes sense when we consider that sex differences in general intelligence are not found in the population at large. A few early studies did report IQ elevation, relative to population norms, in groups of patients exposed to natural or synthetic progestins in utero (e.g., Ehrhardt and Money 1967). For a time, this raised the possibility that progestins might exert favorable effects on intelligence. The error of this interpretation became clear when it was discovered that elevated IQ was also present in unaffected members of the same families who did not have atypical hormone exposure (e.g., Reinisch and Karow 1977). This illustrates the importance of appropriate control groups. The currently accepted explanation is that the "IQ effect" was nothing more than an artifact of selection bias in the groups of patients who took part in the early research. In other words, better educated or brighter patients might have disproportionately been aware of or able to afford treatment at the prestigious specialty clinics where these studies were done, or else were willing to take part in IQ-related research projects in disproportionate numbers.

A different picture is emerging from recent studies of sexually differentiated cognitive functions. Increasingly, there is support for an organizing effect of early androgen on spatial ability. It is possible that other cognitive functions are organized by early androgens, too, but so far spatial abilities have received the most intensive study.

CONGENITAL ADRENAL HYPERPLASIA

Some of the best evidence for an organizational effect on spatial abilities comes from studies of females who have CAH. Because of their malelike early hormone environment, we might expect to see improved spatial abilities in girls with CAH relative to control girls, if spatial functions are organized by early androgens. Two studies do confirm this prediction. Resnick and colleagues (1986) found that young women with CAH outperformed their unaffected female relatives on three tests of spatial abilities. This effect was seen only on spatial measures. Recently Hampson, Rovet, and Altmann (1998) found that pre-pubertal girls with CAH scored higher than female sibling controls on a standardized test of spatial visualization (figure 15.5). A double dissociation was found in the Hampson study in that the girls with CAH also got *poorer* scores than control girls on a test of perceptual speed, a function

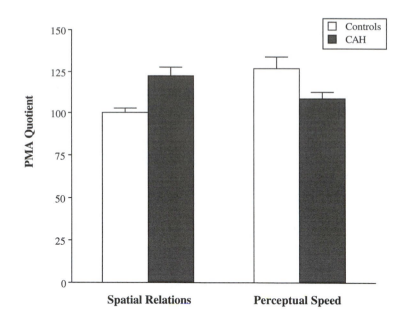

Figure 15.5 Cognitive abilities in girls with CAH may be altered as a result of their early life exposure to high levels of androgens. We gave a test of spatial ability to girls with CAH and their sisters. The girls with CAH had significantly better spatial ability, but they scored lower on a test of perceptual speed than their unaffected sisters. This type of spatial ability—spatial visualization—typically is better in males. (Redrawn from Hampson 2000.)

that normally shows a female advantage. The size of the spatial effect in both studies was large, with CAH girls scoring near the mean of control boys. These two studies support an early organizing effect of androgens, but not all studies of people with CAH have found improved spatial ability (e.g., Baker and Ehrhardt 1974; McGuire, Ryan, and Omenn 1975). Methodological factors are the likely reason for the differing results, including small sample sizes, use of atypical spatial tests, or factors related to the general health of the CAH groups.

Spatial abilities may not be the only abilities affected by prenatal hormones in CAH. A deficit on arithmetic tests in females with CAH has also been reported (Baker and Ehrhardt 1974; Perlman 1973). This might seem paradoxical at first glance because mathematical reasoning is an ability at which males normally excel. If anything, however, females have the advantage in performing arithmetic operations and computations (Jensen 1988). The two studies finding a numerical deficit in CAH used tests emphasizing calculations and procedural knowledge, not mathematical problem-solving. Further studies are needed to clarify which cognitive skills are actually affected in CAH. The deficit could be due to a decrease in arithmetic aptitude, or it could be a deficit in perceptual speed and accuracy, or something else. Perceptual speed favors females, so it would come as no surprise if it were adversely affected by excess androgens in girls with CAH.

EXPOSURE TO EXOGENOUS HORMONES

A few studies have examined spatial abilities in people exposed to diethylstilbestrol (DES) in utero. DES is a synthetic estrogen that has masculinizing or defeminizing effects in the CNS in other species. Investigating people with DES exposure is important for helping to clarify whether the organizing effects of early androgens on spatial abilities might occur by the aromatization route. The role of estrogen in the differentiation of the primate brain is less certain than in rodents, but the possible involvement of estrogen in cortical differentiation is suggested by the fact that aromatase activity is found in the association cortex of developing rhesus monkey brains (MacLusky, Naftolin, and Goldman-Rakic 1986). With respect to spatial abilities, the evidence from DES studies is inconclusive so far. Yalom and colleagues (1973) found that boys exposed to DES and small amounts of synthetic progestins were less aggressive, less athletic, and had lower scores on the Embedded Figures Test than two comparison groups. In an analysis of 10 pairs of brothers, one of whom was DES-exposed, Reinisch and Sanders (1992) found the exposed brothers achieved lower scores than controls on an index of spatial ability. Hines and Shipley (1984) found that DES-exposed women showed no advantage on a spatial measure. More recently, Hines and Sandberg (1996) failed to find any effect of DES in women on six spatial tests assessing four different types of spatial ability. There were indications, however, that the timing of DES exposure might be an important consideration. Hines found that being exposed to DES late in gestation was associated with higher scores on a composite measure of spatial ability.

The confusing results from DES studies may be telling us something important. An intriguing possibility is that the effects of DES exposure may depend on an individual's sex. A few studies in animals have hinted that excessive levels of androgens or estrogens in early development can demasculinize behavior in males (Baum and Schretlen 1975; Diamond et al. 1973). Consistent with this, in the CAH study by Hampson and colleagues (1998), boys with CAH showed reduced spatial scores compared with their brothers, a change in the demasculinized direction despite their increased androgen production in utero. Lower spatial ability in boys as a result of exposure to DES is therefore not altogether out of the question. But if DES is, in fact, neuroactive, why haven't women exposed to DES been found to show the expected masculinization of spatial functions? The findings by Hines and Sandberg (1996) suggest it may be profitable to study women who were exposed to DES very late in gestation. If DES does prove to have effects on spatial abilities in both men and women, we will not only have evidence for sexual differentiation of a cognitive function by the aromatization route, but we will also have a tool that can shed light on the *timing* of the sensitive period. By carefully studying the timing of DES exposure that does and does not lead to cognitive effects, we can begin to delimit the critical period when these effects can occur.

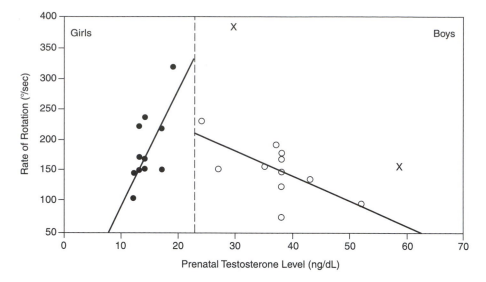

Figure 15.6 Grimshaw et al. (1995) studied the relationship between prenatal testosterone (T) and later spatial abilities. Testosterone was measured in amniotic fluid obtained 14 to 20 weeks after conception. Mental rotation was tested in the same children when they reached 7 years of age. Prenatal T was positively correlated with spatial scores in girls, but negatively correlated with spatial scores in boys. (Redrawn from Grimshaw, Sitarenios, and Finegan 1995.)

In the next section, we will return to the issue of the paradoxical effects of androgens. Meanwhile, you might contemplate the implications that such effects could have for other behaviors. What are the implications for hormonal theories of sexual orientation in males?

EVIDENCE FROM THE NEW TECHNIQUES
Support for organizational effects of early androgens on spatial abilities is starting to emerge from other paradigms too. In one of the rare studies where prenatal androgens were measured directly, Grimshaw and colleagues (1995) found a positive correlation in girls between levels of T in amniotic fluid at 14 to 20 weeks gestation and later proficiency on a mental rotation test. Girls with higher prenatal T had faster mental rotation times. Boys showed a tendency for the opposite effect; in boys, rotation time was negatively correlated with prenatal T levels (figure 15.6). It should be stressed that Grimshaw's study does not necessarily identify weeks 14 to 20 as the critical period for differentiation of spatial functions. This is when amniotic fluid was taken, but roughly the same individual ranking of T could be present at many other points in development.

Only one study so far has used the twin method to assess spatial ability. Cole-Harding and colleagues (1988) found that females who had a male twin showed higher scores on a mental rotation test than females with a female twin, and showed faster spatial learning over repeated administrations of the test. Unfortunately, the authors did not control for the environmental effects of having a male sibling.

A Cautionary Note

Most of the studies that we've described in this section share a common assumption. They assume that if the human CNS is sensitive to the organizing influence of sex steroids, the critical period for sexual differentiation is most likely to occur during prenatal development. Although this is a reasonable working hypothesis, we should not be blind to other possibilities. Hier and Crowley (1982), for example, reported impaired spatial ability in men with severely low androgen levels due to a lifelong deficiency in gonadotropin-releasing hormone. This condition typically manifests itself as the failure to undergo puberty. However, these males are believed to undergo normal masculinization in utero, thanks to the presence of maternal gonadotropins. In Hier and Crowley's study, administration of androgens to a small group of these men as adults did not improve their spatial ability. Interestingly, men with a similar disorder acquired after a normal puberty as a result of a brain tumor or other causes did not show any spatial deficit, despite having severely low androgen levels. These data raise the possibility of a postnatal organizing influence of androgens on spatial ability that is exerted at or before the time of puberty.

Summary

To summarize, studies of the effects of prenatal hormones on cognitive abilities have produced suggestive results. There is no good evidence that general IQ is at all affected by sex steroids during early development. But an organizational effect is possible for spatial abilities and perhaps other sexually differentiated cognitive functions. Currently, evidence favoring an organizing influence is strongest for spatial functions. Even here, inconsistencies in the literature abound. The possibility of organizing effects in the human CNS is supported by data from other behavioral domains, including sex-typed gender role behaviors. Because of advances in medical care, our resources for studying organizational effects are dwindling. The advent of prenatal therapy for CAH and the discontinuation of widespread use of DES and other synthetic steroids during pregnancy mean that our children are healthier, but we need to find creative new tools for doing organizational studies in human beings.

Activational Effects of Sex Steroids on Cognition

In the last 10 years, researchers have begun to test the hypothesis that sex hormones might have activational influences on human cognition. Again, our scope for manipulating hormones is limited by ethical concerns. We must rely on natural biorhythms in hormone-secretion patterns or on medical conditions that involve hormonal interventions to obtain scientific data.

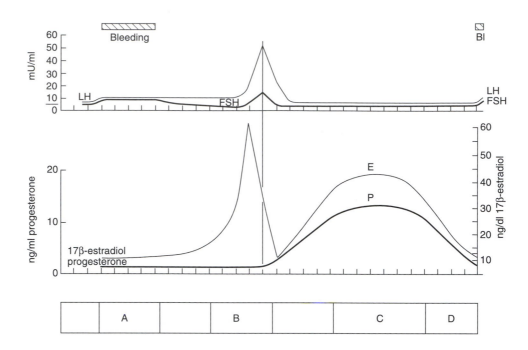

Figure 15.7 Schematic representation of the human menstrual cycle. By convention, the first day of menstruation is day 1, and the other days are numbered consecutively from that point. Day of cycle is depicted on the horizontal axis. *Top:* The pattern of changes in LH and FSH secretion, *Bottom:* Changes in the secretion of estradiol and progesterone. The vertical line between panels indicates the timing of the LH peak. Notice that estradiol and progesterone are lowest during menstruation (menses). There is a peak in estradiol just before ovulation and a more gradual rise in the week after ovulation. A, menses (menstrual phase), B, preovulatory phase, C, midluteal phase, D, premenstrual phase. (Redrawn from Ganong 1977.)

Initially, studies of activational effects on cognition relied on the menstrual cycle as a way to study the effects of large changes in ovarian steroids. Findings from the menstrual-cycle literature will be summarized below. More recently, other methods have been added. While ovarian hormones have begun to receive serious attention, we still know very little about the effects of androgens in the adult CNS.

Evidence From the Menstrual Cycle

Figure 15.7 shows the terms we will use to label the phases of the menstrual cycle. You will need to be familiar with these to understand the following discussion.

AFFECTIVE CHANGES OVER THE MENSTRUAL CYCLE

Until recently, studies of the menstrual cycle focused on mood changes, specifically the negative changes in affect reported premenstrually. Such changes have been reported in ordinary women and to a magnified extent in women who have premenstrual syndrome (PMS). Typically, self-reported depression, anxiety, and hostility peak in the premenstrual or early menstrual days (Ivey and Bardwick 1968; May 1976). But not all women experience emotional changes at this time, and the severity of changes can vary markedly from woman to woman and cycle to cycle. The term "**premenstrual syndrome**" is applied to the most severe premenstrual affective and physical changes.

Many theories of the origins of PMS have been proposed but so far researchers have failed to identify any consistent difference in endocrine variables between women who do and women who do not report emotional changes. The inconsistency of symptoms and the absence of visible differences in hormonal profiles have contributed to the view, still held by some medical professionals, that premenstrual distress has a psychological origin, not a physical one. This view, however, is increasingly difficult to sustain. In favor of a physiological basis, recent studies have reported behavioral changes suggestive of a PMS-like state in nonhuman primates during the few days prior to menstruation (Hausfater and Skoblick 1985). Personality variables, diet, and environmental factors may sharpen or reduce the symptoms in humans, but a hormonal trigger of some kind seems likely. The literature on PMS is complicated by methodological problems in many studies and by a lack of consensus on how to define the concept itself.

Partly because research has emphasized the premenstrual phase, and partly because most instruments designed to assess mood are heavily weighted toward negative items, increased feelings of well-being around ovulation have been less thoroughly documented. These feelings apparently do occur, at least in some women (Abplanalp et al. 1979; Rossi 1980; Sanders 1983). In our own work, we confirmed an enhancement in positive affect during the preovulatory peak in estrogen (Hampson 1990b). There are also reports of a buoyant effect of exogenous estrogens on mood. For example, Sherwin and Gelfand (1985), in a double-blind crossover study, reported amelioration of depression in surgically menopausal women during periods when they were on hormone replacement therapy. This seems to confirm the theory that mood changes are tied to the presence of hormones.

To summarize, mood alterations over the menstrual cycle are common knowledge among laymen. Yet in the laboratory, it has been remarkably difficult to confirm that mood changes *are* linked to the menstrual cycle, or that any linkage is due to ovarian hormones rather than psychological factors (e.g., expectancy effects) or other nonhormonal causes. Complicating the problem is the fact that mood states are not directly observable and can only be quantified by self-report. Even if we do accept that ovarian hormones can affect mood, the mechanism for this is unclear. Two kinds of mechanisms have been proposed: (1) direct hormone-induced changes in neurochemistry, possibly in catecholamine- or serotonin-containing transmitter systems, and (2) mood changes that are secondary to physical discomfort or indirect metabolic alterations caused by steroids (e.g., alterations in calcium balance)

(Thys-Jacobs and Alvir 1995). There is evidence to support both types of mechanism.

SPATIAL ABILITIES

In recent years, researchers have begun to consider whether ovarian hormones might have regulatory effects on spatial abilities. Several labs have discovered modest variations across the menstrual cycle in women's performance on spatial tests. The variations are believed to be linked to estrogen levels.

Only in the last 10 years have studies been explicitly designed to test the activational hypothesis. At least three earlier studies, though, indicated that spatial functions might vary over the menstrual cycle, even though they did not conceptualize their own findings in this way. Studies by Komnenich and colleagues (1978) and Broverman and colleagues (1981) detected lower scores in the week before ovulation on the Embedded Figures Test (EFT). These researchers chose the EFT to measure "perceptual restructuring," a central concept in a theory proposed by Broverman and colleagues (1968). However, a case could be made that the EFT is really a spatial test, because it involves finding a simple figure hidden inside a set of more complex patterns (see figure 15.1). An earlier study of aptitude test scores of women in the British Armed Forces suggested better performance at menses on a test that involved assembling parts into a model with the aid of diagrams (Wickham 1958). All three studies had weak methodology but their findings did lay the groundwork for later systematic research.

Our own studies were the first to explicitly test the possibility of an activational effect of ovarian hormones on cognitive processes. In three studies, we observed modest changes in women's scores on spatial tests that depended on the phase of the menstrual cycle (Hampson and Kimura 1988; Hampson 1990a, 1990b). Scores were discernibly higher at menses than at either the midluteal peak in estrogen and progesterone or the preovulatory peak in estradiol. Three spatial tests were included. The results from these three tests supported the idea that spatial ability is diminished at very high levels of estradiol in women. Since progesterone is still low during the preovulatory estrogen peak, the finding of lower spatial scores in the preovulatory phase implicated estrogen as the active hormone.

These findings have been confirmed by subsequent researchers (e.g., McCourt et al. 1997; Moody 1997; Phillips and Silverman 1997; Silverman and Phillips 1993). Example results are shown in figure 15.8. A few studies, however, failed to detect any menstrual cycle effects (Gordon and Lee 1993; Peters et al. 1995). Therefore, whether there are true cycle-related changes in spatial ability is still a matter of some debate. It seems likely, however, that methodological factors can explain the different findings. Studies that use group testing where women are tested in large groups without any independent confirmation of hormone status are unlikely to succeed because verbal self-reports are not a very accurate indicator of the stage of the cycle. More

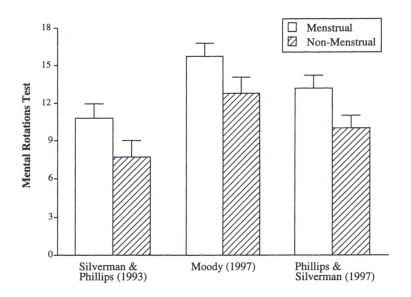

Figure 15.8 Studies of the menstrual cycle have suggested that women's scores on spatial tests are at their best during the menstrual phase, when their estrogen levels are lowest. The results shown here come from several studies that used the Mental Rotations Test to measure spatial ability. This is the test of spatial orientation you saw earlier, in box 15.1. The fact that spatial ability changes over the menstrual cycle is one piece of evidence for an activational influence of estrogen on human cognition.

subtle factors might also be at work. One possibility that has not been explored is that age might enter the equation. Full adult levels of ovarian output are not reached until the early to mid 20s (Ellison 1993). It is possible that any menstrual cycle effect might not be fully apparent in younger women. The type of spatial test might also be important. Phillips and Silverman (1997) argued that tasks involving visualization in three dimensions may be more sensitive to ovarian hormones than simple two-dimensional tasks because they have greater ecological validity, that is, more resemblance to the natural world in which spatial abilities evolved as an adaptation to our three-dimensional environment. Whether this turns out to be correct or not, it is a thought-provoking hypothesis.

PERCEPTUAL SPEED AND ACCURACY

If high levels of estrogen are associated with reduced spatial scores, do other cognitive functions show the same pattern of variation over the menstrual cycle? The answer seems to be no. Fewer studies have looked at abilities that favor women, but the data available so far suggest that if these abilities do vary, the pattern may be very different from what's seen for spatial ability.

Snyder (1977) noted faster performance during days 17 to 22 of the cycle than during the premenstrual and early menstrual days on the Matching Familiar Figures Test. This test has a strong perceptual speed component, in that it requires fine visual discriminations to be made as quickly as possible among sets of similar-appearing stimuli. Similarly, Anderson (1972) found better performance on a measure of perceptual speed during the luteal phase of the cycle than during the early follicular days. However, almost all of Anderson's tests exhibited better luteal-phase performance, including two spatial tests. In our own studies, we found weak evidence of better perceptual speed at the midluteal phase (Hampson 1990a) but no difference between the menstrual and pre-ovulatory phases (Hampson 1990b). A study by Arushanyan and Borovkova (1993) found maximum performance on a proofreading test in 9 of 11 young women at either the mid- or late-luteal phase. In summary, the existing studies imply luteal-phase facilitation in perceptual speed, but due to the scarcity of studies, the issue is far from settled.

VERBAL ABILITIES AND ARTICULATION OF SPEECH
Several investigators have found faster luteal-phase performance on simple verbal-articulatory tasks, such as reading words aloud, naming colors, counting, or repeating syllables (e.g., Anderson 1972). Broverman and colleagues (1981) reported that performance on one such task was faster during the presumed estrogen surge just prior to ovulation than during the luteal phase. More complex verbal tasks have seldom been studied. Wickham (1958), in a large sample, found slightly poorer scores during the menstrual phase than on other days of the cycle on a test involving comprehension of complex instructions. Hampson (1990a) found small changes across the menstrual cycle in verbal fluency, as assessed by tasks requiring women to think of either single words or whole sentences fitting particular phonetic criteria. Performance was better at the midluteal estrogen and progesterone peak than at the menstrual phase when ovarian hormones are low. In another study, we failed to find any facilitation in fluency during the peak in estradiol just prior to ovulation (Hampson 1990b). Both of our studies, however, did reveal a highly significant enhancement at higher estrogen levels of the types of simple verbal-articulatory skills mentioned above (e.g., syllable repetition and speeded counting).

A different measure of verbal output was examined by Silverman, who observed a premenstrual increase in speech errors in a group of women stutterers, compared to their speech quality at midcycle (Silverman, Zimmer, and Silverman 1974). In a later study of nonstutterers, Silverman and Zimmer (1975) counted incidents of speech dysfluency while the women spoke on designated topics. Though ovulation was not always targeted successfully, 9 of 12 women produced more dysfluencies premenstrually than at midcycle. In the work of Silverman and his colleagues, the premenstrual and periovulatory phases were selected for study to maximize state differences in anxiety, which was thought to be the mechanism responsible for the changes. In light of other work, the changes in articulatory accuracy may have reflected changes in sex steroid concentrations per se.

One piece of evidence that favors an effect of ovarian hormones on language-related behaviors is truly unique. It comes from studies of Koko, a

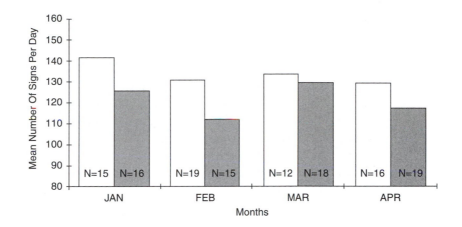

Figure 15.9 A unique piece of evidence that supports an influence of ovarian hormones on cognition comes from Koko, a female lowland gorilla. Koko has been taught to use American Sign Language, the language of the deaf. Koko's output of signs has been found to vary with her estrous cycle. As in human studies of verbal behavior, Koko's signing fluency increases during the week before ovulation when her estrogen levels are rising. (Redrawn from Patterson, Holts, and Saphire 1991.)

female lowland gorilla that has been trained to communicate using American Sign Language. Koko's menstrual cycle has been monitored in captivity since she achieved menarche (onset of menstrual cyclicity at puberty). Detailed records of Koko's signing behaviors have also been kept for many years. In a retrospective analysis of records, Patterson and colleagues (1991) found an association between rises in Koko's estrogen and her level of signed output. Both the number of discrete signs used and the total number of signs per day rose during periovulatory periods, when Koko's estrogen concentrations were raised (figure 15.9).

To summarize, only a few studies have investigated menstrual cycle changes in verbal abilities or perceptual speed. The data available suggest that simple verbal output tasks, such as speed and accuracy of articulation, may be improved at phases of the menstrual cycle characterized by high concentrations of estrogen. The picture for complex verbal functions and perceptual speed is still unclear.

BASIC SENSORY PROCESSES

Are there changes in basic sensory thresholds over the menstrual cycle? There is a small research literature on this topic that has been reviewed by Parlee (1983) and others. Evidence suggests that women's visual sensitivity increases around ovulation (e.g., Diamond, Diamond, Mast 1972; Friedman and Meares 1978; Wong and Tong 1974), as does olfactory sensitivity to certain volatile compounds (Doty et al. 1981). Visual sensitivity is lowest during menstruation. An important point to note is that the changes in visual sensitivity do not parallel the changes in spatial abilities observed across the menstrual cycle. If anything, the two types of functions show opposite patterns, suggesting that alterations in spatial ability are not reducible to changes in basic visual function.

MOTOR BEHAVIORS

Quite a few studies, old and new, have sought to discover whether there are changes in motor behavior across the menstrual cycle. One impetus for this line of research has been self-reports by some Olympic women athletes (Zaharieva 1965) and other sportswomen (Erdelyi 1962) of menstrual or premenstrual declines in athletic performance. Furthermore, Dalton (1960) reported that among women, more than half of all accidents requiring hospitalization or immediate medical care occurred during menstruation or the 4 days preceding it, a finding she suggested might be related to a slowing of reaction times.

Prior to our own work on motor behavior, a few studies showed trends suggesting a menstrual or premenstrual decrement (Stocker 1973; Wearing et al. 1972). These effects appear to be specific to only certain types of motor tasks. Zimmerman and Parlee (1973) reported that arm-hand steadiness was greater during the early luteal phase than premenstrually. A premenstrual decrease in hand steadiness was confirmed by Hudgens and colleagues (1988). In that study, women on average showed greater hand steadiness than men, both on a conventional steadiness task and in holding firearms (!). Becker et al. (1982) found that during menses the total time needed to trace a line was longer, and preferred tapping speed was slower, than during the follicular phase. Three studies have looked at the frequency of spontaneous limb movement across the menstrual cycle (Billings 1934; Morris and Udry 1970; Stenn and Klinge 1972). All reported variations in activity, although aspects of the methodology are open to question. Stenn and Klinge (1972) found that 2 of 7 women examined over several menstrual cycles showed systematic changes in arm movement activity, with peak activity most likely to occur in the late luteal phase and least likely in the menstrual phase. Billings (1934) reported a burst of physical activity around the expected time of ovulation in a small group of psychiatric in-patients. Morris and Udry (1970) obtained a midcycle peak in physical activity as recorded by a pedometer.

Our own menstrual-cycle studies revealed changes in manual dexterity across the cycle. Hampson and Kimura (1988) found better midluteal than menstrual performance on several measures of manual speed and coordination, including the Manual Sequence Box described earlier (figure 15.3). In another study, we found that women performed better on the same motor tasks at the preovulatory estrogen peak than at menstruation (Hampson 1990b). These findings suggest that high levels of ovarian hormones are associated with improved manual performance, at least on the sorts of small-amplitude motor tasks used in our studies. The type of motor behavior examined is probably a critical determinant of whether any facilitative effects of ovarian hormones are seen. In recent work, Saucier and Kimura (1998) observed facilitation at the midluteal phase on the Manual Sequence Box, but not on a gross motor task that involved throwing balls at a remote target. Szekely and colleagues (1998) found effects in oral contraceptive users on the Manual Sequence Box but not on measures of visually guided reaching toward nearby targets. It may be the case that one of the neural systems regulated by estrogen in humans is the left hemisphere "praxis" system we alluded to earlier.

With respect to reaction times, studies have consistently failed to find significant cyclic variations in either simple or choice reaction time (e.g., Hutt et al. 1980; Jensen 1982; Pierson and Lockhart 1963; Zimmerman and Parlee 1973). This is contrary to Dalton's (1960) speculation that reaction times may be slower around the time of menstrual onset and thus contribute to an increase in accidents.

Summary of Menstrual-Cycle Results

Evidence that ovarian hormones can affect the expression of sexually differentiated cognitive and motor functions continues to mount. Evidence also comes from nonmenstrual-cycle paradigms. We will discuss those findings in the next section. Most menstrual-cycle studies suggest the following generalization: *High levels of estrogen may adversely affect certain spatial abilities that normally show a male advantage. High levels of ovarian hormones may improve some abilities that normally show a female advantage, especially abilities related to speech and manual coordination.*

Some researchers have assumed that if changes in cognitive function do occur, they must be a result of changes in mood states across the menstrual cycle. The existing data do not support this interpretation. First of all, reciprocal changes in different functions seem to occur at the same points in the menstrual cycle, which is hard to reconcile with explanations in terms of mood. Second, many studies reporting alterations across the menstrual cycle in cognition or motor function have tried but failed to find concurrent changes in women's self-reported mood states. In a few studies, even though variations in affect did occur, they could not be related in any obvious way to scores on cognitive tests. For example, in one of our own studies, women reported periovulatory *enhancement* in vigor and well-being, yet at the same stage of the cycle, they actually showed *poorer*, not better, scores on spatial measures (Hampson 1990b). Statistically, scores on mood inventories do not appear able to explain the cognitive or motor changes. We should not be surprised. If mood changes arise from alterations in neurochemistry induced by sex steroids, there is no reason why cognitive changes could not occur independently through similar mechanisms.

One last type of explanation must be considered. Is it possible that the variations in cognition and variations in hormone output only *appear* to be linked because they are both a function of some central pacemaker in the CNS? There are several reasons to believe a pacemaker is not responsible. First of all, we know from animal studies that sex steroids have numerous direct effects at the cellular level that can affect neural functioning. It is more parsimonious to assume these can generalize to humans than to invoke a hypothetical pacemaker. Second, a single pacemaker could not explain the divergent pattern of changes shown by different cognitive abilities across the menstrual cycle. At the very least, we would have to hypothesize multiple pacemakers or, in a worst case scenario, a separate pacemaker for each distinct type of ability. This rapidly becomes implausible. Third, the ovarian cycle is a self-perpetuating feedback process regulated by the hypothalamus-pituitary-gonadal axis. In primates, it can proceed with little intervention from higher brain areas. It is not clear that a pacemaker is important for producing the endocrine events associated with the menstrual cycle. Finally, studies involving exogenous administration of estrogens, either in laboratory animals or in humans, have started to confirm the effects on spatial and motor functions seen in menstrual-cycle studies. This seems to rule out intrinsic biorhythms generated by the CNS as the basis of the effects. We'll return to this point later.

Correlates of Hormonal Variation in Men

Recently researchers have begun to investigate whether there are activational effects of androgens in men. Two approaches have been adopted. One is to study behavioral changes in men undergoing androgen treatments or androgen suppression for medical purposes. The other approach uses naturally occurring biorhythms in androgen production, based on the same logic as the menstrual-cycle studies we just discussed. The initial results suggest that androgens or their derivatives may regulate certain cognitive abilities in men.

Spatial abilities are natural candidates for such regulation. We know that there is a male advantage in many spatial functions. We also suspect that early androgen exposure may contribute to sexual dimorphism within spatial-processing systems. A reasonable hypothesis, therefore, is that if any activating effect of adult T does exist, it would accentuate the behavioral dimorphism. The working hypothesis in most studies, therefore, is that higher adult T concentrations will be associated with better spatial abilities *within* the male sex. This does seem to be true, within limits. But for reasons that we don't yet understand, research suggests that further increases in T beyond a certain optimum concentration might actually be linked to diminished spatial abilities in men. The optimum is fairly high, with several studies suggesting an optimum T concentration near the mid to lower end of the young adult range. Thus, in the studies we are about to review, it is often found that men with low T benefit from an increase in T, but that men with the very highest levels of T, such as young men in the prime of their lives, experience improvement in spatial function during periods when their T levels are temporarily lowered.

Not all studies have tried to manipulate T concentrations. Some have just observed the relationship across a number of individuals between scores on spatial measures and circulating T levels, as measured by serum or saliva RIAs. Saliva is a direct measure of the component of T that is free or bioavailable. Women with high concentrations of androgens in serum or saliva seem to do better on spatial tests than women with low androgens, while men with high androgens perform worse than their male counterparts with lower androgens. The studies have been done in healthy people whose androgen concentrations fell within the normal physiological range. This pattern has been found on tests of spatial visualization (Gouchie and Kimura 1991; Moffat and Hampson 1996; Shute et al. 1983), spatial orientation (Gouchie and Kimura 1991; Moffat and Hampson 1996), and mixed indices of spatial functioning (e.g., Gouchie and Kimura 1991; Moffat and Hampson 1996). Using the same approach, Christiansen (1993) found a positive association in the !Kung San of Namibia between free T and scores on the Rod-and-Frame test, but T values in that study fell at the lower end of the normal range for young men in Western countries. In all studies, measures of verbal performance were used as controls, and were either unrelated to T or showed the opposite pattern of relationships. Without manipulating androgens, observational studies only provide a snapshot glimpse of relationships between hormones and cognitive abilities. Any relationships revealed could be activational in origin, but the studies contain no way to verify this.

Recent studies based on biorhythms in T secretion suggest that at least part of the observed correlations may indeed be due to activational influences. In men, T secretion shows a diurnal rhythm. Plasma or saliva T concentrations in the early morning are about 20 to 50% higher than in the evening. Two studies now suggest that diurnal variations in spatial proficiency might occur in men, related to the daily rhythm in T secretion. An old study by Mackenberg and colleagues (1974) found that morning performance on a naming task was significantly faster in men than their afternoon performance, whereas a reverse pattern was seen on the EFT. Infusion of intravenous T partly but significantly reversed the afternoon decline in simple automatized skills (Klaiber et al. 1974). Moffat and Hampson (1996) found that from early to late morning, men's scores on the Mental Rotations Test improved but women's deteriorated, as we might predict from the typical drop in testosterone levels that occurs over this time period. Time-of-day effects were found only on spatial measures and not on two verbal fluency tests used as controls. Further hints that circulating T might have reversible effects on spatial ability in men comes from recent work on circannual cycles. Men living at northern latitudes have higher T, on average, in autumn than in spring. We verified this in our lab (figure 15.10A). Kimura and Hampson (1994) found that men's performance on a composite index of spatial ability was better in spring, when T was lower, than in autumn (figure 15.10B). Female controls showed no significant seasonal changes, either in T or in spatial proficiency.

These studies are new and must be replicated and expanded. Still, it seems safe to argue that the expression of spatial abilities in men, just as in women, might fluctuate with changes in ambient levels of sex steroids. Support for an activational effect of androgens comes from studies in which T levels were altered for medical reasons. Let's turn to these now.

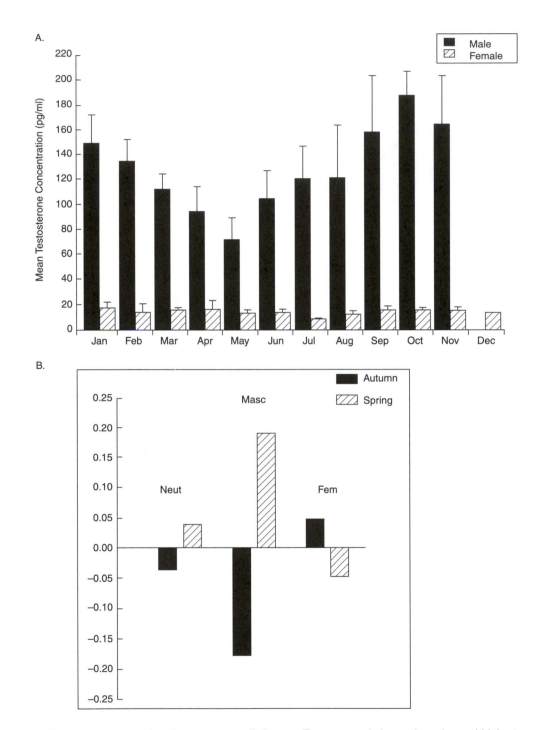

Figure 15.10   (*A*) Testosterone secretion changes seasonally in men. Testosterone is lowest in spring and highest in autumn for men living at northern latitudes. (Redrawn from Moffat and Hampson 2000.) (*B*) Some evidence suggests that there may be corresponding changes in spatial ability. Kimura and Hampson (1994) found that men performed better on spatial tests (Masc) in spring than in fall. Seasonal changes were not found in other abilities (Fem, Neut), nor did women show any seasonal changes. (Redrawn from Kimura and Hampson 1994.)

Other Nonmenstrual Studies

EFFECTS OF THERAPEUTIC MANIPULATIONS OF HORMONES
Additional evidence for the reversible effects of hormones on human cognitive functions comes from recent medical research. In these studies, sex hormones were either administered or suppressed for therapeutic reasons. A special case of this is the use of estrogen replacement therapy (ERT) after menopause, which we shall mention below. Otherwise, studies involving direct interventions are still pretty rare.

Estrogen is used therapeutically to treat girls with Turner's syndrome or in cases of transsexuality where a formal sex change is desired. Turner's syndrome is a condition in which one of the two sex chromosomes is missing or structurally abnormal. The ovaries do not develop normally in girls with Turner's syndrome and consequently, estrogen therapy must be given at puberty to induce the development of secondary sex characteristics. Girls with Turner's syndrome do not make a good research population for activational studies because the chromosomal defect alters many aspects of development and because their organizational history of early-life hormone exposure is likely to be unusual. In a report by Van Goozen and colleagues (1995), however, 15 male-to-female transsexuals in the Netherlands received treatment with anti-androgens and estrogens on a daily basis as a prelude to sex reassignment surgery. After 3 months of cross-sex hormone treatment, spatial ability had declined and verbal fluency had improved, although the changes were fairly small.

Androgen treatments have been examined for their effects on cognition, and again, evidence of an activational influence has been obtained. As a complement to the data described above, Van Goozen and colleagues (1994, 1995) studied cognitive abilities in female-to-male transsexuals being treated with T esters. After 3 months of cross-sex hormones, performance on a mental rotation test had increased relative to pretreatment baseline and relative to controls who were not treated with hormones. Scores on verbal fluency tests deteriorated (Van Goozen et al. 1995; Van Goozen et al. 1994). Of course, transsexuals may not be very representative of ordinary males or females. But there's no reason to think their brains would be especially susceptible to the activation of cognitive circuits. This is the only scenario where we can gather data on hormonal treatments in the opposite sex.

A recent study by Janowsky and colleagues (1994) supports the transsexual findings. Janowsky found improved spatial ability under androgen treatment in healthy normal men. They were treated with T on an experimental basis to rectify age-related decline in T. Treated men showed a selective improvement in spatial ability after 3 months of T treatment, whereas this was not seen in placebo-treated controls. In both Van Goozen's and Janowsky's studies, T concentrations before treatment were extremely low. Under these circumstances we expect, if anything, to see improvement in spatial scores with increases in T. You should be aware, however, that not all studies support an effect of T on spatial ability. Alexander and colleagues (1998), for example, failed to detect any changes in spatial scores in a group of hypogonadal men following T treatment, but did find that verbal fluency improved. T levels increased with treatment, but were still well below the normal male range. This might have had a bearing on Alexander's results. It is possible that other factors associated with hypogonadism also make it less likely that T treatments will be effective.

To summarize, data from various sources is starting to support the view that circulating sex steroids in adults can modify the expression of specific cognitive functions. This may apply to androgens in men as well as to estrogens in women.

ESTROGENS AND MEMORY AFTER MENOPAUSE

In the last few years, a great deal of research has been done on cognitive functioning in post-menopausal women receiving hormone replacement therapy (HRT). These studies are pertinent to the question of activational effects of estrogens but do not enlighten us about spatial abilities because they have focused almost exclusively on memory. Estrogen, combined in most cases with progestin, is given to menopausal women who are at risk for osteoporosis or who have other medical indications. Estrogen is also given to women who are surgically post-menopausal, that is, who have had a complete hysterectomy including removal of the ovaries. On average, surgically menopausal women are younger than naturally menopausal women and in better health.

One of the most consistent findings is that estrogen might help to maintain verbal memory in women following menopause. This is interesting because, as we saw earlier, verbal memory is a function for which there is a female advantage in young adults. For example, in a group of 12 women who underwent a complete hysterectomy with ovarian removal, Sherwin and Phillips (1990) found that women who were treated with estrogen postoperatively showed higher scores on two verbal memory tests at a 2-month follow-up than women who were treated with placebos. There had been no difference in memory in the two groups before the surgery. Interestingly, memory decline is a common complaint among menopausal women, a complaint often dismissed as a natural part of aging. Beneficial effects of estrogen replacement on verbal memory have now been replicated in quite a few studies (for a review, see Sherwin 1996).

Recent work suggests that estrogen might benefit other cognitive functions, too. Kimura (1995) found that long-term users of estrogen replacement had better scores than postmenopausal women who did not use estrogen replacement on several sexually differentiated functions other than verbal memory. Estrogen users had better scores, on average, regardless of whether the cognitive functions favored men or women, suggesting an across-the-board effect. In an epidemiological study, Paganini-Hill and Henderson (1994) found that the use of estrogen was associated with a reduced risk of contracting Alzheimer's disease in aging women. Although these findings are new and controversial, a plausible mechanism has been identified biochemically that could mediate an anti-Alzheimer's effect. In vitro, estrogen reduces the likelihood that an abnormal peptide will be formed, amyloid βA4, which is the central component of senile plaques, one of the characteristic pathological features of Alzheimer's brains (Jaffe et al. 1994).

Research on the role of estrogen in the aging brain is extremely important. We can anticipate exciting new developments over the next few years. Right now, a growing body of evidence suggests that estrogen may have a protective effect on certain elements of brain function in aging women. Because only a few researchers have studied cognitive abilities outside the memory domain, further work is needed to evaluate whether the effects of estrogen on cognition are more widespread. It will also be important to verify that mood changes are not the mediating mechanism for any across-the-board improvements in cognitive function. At the doses used to treat menopausal symptoms, estrogen can have elevating effects on mood, although these may be partially offset by the progestin component of HRT (Sherwin 1994). As for the role of T in aging men and its potential for maintaining cognitive function, virtually nothing is known.

PREGNANCY

You may have noticed that we haven't discussed one of the major changes in endocrine function that marks the life of most women—pregnancy. Estrogen concentrations increase dramatically during pregnancy, especially in the third trimester. In principle, this could affect cognitive function. But pregnancy is enormously complex from an endocrine viewpoint. There are changes in other hormones, plus a host of psychological, physical, and lifestyle changes at that time. This makes it very difficult to pinpoint which factors are responsible for any cognitive changes observed.

For these and other reasons, there has been little effort to study the neuroendocrinology of pregnancy. Complaints of memory difficulties are fairly common in pregnant women, and a few recent studies have reported impairments during pregnancy on objective memory tests (e.g., Buckwalter et al. 1999). So far, any impairments have not been convincingly related to the elevations in sex steroids. A study by Woodfield (1984) found lower scores on the EFT during the 38 to 40th weeks of pregnancy than six weeks after childbirth, when circulating sex steroids had declined. A nonspatial control test showed no changes over the same interval. Whether sex hormones were responsible for the cognitive change is far from clear.

Summary

Our goal in this section was to describe some of the emerging evidence that human cognitive and motor behaviors are modulated by sex steroids in adults. Most of the early data on activational influences came from studies of the menstrual cycle. Support has now been added from new paradigms. The pattern emerging from numerous studies is that circulating hormones can affect the expression of certain cognitive and motor functions. Current evidence implicates estrogen in females (although progesterone cannot be ruled out as also having some effects) and, more tentatively, T in males. Effects appear to be restricted to, or at least most pronounced among, cognitive functions that show sex differences. Either high or low concentrations of steroids can promote better performance: the direction of the effects depends on the sex of the individual, the exact function being studied, and probably other factors yet to be identified.

Discussion and Conclusions

If sex steroids do influence the organization and function of the human brain, then (1) what are the mechanisms responsible, and (2) what implications do the effects have for our everyday lives?

A Question of Mechanism

Human research in neuroendocrinology is still fairly new. This is especially true for higher-order brain functions such as cognition. Researchers have been preoccupied with elementary questions such as establishing whether or not hormone-behavior relationships do exist, and with ruling out nonhormonal factors that could provide competing explanations. As you already know, there are technical and ethical constraints on the kinds of research that can be accomplished in humans. For these and other reasons, we still know little about what mechanisms are responsible for the effects we've described. To make inferences about neural systems and molecular mechanisms, researchers must be guided by research in other species.

ORGANIZATIONAL EFFECTS

In other species, we know that prenatal or perinatal exposure to androgens or their metabolites can cause long-lasting structural changes in some brain regions. The SDN-POA in the rodent brain and the nuclei that control birdsong in passerines are examples of sites where such effects occur. As we saw earlier, sex differences in human brain organization are increasingly being reported. These have been found in in vivo studies using brain-imaging techniques and in conventional neuroanatomy studies. Unfortunately, we lack evidence that any of these sex differences result from the actions of hormones. Alternative possibilities are that the sex differences arise because of the different environmental experiences of the two sexes—that is, they are a result instead of a cause of behavioral differences. Or it is possible that some might have a genetic origin. Given the marked effects of sex steroids in sexual differentiation of the brain in other species, it would be surprising if some analogous effects did not occur in the human brain. But which sex differences are, and which are not, attributable to hormonal induction, is an open question.

One way to study this without having to manipulate hormones in developing infants is to study brain morphology in people who have atypical endocrine histories, such as CAH. For example, we know the volume of the SDN-POA, and the number and size of the neurons it contains are strongly determined in the rat by the level of androgen or estrogen exposure in the perinatal period. This is a plausible site for sex steroids to have organizational effects in humans, too. In fact, homologous cell groups in the human anterior hypothalamus have already been discovered which have a larger volume in men than in women (Allen et al. 1989; Swaab and Fliers 1985). If the same nuclei were found to be consistently larger in females with CAH, for example, than in control women, we would have circumstantial grounds for believing that sex hormones do contribute to this sexual dimorphism. Such studies have not yet been done.

In fact, there have been remarkably few attempts to study the brain organization of people with endocrine abnormalities, even using indirect methods. One exception is the report by Hines that DES-exposed women show a more masculine pattern of lateralization on a verbal dichotic listening test than their unexposed sisters (Hines and Shipley 1984). This raises the possibility of effects in the cerebral language zones. Before this hypothesis can be seriously entertained, though, greater confirmation would be needed, preferably from direct anatomical studies. Recent work by Plante and colleagues (1996) using MRI may be a first step in that direction. They found that five of six girls with CAH had atypical patterns of asymmetry in the perisylvian cortex, a region believed to be linked with language lateralization. Much further research needs to be done.

ACTIVATIONAL EFFECTS

Human studies of the past 10 to 15 years have established that sex steroids modulate a variety of cognitive and motor processes in the adult brain. At the same time, studies in the rat and other species have made gains in identifying the effects of sex steroids at the molecular and systems levels that could mediate behavioral effects in adult animals. We know, for example, that sex steroids interact with, and alter activity levels in, neurotransmitter systems projecting throughout the forebrain. Ironically, only a few years ago, when human studies first began to report the effects of ovarian hormones on cognitive and motor functions, skeptics claimed that such effects were impossible because sex hormones could not affect brain tissue outside the pituitary and hypothalamus. Now our challenge is to identify which of an ever-expanding array of neurochemical effects are responsible for the behavioral alterations we see in human studies.

Many effects on human behavior and cognition are probably mediated by the classical actions of sex steroids on the genome. In the classical model, steroids bind to ligand-specific receptors located in the cytoplasm or nucleus of target cells. Once transported to the nucleus they bind to acceptor sites on the genome (DNA) and activate RNA transcription. By altering protein synthesis, estradiol as well as other sex steroids are able to alter the concentrations of enzymes that participate in neurotransmitter synthesis or breakdown, and can alter receptor densities. Estradiol, for example, alters the expression of several different enzymes, affecting levels of activity in catecholamine, serotonin, and acetylcholine pathways (McEwen et al. 1997; McEwen et al. 1995). A given hormone may be capable of affecting multiple parameters related to the synthesis, release, re-uptake, degradation, or responsiveness to neurotransmitters, and may have effects in several different neurotransmitter systems simultaneously. Therefore, a single hormone may be able to alter multiple behavioral systems.

In humans, one of the most widely accepted effects of estrogens is their effect on mood in adult women. High estradiol levels, such as the preovulatory peak in estrogen, are associated with positive mood. Loss of estradiol is associated in some women with flattened mood or even depression. Estradiol has several effects on neurochemistry that could generate mood effects through genomic mechanisms. Animal studies, for example, indicate that central levels of monoamine oxidase (MAO) are reduced by exposure to estradiol. MAO is an enzyme that deactivates monoamines. MAO is probably hormone-dependent in humans, too, since MAO activity in plasma has been found to vary with the estrogen state in women (Klaiber et al. 1972). (MAO is present in the blood to help metabolize catecholamines and serotonin released peripherally.) Another of estradiol's actions is to increase the density of serotonin-binding sites in the forebrain (Fink et al. 1996). Both serotonin and norepinephrine systems have been implicated in clinical depression, and the fact that activity in these same systems is modulated in a positive fashion by estradiol is consistent with its antidepressive effects on mood.

Some activational effects of estrogens and progestins in the CNS seem to occur in brain areas that are devoid of classical intracellular receptors. One example of this is the action of estradiol on neostriatal functioning. Estradiol in this region alters dopaminergic activity in a complex manner and modulates motor output in both rats (chapter 13) and, tentatively, human beings. For example, we measured the degree of turning bias (toward the left or right) in women under high and low estrogen conditions. As discussed in chapter 13, rotational behavior is considered to be an index of striatal dopamine activity in the rat, with animals turning toward the side with lower dopamine concentrations. We found the strength of turning bias in humans, just as in rats, was altered by estrogen levels (Mead and Hampson 1997). Using a different index of striatal function that had been validated in patients with Parkinson's disease, Jennings and colleagues (1998) also found evidence of behavioral modulation by estrogen in women. In both studies, scores on the behavioral measures were correlated with women's estradiol levels but not with other hormones. In women with disorders of the motor system, the severity of extrapyramidal symptoms is said to vary with the estrogen state (Quinn and Marsden 1986). At present, membrane receptors are the best explanation for how activational phenomena can arise in brain regions that lack conventional intracellular receptors. (See chapters 2 and 13 for more discussion.)

The effects we have described don't exhaust the range of possible mechanisms by which sex steroids could produce activational effects on behavior. It is possible, for example, that hormones may evoke secondary effects on neural activity in brain areas that are synaptically connected with regions that are directly sensitive to sex steroids. We also know that estrogen can be hydroxylated in the brain, conferring a catechol structure on the molecule. It is still inconclusive whether the so-called catechol-estrogens are biologically active. Their potential interaction with enzymes involved in catecholamine metabolism, and possibly even with catecholamine receptors themselves, must be considered (Goy and McEwen 1980; McEwen et al. 1979). Finally, recent evidence suggests that sex steroids might help to regulate important glial cell functions, and we are just beginning to appreciate what this might mean (Baulieu et al. 1996; Garcia-Segura et al. 1996).

Techniques for Localizing Adult Hormone Effects

To summarize, human researchers are seldom able to make inferences about neural mechanisms at a cellular level. On the other hand, making inferences about *where* in the brain the effects might occur is more open to study. Currently, three approaches are being used to provide insights into localization: the neuroanatomical approach, the neuropsychological approach, and the neuroimaging approach.

THE NEUROANATOMICAL APPROACH

This approach uses brain tissue, usually obtained from biopsies or from neurosurgery, to identify specific steroid receptors and their densities in different brain areas, or to map out the distribution of the binding sites of specific hormones. For example, androgen receptors in human temporal neocortex have been detected in ligand-binding (Sarrieau et al. 1990) and in immunocytochemical studies (Puy et al. 1995) using brain tissue from young men. The men had a type of surgery in which parts of the temporal lobes were removed to treat severe epilepsy. Bixo and colleagues (1995) used female brain specimens from cadavers to examine the regional distribution of estradiol accumulation across 17 brain sites. One finding of interest, in light of our discussion of the possible effects of estrogen on dopamine activity in the basal ganglia, was the high concentration of estradiol observed in the substantia nigra.

Studies using the neuroanatomical approach are still rare. This type of work is limited by the lack of widely available receptor antibodies that work well in neural tissue, and by the unavailability of suitable brain specimens. There is rapid degradation in postmortem tissue, so specimens obtained from biopsies or neurosurgeries are the preferred option. But in these cases, tissue is often abnormal. Greater attention needs to be paid to subject characteristics in these studies, such as whether donors are taking medications like anti-convulsants or oral contraceptives that are known to affect steroid profiles.

THE NEUROPSYCHOLOGICAL APPROACH

This approach uses tests of perception, motor function, or cognition that have been demonstrated to assess the functionality of particular neural systems. Many of these tests have been validated by administering them to people with localized brain damage or other kinds of neuropathology. One example of a neuropsychological test is the Manual Sequence Box used by Hampson and Kimura (1988). This test is known to assess the integrity of a specific motor programming system located in the left cerebral hemisphere in most people. Several studies now indicate that performance on the Manual Sequence Box is reliably affected by estrogen status in women. This suggests that the praxis system is one neural system that may be steroid-sensitive in the human brain.

One drawback of the neuropsychological approach is that inferences based on behavioral tests are necessarily indirect; the underlying anatomy is never directly visualized. Therefore, researchers using this approach seek convergent evidence from several sources before drawing conclusions, and they must include intelligent controls in their studies to rule out competing explanations. In the case of the Manual Sequence Box, we know that the praxis system is responsible not just for programming of arm movements but also for programming sequential movements of the mouth and lower face. As expected, oral movements, too, are influenced by the level of ovarian hormones in women (Hampson 1990a, 1990b; Silverman et al. 1974).

THE NEUROIMAGING APPROACH

Recently, a few neuroimaging studies have begun to identify brain regions whose activation levels are dependent on hormone state. The studies use advanced imaging techniques such as functional MRI or PET. These techniques allow researchers to identify more and less active brain regions while subjects are engaged in mental activities specified by the researchers or while the brain is scanned at rest. Adapting these techniques for endocrine studies typically involves comparing the brain-activation patterns of subjects who are in different endocrine states at the time the brain is scanned. Shaywitz and colleagues (1999), for example, observed changes in patterns of activation in brain regions involved in memory and phonological processing when post-menopausal women were treated with a therapeutic dose of estrogen in a double-blind, placebo-controlled crossover trial. In this study, changes in activity were localized using functional MRI.

Neuroimaging studies are few and far between. The techniques are complex, time-consuming, expensive, and in the case of PET, require that subjects be willing to be injected with a radioactive substance. Only certain types of cognitive tests can be used inside the scanner, and movement on the part of the subject must be minimized. Ambiguities in interpreting the results limit the usefulness of these techniques. For example, does greater activation represent excitatory or inhibitory neuronal activity? Still, the new imaging techniques do permit us to directly visualize brain sites that undergo hormone-related changes in activity.

Visuospatial Ability as a Model Function

We spent a lot of time in this chapter discussing hormonal effects on spatial abilities. Several forms of spatial ability are sensitive to the organizational effects of steroids, activational effects, or both. Effects reminiscent of this are seen in the rat on several maze-learning tasks that have been designed to mimic the kinds of spatial demands an animal might encounter in its natural habitat. These include the radial-arm maze (RAM) and Morris water maze (WM), as discussed in chapter 14. In general, maze-learning tasks require that animals learn to navigate quickly and accurately in unfamiliar spatial surroundings.

Parallel findings have led some researchers to wonder if maze-learning in the rat is a suitable model for studying sex steroid effects on human spatial ability. This is controversial. While maze learning does require spatial information to be processed, there are major differences between spatial navigation and the kinds of spatial functions typically assessed in human studies. Can we legitimately generalize from one set of spatial functions to another, very diverse set of functions?

In the rat, performance in the WM and many versions of the RAM is sexually differentiated. Normally, males show faster maze-learning than females. However, this sex difference can be altered by manipulating exposure to sex steroids. In a classic series of experiments, Williams and colleagues (1990) found that adult sex differences in the RAM could be reversed if female rats were exposed neonatally to estradiol or if male rats were castrated in the first few days of life. These experiments confirmed an organizing effect of early steroid exposure, and implicated aromatization of testosterone to estradiol as the likely mechanism by which RAM performance becomes masculinized in the rat.

As in humans, adult hormones might also affect an animal's ability to process spatial information. Although the evidence so far is mixed, some studies suggest a suppressant effect of adult estrogens on spatial learning in intact females. Recent studies using the WM as a spatial measure found diminished spatial learning at high estrogen phases of the estrous cycle in female rats (Frye 1995; Warren and Juraska 1997), or in female voles or deer mice tested in the high-estrogen breeding state (Galea et al. 1994; Galea et al. 1995). There is evidence from gene knockout mice that this effect is mediated by the ERα receptor (Fugger et al. 1998). Less consistent effects have been found using the RAM and in adult rats treated with supra-physiological doses of estradiol.

Since different spatial functions are mediated by different neural systems, we must be careful not to overextend the rodent model. The hippocampus is believed to be important in mediating spatial-navigational behavior in the rat. Changes in hippocampal morphology have been identified in female rats treated neonatally with androgens (Roof and Havens 1992). In the adult rat, Woolley and McEwen (1992) discovered that synaptic connections in part of the hippocampus called CA1 undergo periodic remodeling in females, in conjunction with changes in estradiol levels over the estrous cycle. The number of synapses is about 32% larger at proestrus than 24 hours later at estrus. This provides one possible mechanism for alterations in the rat's spatial proficiency across the estrous cycle. Definite links have yet to be confirmed, though, between the hippocampal effects of steroids and their effects on spatial behaviors.

Whether hormones have any effect on the human hippocampus is not known. Even if they do, we couldn't infer that this is the basis for hormone-related alterations in human spatial abilities, because we lack evidence that the hippocampus is involved in the types of spatial functions typically measured in human neuroendocrine work (e.g., mental rotation). Regions of the neocortex, especially the association cortex of the parietal and frontal lobes, are responsible for a range of spatial processes in primates. We also know that the right hemisphere in humans is more adept than the left at many kinds of perceptual and spatial analysis, including mental rotation (Ditunno and Mann 1990). Because of the differences in the responsible neural structures, generalizing from rodent studies of navigation to human spatial abilities is complex. As far as organizational effects are concerned, aromatization may be a less widespread process in the sexual differentiation of the primate brain than in rodent species.

Implications

The study of hormone-brain-behavior relations in humans is difficult and often controversial. To keep things in perspective, you need to understand that reproductive hormones represent only one of a complex and often interactive multitude of biological and environmental factors that are able to influence human abilities and behaviors. To find an effect of sex steroids on performance does not mean that our abilities are determined by biology. Nor does it diminish the role of environmental or social factors. You must realize that the size of hormonal effects is variable. Some are large and easily visible in everyday experience. For example, the effect size for the difference in spatial ability between CAH girls and control girls is the same as the difference in height between 13- and 18-year-old girls (Cohen 1988). On the other hand, some of the most contentious effects observed so far are fluctuations in performance across the menstrual cycle in healthy women, yet these effects are mostly modest in size.

The menstrual-cycle effects deserve special comment. Women are understandably nervous about such findings because it is only in recent decades that they've achieved workplace equality with men. Several points should be stressed. First, recent work shows that sex steroids may also affect cognitive profiles in men. Second, no phase of the menstrual cycle has been identified that is characterized by either across-the-board improvement or across-the-board deterioration in performance. The picture is one of minor trade-offs among different abilities, many of which are enhanced, not diminished by high estrogen. For a few women, these variations are large enough to be of practical importance, either because of the nature of their work, or because they are unusually reactive to hormones. But in everyday life, most women spend their time in activities that involve many different abilities that may be differently affected by hormones, resulting in little net change in efficiency from one hormone state to another. This is different from the lab setting, where researchers go out of their way to choose tests that can best isolate, or form a particularly pure measure of, specific abilities. Finally, the fact that the effects vary considerably in size from woman to woman emphasizes the inappropriateness of judging any particular woman on the basis of the group results. The same can be said of the cognitive correlates of differing testosterone levels in men.

Why study sex steroids? There are theoretical and applied benefits to neuroendocrine work in humans. Endocrine abnormalities, for example, may provide valuable insights into the role of fetal hormones in normal cognitive development, including the types of cognitive functions affected, and the extent, direction, and timing of influence. If early hormones alter future intellectual capacities, there are important implications for medical control of hormone deficiencies or excesses in utero, for use of exogenous hormones to prevent miscarriage, and for detecting abnormalities through neonatal or even prenatal screening programs. Are there central nervous system effects in women who undergo medical procedures, such as in vitro fertilization, that involve major perturbations of hormones? If a woman has schizophrenia, will taking oral contraceptives diminish or magnify the clinical symptoms of her disease? Does androgen suppression for prostate cancer affect a man's cognitive capacities? Already the research described in this chapter has expanded our understanding of sex differences in one important and surprising way—by encouraging us to think of sex differences as dynamic entities rather than fixed static traits. If our cognitive profiles are modified by circulating levels of sex steroids, then sex differences probably wax and wane at different stages of the lifespan, with seasonal changes in men's testosterone level, or with medications that affect the reproductive hormones. These and many other applied questions still need to be explored.

Study Questions

1. Describe some of the sex differences in cognitive abilities found in humans.
2. Until recently, neuroanatomists believed there were no sex differences of any note in the human brain, with the possible exception of a small difference in total brain weight. Describe some findings that have brought this view into question.

3. What techniques are used in human studies to investigate whether early exposure to gonadal steroids affects sexual differentiation of the brain and behavior? What are the relative advantages and disadvantages of the various techniques?

4. What have we learned from menstrual-cycle studies about the impact of ovarian hormones on cognitive and motor functions?

5. Hormones can normally be administered to human beings only if they are being used to treat a medical condition. What have we learned about the reversible effects of sex steroids on cognition from recent studies involving exogenous hormone administration, either in men or women?

6. What three major approaches are being used to study where sex steroids have their effects in the adult brain?

7. What ethical and practical issues arise when doing neuroendocrine studies in humans?

8. How might the findings from human neuroendocrine studies be useful in improving the medical treatment of people with disorders of the reproductive system?

Acknowledgments

I wish to thank K. Chipman, S. J. Duff, and J. B. Becker for helpful comments on earlier drafts of this chapter.

References

Abplanalp, J. M., Rose, R. M., Donnelly, A. F., and Livingston-Vaughan, L. (1979) Psychoendocrinology of the menstrual cycle: II. The relationship between enjoyment of activities, moods, and reproductive hormones. *Psychosom. Med.* 41: 605–615.

Alexander, G. M., Swerdloff, R. S., Wang, C., Davidson, T., McDonald, V., Steiner, B., and Hines, M. (1998) Androgen-behavior correlations in hypogonadal men and eugonadal men II. Cognitive abilities. *Horm. Behav.* 33: 85–94.

Allen, L. S., Hines, M., Shryne, J. E., and Gorski, R. A. (1989) Two sexually dimorphic cell groups in the human brain. *J. Neurosci.* 9: 497–506.

Anderson, E. I. (1972) Cognitive performance and mood change as they relate to menstrual cycle and estrogen level. *Dissert. Abst. Int.* 33: 1758–B.

Arushanyan, E. B., and Borovkova, G. K. (1993) Differences in monthly fluctuations of mental efficiency in healthy women depending on introversion/extraversion factor. *Hum. Physiol.* 19: 68–70.

Baker, S. W., and Ehrhardt, A. A. (1974) Prenatal androgen, intelligence, and cognitive sex differences. In R. C. Friedman, R. M. Richart, and R. L. Vande Wiele (Eds.), *Sex Differences in Behavior*. New York: Wiley, pp. 53–76.

Baulieu, E. E., Schumacher, M., Koenig, H., Jung-Testas, I., and Akwa, Y. (1996) Progesterone as a neurosteroid: Actions within the nervous system. *Cell. Molec. Neurobiol.* 16: 143–154.

Baum, M. J., and Schretlen, P. (1975) Neuroendocrine effects of perinatal androgenization in the male ferret. *Prog. Brain Res.* 42: 343–355.

Becker, D., Creutzfeldt, O. D., Schwibbe, M., and Wuttke, W. (1982) Changes in physiological, EEG and psychological parameters in women during the spontaneous menstrual cycle and following oral contraceptives. *Psychoneuroendocrinology* 7: 75–90.

Berenbaum, S. A., and Hines, M. (1992) Early androgens are related to childhood sex-typed toy preferences. *Psychol. Sci.* 3: 203–206.

Berenbaum, S. A., and Resnick, S. M. (1997) Early androgen effects on aggression in children and adults with congenital adrenal hyperplasia. *Psychoneuroendocrinology*, 22: 505–515.

Billings, E. G. (1934) The occurrence of cyclic variations in motor activity in relation to the menstrual cycle in the human female. *Bull. Johns Hopkins Hosp.* 54: 440–454.

Bixo, M., Bäckström, T., Winblad, B., and Andersson, A. (1995) Estradiol and testosterone in specific regions of the human female brain in different endocrine states, *J. Steroid Biochem. Mol. Biol.* 55: 297–303.

Broverman, D. M., Klaiber, E. L., Kobayashi, Y., and Vogel, W. (1968) Roles of activation and inhibition in sex differences in cognitive abilities. *Psychol. Rev.* 75: 23–50.

Broverman, D. M., Vogel, W., Klaiber, E. L., Majcher, D., Shea, D., and Paul, V. (1981) Changes in cognitive task performance across the menstrual cycle. *J. Comp. Physiol. Psychol.* 95: 646–654.

Bryden, M. P. (1979) Evidence for sex-related differences in cerebral organization. In M. Wittig and A. C. Petersen (Eds.), *Sex-Related Differences in Cognitive Functioning*. New York: Academic Press, pp. 121–143.

Buckwalter, J. G., Stanczyk, F. Z., McCleary, C. A., Bluestein, B. W., Buckwalter, D. K., Rankin, K. P., Chang, L., and Goodwin, T. M. (1999) Pregnancy, the postpartum, and steroid hormones: Effects on cognition and mood. *Psychoneuroendocrinology* 24: 69–84.

Cappa, S. F., and Vignolo, L. A. (1988) Sex differences in the site of brain lesions underlying global aphasia. *Aphasiology* 2: 259–264.

Choi, J., and Silverman, I. (1997) Sex dimorphism in spatial behaviors: Applications to route-learning. *Evol. Cognit.* 2: 165–171.

Christiansen, K. (1993) Sex hormone-related variations of cognitive performance in !Kung San hunter-gatherers of Namibia. *Neuropsychobiology* 27: 97–107.

Cohen, J. (1988) *Statistical Power Analysis for the Behavioral Sciences.* 2nd edition. Lawrence Erlbaum, Hillsdale, NJ.

Cole-Harding, S., Morstad, A. L., and Wilson, J. R. (1988) Spatial ability in members of opposite-sex twin pairs. *Behav. Genet.* 18: 710.

Dalton, K. (1960) Menstruation and accidents. *Br. Med. J.* 2: 1425–1426.

Desmond, D. W., Glenwick, D. S., Stern, Y., and Tatemichi, T. K. (1994) Sex differences in the representation of visuospatial functions in the human brain. *Rehab. Psychol.* 39: 3–14.

Diamond, M., Diamond, L., and Mast, M. (1972) Visual sensitivity and sexual arousal levels during the menstrual cycle. *J. Nerv. Ment. Dis.* 1555: 170–176.

Diamond, M., Llacuna, A., and Wong, C. L. (1973) Sex behavior after neonatal progesterone, testosterone, estrogen or antiandrogens. *Horm. Behav.* 4: 73–88.

Ditunno, P. L., and Mann, V. A. (1990) Right hemisphere specialization for mental rotation in normals and brain damaged subjects. *Cortex* 26: 17–188.

Doty, R. L., Snyder, P. J., Huggins, G. R., and Lowry, L. D. (1981) Endocrine, cardiovascular, and psychological correlates of olfactory sensitivity changes during the human menstrual cycle. *J. Comp. Physiol. Psychol.* 95: 45–60.

Eals, M., and Silverman, I. (1994) The hunter-gatherer theory of spatial sex differences: Proximate factors mediating the female advantage in recall of object arrays. *Ethol. Sociobiol.* 15: 95–105.

Ehrhardt, A. A., and Baker, S. W. (1974) Fetal androgens, human central nervous system differentiation, and behavior sex differences. In R. C. Friedman, R. M. Richart, and R. L. Vande Wiele (Eds.), *Sex Differences in Behavior*. New York: Wiley, pp. 33–51.

Ehrhardt, A. A., Epstein, R., and Money, J. (1968) Fetal androgens and female gender identity in the early-treated adrenogenital syndrome. *Johns Hopkins Med. J.* 122: 160–167.

Ehrhardt, A. A., and Money, J. (1967) Progestin-induced hermaphroditism: IQ and psychosexual identity in a study of ten girls. *J. Sex. Res.* 3: 83–100.

Ellison, P. T. (1993) Measurements of salivary progesterone, *Ann. N.Y. Acad. Sci.* 694: 161–176.

Erdelyi, G. J. (1962) Gynecological survey of female athletes. *J. Sports Med. Phys. Fitness* 2: 174–179.

Finegan, J. K., Niccols, G. A., and Sitarenios, G. (1992) Relations between prenatal testosterone levels and cognitive abilities at 4 years. *Devel. Psychol.* 28: 1075–1089.

Fink, G., Sumner, B. E. H., Rosie, R., Grace, O., and Quinn, J. P. (1996) Estrogen control of central neurotransmission: Effect on mood, mental state, and memory. *Cell. Mol. Neurobiol.* 16: 325–344.

Friedman, J., and Meares, R. A. (1978) Comparison of spontaneous and contraceptive menstrual cycles on a visual discrimination task. *Aust. New Zeal. J. Psychiat.* 12: 233–239.

Frye, C. (1995) Estrus-associated decrements in a water maze task are limited to acquisition. *Physiol. Behav.* 57: 5–14.

Fugger, H. N., Cunningham, S. G., Rissman, E., and Foster, T. C. (1998) Sex differences in the activational effect of ERα on spatial learning. *Horm. Behav.* 34: 163–170.

Galea, L. A. M., Kavaliers, M., Ossenkopp, K.-P., and Hampson, E. (1995) Gonadal hormone levels and spatial learning performance in the Morris water maze in male and female meadow voles, *Microtus pennsylvanicus*. *Horm. Behav.* 29: 106–125.

Galea, L. A. M., Kavaliers, M., Ossenkopp, K.-P., Innes, D., and Hargreaves, E. L. (1994) Sexually dimorphic spatial learning varies seasonally in two populations of deer mice. *Brain Res.* 635: 18–26.

Galea, L. A. M., and Kimura, D. (1993) Sex differences in route-learning. *Person. Indiv. Diff.* 14: 53–65.

Garcia-Segura, L. M., Chowen, J. A., Dueñas, M., Parducz, A., and Naftolin, F. (1996) Gonadal steroids and astroglial plasticity. *Cell. Mol. Neurobiol.* 16: 225–237.

Gaulin, S. J. C., and Fitzgerald, R. W. (1986) Sex differences in spatial ability: An evolutionary hypothesis and test. *Am. Nat.* 127: 74–88.

Gordon, H. W., and Lee, P. A. (1993) No difference in cognitive performance between phases of the menstrual cycle. *Psychoneuroendocrinology* 18: 521–531.

Gouchie, C., and Kimura, D. (1991) The relationship between testosterone levels and cognitive ability patterns. *Psychoneuroendocrinology* 16: 323–334.

Goy, R. W., and McEwen, B. S. (1980) *Sexual Differentiation of the Brain.* Cambridge, Mass.: MIT Press.

Grimshaw, G. M., Sitarenios, G., and Finegan, J. K. (1995) Mental rotation at 7 years: Relations with prenatal testosterone levels and spatial play experiences. *Brain Cognit.* 29: 85–100.

Halpern, D. F. (1992) *Sex Differences in Cognitive Abilities.* Hillsdale, N.J.: Erlbaum.

Hampson, E. (1990a) Variations in sex-related cognitive abilities across the menstrual cycle. *Brain Cognit.* 14: 26–43.

Hampson, E. (1990b) Estrogen-related variations in human spatial and articulatory-motor skills. *Psychoneuroendocrinology* 15: 97–111.

Hampson, E., and Kimura, D. (1988) Reciprocal effects of hormonal fluctuations on human motor and perceptual-spatial skills. *Behav. Neurosci.* 102: 456–459.

Hampson, E., Rovet, J. F., and Altmann, D. (1998) Spatial reasoning in children with congenital adrenal hyperplasia due to 21-hydroxylase deficiency. *Devel. Neuropsychol.* 14: 299–320.

Harshman, R. A., and Remington, R. (1976) Sex, language, and the brain, Part I: A review of the literature on adult sex differences in lateralization. *UCLA Working Papers in Phonetics* 31: 86–103.

Hausfater, G., and Skoblick, B. (1985) Perimentrual behavior changes among female yellow baboons: Some similarities to premenstrual syndrome (PMS) in women. *Am. J. Primat.* 9: 165–172.

Henderson, B. A., and Berenbaum, S. A. (1997) Sex-typed play in opposite-sex twins. *Devel. Psychobiol.* 31: 115–123.

Hier, D. B., and Crowley, W. F. (1982) Spatial ability in androgen-deficient men. *N. Engl. J. Med.* 306: 1201–1205.

Hier, D. B., Yoon, W. B., Mohr, J. P., Price, T. R., and Wolf, P. A. (1994) Gender and aphasia in the stroke data bank. *Brain Lang.* 47: 155–167.

Hines, M. (1990) Gonadal hormones and human cognitive development. In J. Balthazart (Ed.), *Hormones, Brain and Behaviour in Vertebrates.* Basel: Karger, pp. 51–63.

Hines, M., and Kaufman, F. R. (1994) Androgen and the development of human sex-typical behavior: Rough-and-tumble play and sex of preferred playmates in children with congenital adrenal hyperplasia (CAH). *Child Devel.* 65: 1042–1053.

Hines, M., and Sandberg, E. C. (1996) Sexual differentiation of cognitive abilities in women exposed to diethylstilbestrol (DES) prenatally. *Horm. Behav.* 30: 354–363.

Hines, M., and Shipley, C. (1984) Prenatal exposure to diethylstilbestrol (DES) and the development of sexually dimorphic cognitive abilities and cerebral lateralization. *Devel. Psychol.* 20: 81–94.

Hudgens, G. A., Fatkin, L. T., Billingsley, P. A., and Mazurczak, J. (1988) Hand steadiness: Effects of sex, menstrual phase, oral contraceptives, practice, and handgun weight, *Hum. Factors* 30: 51–60.

Hutt, S. J., Frank, G., Mychalkiw, W., and Hughes, M. (1980) Perceptual-motor performance during the menstrual cycle. *Horm. Behav.* 14: 116–125.

Hyde, J. S., and Linn, M. C. (1988) Gender differences in verbal ability: A meta-analysis. *Psychol. Bull.* 104: 53–69.

Ivey, M. E., and Bardwick, J. M. (1968) Patterns of affective fluctuation in the menstrual cycle. *Psychosom. Med.* 30: 336–345.

Jacklin, C. N., Wilcox, K. T., and Maccoby, E. E. (1988) Neonatal sex-steroid hormones and cognitive abilities at six years. *Devel. Psychobiol.* 21: 567–574.

Jaffe, A. B., Toran-Allerand, C. D., Greengard, P., and Gandy, S. E. (1994) Estrogen regulates metabolism of amyloid β precursor protein. *J. Biol. Chem.* 269: 13065–13068.

James, T. W., and Kimura, D. (1997) Sex differences in remembering the locations of objects in an array: Location-shifts versus location-exchanges. *Evol. Hum. Behav.* 18: 155–163.

Janowsky, J. S., Oviatt, S. K., and Orwoll, E. S. (1994) Testosterone influences spatial cognition in older men. *Behav. Neurosci.* 108: 325–332.

Jarvik, L. F. (1975) Human intelligence: Sex differences. *Acta Genet. Med. Gemell.* 24: 189–211.

Jennings, P. J., Janowsky, J. S., and Orwoll, E. (1998) Estrogen and sequential movement. *Behav. Neurosci.* 112: 154–159.

Jensen, A. R. (1988) Sex differences in arithmetic computation and reasoning in prepubertal boys and girls. *Behav. Brain Sci.* 11: 198–199.

Jensen, B. K. (1982) Menstrual cycle effects on task performance examined in the context of stress research. *Acta Psychol.* 50: 159–178.

Jones, H. E. (1947) Sex differences in physical abilities. *Human Biol.* 19: 12–25.

Kerns, K. A., and Berenbaum, S. A. (1991) Sex differences in spatial ability in children. *Behav. Genet.* 21: 383–396.

Kimura, D. (1982) Left-hemisphere control of oral and brachial movements and their relation to communication. *Phil. Trans. R. Soc. Lond.* B298: 135–149.

Kimura, D. (1983) Sex differences in cerebral organization for speech and praxic functions. *Canad. J. Psychol.* 37: 19–35.

Kimura, D. (1995) Estrogen replacement therapy may protect against intellectual decline in postmenopausal women. *Horm. Behav.* 29: 312–321.

Kimura, D., and Hampson, E. (1994) Cognitive pattern in men and women is influenced by fluctuations in sex hormones. *Curr. Dir. Psychol. Sci.* 3: 57–61.

Klaiber, E. L., Broverman, D. M., Vogel, W., Kobayashi, Y., and Moriarty, D. (1972) Effects of estrogen therapy on plasma MAO activity and EEG driving responses of depressed women. *Am. J. Psychiat.* 128: 42–48.

Klaiber, E. L., Broverman, D. M., Vogel, W., and Mackenberg, E. J. (1974) Rhythms in cognitive functioning and EEG indices in males. In M. Ferin, F. Halberg, R. M. Richart, and R. L. Vande Wiele (Eds.), *Biorhythms and Human Reproduction*. New York: Wiley, pp. 481–493.

Komnenich, P., Lane, D. M., Dickey, R. P., and Stone, S. C. (1978) Gonadal hormones and cognitive performance. *Physiol. Psychol.* 6: 115–120.

Kramer, J. H., Delis, D. C., and Daniel, M. (1988) Sex differences in verbal learning. *J. Clin. Psychol.* 44: 907–915.

Lansdell, H. (1961) The effect of neurosurgery on a test of proverbs. *Am. Psychol.* 16: 448.

Leveroni, C. L., and Berenbaum, S. A. (1998) Early androgen effects on interest in infants: Evidence from children with congenital adrenal hyperplasia. *Devel. Neuropsychol.* 14: 321–340.

Maccoby, E. E., and Jacklin, C. N. (1974) *The Psychology of Sex Differences*. Stanford, Ca.: Stanford Univerity Press.

Mackenberg, E. J., Broverman, D. M., Vogel, W., and Klaiber, E. L. (1974) Morning-to-afternoon changes in cognitive performances and in the electroencephalogram. *J. Educ. Psychol.* 66: 238–246.

MacLusky, N. J., Naftolin, F., and Goldman-Rakic, P. S. (1986) Estrogen formation and binding in the cerebral cortex of the developing rhesus monkey. *Proc. Natl. Acad. Sci. USA* 83: 513–516.

Mann, V. A., Sasanuma, S., Sakuma, N., and Masaki, S. (1990) Sex differences in cognitive abilities: A cross-cultural perspective. *Neuropsychologia* 28: 1063–1077.

Mateer, C. A., Polen, S. B., and Ojemann, G. A. (1982) Sexual variation in cortical localization of naming as determined by stimulation mapping. *Behav. Brain Sci.* 5: 310–311.

May, R. R. (1976) Mood shifts and the menstrual cycle. *J. Psychosom. Res.* 20: 125–130.

McBurney, D. H., Gaulin, S. J. C., Devineni, T., and Adams, C. (1997) Superior spatial memory of women: Stronger evidence for the gathering hypothesis. *Evol. Hum. Behav.* 18: 165–174.

McCourt, M. E., Mark, V. W., Radonovich, K. J., Willison, S. K., and Freeman, P. (1997) The effects of gender, menstrual phase, and practice on the perceived location of the midsagittal plane. *Neuropsychologia* 35: 717–724.

McEwen, B. S., Alves, S. E., Bulloch, K., and Weiland, N. G. (1997) Ovarian steroids and the brain: Implications for cognition and aging. *Neurology* 48(Suppl 7): S8–S15.

McEwen, B. S., Davis, P. G., Parsons, B., and Pfaff, D. W. (1979) The brain as a target for steroid hormone action. *Annu. Rev. Neurosci.* 2: 65–112.

McEwen, B. S., Gould, E., Orchinik, M., Weiland, N. G., and Woolley, C. S. (1995) Oestrogens and the structural and functional plasticity of neurons: Implications for memory, ageing and neurodegenerative processes. In G. R. Bock and J. A. Goode (Eds.), *Non-Reproductive Actions of Sex Steroids*. New York: Wiley, pp. 52–73.

McFadden, D. (1993) A masculinizing effect on the auditory systems of human females having male co-twins. *Proc. Natl. Acad. Sci. USA* 90: 11900–11904.

McGlone, J. (1977) Sex differences in the cerebral organization of verbal functions in patients with unilateral brain lesions. *Brain* 100: 775–793.

McGlone, J. (1980) Sex differences in human brain asymmetry: A critical survey. *Behav. Brain Sci.* 3: 215–263.

McGuinness, D., and Morley, C. (1991) Sex differences in the development of visuo-spatial ability in pre-school children. *J. Ment. Imagery* 15: 143–150.

McGuire, L. S., Ryan, K. O., and Omenn, G. S. (1975) Congenital adrenal hyperplasia. II. Cognitive and behavioral studies. *Behav. Genet.* 5: 175–188.

Mead, L. A., and Hampson, E. (1997) Turning bias in humans is influenced by phase of the menstrual cycle. *Horm. Behav.* 31: 65–74.

Moffat, S. D., and Hampson, E. (1996) A curvilinear relationship between testosterone and spatial cognition in humans: Possible influence of hand preference. *Psychoneuroendocrinology* 21: 323–337.

Moody, M. S. (1997) Changes in scores on the Mental Rotations Test during the menstrual cycle. *Percept. Mot. Skills* 84: 955–961.

Morris, N. M., and Udry, J. R. (1970) Variations in pedometer activity during the menstrual cycle. *Obst. Gynecol.* 35: 199–201.

Nicholson, K. G., and Kimura, D. (1996) Sex differences for speech and manual skill. *Percept. Mot. Skills* 82: 3–13.

Paganini-Hill, A., and Henderson, V. W. (1994) Estrogen deficiency and risk of Alzheimer's disease in women. *Am. J. Epidemiol.* 140: 256–261.

Parlee, M. B. (1983) Menstrual rhythms in sensory processes: A review of fluctuations in vision, olfaction, audition, taste, and touch. *Psychol. Bull.* 93: 539–548.

Paivio, A. (1971) *Imagery and Verbal Processes*. New York: Holt, Rinehart and Winston.

Patterson, F. G. P., Holts, C., and Saphire, L. (1991) Cyclic changes in hormonal, physical, behavioral, and linguistic measures in a female lowland gorilla. *Am. J. Primat.* 24: 181–194.

Perlman, S. M. (1973) Cognitive abilities of children with hormone abnormalities: Screening by psychoeducational tests. *J. Learn. Disabil.* 6: 26–34.

Peters, M., Laeng, B., Latham, K., Jackson, M., Zaiyouna, R., and Richardson, C. (1995) A redrawn Vandenberg and Kuse Mental Rotations Test: Different versions and factors that affect performance. *Brain Cognit.* 28: 39–58.

Phillips, K., and Silverman, I. (1997) Differences in the relationship of menstrual cycle phase to spatial performance on two- and three-dimensional tasks, *Horm. Behav.* 32: 167–175.

Pierson, W. R., and Lockhart, A. (1963) Effect of menstruation on simple reaction and movement time. *Brit. Med. J.* 1: 796–797.

Plante, E., Boliek, C., Binkiewicz, A., and Erly, W. K. (1996) Elevated androgen, brain development and language/learning disabilities in children with congenital adrenal hyperplasia. *Devel. Med. Child Neurol.* 38: 423–437.

Puy, L., MacLusky, N. J., Becker, L., Karsan, N., Trachtenberg, J., and Brown, T. J. (1995) Immuno-cytochemical detection of androgen receptor in human temporal cortex: Characterization and application of polyclonal androgen receptor antibodies in frozen and paraffin-embedded tissues. *J. Steroid Biochem. Mol. Biol.* 55: 197–209.

Quinn, N. P., and Marsden, C. D. (1986) Menstrual-related fluctuations in Parkinson's disease. *Mov. Disord.* 1: 85–86.

Reinisch, J. M. (1981) Prenatal exposure to synthetic progestins increases potential for aggression in humans. *Science* 211: 1171–1173.

Reinisch, J. M., and Karow, W. G. (1977) Prenatal exposure to synthetic progestins and estrogens: Effects on human development. *Arch. Sex. Behav.* 6: 257–288.

Reinisch, J. M., and Sanders, S. A. (1992) Effects of prenatal exposure to diethylstilbestrol (DES) on hemispheric laterality and spatial ability in human males. *Horm. Behav.* 26: 62–75.

Resnick, S. M., Berenbaum, S. A., Gottesman, I. I., and Bouchard, T. J. (1986) Early hormonal influences on cognitive functioning in congenital adrenal hyperplasia. *Devel. Psychol.* 22: 191–198.

Resnick, S. M., Gottesman, I. I., and McGue, M. (1993) Sensation seeking in opposite-sex twins: An effect of prenatal hormones? *Behav. Genet.* 23: 323–329.

Roof, R. L., and Havens, M. D. (1991) Testosterone improves maze performance and induces development of a male hippocampus in females. *Brain Res.* 572: 310–313.

Rossi, A. S. (1980) Mood cycles by menstrual month and social week. In A. J. Dan, E. A. Graham, and C. P. Beecher (Eds.), *The Menstrual Cycle*, vol. 1. *A Synthesis of Interdisciplinary Research*. New York: Springer, pp. 56–71.

Sanders, B., Soares, M. P., and D'Aquila, J. M. (1982) The sex difference on one test of spatial visualization: A nontrivial difference. *Child Devel.* 53: 1106–1110.

Sanders, D., Warner, P., Bäckström, T., and Bancroft, J. (1983) Mood, sexuality, hormones and the menstrual cycle. I. Changes in mood and physical state. *Psychosom. Med.* 45: 487–501.

Sandstrom, N. J., Kaufman, J., and Huettel, S. A. (1998) Males and females use different distal cues in a virtual environment navigation task. *Cognit. Brain Res.* 6: 351–360.

Sarrieau, A., Mitchell, J. B., Lal, S., Olivier, A., Quirion, R., and Meaney, M. J. (1990) Androgen binding sites in human temporal cortex. *Neuroendocrinology* 51: 713–716.

Saucier, D. M., and Kimura, D. (1998) Intrapersonal motor but not extrapersonal targeting skill is enhanced during the midluteal phase of the menstrual cycle. *Devel. Neuropsychol.* 14: 385–398.

Schlaepfer, T. E., Harris, G. J., Tien, A. Y., Peng, L., Lee, S., and Pearlson, G. D. (1995) Structural differences in the cerebral cortex of healthy female and male subjects: A magnetic resonance imaging study. *Psychiat. Res: Neuroimaging* 61: 129–135.

Shaywitz, B. A., Shaywitz, S. E., Pugh, K. R., Constable, R. T., Skudlarski, P., Fulbright, R. K., Bronen, R. A., Fletcher, J. M., Shankweiler, D. P., Katz, L., and Gore, J. C. (1995) Sex differences in the functional organization of the brain for language. *Nature* 373: 607–609.

Shaywitz, S. E., Shaywitz, B. A., Pugh, K. R., Fulbright, R. K., Skudlarski, P., Mencl, W. E., Constable, R. T., Naftolin, F., Palter, S. F., Marchione, K. E., Katz, L., Shankweiler, D. P., Fletcher, J. M., Lacadie, C., Keltz, M., and Gore, J. C. (1999) Effect of estrogen on brain activation patterns in postmenopausal women during working memory tasks. *JAMA* 281: 1197–1202.

Sherwin, B. B. (1994) Sex hormones and psychological functioning in postmenopausal women. *Exp. Gerontol.* 29: 423–430.

Sherwin, B. B. (1996) Hormones, mood, and cognitive functioning in postmenopausal women. *Obstet. Gynecol.* 87(Suppl.): 20S–26S.

Sherwin, B. B., and Gelfand, M. M. (1985) Sex steroids and affect in the surgical menopause: A double-blind, crossover study. *Psychoneuroendocrinology* 10: 325–335.

Sherwin, B. B., and Phillips, S. (1990) Estrogen and cognitive functioning in surgically menopausal women. *Ann. New York Acad. Sci.* 592: 474–475.

Shute, V. J., Pellegrino, J. W., Hubert, L., and Reynolds, R. W. (1983) The relationship between androgen levels and human spatial abilities. *Bull. Psychonom. Soc.* 21: 465–468.

Silverman, E. M., and Zimmer, C. H. (1975) Speech fluency fluctuations during the menstrual cycle. *J. Speech Hear. Res.* 18: 202–206.

Silverman, E. M., Zimmer, C. H., and Silverman, F. H. (1974) Variability of stutters' speech disfluency: The menstrual cycle. *Percept. Mot. Skills* 38: 1037–1038.

Silverman, I., and Eals, M. (1992) Sex differences in spatial abilities: Evolutionary theory and data. In J. H. Barkow and L. Cosmides (Eds.), *The Adapted Mind*. New York: Oxford, pp. 533–549.

Silverman, I., and Phillips, K. (1993) Effects of estrogen changes during the menstrual cycle on spatial performance. *Ethol. Sociobiol.* 14: 257–270.

Snyder, D. A. B. (1978) The relationship of the menstrual cycle to certain aspects of perceptual cognitive functioning. *Dissert. Abstr. Int.* 39: 962B–963B.

Stenn, P. G., and Klinge, V. (1972) Relationship between the menstrual cycle and bodily activity in humans. *Horm. Behav.* 3: 297–305.

Stocker, J. M. (1973) Motor performance and state anxiety at selected stages of the menstrual cycle. *Dissert. Abst. Int.* 34: 3971–A.

Swaab, D. F., and Fliers, E. (1985) A sexually dimorphic nucleus in the human brain. *Science* 228: 1112–1115.

Szekely, C., Hampson, E., Carey, D. P., and Goodale, M. A. (1998) Oral contraceptive use affects manual praxis but not simple visually guided movements. *Devel. Neuropsychol.* 14: 399–420.

Thys-Jacobs, S., and Alvir, M. J. (1995) Calcium-regulating hormones across the menstrual cycle: Evidence of a secondary hyperparathyroidism in women with PMS. *J. Clin. Endocrin. Metab.* 80: 2227–2232.

Tyler, L. E. (1965) *The Psychology of Human Differences*, 3rd edition. New York: Appleton-Century-Crofts.

Udry, J. R., Morris, N. M., and Kovenock, J. (1995) Androgen effects on women's gendered behaviour. *J. Biosoc. Sci.* 27: 359–368.

Van Goozen, S. H. M., Cohen-Kettenis, P. T., Gooren, L. J. G., Frijda, N. H., and Van de Poll, N. E. (1994) Activating effects of androgens on cognitive performance: Causal evidence in a group of female-to-male transsexuals. *Neuropsychologia* 32: 1153–1157.

Van Goozen, S. H. M., Cohen-Kettenis, P. T., Gooren, L. J. G., Frijda, N. H., and Van de Poll, N. E. (1995) Gender differences in behaviour: Activating effects of cross-sex hormones. *Psychoneuroendocrinology* 20: 343–364.

Vignolo, L. A., Boccardi, E., and Caverni, L. (1986) Unexpected CT-scan findings in global aphasia. *Cortex* 22: 55–69.

Voyer, D., Voyer, S., and Bryden, M. P. (1995) Magnitude of sex differences in spatial abilities: A meta-analysis and consideration of critical variables. *Psychol. Bull.* 117: 250–270.

Warren, S. G., and Juraska, J. M. (1997) Spatial and nonspatial learning across the rat estrous cycle. *Behav. Neurosci.* 111: 259–266.

Wearing, M. P., Yuhosz, M. D., Campbell, R., and Love, E. J. (1972) The effect of the menstrual cycle on tests of physical fitness. *J. Sports Med.* 12: 38–41.

Wickham, M. (1958) The effects of the menstrual cycle on test performance. *Br. J. Psychol.* 49: 34–41.

Williams, C. L., Barnett, A. M., and Meck, W. H. (1990) Organizational effects of early gonadal secretions on sexual differentiation in spatial memory. *Behav. Neurosci.* 104: 84–97.

Wilson, J. R., and Vandenberg, S. G. (1978) Sex differences in cognition: Evidence from the Hawaii family study. In T. E. McGill, D. A. Dewsbury, and B. D. Sachs (Eds.), *Sex and Behavior: Status and Prospectus.* New York: Plenum Press, pp. 317–335.

Witelson, S. F., Glezer, I. I., and Kigar, D. L. (1995) Women have greater density of neurons in posterior temporal cortex. *J. Neurosci.* 15: 3418–3428.

Wong, S., and Tong, J. E. (1974) Menstrual cycle and contraceptive hormonal effects on temporal discrimination. *Percept. Mot. Skills* 39: 103–108.

Woodfield, R. L. (1984) Embedded figures test performance before and after childbirth. *Br. J. Psychol.* 75: 81–88.

Woolley, C. S., and McEwen, B. S. (1992) Estradiol mediates fluctuation in hippocampal synapse density during the estrous cycle in the adult rat. *J. Neurosci.* 12: 2549–2554.

Yalom, I. D., Green, R., and Fisk, N. (1973) Prenatal exposure to female hormones: Effect on psychosexual development in boys. *Arch. Gen. Psychiat.* 28: 554–561.

Zaharieva, E. (1965) Survey of sportswomen at the Tokyo Olympics. *J. Sports Med. Phys. Fitness* 5: 215–219.

Zimmerman, E., and Parlee, M. B. (1973) Behavioral changes associated with the menstrual cycle: An experimental investigation. *J. Applied Social Psychol.* 3: 335–344.

V Reciprocal Regulation of Hormones and Behavior

Now we begin to consider how hormones and behaviors travel a two-way street. Changing an animal's hormonal levels can affect its subsequent behavior, as we have seen in previous chapters. But if they are to survive, organisms must be very sensitive to environmental cues such as those that help predict food availability, coming bad weather, and the presence of potential mates. The individual must also attend to internal cues, such as whether there are sufficient body stores of food, water, and other nutrients. These are just a few of the hundreds of stimuli to which animals must attend. All these cues, plus hundreds of others, affect hormone secretion to prepare the body physiologically for the future. In other words, experience can alter hormone secretion and, because the animal's behavior often determines whether it will be exposed to stimuli such as daylight, odors, tastes, and so on, changes in behavior can cause changes in hormone secretions.

This reciprocal relationship between hormones and behavior has come up in previous chapters. For example, in chapter 11 we learned how the perception of danger, whether it is real or imagined, can maintain the secretion of "stress hormones." In chapter 12 we saw how the timing of hormonal secretion is coordinated by biological rhythms, many of which are set by external events. However, for the most part, we have spoken as though hormones alter behavior but not vice versa. This is a convenient manner of thinking that allows us to understand a great many of the relationships between hormones and behavior, but it is clearly an oversimplification. Therefore, in this final portion of the text we dwell further upon this additional complication to our study of behavioral endocrinology.

Why have hormones and behavior come to affect each other in this reciprocal fashion? Evolution has not conspired to confuse would-be students. Rather, as we suggested above, it is absolutely crucial that organisms carefully respond to external and internal cues so that they can survive. Often the optimal response to such cues is to alter hormonal secretions to prepare the body and the brain for what lies ahead. Chapter 16 covers the relations between the substances ingested and the internal levels of water, salt, and calories. Hormones play a role in maintaining a balance in these elements, both in response to behavior (food intake, for example) and in response to the nutrients ingested. Chapter 17 reviews work with invertebrates, which shows that photoperiod affects hormone release, which affects behavior, which then affects subsequent hormone release, and so on, resulting in the metamorphosis of the caterpillar to the moth. Finally, chapter 18 concludes with a discussion of how our environment impacts our hormones in as many ways as you can imagine. Sensory input (sight, touch, taste, and smell) provide important cues for the reproductive future of animals and therefore can have powerful effects on hormones and behavior.

16 Hormonal Regulation of Ingestive Behaviors

S. Marc Breedlove

The thousands of chemical processes that take place in our bodies every day rely on the careful maintenance of internal chemistry and the continuous flow of nutrients and energy to sustain that chemistry. The brain provides the control center that monitors internal conditions and directs the activity of major organs such as the heart, liver, and kidneys as well as the ingestive behavior of the animal to maintain the internal milieu. Hormones act as messengers that direct information from various organs to the brain and deliver the brain's orders back to those organs to conserve needed nutrients. Furthermore, there is at least one instance in which hormones may act directly on the brain to affect ingestive behaviors.

Which hormones help maintain energy and fluid balance, and what happens to that balance when there is a loss of these hormones? How do changes in these hormones indirectly affect ingestive behavior and what is the evidence that hormones can also act directly on the nervous system to affect ingestive behavior?

Introduction

Life is precarious, because every cell in our body can function only within very particular conditions. The chemical reactions taking place inside cells can work properly only when the concentrations of various ions and other chemicals fall within a very narrow range. For this reason, the internal conditions of our body, or **internal milieu**, is tightly regulated by a host of physiological mechanisms. In other words, the body works to keep the internal milieu fairly constant. We call this tendency of the body's interior to stay the same **homeostasis**. Whenever something happens to perturb internal conditions, the body must compensate to return to homeostasis to keep cells alive.

General Principles of Homeostasis

Among the many ingredients needed to maintain homeostasis are water, nutrients, and energy. In this chapter we will discuss the role that hormones play in regulating the ingestive behaviors, drinking and eating, that provide these ingredients. Each organism must carefully balance the amount of water inside the body to keep its cells functioning properly, and the organism must also gather the chemicals it needs to grow and repair itself. Finally, each organism must also gather chemicals to provide the energy it needs to fuel the chemical reactions inside its cells. The need for chemical energy is especially urgent for birds and mammals, because their cells also require a narrow range of body temperature, and a great deal of food must be broken down simply to generate heat so those cells will continue to function.

Homeostasis and Negative Feedback

One general principle the body uses to maintain homeostasis of fluid, nutrients, and energy is the same **negative feedback** we described in chapter 1 when we discussed hormone levels. You recall that the brain directs endocrine organs to produce hormones and each of these hormones in turn feeds back to the brain to inhibit any further call for that hormone. Because the hormone exerts a negative feedback effect, levels of the hormone do not get too high. If hormone levels fall, the negative feedback is lifted and the brain calls for more of the hormone to prevent levels from getting too low. Negative feedback effects are also seen in the regulation of drinking and eating. When we are thirsty, the brain directs us to drink water, which reduces, temporarily, our tendency to drink further. Eating reduces, for a time, our tendency to eat more. As we lose water and use up energy, we seek out water and food. This perspective helps to frame questions about hunger and thirst: how does the brain know whether the supplies of water or food are low, and what happens in the brain to cause the organism to conserve present supplies and seek out more?

As we'll see, hormones play crucial roles in these behaviors for several reasons: (1) because hormones often signal the brain about body stores of fluid and energy, and (2) because the brain often uses hormones to direct how we use and conserve our present supplies of water, nutrients, and chemical energy.

First we'll discuss the role of hormones in fluid regulation, which will also entail a brief discussion of salt balance, and then we'll discuss the role of hormones in eating and body-weight regulation.

Fluid Regulation

Fluid Compartments and Osmolality

To understand how the body regulates fluid, we must think about the various body compartments that contain water. When we drink water, it first moistens the mouth and then enters the stomach. Technically, the water is not yet inside the body because it is not yet available to the cells there. But once the water has crossed the walls of the stomach or intestines, it becomes available in one of two compartments: either inside cells (**intracellular compartment**) or between cells (**extracellular compartment**). You can think of the extracellular compartment as surrounding the intracellular compartment, since only a tiny minority of cells form the body surface. The amount of fluid in the extracellular compartment can vary in the course of a day, but the amount of fluid in the intracellular compartment must be tightly regulated. If a cell has too little water, intracellular processes will be disrupted, and a given cell can only take in so much water before it will rupture. Thus, you may think of the extracellular fluid compartment as a buffer zone, a compartment that can take up water or release it in order to ensure the relative stability of the intracellular compartment.

Hypovolemic versus Osmotic Thirst

HYPOVOLEMIC THIRST

Sometimes a great deal of water may be lost from the extracellular fluid compartment, as when we vomit, have diarrhea, or lose blood. Even in the absence of these distressing events, we lose a great deal of water constantly through evaporation through our skin. When you are sweating this water loss is obvious, but even when you are not sweating, water is passing through your skin and evaporating. Several factors can affect the rate of this evaporation: high temperature, low ambient humidity, or low atmospheric pressure (as at high altitudes) all accelerate this evaporative loss of water. No matter how water is lost from the extracellular compartment, we call such loss **hypovolemia**, meaning reduced volume. When the extracellular fluid compartment is sufficiently depleted, you will actively seek out water to drink. In the laboratory, hypovolemia causes an animal to change its behavior and it will work—for example, by pressing a bar or walking a great distance—to gain water, so we say it is **thirsty**. Presumably the animal's *experience* of thirst is much like ours. But because we cannot easily prove that, we will simply assume that an animal seeking water is thirsty. An animal made thirsty by loss of extracellular water is said to display **hypovolemic thirst**.

Because your experience of thirst includes the feeling of a dry mouth, you might think, reasonably enough, that animals learn they're thirsty by experiencing a dry mouth. Surely the sensation of having a dry mouth makes some contribution to thirst, but it was fairly easy to demonstrate that other factors can drive thirst. If surgery is done to prevent the water the animal drinks from entering its stomach (a "sham-drinking" preparation), the animal does not stop drinking once its mouth is wetted. Rather, the animal continues to drink, so some other cues from the body must be driving thirst. One internal cue that drives thirst is directly related to hypovolemia. If the extracellular fluid compartment gets low, then there is a reduced volume of blood. That means blood pressure will drop. In the major blood vessels, especially those directly connected to the heart, and in the heart itself, neurons are embedded in the walls that detect whether they are taut (indicating high blood pressure) or slack (indicating low blood pressure). We call these neurons **baroreceptors**, meaning pressure detectors. If the baroreceptors detect a drop in blood pressure, they then send a signal through the autonomic nervous system to the brain, triggering thirst so the animal will seek water to restore extracellular volume. So one internal cue that drives thirst comes from baroreceptors monitoring extracellular volume. But there is an additional cue driving thirst and to understand that cue, we must consider osmosis and osmolality.

OSMOTIC THIRST

Water passes rather freely across cell membranes, which means that water molecules move passively back and forth between the intracellular and extracellular fluid compartments in a process known as **osmosis**. But among those water molecules are dissolved substances (called **solutes**) such as sodium (Na^+) ions, which do not pass across cell membranes readily. Mammalian cells have the equivalent of approximately 0.9 grams of salt (sodium chloride; Na^+Cl^-) per 100 ml of fluid, a so-called 0.9% solution. Any solution with an equivalent concentration of solutes is said to be **isotonic**. If the concentration of salt is higher than 0.9%, it is said to be **hypertonic**; if lower than 0.9%, it is **hypotonic**. We say the cell membrane is **semipermeable** because it allows some molecules, such as water, to pass readily while it resists the passage of other molecules, such as Na^+ ions. Because molecules have a tendency to distribute themselves evenly, the semipermeable nature of the cell membrane can result in **osmotic pressure**. If there is a greater concentration of Na^+ ions on one side of the membrane than the other, then osmotic pressure will push water molecules across to try to equalize the Na^+ concentrations on the two sides.

Figure 16.1 depicts a simple case of a semipermeable membrane that permits water, but not Na^+, to cross. Initially, the amount of water and the concentration of Na^+ in the water are the same on both sides of the membrane (A). We can consider this analogous to the intracellular and extracellular water compartments. But if we add salt to the extracellular compartment (as, say, when we eat a very salty meal), making it hypertonic, the salt cannot readily enter the intracellular compartment (B). But osmotic pressure will pull water molecules across the membrane, making the two sides more isotonic, so that soon there will be less water in the intracellular compartment (C). For cells, such an intracellular fluid loss would be disastrous. So after we build up extracellular Na^+ with a salty meal, we quickly become thirsty, as the body tries to keep intracellular and extracellular compartments equal in osmolality. We call such thirst **osmotic thirst** to distinguish it from hypovolemic thirst. Eventually the water we drink will be used to flush the excess Na^+ out in urine, returning the two fluid compartments to homeostasis.

Baroreceptors and Osmoreceptors

Just as baroreceptors monitor fluid volume, there must be specialized receptors, called **osmoreceptors**, that monitor extracellular osmolality. The osmoreceptors are almost certainly neurons in the brain, because infusions of tiny amounts of hypertonic saline into some brain regions induces thirst even when the animal has plenty of water. The most effective site for such infusions is in brain regions named for their position around brain ventricles: **circumventricular organs**. The blood-brain barrier is especially weak among the circumventricular organs, which means that neurons there have greater access to blood-borne characteristics such as tonicity and hormone concen-

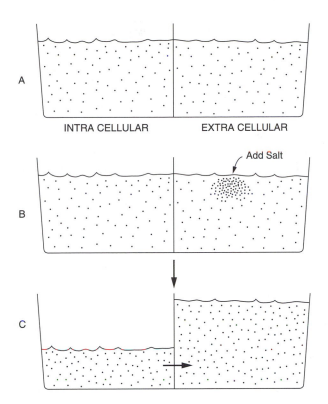

INTRA CELLULAR   **EXTRA CELLULAR**

Figure 16.1 Osmosis and osmotic pressure. Internal water stores are either inside cells (the intracellular compartment) or outside cells (extracellular compartment). Water molecules readily move across the cell membranes between the two compartments, but most ions, such as salt, do not. Because molecules tend to move from regions of high concentration to regions of low concentration, adding salt to the extracellular compartment (e.g., after eating a very salty meal) will induce water molecules to leave the intracellular compartment. This movement of fluid out of the intracellular compartment will induce thirst, specifically, osmotic thirst.

trations. Among circumventricular organs are the **subfornical organ**, the **area postrema**, and the sesquipedalian **organum vasculosum of the lamina terminalis**, **OVLT** for short. The OVLT may be the site of osmoreceptor neurons, because hypertonic infusions work best there, and lesions of the OVLT and nearby regions greatly reduce osmotic thirst (Johnson and Edwards 1990). OVLT neurons in turn send axons to the preoptic area (POA), which will be discussed shortly.

Hormonal Regulation of Fluids

Vasopressin System

Two hypothalamic nuclei, the paraventricular nucleus (PVN) and supraoptic nucleus (SON) contain neuroendocrine cells that project their axons down the pituitary stalk, ending in the posterior pituitary. As we described in chapter 1, these neuroendocrine cells receive synapses from various brain neurons. With sufficient synaptic stimulation, these neuroendocrine cells generate an action potential which spreads to the end of the axon and causes one of two peptide hormones to be released: either oxytocin or vasopressin. You have already learned about the role of oxytocin in sexual behavior (chapter 4) and in parental behavior (chapter 9). Vasopressin plays a central role in fluid regulation. The vasopressin peptide is 9 amino acids long and the exact sequence of amino acids varies slightly across vertebrates, with the mammalian version designated as **arginine vasopressin** (**AVP**). The name vasopressin reflects the ability of this hormone to cause blood vessels to constrict, increasing blood pressure. This is one way to temporarily compensate for a loss of extracellular fluid—by reducing the size of the vasculature, AVP maintains blood pressure and avoids activating the baroreceptors. But the peptide we are calling AVP is also known under a different name: **anti-diuretic hormone** (**ADH**). A diuretic is a compound that encourages the loss of water through urination, so an anti-diuretic is a compound that discourages water loss through urination. After release from the posterior pituitary, ADH acts on the kidneys to decrease water loss by increasing the concentration of the urine. By making the urine more concentrated, less water is required to dispose of the various waste products found in it. Note that these two actions are similar: each serves to conserve and make good use of water when the extracellular compartment is low. (To avoid confusion from now on we will use only the term AVP.)

The neuroendocrine cells manufacturing and releasing AVP respond to both neural and hormonal signals. We don't know much about the source of those neurons that synaptically excite AVP-releasing neuroendocrine cells, but presumably they represent a significant integration of information about body fluids, because both hypovolemic and osmotic thirst can trigger AVP release. The hormone favoring release of AVP is angiotensin II, to be discussed shortly.

Sometimes individuals fail to produce AVP, either from birth or abruptly in adulthood. A spontaneous mutation disrupting the AVP gene arose in a colony of rats in Brattleboro, Vermont, so these rats are known as "**Brattleboro rats**." The absence of AVP means that the kidneys fail to concentrate urine and so the animals urinate copious amounts of very dilute fluid. Because they urinate so much, they must drink constantly, up to 10 times as much water as normal rats. Treating the animals with AVP causes their kidneys to produce more concentrated urine, and the animals therefore urinate and drink normal amounts of fluid. A failure to produce or respond to AVP, in both rats or humans, produces a condition known as **diabetes insipidus** (which means passing dilute [urine]). Today, treating diabetes insipidus in humans is rather straightforward: a nasal spray containing AVP is used several times a day. The same spray is sometimes used before bedtime to treat people, mostly children, who do not suffer from diabetes insipidus but wet the bed. Later we'll learn about another, quite distinct disorder, diabetes mellitus, that concerns sugar metabolism.

Angiotensin System

The liver produces a protein called **angiotensinogen**, making angiotensinogen constantly available in blood plasma. By itself, angiotensinogen has little physiological effect. But when baroreceptors in the kidneys, which constantly monitor the blood passing through, detect reduced blood flow indicating hypovolemia, they send a signal through the autonomic nervous system. The sympathetic division of the autonomic nervous system then stimulates the kidneys to release a hormone called **renin** (named after the kidneys, also known as renal glands). Presumably this sympathetic activation of renin release can also be triggered in response to brain osmoreceptors and baroreceptors associated with the heart, as well as to the kidney baroreceptors. Once released into plasma, renin converts the angiotensinogen there into another hormone, **angiotensin I**. As the angiotensin I passes through capillaries, it is converted to an active form, **angiotensin II**, which has 4 effects (figure 16.2). Outside the brain, angiotensin II has two effects: (1) it causes blood vessels to constrict (an action much like that of AVP) to increase blood pressure; and (2) it causes the adrenal glands to release another hormone, the steroid aldosterone, which also increases blood pressure, as will be discussed below.

Angiotensin II also enters the brain, specifically a collection of brain regions in which the blood-brain barrier is rather weak, the circumventricular organs we discussed earlier. Once inside the brain, angiotensin has two additional effects: (1) it indirectly activates neuroendocrine cells in the paraventricular nucleus and supraoptic nucleus to release AVP, to further conserve current water supplies, as we discussed earlier; and (2) it acts in the circumventricular organs, especially the SFO (Lebrun et al. 1995), to trigger thirst, so the organism seeks out water.

We know that infusions of angiotensin most effectively trigger thirst when placed in the SFO, but presumably the resulting thirst behavior is mediated not just by the SFO alone but by a network of brain sites activated by the SFO. One of the major projections of SFO neurons is to the preoptic area (POA), and lesion and electrical stimulation experiments confirm the idea that the POA is a part of the thirst system.

Figure 16.3 summarizes what we know about the various cues for thirst and where that information enters the brain.

The Role of Sodium in Fluid Balance

SODIUM HUNGER

We have already discussed how the osmolality of extracellular fluid must be kept within a certain range in order to protect intracellular fluid levels.

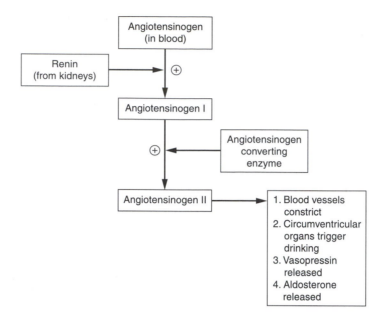

Figure 16.2 Hormonal regulation of fluid balance. A loss of blood volume (hypovolemia) will be detected by baroreceptors in the heart and kidney. In response, the kidneys release renin, which converts circulating angiotensinogen into angiotensin I, which is converted into angiotensin II. Angiotensin II then causes blood vessels to constrict (to maintain blood pressure), and causes the brain to initiate thirst and release vasopressin (to further constrict blood vessels and to induce water conservation of the kidneys), and causes the adrenal cortex to release aldosterone (which stimulates the kidneys to retain sodium).

It turns out that the major solute determining how much water we can keep in the extracellular compartment is sodium (Na^+). Without sodium, we cannot retain extracellular water. However, because some loss of sodium is unavoidable in producing urinary waste products, animals must carefully regulate sodium stores to avoid dehydration. When animals are deprived of sodium, they display a very specific **sodium hunger**, seeking out salty foods. Normally we know when we are in need of sodium, because salty foods taste especially good at those times. Presumably, animals displaying sodium hunger also find salty foods especially palatable.

Thus, animals must walk the fine line of procuring sufficient Na^+ to retain extracellular fluid, but not gather so much extracellular Na^+ that they risk reducing intracellular fluid. So there are at least two major systems to regulate the loss of Na^+: an adrenal system to slow Na^+ loss, and a cardiac system to favor Na^+ loss.

THE ROLE OF ALDOSTERONE IN SODIUM AND FLUID BALANCE
In chapter 1 we learned that the adrenal cortex produces two classes of steroid hormones: glucocorticoids that, among other things, regulate glucose, and **mineralocorticoids**, named for their regulation of minerals, specifically

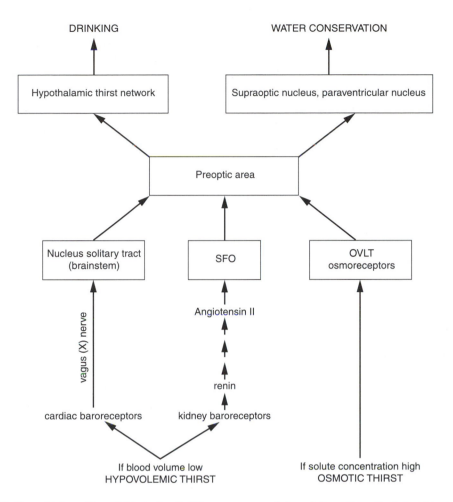

Figure 16.3 Neural integration of thirst signals. The vagus nerve brings information about heart baroreceptors to the brain. Kidney baroreceptors trigger a cascade of hormones, eventually sending angiotensin II to the subfornical organ (SFO). Meanwhile, osmoreceptors in the organum vasculosum of the lamina terminalis (OVLT) can detect increased solutes in circulation. The preoptic area (POA) seems to integrate these various signals and trigger both thirst and the release of vasopressin to conserve present water stores.

Na^+. The major mineralocorticoid is **aldosterone**. As we described above, the formation of angiotensin II in plasma stimulates the release of aldosterone from the adrenals. Following the steps in the hormonal regulation of aldosterone illustrates the coordination of water conservation with Na^+ conservation. Reduced blood volume causes the release of renin from the kidneys, and the renin catalyzes the formation of angiotensin II in plasma. Angiotensin II triggers both thirst in the brain and the release of aldosterone from the adrenals. The aldosterone then binds to mineralocorticoid receptors in the kidneys, causing them to conserve Na^+. While angiotensin II is responsible for significant *changes* in aldosterone release, the anterior pituitary hormone adrenocorticotropic hormone (ACTH) has a smaller role, stimulating *tonic* aldosterone release. ACTH plays the primary role in regulating the other adrenal steroids, the glucocorticoids, as we'll discuss later in this chapter.

While aldosterone promotes Na^+ retention, another hormone promotes Na^+ loss. The upper chambers of the heart, the atria, produce a hormone that favors the passage of sodium into urine. The hormone is called **atrial natriuretic peptide** (**ANP**) because it originates in the atria and because natriuretic means sodium-passing. (The hormone is also known as atriopeptin.) ANP has four major actions: (1) it reduces the release of renin from the kidneys, (2) it reduces the production of aldosterone from the adrenal glands, (3) it inhibits AVP release, and (4) it relaxes blood vessel walls. These actions together lower blood pressure and increase the production of urine and the amount of sodium lost through the urine. After ANP was isolated, similar peptides, each exerting similar effects, were found to be released from the brain, but they have not been as well studied as ANP. Since ANP favors the loss of both water and sodium, it tends to be released only when the organism has ample reserves of fluid and sodium. Together, ANP and aldosterone regulate Na^+ levels to maintain the extracellular fluid compartment, which in turn protects intracellular fluid.

Body-Weight Regulation

Energy Balance, Thermoregulation, and Metabolic Rate

Nutrients are chemical building blocks, such as amino acids, minerals, and vitamins, which are needed for basic cellular functions. But cells also need some chemicals simply to generate energy to drive the many chemical reactions taking place within them. Mammals and birds have evolved a characteristic that makes chemical energy from food even more important: a regulated body temperature. The cells of mature birds and mammals quickly die when subjected to temperatures much above or much below body temperature. So when we break down food, only a small minority of it provides nutrients; the vast majority is used simply to release heat (from the breakdown of molecular bonds) to maintain body temperature to keep our cells functioning. This is why, pound for pound, a pet dog must be fed much more food than a pet lizard or snake, which allows its body temperature to change with the environment.

We can't know what an animal feels when it is eating, but we can assume that an animal which will work, by pressing a bar or running a maze or digging up seeds, to gain and eat food is experiencing hunger. Probably under such conditions the animal feels much as we do when we are hungry, but we needn't make any assumptions about that. Alternatively, when an animal shows no interest in eating we say it is not hungry and if it has eaten a reasonable amount lately we may assume it is full (satiated or sated).

What we may not realize is that, because it takes time to break down food to provide the raw materials cells need, each organism must gather food prospectively and not just in response to present shortages, because a shortage of energy would be fatal. Rather, the organism must carefully monitor energy stores to anticipate future needs and gather food well in advance of those needs. Obviously, these circumstances mean that animals must have a system of short- and long-term storage for nutrients and energy, and much of our discussion of body-weight regulation will deal with the shuttling of resources into storage and the release of stored resources for immediate use. Because the decision about when to gather and when to store energy must take into account many different parameters, the brain plays the central role in body-weight regulation. Because hormones can coordinate different systems within the body, they play important roles in both informing the brain about internal conditions and implementing brain commands about energy distribution.

Energy Sources for the Body and Brain

GLUCOSE, GLYCOGEN, AND FAT AS ENERGY SOURCES
The most readily usable form of chemical energy in the body is the sugar molecule **glucose**. Glucose can be quickly metabolized to provide energy for almost all cellular processes, and so the body works hard to make sure there is a certain level of glucose in circulation at all times (figure 16.4). But too much glucose in circulation can have very deleterious effects on a wide variety of tissues, so we cannot keep much of a reserve of glucose in circulation at any one time. So organisms maintain both short-term and long-term storage depots of glucose. Linking a few glucose molecules together, the body forms the molecule **glycogen**. Glycogen can be readily broken down to form glucose molecules, so it offers a short-term depot of glucose. Two hormones from the **pancreas** control the transformation back and forth from glycogen to glucose. The **alpha cells** of the **islets of Langerhans** in the pancreas produce the peptide hormone **glucagon**, which catalyzes the conversion of glycogen to glucose, providing ready energy.

THE CENTRAL ROLE OF INSULIN IN ENERGY BALANCE
Conversely, the **beta cells** of the pancreatic islets of Langerhans produce the peptide hormone **insulin**, which favors the conversion of glucose into glycogen storage. Insulin also promotes the formation of long-term storage of glucose molecules as **lipid** (or fat) molecules in the liver and **adipose tissues**. After a meal, glucose liberated from the food enters the circulation and triggers the release of insulin. One of the things insulin does with the glucose is promote its storage as glycogen and/or lipid. You can regard the shuttling of energy back and forth from glucose to glycogen/fat storage as reflecting an energy balance. When the body has taken in more energy than it is using at present, it directs glucose into storage and the insulin released after a meal facilitates this transfer. After the food is absorbed and insulin levels fall, the body is using up more energy than it is taking in, so glucose is liberated from various stores.

But another vital role of insulin is to activate a variety of **glucose transporters** that transfer glucose molecules to the inside of cells where they can

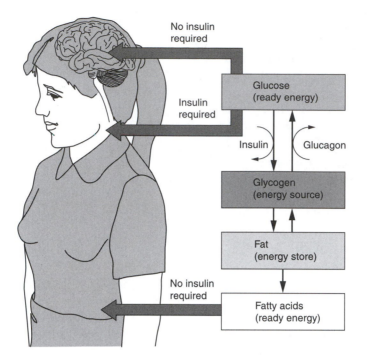

Figure 16.4 Hormonal regulation of glucose availability and storage. Most of the body requires insulin to utilize the sugar glucose, while the brain can use glucose without insulin. Ingestion of food brings a rise in circulating glucose and the pancreas releases insulin in response so the body can make use of the sugar. During such times of plentiful glucose, the insulin also promotes storage of glucose as glycogen, which may later be turned into long-term energy stores as fat. Glucagon, on the other hand, is released when glucose levels are low and promotes the conversion of glycogen energy stores into glucose.

be used for energy. Most of the body cannot use glucose for energy without this action of insulin, so the hormone is crucial for providing energy to muscles and other tissues. Most of the body can also use an alternate molecular source of energy, the so-called **fatty acids** that can be broken down from lipids. Fatty acids can be used for energy without the assistance of insulin, but they do not provide an efficient energy source, so glucose is preferred. One important exception to this dependence on insulin for glucose use is the brain—tissues there can utilize glucose molecules without the aid of insulin. In fact, brain cells are quite dependent on glucose, because they cannot readily make use of fatty acids for energy. This means that brain function is critically dependent on circulating glucose.

Diabetes

What we've learned so far about insulin's actions can help us to understand what happens when the hormone is not available. **Diabetes mellitus** results when a person either slows or stops insulin production or becomes less responsive to insulin. Without insulin, glucose liberated from food can be used by the brain, but not by the body. Furthermore, without insulin, little of the glucose is taken from circulation to be stored in glycogen or fat. This means that circulating levels of glucose become too high, which has many unfavorable consequences. For one thing, the kidneys become unable to filter out all the glucose, so considerable glucose spills out in the urine. This symptom provided the name diabetes mellitus ("passing honeylike urine"). The kidneys also produce copious amounts of urine (as also happens with diabetes insipidus, but in that case the urine is dilute and "tasteless"), and therefore the person is often thirsty. More seriously, excess glucose, especially the buildup of various glucose metabolites, also damages the kidneys, retina, peripheral nerves, and cardiovascular system. A grim irony of a person with untreated diabetes mellitus is that they are constantly hungry and may eat great amounts, yet because their bodies can make little use of the energy, they lose weight.

A person who fails to produce insulin is said to display insulin-dependent, or **type I diabetes**, also sometimes called juvenile diabetes because it tends to occur early in life. Insulin supplements can treat the symptoms, directing glucose out of circulation into tissues that need it, and even into storage. But insulin injections are not a perfect treatment, because we do not yet have the technology to deliver exactly the right amounts of insulin in exactly the same pattern as the pancreas normally does. **Type II diabetes**, also called non-insulin–dependent diabetes, is not characterized by a complete loss of insulin production but rather by a significant loss of insulin *sensitivity*. This also leads to high circulating levels of glucose, which can be averted by oral drugs that improve the function of the insulin receptors. Type I diabetes is known to have a heritable component, which is probably a vulnerability to an environmental insult, like a viral infection, that causes the immune system to attack and destroy the beta cells of the pancreas. Obesity can lead to type II diabetes, as if the increased release of insulin caused by overeating somehow leads to reduced insulin sensitivity. In mild cases, type II diabetes can be effectively treated by weight loss without drug treatment.

Glucodetectors
What normally regulates pancreatic release of insulin? One set of cues comes from the intestines, which will be discussed shortly. But another important factor regulating insulin release is the amount of glucose in circulation. Probably the most important **glucodetectors**, cells specialized to detect circulating glucose, are in the liver. Cells there send information about circulating glucose through the vagus nerve to the brain. The brain, in turn, integrates this information with other cues (including time-of-day, time-of-year, odors, and so on) and activates the autonomic nervous system to stimulate the pancreas. But glucose is not the only cue controlling insulin release. If you show a person, especially a hungry person, some attractive food, they will soon experience a rise in insulin levels. So the brain anticipates the glucose that will soon be added to the blood and orders up some insulin to put the glucose to good use.

The liver glucodetectors also help modulate hunger, since local infusions of glucose to the liver can cause an animal to stop eating, even if overall glucose levels are low. We know this information from the liver enters the brainstem through the nucleus of the solitary tract, and eventually reaches the hypothalamus, including the arcuate nucleus, the paraventricular nucleus, and the lateral hypothalamus (Watts 2000).

BODY FAT REGULATION AND LEPTIN

Several mutations in mice result in obesity, including mutations named *obese (ob/ob)* and *diabetic (db/db)*. In addition to demonstrating the potential importance of heritable factors in body weight, these mutants also indicated that hormones play a role in obesity. When Coleman and Hummel (1973) joined mice through **parabiosis**, allowing circulating factors from two mice to pass back and forth between them, they found an interesting pattern of results. Parabiosis of a normal (wild-type) animal with an *ob/ob* mouse kept the *ob/ob* mouse from becoming obese, as if the wild-type animal provided some hormone that the mutant was missing. We now know that the hormone that is missing in *ob/ob* mice is a protein called **leptin** (Zhang et al. 1994), named after the Greek word for "thin." Injecting *ob/ob* mice with leptin causes them to lose weight. Parabiosis experiments show that the *db/db* mice produce normal leptin because joining a *db/db* mouse to an *ob/ob* mouse causes the *ob/ob* mouse to lose weight. But in such pairs, the *db/db* animals do not lose weight. In fact, pairing a wild-type animal with a *db/db* mouse had no effect on the mutants, suggesting that their problem was a failure to respond to some hormone. We now know that *db/db* mice have a defective leptin receptor (Tartaglia et al. 1995), usually designated as **Ob-R** (i.e., as the receptor for the *obese* gene product, which is leptin). As you would predict, leptin treatment does not affect *db/db* mice.

Leptin is secreted from **adipocytes**, cells specialized to store large amounts of fat (hence they are also called fat cells) (figure 16.5). Adipocytes manufacture and secrete leptin, so circulating levels of leptin offer a gauge of total body fat. Leptin receptors (Ob-R) are found primarily in the brain, especially in the hypothalamic **arcuate nucleus** (Baskin et al. 1999). Recall that the arcuate also receives information, via the autonomic nervous system, about circulating glucose monitored by liver glucodetectors. So the neuroanatomy alone suggests that the arcuate nucleus is integrating information relevant to energy stores. The arcuate in turn projects widely, to the brainstem and forebrain in addition to various hypothalamic sites. One of the effects of leptin arrival at the arcuate is a reduction in the hypothalamic synthesis and release of **neuropeptide Y (NPY)**. In fact, many NPY-releasing arcuate neurons possess Ob-R, and exogenous leptin treatment reduces their NPY production (Baskin et al. 1999), so leptin probably acts directly on these cells to reduce NPY release. Activation of hypothalamic NPY receptors induces sated animals to eat. So leptin arrival at the arcuate causes neurons there to reduce the release of NPY, thereby reducing eating. Because the leptin indicates there

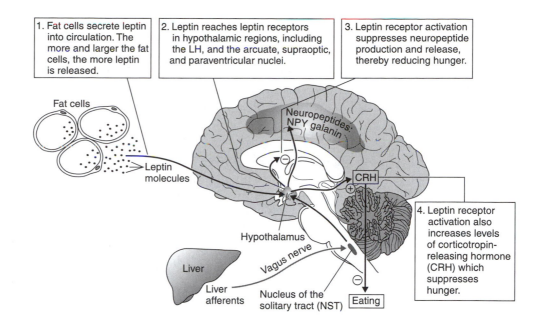

Figure 16.5 Leptin regulation of food intake. Fat cells release the hormone leptin into circulation. The leptin is detected by cells in the arcuate nucleus of the hypothalamus. Leptin promotes the release of melanocyte stimulating hormone (MSH) which normally inhibits eating. Leptin also inhibits the release of neuropeptide Y (NPY), which normally promotes feeding. Each of these two effects of leptin decrease eating, as if the brain interprets leptin as an indicator of adequate fat stores.

are ample fat supplies, that seems a reasonable response. Lactating rats display reduced levels of leptin (Woodside et al. 2000), which probably contributes to the increased eating that is necessary to sustain lactation.

While leptin reduces the release of NPY, which normally activates hunger, it seems to excite the release of another group of peptides, the **melanocortins** (**MC**), which seem to inhibit hunger. MC (which include the alpha-melanocyte-stimulating hormone, alpha MSH) are produced in the hypothalamus, especially the arcuate nucleus, and project widely through the hypothalamus and brainstem (Delbende et al. 1985). There are at least four melanocortin receptors; MC receptor numbers 3 and 4 are expressed in the brain, especially the arcuate and paraventricular nuclei (Mountjoy et al. 1994). There is also an endogenous MC **antagonist**, called agouti-related peptide, which is made almost exclusively in the arcuate nucleus (Broberger 1998) and distributed across the hypothalamus and brainstem. So there appears to be a complex system of hunger-modulating neuropeptides, including NPY and MC agonists and antagonists, influenced by leptin.

There was great hope that the discovery of leptin would reveal the cause of obesity in humans, but that hope has not yet been realized. For one thing, it turned out that obese humans, unlike *ob/ob* mice, had *more* leptin in circulation than nonobese people. Exhaustive, worldwide screening of obese humans detected only two people with defective leptin genes. So defective leptin secretion cannot significantly account for human obesity, and treating obese people with leptin would not be expected to solve their problem. In fact, some obese people may be relatively insensitive to leptin, which would also lessen the effectiveness of leptin treatment. Obesity research now is concentrating on looking for individual differences in leptin sensitivity and for drugs to modulate the responsiveness of the leptin receptor.

OREXIN

The name of the peptide **orexin** means "to desire," because orexin injections into the brain cause animals that were full to want to eat. Orexins (also called hypocretins) are produced almost exclusively in the lateral hypothalamus (Sakurai et al. 1998) and project to several hypothalamic areas, including the arcuate, paraventricular, and mammillary nuclei, where two different orexin receptors are found (Lu et al. 2000). Thus, orexins seem to focus on the same hypothalamic nuclei that detect leptin, but how orexins are regulated by, or regulate, leptin is still unknown. Evidence that orexins play a role in narcolepsy suggests that they may play a complicated role in behavior.

GONADAL STEROIDS AND BODY-WEIGHT REGULATION

It is easy to demonstrate that gonadal steroids play a role in determining body weight. Castrating adult male rats will cause them to gain weight more slowly than gonadally intact controls, while castrating adult female rats will cause them to gain weight more rapidly than control females (Wade 1986) (also see chapter 13). What is more difficult to determine is whether steroids affect feeding and body weight by influencing the brain directly. The alternative possibility is that the steroids directly influence the body and the brain detects changes in the body and directs feeding to compensate. For example, androgens such as testosterone are famous for their **anabolic** effect: they cause several tissues, especially muscles, to amass protein and thereby grow larger (Kochakian 1935). Muscles have androgen receptors (Jung and Baulieu 1992), and androgen can act directly on muscles to cause them to grow (Rand and Breedlove 1992). Androgen treatment also causes male rats to eat more food, but is that simply a response to the shuttling of more of the ingested protein into muscle? Implants of dihydrotestosterone, a nonaromatizable androgen, into the hypothalamus had no effect on food intake, while testosterone implants reduced feeding (Nunez et al. 1980). So there is little evidence that androgen acts centrally to increase hunger.

Why would testosterone implants in the brain decrease feeding? Perhaps because the hormone was aromatized to estrogen, which seems to act centrally to reduce feeding (Wade 1986). We said earlier that ovariectomy of adult rats leads to increased eating and weight gain. Estrogen acts centrally, since hypothalamic implants of the steroid reduce food intake and body weight (Wade and Zucker 1970). But ovarian hormones also act directly on fat cells. Estrogen treatment of ovariectomized female rats causes fat cells to produce progesterone receptors. Subsequent treatment of the rats with progesterone then activates those receptors and augments the uptake of fat by adipocytes (Gray and Wade 1979). This sequential effect of ovarian steroids may encourage the buildup of fat stores during pregnancy, because pregnancy and the subsequent lactation present a tremendous energy demand for the mother.

Summary

1. Homeostasis is the tendency of the body to maintain physiological variables within a particular range. The same principles of negative feedback that maintain circulating hormone levels within certain values also act to maintain internal fluid and energy balance. The brain integrates a wide variety of information about the environment, circulating hormones, and other internal conditions. The brain then induces the release of various hormones and the activation of ingestive behaviors to maintain homeostasis, often in anticipation of future needs.

2. Water freely moves from two internal compartments: the intracellular and extracellular compartments. The brain can detect low fluid levels in the extracellular compartment (hypovolemia) through baroreceptors in blood vessels. Loss of extracellular fluid or increases in extracellular salt will draw fluid out of the intracellular compartment. Osmoreceptors in the hypothalamus detect such osmolality and trigger thirst.

3. Three hormonal systems conserve internal water stores: (a) vasopressin (antidiuretic hormone), from the posterior pituitary, constricts blood vessels and reduces the loss of water in urine; (b) aldosterone, released from the adrenal cortex, induces the kidneys to retain sodium and therefore retain water; and (c) angiotensin II, produced in the blood in response to renin release from the kidneys, constricts blood vessels, facilitates the release of vasopressin and aldosterone, and enters circumventricular organs to induce thirst.

4. The most readily usable circulating source of energy is the sugar glucose. The pancreatic hormone insulin is needed for the body to readily use glucose. Insulin also facilitates the conversion of glucose to glycogen for short-term storage. Another pancreatic hormone, glucagon, converts glycogen back to glucose. Thus, pancreatic hormones regulate energy balance in the body.

5. The hormone leptin is released from fat cells and affects cells in the arcuate nucleus. In response to leptin, these cells increase the hypothalamic release of peptides such as melanocortin, which normally suppresses eating, and decrease the release of other peptides, such as neuropeptide Y, which normally activate eating. Thus, fat-cell release of leptin seems to suppress hunger through a brain pathway that begins in the hypothalamus.

Study Questions

1. In this chapter we again encounter negative feedback regulation. What other instances of negative feedback do you encounter in nature? What function

does negative feedback seem to serve? Can you find examples of positive feedback effects?

2. Why is it important to maintain a particular level of intracellular fluid? Why do cells require a particular level of salinity to function properly? What evolutionary history is reflected in the normal intracellular levels of salinity? In what way is the extracellular fluid compartment a buffer for the intracellular compartment?

3. What are the three major hormonal systems that serve to conserve internal water stores? How do these three systems interact? How does the brain modulate each of the three systems?

4. What is the role of insulin in controlling energy balance? What happens when insulin levels become too high or too low? How does the brain monitor circulating levels of glucose?

5. What is the hypothesized role of the hormone leptin in body-weight regulation? Can most cases of human obesity be ascribed to abnormal levels of circulating leptin? What other alteration of the leptin system could cause obesity?

References

Baskin, D. G., Schwartz, M. W., Seeley, R. J., Woods, S. C., Porte, D. Jr., Breininger, J. F., Jonak, Z., Schaefer, J., Krouse, M., and Burghardt, C. (1999) Leptin receptor long-form splice-variant protein expression in neuron cell bodies of the brain and co-localization with neuropeptide Y mRNA in the arcuate nucleus. *J. Histochem. Cytochem.* 47: 353–362.

Broberger, C., Johansen, J., Johansson, C., Schalling, M., and Hokfelt, T. (1998) The neuropeptide Y/agouti gene-related protein (AGRP) brain circuitry in normal, anorectic, and monosodium glutamate-treated mice. *Proc. Natl. Acad. Sci. USA* 95: 15043–15048.

Coleman, D. L., and Hummel, K. P. (1973) The influence of genetic background on the expression of the obese (Ob) gene in the mouse. *Diabetologia* 9: 287–93.

Delbende, C., Jegou, S., Tranchand-Bunel, D., Leroux, P., Tonon, M. C., Mocaer, E., Pelletier, G., and Vaudry, H. (1985) Role of alpha-MSH and related peptides in the central nervous system. *Rev. Neurol.* 141: 429–439.

Gray, J. M., and Wade, G. N. (1979) Cytoplasmic progestin binding in rat adipose tissues. *Endocrinology* 104: 1377–1382.

Johnson, A. K., and Edwards, G. L. (1990) The neuroendocrinology of thirst. *Curr. Topics Neuroendocrinol.* 10: 149–190.

Jung, I., and Baulieu, E. E. (1972) Testosterone cytosol "receptor" in the rat levator ani muscle. *Nat. New Biol.* 237: 24–26.

Kochakian, C. D. (1935) Effect of male hormone on protein metabolism of castrate dogs. *Proc. Exp. Biol. Med.* 32: 1064–1065.

Lebrun, C. J., Blume, A., Herdegen, T., Seifert, K., Bravo, R., and Unger, T. (1995) Angiotensin II induces a complex activation of transcription factors in the rat brain: Expression of Fos, Jun and Krox proteins. *Neuroscience* 65: 93–99.

Lu, X. Y., Bagnol, D., Burke, S., Akil, H., and Watson, S. J. (2000) Differential distribution and regulation of OX1 and OX2 orexin/hypocretin receptor messenger RNA in the brain upon fasting. *Horm. Behav.* 37: 335–344.

Mountjoy, K. G., Mortrud, M. T., Low, M. J., Simerly, R. B., and Cone, R. D. (1994) Localization of the melanocortin-4 receptor (MC4-R) in neuroendocrine and autonomic control circuits in the brain. *Mol. Endocrinol.* 8: 1298–1308.

Nunez, A. A., Gray, J. M., and Wade, G. N. (1980) Food intake and adipose tissue lipoprotein lipase activity after hypothalamic estradiol benzoate implants in rats. *Physiol. Behav.* 25: 595–598.

Rand, M. N., and Breedlove, S. M. (1992) Androgen locally regulates rat bulbocavernosus and levator ani size. *J. Neurobiol.* 23: 17–30.

Sakurai, T., Amemiya, A., Ishii, M., Matsuzaki, I., Chemelli, R. M., Tanaka, H., Williams, S. C., Richardson, J. A., Kozlowski, G. P., and Wilson, S. (1998) Orexins and orexin receptors: A family of hypothalamic neuropeptides and G protein-coupled receptors that regulate feeding behavior. *Cell* 92: 573–585.

Tartaglia, L. A., Dembski, M., Weng, X., Deng, N., Culpepper, J., Devos, R., Richards, G. J., Campfield, L. A., Clark, F. T., and Deeds, J. (1995) Identification and expression cloning of a leptin receptor, OB-R. *Cell* 83: 1263–1271.

Wade, G. N. (1986) Sex steroids and energy balance: Sites and mechanisms of action. *Ann. NY Acad. Sci.* 474: 389–399.

Wade, G. N., and Zucker, I. (1970) Modulation of food intake and locomotor activity in female rats by diencephalic hormone implants. *J. Comp. Physiol. Psychol.* 72: 328–336.

Watts, A. G. (2000) Understanding the neural control of ingestive behaviors: Helping to separate cause from effect with dehydration-associated anorexia. *Horm. Behav.* 37: 261–283.

Woodside, B., Abizaid, A., Walker, C. (2000) Changes in leptin levels during lactation: Implications for lactational hyperphagia and anovulation. *Horm. Behav.* 37: 353–365.

Zhang, Y., Proenca, R., Maffei, M., Barone, M., Leopold, L., and Friedman, J. M. (1994) Positional cloning of the mouse obese gene and its human homologue. *Nature* 372: 425–32.

17   Invertebrate Systems for the Study of Hormone Brain-Behavior Relationships

James W. Truman

Invertebrates account for far and away the majority of animal species on this planet. We may tend to ignore them or take them for granted, but there is one process that is common among insects that no mammal or bird has accomplished—metamorphosis. This nearly total reorganization of the body requires the coordinated efforts of several hormones, including both steroids and proteins. We will find that these hormones alter both the body and the nervous system of insects, activating behaviors that are crucial for the successful transition from larva to adult.

What organs control the neuroendocrine systems of invertebrates and how do hormones coordinate behavior with the physiology of reproduction and metamorphosis? What are motor programs and how do hormones activate them?

Introduction

Invertebrates have provided a fruitful ground for the study of the neural basis of behavior. This large assemblage of phyla, which is referred to collectively as the invertebrates, has a rich diversity of body forms and behavior. A comparative approach based on this diversity allows us to define some of the basic principles of brain-behavior interactions. Some invertebrate nervous systems are quite complex. For example, in the cephalopod molluscs (i.e., squid and octopus) the number of neurons and the complexity of brain organization rivals that of their fish competitors. Other invertebrates are quite simple. The nervous system of the nematode, *Caenorhabditis elegans*, has a fixed number of 302 neurons.

Functional studies on invertebrate nervous systems have been aided by this numerical simplicity and also by the presence of nerve cells that can be identified as unique. Since these "identified neurons" can be repeatedly found in successive individuals, the function of a particular neuron can be thoroughly defined and then analyzed in different developmental, physiological, and behavioral contexts. This identified-neuron approach has been a valuable tool in the study of the cellular aspects of nervous-system function. Since many molluscs and arthropods achieve moderate size and possess the large identifiable neurons that facilitate intracellular recording, these animals have been especially popular for neurophysiological studies. More recently, however, both *C. elegans* and the fruitfly, *Drosophila melanogaster*, have emerged as premiere systems for examining the molecular and genetic basis of nervous-system development and function.

The endocrine signals that organize the development, physiology, and behavior of invertebrates are quite diverse and, in general, differ from those found in vertebrates. However, the same classes of regulatory molecules that are used in vertebrates—peptides, amines, steroids, and nitric oxide (NO)—are also used throughout the invertebrates, and the actions of each class of compounds are typically mediated via similar types of receptors in both groups. The ancient origins of many of these signaling systems is attested to by the ubiquitous use of NO (Jacklet 1997), the widespread occurrence of biogenic amines in invertebrate nervous systems, and the existence of specific peptide hormone families that are found in both vertebrates and invertebrates. For some of these peptide families, physiological function as well as chemical structure appears to have been conserved across a wide array of phyla (Hoyle 1998). For example, the insulin-like molecules are widely associated with carbohydrate metabolism, and the vasopressin-like peptides with water relations in both vertebrates and invertebrates.

A single chapter devoted to the invertebrates cannot capture the rich diversity of hormone-brain-behavior relationships shown by these animals. Also, for many phyla, a detailed understanding of their endocrinology lags behind our knowledge of their nervous systems. This is not true, though, for the arthropods and the molluscs, because we know a considerable amount about their endocrine and neuroendocrine systems. Rather than being comprehensive, though, the goal of this chapter is to focus in depth on a few invertebrate systems that illustrate some basic principles of hormone-brain-behavior relationships.

Organizational Effects of Hormones on the Nervous System of Invertebrates

In vertebrates, hormones are known both for their ability to direct the development of the nervous system and for regulating contemporary changes in behavior. The developmental effects, often called organizational effects, are especially evident in the role of androgens in directing the sexual differentiation of the brain and spinal cord (see chapter 3). In invertebrates, there is considerable variation in the importance of hormones in directing the sexual differentiation of brain and behavior. Androgens and estrogens have been isolated from many invertebrates but their sex-dependent production and their developmental roles continue to be in debate. A clear role for the hormonal control of sexual differentiation is seen in crustaceans. Here, an androgenic gland associated with the developing reproductive tract produces a hormone that controls differentiation of the testis and the production of male secondary sex characteristics (Charniaux-Cotton and Payen 1988). But rather than being a steroid, this androgenic hormone is a glycosylated protein (Martin et al. 1999). The effects of this androgenic hormone on behavior and nervous system development, however, still need to be explored.

Sex hormones appear to be absent in insects, and sex is determined chromosomally on a cell-by-cell basis. Thus, it is possible to have gynandromorphic individuals, which means that in the same individual some tissues are fully male and others are fully female, with sharp boundaries in between. While the choice of sex in insects appears to be cell autonomous, there are a few situations in which cell-cell interactions have been shown to establish the sexual identity of developing brain structures. The most dramatic example is seen in the moth, *Manduca sexta*, after grafting a male antennal primordium onto the head of a female caterpillar. During metamorphosis, this male antenna induces the formation of male-specific glomeruli in the antennal lobe of the female's brain. These females then display some malelike behaviors, such as tracking an odor plume of the female sex pheromone (Schneiderman et al. 1986).

Although hormones in insects do not control the development of sexual dimorphisms, these animals show other developmental polymorphisms that are profoundly influenced by hormones. This is especially evident in the social insects in which the social caste of an individual is associated with strikingly different morphologies and behaviors, such as is seen for the soldier, worker, and reproductive castes of termites. These caste differences are established by the sesquiterpenoid hormone, juvenile hormone (JH), and the presence or absence of JH during certain critical periods of nymphal life results in irreversible shifts in the development of the individual (Nijhout and Wheeler 1982).

Even within a particular caste, hormones can influence the progression of tasks that an individual performs for the colony. This is best seen in worker honeybees, in which the worker goes from brood care, to nest guarding, to foraging during its lifespan. This behavioral progression is regulated by increasing levels of JH (Robinson and Vargo 1997).

Besides polymorphisms between individuals, a single individual can go through a sequential polymorphism, as is seen in the case of metamorphosis. In the most familiar examples of amphibians and higher insects, the animal begins its life as a larval morph with behavioral and morphological adaptations directed towards feeding and growth. After sufficient growth, it transforms into the adult morph with a completely different morphology and with behaviors directed towards reproduction. In amphibians, these metamorphic changes are driven by thyroid hormone, whereas in insects a family of steroid hormones, the ecdysteroids, is responsible for this transition. Although chemically unrelated, these two types of hormones have remarkably similar modes of action, and many mechanistic parallels exist between the amphibian and the insect systems (Tata 1993; Gilbert et al. 1996). The action of ecdysteroids in orchestrating the metamorphosis of the insect nervous system will be the focus for our examination of the organizational actions of hormones.

Metamorphosis of the Insect Nervous System

The tobacco hornworm moth, *Manduca sexta*, is typical for an insect that undergoes complete metamorphosis (figure 17.1). In its larval form as a caterpillar, it is relatively sedentary and is adapted for feeding. Locomotion is by crawling, which is produced primarily by movements of the abdomen.

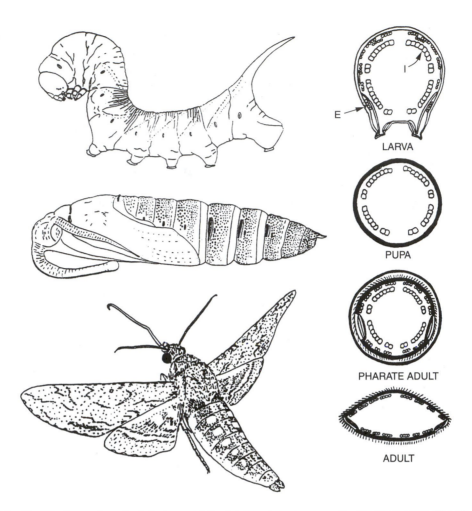

Figure 17.1 The larval, pupal, and adult stages of the tobacco hornworm moth, *Manduca sexta*. The diagrams show a cross-section through the abdominal region of a larva, a new pupa, a "pharate adult" which has completed adult development but has not yet shed its pupal cuticle, and an adult. The larva has both internal (I) and external (E) muscle groups. Most external muscles degenerate soon after pupal ecdysis, leaving the pupa with only some of the internal set. These persist during adult development while the adult-specific muscles form, but they die soon after adult emergence, leaving the abdomen with its new adult musculature.

Mechanoreception and contact chemoreception are the animal's dominant sensory modalities, and vision and olfaction are reduced and directed towards close-range stimuli. As the insect grows, it progresses through a number of larval stages (instars), the transition from one to the next occurring during a molt. Molting starts with the detachment of the epidermis from the old cuticle, progresses through a complex program of new cuticle synthesis and secretion, and ends with the shedding of the old cuticle, a process termed ecdysis.

At the end of larval growth, the larva stops feeding, searches for an appropriate site for metamorphosis, and then undergoes a molt to the pupal stage. Except for its abdomen, the pupa of *Manduca* is incapable of movement. The form of the pupa prefigures that of the adult, and the adult then develops within the mold formed by the pupal cuticle.

The adult is typically the most active life stage and its behaviors are directed towards reproduction. Locomotory function shifts to the thorax and the animal has well-developed thoracic legs and wings, which are used for walking and flight, respectively. The adult sensory systems are modified for fast response times and for the detection of distant stimuli, both of which are modifications befitting a flying insect that can move rapidly through its environment. This transformation of the motor and sensory capacities of the insect is accompanied by dramatic changes in its nervous system (Truman 1996).

REORGANIZATION OF THE NEUROMUSCULAR SYSTEM

On a gross level, the transition of the central nervous system (CNS) from its larval to its adult form involves the growth of some regions of the nervous system, the regression of others, and the fusion of particular ganglia. Ganglionic fusion is especially common in the thoracic area and is associated with flight. Presumably the ganglionic fusion reduces the time for interganglionic coordination, and thus facilitates the participation of abdominal neurons in thoracic-based behaviors such as flight.

Metamorphic changes are also seen at the level of individual neurons. These are best understood for the neuromuscular system of *Manduca* (figures 17.1 and 17.2), which has been reviewed a number of times (Levine and Weeks 1990; Truman 1992a; Levine et al. 1995). The larval bodywall musculature can be divided into external and internal muscle groups (figure 17.1). During the transition from the larva to the pupa, the external muscles and some of the internal muscles degenerate, leaving the pupa with only a set of functional internal muscles in its abdomen. The motoneurons that supply these internal muscles stay relatively unchanged through metamorphosis and provide a core of functional circuitry that controls the limited behavior of the pupa as the rest of the neuromuscular system is rebuilt. Depending on the region of the body, the musculature of the adult arises during metamorphosis either *de novo* (the legs), or from the remains of the old external muscle set (the abdomen). In the latter case, the motoneurons that supplied the larval muscles remain after their larval target degenerates during the transformation

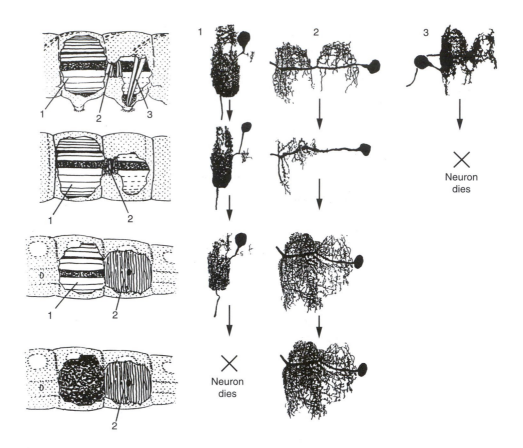

Figure 17.2 Changes in the abdominal neuromuscular system of *Manduca sexta* during metamorphosis. The left shows cutaway views of the abdominal segments A5 and A6 in the larva, pupa, newly ecdysed adult, and 2-day-old adult, respectively. The ventral internal muscles of the larva (1) persist through metamorphosis and adult emergence but then degenerate within the next day. The motoneuron VIO supplies some of the internal muscle fibers and maintains a stable morphology through metamorphosis but dies after adult emergence. The larval tergopleural muscles (2) degenerate but are replaced by a sheet of tergosternal muscles in the adult. The tergopleural motoneuron, MN3, prunes back its larval dendrites after the formation of the pupa and then grows adult-specific dendrites as it controls its new muscle. The larval muscle PPRM (3) controls the retraction of the larval-specific proleg. The muscle dies during the larval-pupal transition and is not replaced. Its motoneuron likewise degenerates after the formation of the pupal stage.

to the pupa. The neurons show a dramatic pruning back of axonal and dendritic arbors (figure 17.2), but their axons stay associated with the regrowing adult muscles and later richly innervate them. During the pupal-adult transition, these neurons also sprout new dendritic arbors and acquire the new morphologies and synaptic connections appropriate for their role in the adult (figure 17.2).

GENERATION OF ADULT SENSORY SYSTEMS

While the strategy on the motor side is that of recycling of larval components, the sensory system is built primarily from new, adult-specific neurons. The vast majority of primary sensory neurons arise in the periphery during metamorphosis in conjunction with the development of the adult legs, wings, compound eyes, and so on. Most of the central neurons that deal with this expanded sensory input also appear to be adult specific and arise from neuronal stem cells (neuroblasts) that are scattered throughout the medial brain and thoracic ganglia (Booker and Truman 1987a). There are also discrete neural proliferation zones that produce the tens of thousands of visual interneurons that are found in the optic lobes. Many of these adult-specific neurons are born during larval life but they remain arrested, immature neurons until exposed to the hormonal signals that cause metamorphosis.

One of the most complex of adult sensory structures that arises during metamorphosis is the compound eye. Larvae are equipped with only a small number of simple eyes, called stemmata, but the adult possesses a pair of large, elaborate compound eyes that may have many hundreds to thousands of individual photoreceptor units termed ommatidia (figure 17.3). In *Manduca* the adult eye begins forming in the last larval stage when a zone of epidermis immediately anterior to the larval eyes invaginates and begins to grow to form an eye imaginal disc. When metamorphosis begins, the eye imaginal disc begins to pattern itself as a morphogenetic furrow arises at the posterior boarder of the disc and slowly moves anteriorly. In the wake of the furrow, cells acquire their final identity of pigment cells, photoreceptors, and so on, and organize into immature ommatidial units. After the eye disc is completely patterned, the cells of the ommatidia then undergo a final maturation to become the functional units of the adult compound eye.

Given the size of the adult eye, it is not surprising that the most dramatic growth in the brain occurs in the optic lobes (Meinertzhagen and Hansen 1993). The progressive posterior to anterior development of the eye results in a progressive wave of photoreceptor axons that grow into the developing optic lobe. These in-growing axons direct proliferation in the lamina portion of the outer proliferation zone and also support the survival of neurons in the first two optic neuropils, the lamina and the medulla. Gradients of proliferation, selection of synaptic partners, and cell death are evident throughout these regions through the first half of metamorphic development.

The cellular strategies used in the nervous system of insects during their metamorphosis are also employed by other organisms that have metamorphic

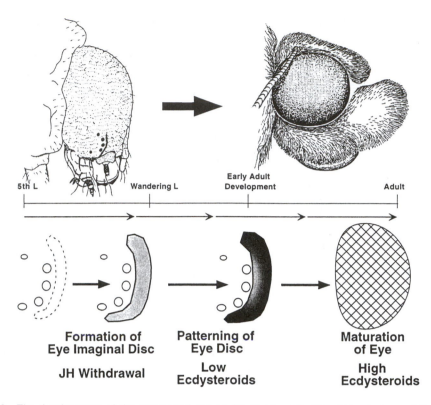

Figure 17.3 The development of the compound eye of *Manduca sexta. Top:* Lateral views of the head of the larva and the adult. The eyes of the larva include five to six simple eyes located just dorsal to the antenna and mouthparts; the compound eye of the adult is the dominant feature of the head. *Bottom:* Timeline for the development of the compound eye. At the start of the last larval stage, the decline in the titer of juvenile hormone allows a crescent-shaped field of cells immediately anterior to the larval eyes to initiate proliferation and grow to form the eye imaginal disc. After the larva stops feeding and begins to search for a site for pupation (the wandering stage), low levels of ecdysteroid support the movement of a morphogenetic wave across the eye disc, resulting in the formation of immature photoreceptor units. The maturation of the structure is then caused by the high levels of ecdysteroids that appear during the differentiation of the adult.

life histories. In frogs and toads, for example, the neurons of the tadpole have varied fates at metamorphosis. Some larval neurons, such as the Mauthner cells which are involved in the startle response of the tadpole, appear to degenerate at metamorphosis (Zottoli 1978). Others, such as the motoneurons to the jaw musculature, are preserved through metamorphosis and remodeled to control the redesigned jaw of the frog (Alley and Omerza 1998). The adult also possesses new, adult-specific sets of neurons that are apparently present but not used in the tadpole stage.

The Endocrine Regulation of Nervous System Metamorphosis
The life cycles of insects are regulated primarily by two families of developmental hormones, the **ecdysteroids** and the **juvenile hormones** (Gilbert

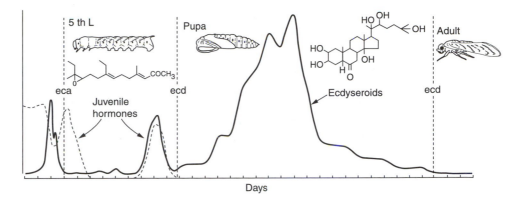

Figure 17.4 The structure of the principal juvenile hormone (JH-I) and the ecdysteroid (20-hydroxyecdysone) found in *Manduca sexta*, and the blood titers of ecdysteroids and juvenile hormones through metamorphosis. ecd, ecdysis.

1989; Nihjout 1994). Titers of these hormones during late larval life and metamorphosis are illustrated in figure 17.4 for *Manduca*. Ecdysteroids are polyhydroxylated steroids that cause the molting process. They are secreted from the prothoracic glands, paired endocrine glands located in the anterior part of the thorax. Ecdysone (E) is liberated into the blood and then converted by peripheral tissues to 20 hydroxyecdysone (20E).

The secretion of ecdysteroids is under tropic control from the brain through a peptide hormone, the prothoracicotropic hormone (PTTH). The nature of the molt—whether it is from one larval stage to the next, or from a larval stage to the pupal stage—is determined by the presence or absence of juvenile hormone (JH). These sesquiterpenoid hormones are produced by paired glands, the corpora allata, situated in the posterior region of the head. JH is maintained at high levels through most of larval life. When ecdysteroids are secreted to cause a molt, the presence of JH results in a "status-quo" molt, in which a larva molts to another larval stage. With the start of the last larval stage, the decline in the JH titer then allows sequential surges of ecdysteroid to evoke the programs of tissue remodeling and maturation that transform the larva into the pupa and then the pupa into the adult.

HORMONES AND THE REMODELING OF LARVAL NEURONS

For the nervous system, as for the animal as a whole, the withdrawal of JH is the prerequisite for metamorphosis to occur, but the metamorphic changes themselves are caused by the surges of ecdysteroids. At a gross level, this requirement for ecdysteroids can be shown for the ganglion migration and fusion that occur early in metamorphosis (Amos et al. 1996). At the level of individual neurons, though, the hormonal regulation of metamorphosis is best understood for the remodeling of the neuromuscular system of *Manduca*. This remodeling occurs in two steps. First, the surge of ecdysteroids that occurs during the larval-pupal transition causes degeneration of most of the larval muscle groups (e.g., Weeks and Truman 1985). It also causes the motoneurons to lose their motor endplates and to prune back both their axonal and dendritic arbors. After the formation of the pupal stage, the prolonged ecdysteroid surge that causes the pupal-adult transformation causes muscle regrowth and the elaboration of adult neuronal arbors and motor endings. Since the steroid exposures cause changes to both the neurons and their targets (i.e., muscle regression and the loss of motor axonal arbors), an important issue is whether the steroid acts directly on the motoneuron or indirectly through steroid-induced changes in the target muscle.

A partial answer to this question was provided by an elegant series of in vitro experiments utilizing *Manduca* motoneurons (Prugh et al. 1992). Larval leg motoneurons were labeled by injecting a retrograde tracer into the leg of the caterpillar. This fluorescent tracer was transported to the cell bodies of the leg motoneurons, where it persisted through metamorphosis. In the early pupal stage, thoracic ganglia were dissociated and the neurons grown in cell culture. The leg motoneurons could be readily identified in the dissociated culture by the presence of the fluorescent tracer. Motoneurons taken from early pupae extended axons and survived well in culture even in the absence of ecdysteroids. The addition of 20E, however, resulted in the extensive growth of dendritelike processes, as would be expected from the response of the cell in situ to 20E exposure (figure 17.5).

Interestingly, when the same neurons were explanted from larval, rather than from pupal, ganglia, exposure to 20E did not induce dendritic growth. If anything, the presence of 20E resulted in a reduction of processes over that seen in the absence of steroid. These experiments show that the ability of neurons to respond to 20E and the stage-specific nature of the response, resides with the neuron itself, rather than with the targets with which the

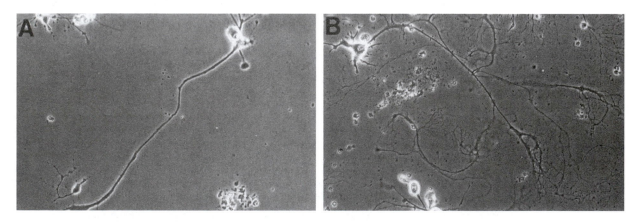

Figure 17.5 Isolated leg motoneurons from *Manduca* show enhanced production of dendritelike processes when exposed to ecdysteroids. The neurons were isolated from early pupal ganglia and maintained in the absence (*A*) or presence (*B*) of 1000 ng/ml of 20 hydroxyecdysone for 7 days. (From Prugh et al. 1992.)

neuron might interact. The results of these and other in vitro studies (reviewed in Levine and Weeks 1996) show that there are three major classes of developmental responses to 20E: process outgrowth, process loss, and programmed cell death. These processes appear to be cell-autonomous responses that neurons show either in vitro or in their normal cellular context when exposed to the appropriate hormonal signal.

HORMONAL REGULATION OF DEVELOPMENT OF ADULT-SPECIFIC NEURONS

Most of the studies on neuronal development during metamorphosis have focussed on fates and responses of larval neurons. The development of the clusters of adult-specific interneurons is less complicated because these neurons have no larval specializations that have to be removed. Ecdysteroids, acting in the absence of JH, are required for these arrested neurons to initiate metamorphic development (Booker and Truman 1987b). The most detailed information on the hormonal control over the development of adult-specific structures comes from the developing visual system—the compound eyes and the optic lobes (figure 17.3).

The withdrawal of JH early in the last larval stage allows the formation and growth of the imaginal disc for the compound eye. A small peak of ecdysteroid, acting in the absence of JH, then causes the larva to stop feeding and also shifts the growing eye imaginal disc into a phase of cell specification and tissue patterning. These processes occur progressively in a wave that begins at the posterior margin of the disc and then gradually moves anteriorly.

In the wake of this "morphogenetic furrow," cells become determined to become photoreceptors; they organize into proto-ommatidial clusters and send axons into the developing optic lobe. At this same time, the outer and inner proliferation zones of the optic lobe produce visual interneurons that will integrate and interpret to input from the photoreceptors. In vivo and in vitro studies on both the developing eye and the optic lobe show that these processes of neuronal birth, tissue patterning, and neuronal maturation are dependent on ecdysteroids. Importantly, though, different levels of steroid drive different types of developmental programs (Champlin and Truman 1998a,b). Moderate levels of 20E ($>$60 ng/ml) are needed for progression of the morphogenetic furrow and the associated processes that organize the immature ommatidia.

Within the brain, similar levels of steroid support the generation of neurons in the optic lobe proliferation zones. These steroid requirements are tonic and the events progress as long as there is 20E in the appropriate concentration range. High levels of 20E ($>$1000 ng/ml), by contrast, irreversibly repress proliferation and evoke cellular maturation in both the eye and the optic lobes. These high levels of 20E evoke the developmental programs that underlie eye maturation, such as formation of the crystaline cones, synthesis of screening pigments, production of photosensitive microvillae in the

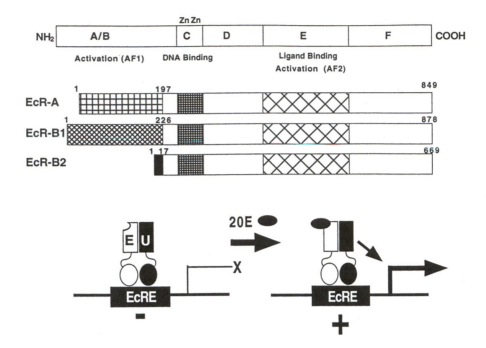

Figure 17.6 The function of nuclear receptors that mediate the action of 20 hydroxyecdysone (20E) in insects. *Top:* The protein sequence of a generalized member of the nuclear hormone receptor family. The receptor protein has discrete functional domains: the C domain contains two "zinc fingers" that are involved in binding to DNA, the E domain is the hormone-binding domain, and both the A/B and E domains contain sites involved in activating the promoters of target genes. *Middle:* The ecdysone receptor (EcR) of *Drosophila* includes three distinct protein isoforms that differ in their A/B regions but have identical DNA- and hormone-binding domains. *Bottom:* The functional ecdysone receptor complex is a heterodimer composed of EcR (E) and another nuclear receptor member, Ultraspiracle (U). This complex binds to specific response elements (EcRE) associated with the promoter of target genes. In the absence of ligand, the receptor complex can suppress transcription but the binding of 20E then stimulates gene transcription.

photoreceptors, and so on. Once these high-threshold programs are initiated, they can continue even if steroid is subsequently removed.

Steroid Receptors and the Regulation of Neuronal Development

Ecdysteroids act through a receptor complex that is a heterodimer of two members of the nuclear receptor superfamily. Members of this superfamily are characterized by a DNA-binding domain that contains two "zinc-fingers" and a hormone-binding domain that forms a pocket that binds the ligand (figure 17.6). The heterodimer includes the ecdysone receptor (EcR) and ultraspiracle (USP). The EcR/USP complex binds to specific DNA sequences in the promoter regions of target genes to regulate their expression (see Riddiford et al. 2000 for a review).

In contrast to this insect steroid hormone, the principal steroid hormones of vertebrates work through a different family of nuclear receptors that typically function as homodimers. This family has thus far been found only in vertebrates. The receptor heterodimer that mediates ecdysteroid action is from two more ancient nuclear receptor families that are represented in both vertebrates and invertebrates. EcR is in a receptor family with the receptors for thyroid hormone, retinoic acid, and vitamin D (Laudet 1997). The latter receptors form heterodimers with the retinoid X receptor (RXR), a nuclear receptor from a different family. USP is the homolog for RXR that is found in higher insects. Thus, the EcR/USP heterodimer represents an ancient relationship between nuclear receptor families which was established before the divergence of the protostome and deuterostome branches that gave rise to arthropods and vertebrates, respectively.

STEROID RECEPTOR ISOFORMS AND THEIR PATTERN OF EXPRESSION DURING METAMORPHOSIS

Many nuclear receptors exist in a number of different forms. In the case of the thyroid hormone and retinoic acid receptors, the various receptor forms arise from different genes. For EcR, by contrast, a single gene produces different receptor isoforms based on promoter and splicing variants (Talbot et al. 1993). There are typically 2 isoforms of EcR that vary in the N-terminal region of the protein, but *Drosophila* has three isoforms, EcR-A, EcR-B1, and EcR-B2 (figure 17.6). At this point, there are only data for the expression of EcR-A and EcR-B1 in the fruit fly. As seen in figure 17.7, these two isoforms exhibit a complex pattern of expression that mirrors the diverse origins and cellular fates seen in central neurons at the outset of metamorphosis (Truman et al. 1994).

During larval life, neurons show little in the way of EcR expression, consistent with a lack of known effects of ecdysteroids on neurons in the larva. EcR starts to be expressed in preparation for metamorphosis, and ecdysteroids now evoke complex responses involved with neuronal growth, remodeling, or death. As shown in figure 17.7, the levels of EcR-A are generally quite similar across the various classes of neurons but EcR-B1 is very dynamic in its fluctuations and varies markedly from one type of neuron to another. The pattern of isoform expression is most complex at the outset of metamorphosis, but by the end of metamorphosis most neurons are showing similar patterns of receptor expression. The early diversity in receptor expression is probably due to the diversity of developmental responses that are directed by ecdysteroids at the start of metamorphosis. By contrast, towards the end of metamorphosis, most neurons show the same types of responses to ecdysteroids as development nears completion.

CORRELATION OF RECEPTOR ISOFORMS TO DEVELOPMENTAL RESPONSES

For many larval neurons, EcR-B1 expression begins midway through the last larval stage, with peak levels occurring during the transition from the larval to the pupal stage. Identified neurons that show this pattern of EcR

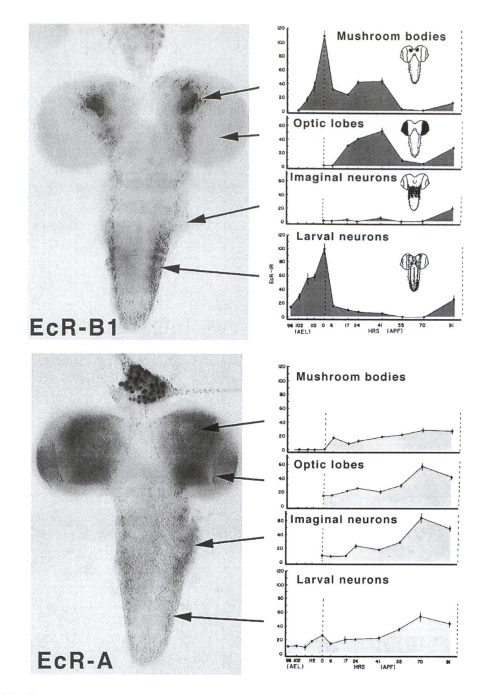

Figure 17.7 Temporal and spatial variation in the expression of ecdysone receptor isoforms in the CNS during the course of metamorphosis in *Drosophila*. (*Left*) Photomicrographs showing the distribution of EcR-B1 and EcR-A in the central nervous system at the start of metamorphosis (puparium formation). Included are the two brain lobes that are connected to the fused ganglia from the thoracic and abdominal regions of the body; the endocrine ring gland is located in front of the brain and is at the top of the picture. (*Right*) Relative levels of the two isoforms, EcR-A and EcR-B1, in various classes of central neurons through metamorphosis, including the mushroom bodies, the optic lobes, the adult-specific neurons in the thorax, and the larval abdominal neurons. Major peaks of ecdysteroid occur at pupariation, and about 24 to 40 hours after puparium formation (APF). Hours 96 to 112 AEL (after egg-laying) are during the last larval stage. (Data modified from Truman et al. 1994.)

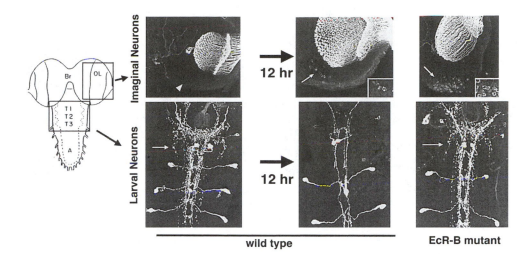

wild type

EcR-B mutant

Figure 17.8 Nervous systems from wild-type and EcR-B mutants showing that the lack of these isoforms allows the early metamorphic development of adult-specific neurons in the optic lobes but not of larval neurons in the thoracic CNS. The images are of wild-type nervous systems at the start of meta-morphosis (white puparium stage) and 12 hours later. The nervous system of the EcR-B mutant is equivalent in time to the 12-hour CNS. (*Top*) Antibodies against the cell surface protein, chaoptin, show that this protein is abundantly expressed in photoreceptor axons that project into the optic lobes. Immature optic lobe visual interneurons do not express chaoptin at pupariation (arrow head), but they then show expression by 12 hours later (arrow, inset). These neurons in the EcR-B mutants also show the induction of choaptin expression (arrow, inset). (*Bottom*) Larval neurons that express the neuropeptide FMRFamide show a dramatic pruning back of their dendritic pro-cesses (arrow) during the first 12 hours of metamorphosis. This fails to occur in larvae that lack the EcR-B isoforms. (Data from Schubiger et al. 1998.)

expression show a marked pruning back of their larval dendritic arbors at the start of metamorphosis. The need for EcR-B isoforms during this transition was examined using *Drosophila* that lacked either EcR-B1 or both EcR-B1 and EcR-B2 (figure 17.8). The larvae lacking EcR-B1 still showed pruning back of larval arbors at the outset of metamorphosis but those lacking both EcR-B1 and B2 were unable to accomplish this response, despite the pres-ence of EcR-A in these neurons (Schubiger et al. 1998).

In contrast to the larval neurons, the early development of imaginal-specific neurons was not blocked by the loss of the EcR-B isoforms (figure 17.8). These data argue that the different EcR isoforms differ in the types of steroid-driven development that they can direct. At this time, it is not known whether the different phenotypes seen for the two classes of EcR-B mutants means that there is a unique function for EcR-B2, or whether EcR-B1 and EcR-B2 isoforms have overlapping functions in mediating the pruning re-sponse so that both forms have to be removed before the response is blocked.

The early patterns of EcR isoform expression in other classes of neurons also conforms to this pattern. The adult-specific neurons in the central brain and thoracic regions of the CNS express only EcR-A early in metamorphosis (figure 17.7), a pattern consistent with these cells being immature neurons that have been arrested and have no larval features to prune back. At first sight, the mushroom body neurons, which are involved in olfactory learning, appear to be an exception because they are born during larval life and yet show high EcR-B1 expression at the start of metamorphosis (figure 17.7). Unlike other neurons that are born postembryonically, though, the mushroom body neurons mature and become functional in the larva. These neurons then prune back their larval axons at the start of metamorphosis (Technau and Heisenberg 1982) as they remodel into their adult form.

The other set of adult-specific neurons that shows early EcR-B1 expression are the neurons of the optic lobes (figure 17.7). They express EcR-B1 relatively late (10 hours after pupariation) and the receptor then persists until midway through metamorphosis. These interneurons are not functional in the larva, so one cannot invoke pruning of larval arbors as the basis of their EcR-B1 expression. This region of the brain, though, has unique developmental requirements. The photoreceptors in the eye imaginal disc are born over a 35 to 40 hr period starting midway through the last larval stage and ending about 10 hours after pupariation.

From the arrival of the last photoreceptor axons until the midpoint of metamorphic development, the photoreceptor axons undergo extensive interactions with optic lobe interneurons to generate the ordered synaptic arrays needed for vision (Meinertzhagen and Hanson 1993). During this period, there are gradients of development seen across the optic lobe, reflecting the earlier gradient of photoreceptor ingrowth. The period of high EcR-B1 expression spans this period when synaptic partners are being selected. It is speculated that the high levels of EcR-B1 are associated with maintaining plasticity in this region of the brain so that appropriate synaptic partners can be selected (Truman et al. 1994). Therefore, this region of the brain is protected from the high levels of ecdysteroids that are driving neuronal maturation in other regions of the CNS.

While EcR-B1 typically disappears during the middle of metamorphosis, it reappears as metamorphosis is nearing completion (figure 17.7). The function of the late appearance of the EcR-B1 isoform has not yet been determined, but it is seen in all neuronal types. The only heterogeneity seen in EcR expression late in metamorphosis is an enhanced expression of EcR-A seen in a group of about 300 neurons (Robinow et al. 1993). Interestingly, these neurons show a steroid-dependent fate that is not exhibited by the other central neurons—they all undergo programmed cell death after the emergence of the adult. How the overexpression of EcR-A relates to the degeneration of these cells still needs to be resolved.

Regulation of EcR Isoform Expression

Considering the pivotal role that the EcR isoforms have in directing cellular responses to ecdysteroids, it is important to understand how isoform expression is regulated. One factor of great importance is the ecdysteroid titers, and there is evidence from both *Drosophila* and the *Manduca* that the rising ecdysteroid titer stimulates EcR expression (Riddiford et al. 2000), with EcR-B1 generally having a lower threshold than EcR-A. Within a given tissue, though, fine-scale patterns of isoform expression may arise from local cell-cell interactions within that tissue.

At this time we do not know if cell-cell interactions play a role in directing EcR isoform expression within the CNS. There is evidence for this, though, in the developing neuromuscular system of *Manduca*. (Hegstrom et al. 1998). In the abdomen, the adult muscles grow from the remains of selected larval muscle fibers. The fate of a given larval muscle fiber, though, depends on the presence or absence of contact with a motoneuron; in the presence of innervation the fiber regrows, whereas in its absence the muscle remnant undergoes programmed cell death. This decision, to regrow or to die, occurs in response to the rising ecdysteroid titer that drives adult development. The rising steroid titer also causes the upregulation of EcR but, importantly, the isoform that is expressed is correlated with whether or not the fiber is innervated.

In the presence of innervation, EcR-B1 is expressed at high levels and proliferation ensues. In the absence of innervation, EcR-A is the major isoform and apoptosis occurs. Early denervation of a muscle remnant prevents the upregulation of EcR-B1 in response to rising ecdysone titers. Denervation at later times, after EcR-B1 has appeared, results in the loss of this isoform within about 24 hours (Hegstrom et al. 1998). Consequently, it appears that factors from the motor neuron are important for determining which EcR isoform is expressed in the muscle. Whether this receptor selection is the switch that directs the ecdysteroid-driven fates remains to be established.

Hormones as Activators and Coordinators of Behavior

Besides their developmental roles, hormones act to adjust behavior to match the physiological or developmental state of the animal. One of the earliest indications that hormones are involved in regulating behavioral states in invertebrates came from observations of reproductive behavior in insects. Experiments by Milburn and Roeder in the late 1960s were based on anecdotal observations that male praying mantises deprived of their heads showed incessant copulatory movements and often successfully mated with the females that decapitated them. In other insects, such as cockroaches, decapitation of males also releases rhythmic movements of the genitalia, suggesting that copulatory motor programs reside in the abdominal ganglia but that they are normally inhibited by centers in the head. This suppression was postulated to be removed during normal mating. Milburn et al. (1960) found that extracts of the corpora cardiaca, a neurohemal structure behind the brain, acted on the nervous systems of intact males to release the copulatory motor pattern, presumably by suppressing the descending inhibition.

Egg-Laying in *Aplysia*

The ability of neuropeptides to evoke complex behavioral responses is also seen in molluscs. Studies on the seahare, *Aplysia californica*, first showed that extracts of a group of abdominal neurons evoked the stereotyped behavior of egg-laying when injected into gravid individuals (Kupfermann 1967). Further work on *Aplysia* and also on the pond snail *Lymnaea stagnalis* showed that a neuropeptide, egg-laying hormone (ELH), is released both into the circulation to induce ovulation and into the CNS to evoke the stereotyped behavioral sequence utilized by the animal for the laying of the egg string (see Geraerts et al. 1988 for a review). Interestingly, ELH initiates the initial phases of the behavioral sequence, but subsequent stimuli such as those provided by the egg string are needed to move the behavior into later phases.

The Stomatogastric Ganglion (STG) of Crabs and Lobsters

The question with ELH is how does this hormone act on neuronal circuits to evoke novel motor patterns? Although we can study the action of ELH on specific, identified neurons, we are still faced with the challenge of relating the change in function of that one neuron to overall shifts in behavior. Over the last decade or so, important insights into how hormones may alter the overall functioning of nervous systems have come from studies of the stomatogastric ganglion (STG) of crabs and lobsters—a small ganglion that contains only about 30 neurons. The STG is associated with the stomach (figure 17.9) and the majority of its neurons are motorneurons. The stomach of these animals is a complex structure that is divided into areas for food storage (the cardiac sac), the chewing of food particles (the gastric mill), and the sorting of these particles (the pylorus).

The STG has provided a simple, but elegant, model system for showing how hormones and other neuromodulators interact with groups of neurons to modify their functional state (Harris-Warrick et al. 1997; Nusbaum et al. 1997). In the absence of modulators, the neurons of the STG generate little in the way of patterned motor output. However, when exposed to a neuromodulator, such as dopamine or serotonin or octopamine, the STG neurons transiently configure into a functional circuit that generates a particular motor pattern. The circuit that is assembled, though, depends on the modulator, and it arises through changes in the membrane properties of selected neurons and/or the strengths of specific synapses. As the modulators change, the neurons dynamically reconfigure themselves into different functional circuits and, hence, different motor patterns are produced (figure 17.9). Therefore, the neuromodulators and hormones serve to control the functional state of the ganglion. These molecules sit in a commanding position for regulating the functional states of the nervous system and the shift from one state to another. Consequently, a key to understanding behavioral changes may lie in understanding how behaviorally important stimuli act on these modulatory systems.

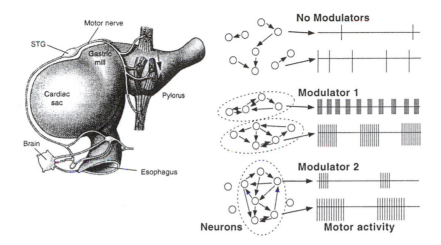

Figure 17.9 The role of neuromodulators and hormones in organizing the activity of the neurons of the stomatogastric ganglion. (*Left*) Diagram showing the structure of the stomach of the lobster and the location of the stomatogastric ganglion (STG). (*Right*) schematic representation of a set of neurons from the STG; arrows show the functional synaptic connections and the motor output of two of the neurons shown to the right. In the absence of modulators, the motor output is weak and unpatterned. Modulator 1 acts on the set of neurons to assemble two functional subnetworks that provide a fast rhythm for the pylorus and a slower rhythm for the gastric mill. Modulator 2 acts on the neurons to configure into a unified network that produces rhythmic coordinated movements that include both the pylorus and the gastric mill.

Antagonistic Behavior in Lobsters

The lesson of how neuromodulators/hormones can control the functioning of a single ganglion, like the STG, can also be extended to the entire CNS and the overall behavior of the organism. The latter situation, though, requires widespread action of the modulator/hormone throughout the nervous system. This spatial domain is appropriate for circulating hormones and also for neuromodulatory systems that extend throughout the CNS. In both cases, activity of these systems can broadly alter the chemical environment of the CNS, thereby resulting in an overall change in the behavioral state. For example, in lobsters, individuals establish dominant-subordinate relationships on the basis of antagonistic interactions. The outcomes of such interactions appear to adjust the output levels of systems of biogenic amines in individuals, enhancing octopamine production in the subordinate lobsters and enhancing 5HT (serotonin) production in the dominant lobsters (Kravitz 1988; Huber et al. 1997). The biogenic amine systems involved are ones that can release amines widely through the CNS and also into the blood, thereby producing a coordinated change in amine levels throughout the organism. The challenge of a complex system such as dominance status in lobsters is in understanding how information about social conflicts is conveyed to the CNS and how this information then alters the output of the appropriate aminergic system.

The Ecdysis Sequence of Insects

The impact of changing levels of neurohormones on the organization of behavior is well illustrated in the ecdysis behaviors of insects. Behavior is markedly altered during the time of molting, when the insect is making a new cuticle, because motor function is compromised and the animal is more vulnerable to predation. Feeding activity is typically also curtailed, the insect is less active, and it may go into hiding. As the molting process nears its end, the insect then prepares to shed the remains of its old exoskeleton. This shedding of the old cuticle involves a stereotyped series of behaviors, the **ecdysis sequence**, which are dedicated to this process and are not performed in any other context. As a prerequisite to begin the ecdysis sequence, the ecdysteroid titer must decline from the high levels that it had reached midway through the molt (Truman et al. 1983) (figure 17.4). The ecdysis sequence itself, though, is orchestrated through a cascade of neuroendocrine interactions.

PRE-ECDYSIS BEHAVIORS

As seen in figure 17.10, the ecdysis sequence is typically comprised of three distinct phases, each of which is composed of unique sets of motor patterns. The **pre-ecdysis phase** includes behaviors that immediately lead up to ecdysis. In a mobile insect, like a molting cricket or grasshopper, this phase

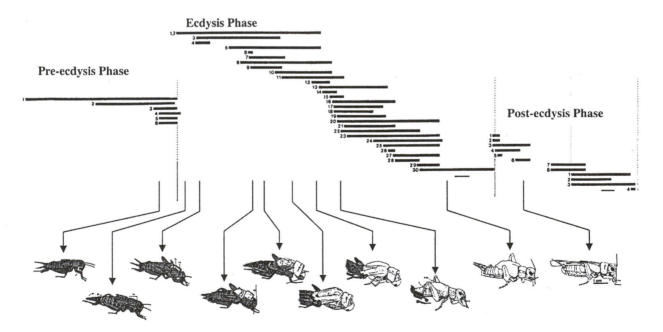

Figure 17.10 The ecdysis sequence of the cricket, *Teleogryllus oceanicus*, showing the temporal organization of the motor patterns that make up the three phases of the ecdysis sequence. Each horizontal line gives the duration of a separate motor pattern. Different motor patterns are characteristic of the pre-ecdysis, ecdysis, and post-ecdysis phases. (Modified from Carlson 1977.)

includes the behaviors involved in searching for a proper ecdysis perch and the motor patterns that loosen the old cuticle (Carlson 1977). For insects that are relatively immobile, such as a molting caterpillar, the ecdysis site was selected days earlier at the start of the molt and the pre-ecdysis movements are confined to rhythmic contractions that loosen the connections between the old and new cuticles.

In larval *Manduca*, the pre-ecdysis behaviors can be divided into two components—pre-ecdysis I and pre-ecdysis II (Zitnan et al. 1999). Pre-ecdysis I involves rhythmical dorsal-ventral contractions along the length of the caterpillar. The pre-ecdysis I movements are driven by a pattern generator in the terminal abdominal ganglion which excites the lateral muscle motorneurons along the length of the body via a pair of ascending interneurons (Novicki and Weeks 1995).

Electrophysiological recordings from the motor roots leading to the larval tergopleural muscles show rhythmical motor bursting occurring synchronously along the length of the abdomen (figure 17.11). Pre-ecdysis II involves two types of rhythmical coordinated movements: constriction/relaxation cycles along the lateral margin of the abdominal segments, and relaxation-extension cycles of the prolegs along the length of the abdomen. The latter movements involve pattern generators that are apparently located in each of the segmental ganglia.

ECDYSIS BEHAVIORS

The **ecdysis phase** includes the motor patterns used for shedding the old cuticle. In *Manduca* larvae, these are primarily anteriorly directed peristaltic waves that move along the body (Weeks and Truman 1984); the motor output from the nervous system shows bursts that move progressively along the chain of ganglia (figure 17.11). Early in the ecdysis process, the old cuticle splits in the thoracic area and the peristaltic movements slide the old cuticle backwards along the length of the body. In insects with long appendages, such as crickets, these movements are accompanied by behavioral subroutines that aid in freeing and withdrawing these appendages from their sheath of old cuticle (figure 17.10).

POST-ECDYSIS PHASE

The insect typically emerges from the old cuticle with a new cuticle that is soft and may be only partially uninflated. The behaviors of the **post-ecdysis phase** are used for inflation of the new cuticle and usually have a period of quiescence to allow time for the hardening of the cuticle. After ecdysis, *Manduca* larvae show a quiescent period of about 90 min although this is not accompanied by any obvious motor patterns associated with the expansion of the new larval cuticle. At the ecdysis to the adult stage, there are stereotyped post-ecdysis behaviors that the moth uses to inflate its wings to their proper size (Truman and Endo 1974).

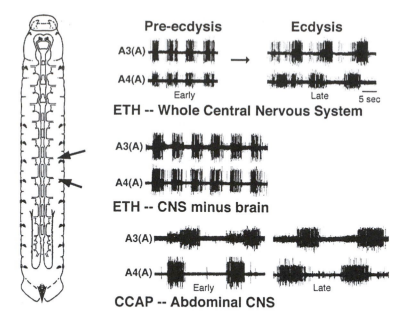

Figure 17.11 The pre-ecdysis and ecdysis motor patterns of larval *Manduca sexta*. *Left:* A dorsal view of a caterpillar just prior to ecdysis showing an exaggerated version of the central nervous system. The electrophysiological records are from isolated CNS preparations from the anterior branch of the intersegmental nerve for ganglia A3 and A4 (arrows). *Right:* Motor activity evoked by exposing the isolated nervous system to various peptide hormones. *Top:* Exposure of the entire isolated CNS to ETH results in the initial performance of the pre-ecdysis motor pattern characterized by synchronous motor bursts from along the nerve cord. The nervous system later switches to the ecdysis motor pattern characterized by bursts progressing anteriorly up the chain of ganglia. *Middle:* If the brain is not included, then only the pre-ecdysis motor program is elicited. *Bottom:* Exposure of the isolated abdominal nervous system to CCAP results in the rapid and sustained performance of the ecdysis motor pattern.

Hormones Involved in Ecdysis Regulation

Our understanding of the neuroendocrine regulation of ecdysis is confined to the first two phases of the ecdysis sequence, the pre-ecdysis and ecdysis phases. Four peptide hormones are known to be involved with coordinating these two phases (figure 17.11): eclosion hormone (EH), ecdysis-triggering hormone (ETH), pre-ecdysis-triggering hormone (PETH), and crustacean cardioactive peptide (CCAP). The first three peptides appear to be dedicated exclusively to ecdysis-related activities, whereas CCAP has the additional function of regulating the heart rate at times other than ecdysis. These peptide hormones and the cells that make them appear to be found in all insects.

ECDYSIS-TRIGGERING HORMONE AND PRE-ECDYSIS TRIGGERING HORMONE
ETH (Zitnan et al. 1996) and PETH (Zitnan et al. 1999) are the most recently identified peptides involved in the ecdysis control. They were first isolated from the moth *Manduca sexta* and are produced by an endocrine cell, called

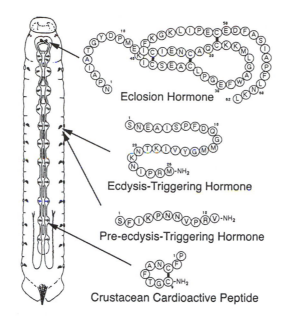

Eclosion Hormone

Ecdysis-Triggering Hormone

Pre-ecdysis-Triggering Hormone

Crustacean Cardioactive Peptide

Figure 17.12 The structure and source of the four peptides that are involved in orchestrating the pre-ecdysis and ecdysis phases of the ecdysis sequence in *Manduca sexta*. Eclosion hormone (EH) is produced by two pairs of brain neurons that send axons through the length of the nervous system and to release sites along the hindgut. Ecdysis-triggering hormone (ETH) and pre-ecdysis-triggering hormone (PETH) are made by endocrine cells (Inka cells) located by each of the lateral spiracles. Crustacean cardioactive peptide (CCAP) is typically produced by two pairs of neurons located in each of the ventral ganglia.

an Inka cell, which is associated with the epitracheal glands located on the tracheal trunks near the spiracles (figure 17.12). ETH and PETH are moderate-sized peptides that are amidated on their C-terminal. The gene encoding these peptides has been sequenced (Zitnan et al. 1999) and the precursor contains one copy of each peptide as well as a peptide of unknown function. Even though they are made from the same precursor, PETH is released in somewhat higher amounts than ETH because of the incomplete processing of the precursor.

A fascinating aspect of the function of ETH and PETH is its cooperative effect in orchestrating the pre-ecdysis behavior. PETH acts on the terminal ganglion to drive the pre-ecdysis I behavior. ETH, by contrast, is needed for pre-ecdysis II behavior. These actions of ETH and PETH are seen both when the peptides are injected into intact animals and also when the isolated CNS is exposed to the appropriate peptide (Zitnan et al. 1999). Besides inducing pre-ecdysis II behavior, ETH also causes the onset of the ecdysis motor pattern, but after a delay of about 35 min. While the ability of ETH to trigger pre-ecdysis behavior is independent of the presence of the brain, the subsequent shift to ecdysis behavior requires that the brain be present (figure 17.11). One known target for ETH in the brain is the neurons that produce EH (Gammie and Truman 1999).

ECLOSION HORMONE

The hormonal control of ecdysis was first established for moths in the early 1970s with the demonstration that the time of ecdysis could be switched between different species by interchanging their brains (Truman and Riddiford 1970). This observation eventually lead to the isolation and purification of EH, the peptide responsible for this control (see Truman 1992 for review). EH has since been found to occur throughout the insects (Horodyski 1996). It is produced by one or two pairs of neurons located in the ventromedial region of the brain (Truman and Copenhaver 1989). The axons from these neurons extend through the length of the ventral nervous system and also project to peripheral neurohemal sites in the head and/or the abdomen.

EH from *Manduca* is a 62 amino acid peptide (figure 17.12). Although long thought to be the sole activator of the ecdysis program (Truman 1992), its function now appears to be intermediate between the action of ETH (the latter perhaps signaling the readiness of the periphery for ecdysis) and the final effector of the ecdysis motor program (Gammie and Truman 1999). A "signature" for EH action is the stimulation of cyclic GMP production in target cells. Using an immunocytochemical approach to monitor cGMP changes in individual cells, researchers found that EH release was accompanied by the abrupt appearance of cGMP in a variety of cells, including a network of central neurons (figure 17.13) (Ewer et al. 1994), the epitracheal glands (Ewer et al. 1997; Kingan et al. 1997), dermal glands, tracheae (Baker et al. 1999), and cells associated with the transverse nerve (Morton 1996). Among the peripheral tissues, the function of the last target is still unknown, but EH stimulates the Inka cells to secrete ETH (Ewer et al. 1997; Kingan et al. 1997), the dermal glands to secrete a waterproofing mixture for the surface of the new cuticle

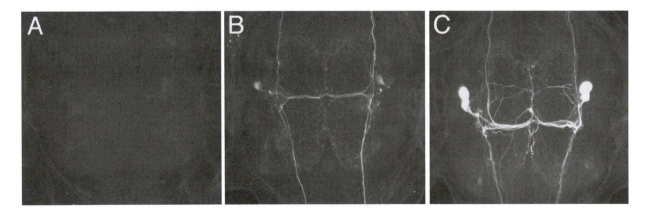

Figure 17.13 Example of using fluorescence immunocytochemical techniques to track the production of cyclic GMP in the network of neurons that contain CCAP during the course of the ecdysis sequence. The images focus on changes in the 4th abdominal ganglion. (*A*) The ecdysis sequence was induced by injecting ETH at time 0. (*B*) 15 minutes later endogenous stores of EH have been released and cGMP begins to appear in the CCAP cells. (*C*) 30 minutes later cGMP levels are high and these cells start to release CCAP to trigger the ecdysis motor program.

(Hewes and Truman 1991), and the newly formed tracheal trunks to become filled with air (Baker et al. 1999).

It took over 25 years to unravel the central effects of EH. For many years the behavioral role of EH appeared straightforward because the injection of EH into competent larvae resulted in the performance of the pre-ecdysis and ecdysis behaviors. Moreover, EH could evoke the complete behavioral programs from isolated nervous systems, but only if the tracheal system supplying the CNS was also included. It was assumed that the requirement for the trachea was to provide adequate oxygen to reach the CNS, but the subsequent discovery of ETH and the fact that the Inka cells are located on the tracheal trunk leading to the CNS immediately suggested an alternative explanation—namely, that EH actually acted on the Inka cells to release ETH and the latter peptide then caused ecdysis (Zitnan et al. 1996). EH was later confirmed to be a potent releaser of ETH, but the relationship became complicated with the demonstration that ETH was also a potent exciter of the neurons that release EH (Ewer et al. 1997; Gammie and Truman 1999).

Understanding the behavioral actions of EH was also complicated by the blood-brain barrier. It had always been curious how EH, a relatively large peptide, could cross the blood-brain barrier in isolated nervous-system preparations. It now seems evident that it cannot. In the absence of a source of ETH, the addition of EH to the bath around an isolated CNS results in no motor response. However, if the CNS is desheathed, then EH is an effective activator of the ecdysis motor pattern, but not of pre-ecdysis (Gammie and Truman 1997b). With the desheathed preparation, the delay between EH addition and the onset of ecdysis is shorter that that between the addition of ETH and the start of the ecdysis phase. This difference is consistent with the idea that EH release is downstream of ETH action. The inability of EH to cross the blood-brain barrier also explains why the EH neurons project widely throughout the CNS as well to neurohemal sites. EH released into the circulation acts on peripheral targets like dermal glands and the trachea, but central targets respond to EH released from descending axons within the CNS (Hewes and Truman 1991). These targets, which include neurons that produce and release CCAP, will be considered in the next section.

Although EH is sufficient to evoke ecdysis behavior, is it necessary? Early experiments with moths that were "debrained" early in adult development showed that they could subsequently shed the old cuticle but that the different phases of the ecdysis sequence no longer appeared as a coordinated unit (Truman 1971). A more refined approach to assessing the need for EH was performed on *Drosophila* by using molecular genetic techniques to express cell-death genes selectively in the EH neurons, thereby selectively killing them (McNabb et al. 1997). *Drosophila* that lacked their EH neurons were typically able to shed their old cuticle, but the ecdysis behavior was weak and often dissociated from other components of the ecdysis sequence such as wing-expansion behavior. In wild-type flies, the injection of ETH elicits EH release followed by ecdysis. In flies that lack their EH neurons, by contrast,

ETH injections are no longer effective in inducing ecdysis behavior. These results support the idea that EH is a crucial intermediate between ETH and ecdysis, but they also show that there are other pathways by which the insect can initiate ecdysis behavior.

CRUSTACEAN CARDIOACTIVE PEPTIDE (CCAP)
Crustacean cardioactive peptide (CCAP) was first found in crustaceans (Stangier et al. 1987), but it has since also been isolated from insects, including grasshoppers and *Manduca* (Cheung et al. 1992). In both insects and crustaceans, the peptide is typically found in 2 pairs of neurons in each ventral ganglion (figure 17.12) (Dircksen 1994). Indeed, these neurons and the peptide that they produce appear to be an ancient feature of the insect-crustacean line. In both insects (Gammie and Truman 1997b) and crustaceans (Phlippen et al. 1999), CCAP appears to be the key peptide in causing the ecdysis motor pattern.

Immunocytochemistry revealed a group of central neurons that showed a prominent increase in cGMP associated with the release of EH (figure 17.13) (Ewer et al. 1994, 1997). These neurons were predominantly the CCAP neurons. Intracellular studies of these neurons showed that they normally have a very high spike threshold and that the rise in intracellular cGMP caused a dramatic increase in their excitability (Gammie and Truman 1997a). The role of CCAP in ecdysis control was then examined in *Manduca* by exposing the isolated chain of abdominal ganglia to CCAP. CCAP exposure causes a rapid onset of ecdysis motor bursts that continue for as long as CCAP is present (figure 17.11). This motor program can be repeatedly turned on and off by addition and removal of the peptide (Gammie and Truman 1997b).

In this regard, the response to CCAP is very different from the response to EH because the latter appears to have a triggering function—added to a desheathed preparation, EH can then be washed out and the ecdysis motor program will still begin later on. The continuing presence of CCAP, by contrast, is necessary for the maintenance of the motor program. In a manner analogous to the stomatogastric ganglion, CCAP probably configures neurons in the ventral CNS into an ecdysis circuit that can be assembled or disassembled depending on the presence or absence of this peptide. CCAP also has the ability to suppress an on-going pre-ecdysis program.

The Neuroendocrine Cascade and Behavioral Sequences

STEROID PRIMING OF THE SYSTEM
An invarient feature of ecdysis is that it occurs at the end of a molt when an insect has an old cuticle that is capable of being shed. For ecdysis to occur, the insect must be exposed to a high titer of ecdysteroids and then the steroid titer has to decline (Truman et al. 1983). Ecdysteroids appear to impact the ecdysis control machinery at multiple levels. The ecdysis motor program itself appears to be available at any time if CCAP is provided. This is indicated by the finding that desheathed nervous systems from animals that are in the

process of molting (steroid primed) or from those in the intermolt period (without steroid exposure) both respond to CCAP by generating the ecdysis motor pattern (Gammie and Truman 1997b). Therefore, the steroid control over the behavior resides in the neuroendocrine circuitry and is upstream of CCAP action.

INTERACTION BETWEEN EH AND ETH IN TIMING THE EARLY PHASES OF THE SEQUENCE

A crucial point for this control appears to reside at the level of the Inka cells. The Inka cells release all their stored peptide at the time of ecdysis and do not begin to resynthesize ETH and PETH until the rising titer of ecdysteroids initiates the next molt (Zitnan et al. 1999). A decline in ecdysteroid titer, though, is then required for the Inka cells to become competent to release their peptides (Zitnan et al. 1999). Besides the Inka cells, ecdysteroids also act at other levels in the neuroendocrine pathway. The declining titer of ecdysteroids enhances excitability in the EH neurons (Hewes and Truman 1994) and also induces novel CNS proteins that are subsequently phosphory-lated in response to EH (Morton and Truman 1986).

Figure 17.14 illustrates how the various peptides interact with one other and how they relate to the underlying behaviors. It is based primarily on the control of the ecdysis sequence in *Manduca*. Some of the points are still

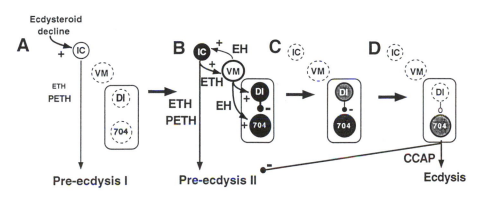

Figure 17.14 The organization of the neuroendocrine cascade that regulates pre-ecdysis and ecdysis behavior for larval *Manduca*. (*A*) The declining levels of ecdysteroids at the end of the molt causes the Inka cells (IC) to begin to secrete ecdysis-triggering hormone (ETH) and pre-ecdysis-triggering hormone (PETH). The higher levels of PETH initiate the pre-ecdysis I behavior. (*B*) As the titer of secreted hormone increase, the rising levels of ETH recruit the pre-ecdysis II behavior and also stimulate the VM neurons in the brain to secrete eclosion hormone (EH). EH acts to excite a number of targets through an elevation in cyclic GMP levels (dark shading); these targets include the Inka cells, evoking additional peptide release, and central neurons that include the abdominal neurons (the cell 704s) that contain crustacean cardioactive peptide (CCAP) and descending interneurons (DI) from the subesophageal ganglion that inhibit cell 704. (*C*) There is then a waiting period after EH release when the influence from the DIs is strong enough to suppress CCAP release from cell 704. (*D*) The waning influence of the DIs eventually allows cell 704 to release CCAP, which initiates the ecdysis phase and suppresses the pre-ecdysis behaviors.

somewhat controversial, and the student is referred to Zitnan et al. (1999) for alternate views of some of the details. One controversial issue is how the sequence is actually initiated. It is clear that a decline in ecdysteroids at the end of the molt is essential for ecdysis to occur. It is likely that the main target for this decline is the Inka cells and that this initiates PETH and ETH release.

A nonbrain site is the most likely target for ecdysteroid action because debrained molting larva initiate pre-ecdysis behavior at the expected time relative to the time course of the molt (Novicki and Weeks 1996). It is not clear, though, if ecdysteroids act directly on the Inka cells to cause secretion or indirectly through steroid-induced changes of the tracheal epidermis on which the cells reside. The blend of peptides released from the Inka cell is composed predominantly of PETH because of incomplete processing of the ETH precursor. Hence, pre-ecdysis I is the first behavior to appear. As the combined PETH/ETH titers rise, ETH begins to recruit the motor programs for the pre-ecdysis II behaviors and also to excite the EH neurons. The appearance of EH, in turn, stimulates further ETH release. This positive feedback loop results in a massive release of both ETH/PETH and EH over the space of a few minutes. The stores of both peptides are completely exhausted well before the ecdysis behavior finally begins.

DESCENDING INHIBITION AND THE REGULATION OF CCAP RELEASE

The circulating EH acts on peripheral tissues to evoke ecdysis-related changes, but it is the centrally released EH that moves the behavioral sequence to the next phase. Working through an increase in intracellular cGMP, EH excites the network of neurons that includes the CCAP cells. However, for larval ecdysis in *Manduca* the release of CCAP and the resultant onset of the ecdysis behavior are delayed for at least 20 minutes after the cells are excited. This delay appears to result from EH coactivating descending inhibitory neurons from the subesophageal ganglion as well as from the CCAP cells in the abdominal ganglia (M. Fuse and Truman, unpublished). Hence, the CCAP neurons are activated but simultaneously suppressed by these descending inhibitory (DI) neurons.

The existence of this descending suppression is inferred from the results of decapitation experiments—the decapitation of the insect at any time during the waiting period between EH release and ecdysis leads to a rapid onset of ecdysis behavior. For the scheme in figure 17.14, we suggest that the EH-induced excitation of the DIs wanes faster than that of the abdominal CCAP cells. With time, the waning inhibition will no longer be able to suppress the primed CCAP cells and CCAP is released to start the ecdysis program. This programmed delay provides time for peripheral tissues to finish EH-initiated processes like dermal gland secretion and tracheal gas filling before the ecdysis behavior actually starts. Also, as discussed below, it opens the way for other stimuli to influence the time of ecdysis.

The amounts of CCAP released into the CNS during ecdysis can only be estimated indirectly by the loss of CCAP immunoreactivity from central processes (Gammie and Truman 1997b). Such measurements suggest that CCAP is released in a tonic low-level fashion, rather than with the massive release that is seen for EH. During a normal ecdysis, only about half the stored CCAP is depleted from the central arbors of the CCAP neurons. Hence, the neurons appear to have a significant safety factor so that additional peptide can be mobilized if the animal encounters problems during the shedding of the old cuticle. Experimental interference with the shedding of the cuticle prolongs the ecdysis pattern for up to an hour before the behavior finally stops. At the end of this time, the central stores of CCAP are severely depleted (Gammie and Truman 1997b). The fact that the animal finally gives up its ecdysis attempt is probably due to an exhaustion of its CCAP stores and the resultant inability to maintain the ecdysis motor pattern.

The above scheme shows that the overall sequencing of the pre-ecdysis and ecdysis behaviors is enforced on at least two levels. Firstly, the endocrine and neuroendocrine cells involved in regulating the behaviors are arranged in a hierarchical manner with ETH stimulating EH release and EH, in turn, causing the release of CCAP. Also, at the level of the responding circuit, there is a hierarchy in responsiveness because the hormone that activates the second behavioral phase (CCAP) also turns off the behavior of the first phase.

Plasticity and Species Variation in Ecdysis Control

Ecdysis is a complex behavior whose timing and coordination depends on the form of the animal that is undertaking the behavior and the nature of the cuticle that is being shed. For example, in the case of *Manduca sexta*, the insect has limited mobility late in the molt with little (larval ecdysis) or no (pupal and adult ecdysis) locomotor capacity. The site for ecdysis was chosen days or weeks earlier, when the animal initiated the molting process, and the timing of the behavior is closely linked with the ecdysteroid decline and the developmental progression of the molt. Indeed, the onset of ecdysis can be predicted with high accuracy based on the sequential appearance of markers in the new cuticle (e.g., Truman et al. 1980). In contrast to *Manduca*, insects like grasshoppers and dragonflies are mobile during the molting process but often require an ecdysis perch from which to hang as they shed the old cuticle (e.g., Hughes 1980) Consequently, even if the insect has completed the formation of the new cuticle, it can delay the onset of ecdysis for hours while it seeks an appropriate perch. In this case, then, the onset of the behavior is somewhat disconnected from the developmental sequence of the molt. We would like to know how the neuroendocrine cascade can be modified to allow this plasticity in behavioral control.

In *Manduca*, the strong link between the ecdysteroid decline and the onset of ecdysis appears to be forged through the Inka cells and their release of ETH (Zitnan et al. 1999). ETH has a strong excitatory action on the EH neurons, and the delay between ETH exposure and EH release is essentially constant, irrespective of stage. Some behavioral plasticity, though, is built into the system between EH release and the following CCAP release and ecdysis. As described above, there is a delay between the two events that varies from 20 minutes (larval ecdysis) to 2 to 3 hours (adult ecdysis). While allowing the completion of EH-initiated physiological events (such as filling of the new trachea) prior to ecdysis, this delay also provides an avenue by which behaviorally relevant stimuli can evoke a rapid ecdysis response.

This concept is best illustrated in *Drosophila*, in which there is a 50-minute delay between EH release and ecdysis of the adult (Baker et al. 1999). Flies that are in this waiting period respond to abrupt signals, like a lights-on signal, with the rapid onset of ecdysis. Within a developing population of flies, this results in a prominent spike of eclosion immediately following the lights-on signal (dawn). The simultaneous emergence of a large number of flies, rather than their "dribbling" out over approximately a 1-hour period would be beneficial in the context of predator swamping. In adult *Manduca*, mechanical agitation, such as one newly emerged animal crawling over a waiting one, likewise results in abrupt ecdysis. Consequently, an extended delay may provide the opportunity for social stimuli to synchronize ecdysis. As indicated in figure 17.15, we speculate that these stimuli act by suppressing the descending inhibition. This speculation is supported by the observation that the removal of the EH neurons in *Drosophila* deletes both the lights-on response and any sign of the descending inhibition (McNabb and Truman, unpublished; Baker et al. 1999).

There may be a different placement of a checkpoint for insects that require an ecdysis perch before they can initiate the behavior. The fact that ecdysis behavior can be separated by many hours from the completion of the molt suggests that factors besides the ecdysteroid decline must come into play. Some insight into the site of this control is provided by the ecdysis of the first nymphal stage of the grasshopper, *Locusta migratoria*. When these insects

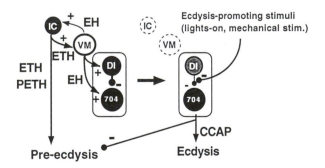

Figure 17.15 Proposed pathway by which sensory stimuli can cause early ecdysis by interrupting the delay between EH release and CCAP release. During the period when the descending inhibitors (DIs) have been activated and they are actively suppressing CCAP release, it is speculated that key stimuli can suppress this inhibition, which may result in the rapid release of CCAP from the cell 704s. (See figure 17.14 for abbreviations.)

hatch from the egg pod that is buried deep in the soil, they are still covered by the cuticle of the last embryonic stage. Only after they dig free of the soil do they initiate ecdysis behavior and shed this cuticle (Bernays 1972). Importantly, ecdysis can be delayed for hours by keeping the animal covered with sand but it commences within 60 seconds after the animal becomes uncovered (Truman et al. 1996).

In terms of the components involved in ecdysis control, we see that digging animals have no air in their trachea and show no cGMP expression in any of the typical EH targets—the CCAP cells, the dermal glands, or the epitracheal glands. Trachea fill with air and cGMP abruptly appears in all of these cells, though, during the brief period between digging free of the soil and the start of ecdysis (Truman et al. 1996). The abrupt appearance of this constellation of EH-related changes suggests that EH release occurs during the brief period after the insect digs free, although this has not been confirmed directly in *Locusta* because of the lack of appropriate reagents. Grasshoppers also have Inka cells and they release their products around the time of ecdysis (O'Brien and Taghert 1998). It is likely that ETH excites the EH neurons in grasshoppers, as is seen in *Manduca*, but in grasshoppers this by itself is not sufficient to evoke EH release. Additional input, associated with release from the soil, is probably required to bring about EH release and the downstream events that cause ecdysis (figure 17.16).

The comparison of grasshopper and *Manduca* indicates that there is flexibility in the control pathway that regulates ecdysis behavior. Depending on the relative importance of developmental and behavioral factors, different portions of the pathway appear to be emphasized. The discovery of this neuromodulatory circuit, though, provides a set of targets for examining how behaviorally relevant stimuli act in the nervous system to bring about changes in behavioral states.

Summary

1. By relying heavily on hormones and neuromodulators, invertebrates have been able to generate rich behavioral repertoires from nervous systems that contain relatively small numbers of neurons.
2. Organizational actions of hormones in invertebrates are illustrated by the role of the steroid hormones, the ecdysteroids, in directing the remodeling of the insect nervous system during metamorphosis. The variety of stage- and cell-specific responses to the steroid signals is associated with the blends of steroid receptors found in particular neurons through metamorphosis. In some of the cases, this relationship has been shown to be causal.
3. Studies of the stomatogastric ganglion (STG) of crabs and lobsters show that neuromodulators and hormones can act to transiently reconfigure neural circuits and thereby change behavioral outputs. This would probably adjust neural activity to match the changing physiological or developmental state of the animal.

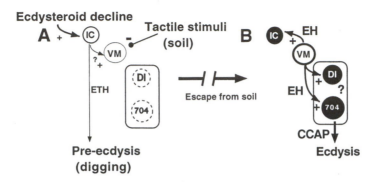

Figure 17.16 Possible modifications of the ecdysis control pathway to accommodate insects such as grass-hoppers that need to select a suitable site before initiating ecdysis. The scheme is based on the control over the shedding of the last embryonic cuticle by newly hatched grasshoppers after they dig to the surface of the soil. The ecdysteroid decline probably acts on the Inka cells (IC) to evoke ETH release, and this may evoke pre-ecdysis behaviors associated with digging to the surface. Despite the likely presence of ETH, the release of EH from the VM neurons appears to be repressed for as long as the insect is buried. Escape from the soil allows the activation of the VM neurons and EH can then evoke the downstream events leading to CCAP release and ecdysis. There appears to be very little delay (< 1 min) between EH release and the onset of ecdysis, so a delay due to activation of descending inhibitors (DI) is negligible. (See figure 17.14 for other abbreviations.)

4. Higher order organization of behavioral sequences is illustrated by the ecdysis sequence in which an insect progresses through a number of discrete behavioral phases as it sheds its old cuticle at the end of a molt. Since each phase is caused by the action of a different hormone, the overall organization of the behavioral sequence is based primarily on the organization of an endocrine circuit that regulates the timing and duration of release of the appropriate neuromodulators.

5. Species- and group-specific changes in the ecdysis sequence may arise by altering the neuroendocrine "circuit," either by altering the strength of the interaction between various components or the role of sensory input into the circuit.

Study Questions

1. By virtue of being released into the circulation, hormones like the ecdysones act on a wide variety of cells, yet these cells may show very different responses to the same hormonal signal. What factors might be involved in sculpting local responses to these global signals?

2. Using the stomatogastric ganglion, discuss the role of hormones and neuromodulators in establishing the plasticity of neuronal responses. What strategy would a ganglion have to use to achieve a similar level of plasticity without neuromodulation?

3. What would be the benefits of a positive feedback system, such as the relationship between ETH and EH, in moving from one phase to the next of a behavioral sequence?

4. How does the organization of the neuroendocrine circuit associated with the ecdysis sequence relate to the particular behavioral phases? At what points does sensory feedback appear to act?

5. Think about other hormonal systems we have studied where there is a switch from negative to positive feedback in the effect of a given hormone: How might lessons from invertebrate systems help us to think or rethink about the possible mechanisms involved in the phenomena we have discussed previously?

References

Alley, K. E., and Omerza, F. F. (1998) Reutilization of trigeminal motoneurons during amphibian metamorphosis. *Brain Res.* 813: 187–190.

Amos, T. M., Gelman, D. B., and Mesce, K. A. (1996) Steroid hormone fluctuations regulate ganglionic fusion during metamorphosis of the moth *Manduca sexta. J. Insect Physiol.* 42: 579–791.

Baker, J. D., McNabb, S. L., and Truman, J. W. (1999) The hormonal coordination of behavior and physiology at adult ecdysis in *Drosophila melanogaster. J. Exp. Biol.* 202: 3037–3048.

Bernays, E. A. (1972) The intermediate moult (first ecdysis) of Schistocerca gregaria (Forskal) (Insecta, Orthoptera). *Z. Morph. Tiere* 71: 160–179.

Booker, R., and Truman, J. W. (1987a) Postembryonic neurogenesis in the CNS of the tobacco hornworm, *Manduca sexta.* I. Neuroblast arrays and the fate of their progeny during metamorphosis. *J. Comp. Neural.* 255: 548–559.

Booker, R., and Truman, J. W. (1987b) Postembryonic neurogenesis in the CNS of the tobacco Hornworm, *Manduca sexta.* II. Hormonal control of imaginal nest cell degeneration and differentiation during metamorphosis. *J. Neurosci.* 7: 4107–4114.

Carlson, J. R. (1977) The imaginal ecdysis of the cricket (*Teleogryllus oceanicus*). I. Temporal structure and organization into motor programmes. *J. Comp. Physiol.* 115: 299–317.

Champlin, D. T., and Truman, J. W. (1998a) Ecdysteroid control of cell proliferation during optic lobe neurogenesis in the moth *Manduca sexta. Development* 125: 269–277.

Champlin, D. T., and Truman, J. W. (1998b) Ecdysteroids govern two phases of eye development during metamorphosis of the moth, *Manduca sexta. Development* 125: 2009–2018.

Charniaux-Cotton, H., and Payen, G. (1988) Crustacean reproduction. In H. Laufer and R. G. H. Downer (Eds.), *Endocrinology of Selected Invertebrate Types.* New York: Liss, pp. 279–303.

Cheung, C. C., Loi, P. K., Sylwester, A. W., Lee, T. D., and Tublitz, N. J. (1992) Primary structure of a cardioactive peptide from the tobacco hawkmoth *Manduca sexta. FEBS Lett.* 313: 165–168.

Dickinson, P., Mecsas, C., and Marder, E. (1990) Neuropeptide fusion of two motor-pattern generator circuits. *Nature* 344: 155–158.

Dircksen, H. (1994) Distribution and physiology of crustacean cardioactive peptide in arthropods. In K. G. Davey, R. E. Peter, and S. S. Tobe (Eds.), *Perspectives in Comparative Endocrinology.* Ottawa: National Research Council of Canada, pp. 139–148.

Ewer, J., de Vente, J., and Truman, J. W. (1994) Neuropeptide induction of cyclic GMP increases in the insect CNS: Resolution at the level of single identifiable neurons. *J. Neurosci.* 14: 7704–7712.

Ewer, J., Gammie, S. C., and Truman, J. W. (1997) Control of insect ecdysis by a positive feed-back endocrine system: Roles of eclosion hormone and ecdysis triggering hormone. *J. Exp. Biol.* 200: 869–881.

Gammie, S. C., and Truman, J. W. (1997a) An endogenous elevation of cGMP increases the excitability of identified insect neurosecretory cells. *J. Comp. Physiol. A* 180: 329–338.

Gammie, S. C., and Truman, J. W. (1997b) Neuropeptide hierarchies and the activation of sequential motor behaviors in the hawkmoth, *Manduca sexta. J. Neurosci.* 17: 4389–43.

Gammie, S. C., and Truman, J. W. (1999) Eclosion hormone provides a link between ecdysis triggering hormone and crustacean cardioactive peptide in the neuroendocrine cascade that controls ecdysis behaviour. *J. Exp. Biol.* 202: 343–352.

Geraerts, W. P. M., Ter Maat, A., and Vreugdenhil, E. (1988) The peptidergic neuroendocrine control of egg-laying behavior in *Aplysia* and *Lymnaea.* In H. Laufer and R. G. H. Downer (Eds.), *Endocrinology of Selected Invertebrate Types.* New York: Liss, pp. 141–231.

Gilbert, L. I. (1989) The endocrine control of molting: The tobacco hornworm, *Manduca sexta*, as a model system. In J. A. Koolman (Ed.), *Ecdysone: From Chemistry to Mode of Action*. Stuttgart: Georg Thieme Verlag, pp. 448–471.

Gilbert, L. I., Atkinson, B. G., and Tata, J. R. (Eds.) (1996) *Metamorphosis: Postembryonic Reprogramming of Gene Expression in Amphibian and Insect Cells*. Orlando: Academic Press, p. 687.

Harris-Warrick, R. M., Baro, D. J., Coniglio, L. M., Johnson, B. R., Levini, R. M., Peck, J. H., and Zhang, B. (1997) Chemical modulation of crustacean stomatogastric pattern generator networks. In P. S. G. Stein, S. Grillner, A. I. Selverston, and D. G. Stuart (Eds.), *Neurons, Networks and Motor Behavior*. Cambridge, Mass.: MIT Press, pp. 209–215.

Hegstrom, C., Riddiford, L. M., and Truman, J. W. (1998) Steroid and neuronal regulation of ecdysone receptor expression during metamorphosis of muscle in the moth Manduca sexta. *J. Neurosci.* 18: 1786–1794.

Hewes, R. S., and Truman, J. W. (1991) The roles of central and peripheral eclosion hormone release in the control of ecdysis behavior in *Manduca sexta*. *J. Comp. Physiol. A* 168: 697–707.

Hewes, R. S., and Truman, J. W. (1994) Steroid regulation of excitability in identified insect neurosecretory cells. *J. Neurosci.* 14: 1812–1819.

Horodyski, F. M. (1996) Neuroendocrine control of insect ecdysis by eclosion hormone. *J. Insect Physiol.* 42: 917–924.

Hoyle, C. H. (1998) Neuropeptide families: Evolutionary perspectives. *Regul. Pept.* 73: 1–33.

Huber, R., Orzeszyna, M., Prokorny, N., and Kravitz, E. A. (1997) Biogenic amines and agression: Experimental approaches in crustaceans. *Brain Behav. Evol.* 50(Suppl 1): 60–68.

Hughes, T. D. (1980) The imaginal ecdysis of the desert locust, Schistocerca gregaria. I. A description of the behaviour. *Physiol. Entomol.* 5: 47–54.

Jacklet, J. W. (1997) Nitric oxide signaling in invertebrates. *Invert. Neurosci.* 3: 1–14.

Kravitz, E. A. (1988) Hormonal control of behavior: Amines and the biasing of behavioral output in lobsters. *Science* 241: 1775–1781.

Kingan, T. G., Gray, W., Zitnan, D., and Adams, M. E. (1997) Regulation of ecdysis-triggering hormone release by eclosion hormone. *J. Exp. Biol.* 200: 3245–3256.

Kupfermann, I. (1967) Stimulation of egg laying: Possible neuroendocrine function of the bag cells of abdominal ganglia of *Aplysia Californica*. *Nature* 216: 814–815.

Laudet, V. (1997) Evolution of the nuclear receptor family: Early diversification from an ancestral orphan receptor. *J. Mol. Endocrinol.* 19: 207–226.

Levine, R. B., and Weeks, J. C. (1990) Hormonally mediated changes in simple reflex circuits during metamorphosis in Manduca. *J. Neurobiol.* 21: 1022–1036.

Levine, R. B., and Weeks, J. C. (1996) Cell culture approaches to understanding the actions of steroid hormones on the insect nervous system. *Devel. Neurosci.* 18: 73–86.

Levine, R. B., Morton, D. B., and Restifo, L. L. (1995) Remodeling of the insect nervous system. *Curr. Biol.* 5: 28–35.

Martin, G., Sorokine, O., Moniatte, M., Bulet, P., Hetru, C., Van Dorsselaer, A. (1999) The structure of a glycosylated protein hormone responsible for sex determination in the isopod *Armadillidium vulgare*. *Eur. J. Biochem.* 262: 727–736.

McNabb, S. L., Baker, J. D., Agapite, J., Steller, H., Riddiford, L. M., and Truman, J. W. (1997) Disruption of a behavioral sequence by targeted death of peptidergic neurons in Drosophila. *Neuron* 19: 813–823.

Meinertzhagen, I. A., and Hanson, T. E. (1993) The development of the optic lobe. In M. Bate and A. Martinez Arias (Eds.), *The Development of Drosophila melanogaster*. Cold Spring Harbor: Cold Spring Harbor Press, pp. 1363–1491.

Milburn, N., Weiant, E. A., and Roeder, K. D. (1960) The release of efferent nerve activity in the roach, *Periplaneta americana*, by extracts of the corpus cardiacum. *Biol. Bull. Mar. Biol. Lab. Woods Hole* 118: 111–119.

Morton, D. B. (1996) Neuropeptide-stimulated cyclic guanosine monophosphate immunoreactivity in the neurosecretory terminals of a neurohemal organ. *J. Neurobiol.* 29: 341–353.

Morton, D. B., and Truman, J. W. (1986) Substrate phosphoprotein availability regulates eclosion hormone sensitivity in an insect CNS. *Nature* 323: 264–267.

Nijhout, H. F. (1994) *Insect Hormones*. Princeton, N.J.: Princeton University Press.

Nijhout, H. F., and Wheeler, D. E. (1982) Juvenile hormone and the physiological basis of insect polymorphisms. *Quart. Rev. Biol.* 57: 109–133.

Novicki, A., and Weeks, J. C. (1995) A single pair of interneurons controls motor neuron activity during pre-ecdysis compression behavior in larval Manduca sexta. *J. Comp. Physiol. A* 176: 45–54.

Novicki, A., and Weeks, J. C. (1996) The initiation of pre-ecdysis and ecdysis behavior in larval *Manduca sexta*: The roles of the brain, terminal ganglion and eclosion hormone. *J. Exp. Biol.* 199: 1757–1769.

Nusbaum, M. P., El Manira, A., Gossard, J.-P., and Rossignol, S. (1997) Presynaptic mechanisms during rhythmic activity in vertebrates and invertebrates. In P. S. G. Stein, S. Grillner, A. I. Selverston, and D. G. Stuart (Eds.), *Neurons, Networks and Motor Behavior*. Cambridge, Mass.: MIT Press, pp. 237–253.

O'Brien, M. A., and Taghert, P. H. (1998) A peritracheal neuropeptide system in insects: Release of myomodulin-like peptides at ecdysis. *J. Exp. Biol.* 201: 193–209.

Phlippen, M. K., Webster, S. G., Chung, J. S., and Dircksen, H. (2000) Ecdysis of decapod crustaceans is associated with a dramatic release of crustacean cardioactive peptide into the haemolymph. *J. Exp. Biol.* 203: 521–536.

Prugh, J., Della Croce, K., and Levine, R. B. (1992) Effects of the steroid hormone, 20-hydroxyecdysone, on the growth of neurites by identified insect motoneurons in vitro. *Devel. Biol.* 154: 331–347.

Riddiford, L. M., Cherbas, P., and Truman, J. W. (2000) Ecdysone receptors and their biological actions. *Vit. Horm.* 60: 1–73.

Robinow, S., Talbot, W. S., Hogness, D. S., and Truman, J. W. (1993) Programmed cell death in the Drosophila CNS is ecdysone-regulated and coupled with a specific ecdysone receptor. *Development* 119: 1251–1259.

Robinson, G. E., and Vargo, E. L. (1997) Juvenile hormone in adult eusocial Hymenoptera: Gonadotropin and behavioral pacemaker. *Arch. Insect Biochem. Physiol.* 35: 559–583.

Schneiderman, A. M., Hildebrand, J. G., Brennan, M. M., and Tumlinson, J. H. (1986) Trans-sexually grafted antennae alter pheromone-directed baheviour in a moth. *Nature* 226: 373–382.

Schubiger, M., Wade, A. A., Carney, G. E., Truman, J. W., and Bender, M. (1998) Drosophila EcR-B ecdysone receptor isoforms are required for larval molting and for neuron remodeling during metamorphosis. *Development* 125: 2053–2062.

Stangier, J., Hilbich, C., Beyreuther, K., and Keller, R. (1987) Unusual cardioactive peptide (CCAP) from pericardial organs of the shore crab *Carcinus maenas*. *PNAS* 84: 575–579.

Talbot, W. S., Swyryd, E. A., Hogness, D. S. (1993) Drosophila tissues with different metamorphic responses to ecdysone express different ecdysone receptor isoforms. *Cell* 73: 1323–1337.

Tata, J. R. (1993) Gene expression during metamorphosis: An ideal model for post-embryonic development. *Bioessays* 15: 239–248.

Technau, G., and Heisenberg, M. (1982) Neural organization during metamorphosis of the corpora pedunculata in *Drosophila melanogaster*. *Nature* 295: 405–407.

Truman, J. W. (1971) Physiology of insect ecdysis. I. The eclosion behaviour of saturniid moths and its hormonal release. *J. Exp. Biol.* 54: 805–814.

Truman, J. W. (1992a) Developmental neuroethology of insect metamorphosis. *J. Neurobiol.* 23: 1404–1422.

Truman, J. W. (1992b) The eclosion hormone system of insects. *Prog. Brain Res.* 92: 361–374.

Truman, J. W. (1996a) Steroid receptors and nervous system morphogenesis in insects. *Devel. Neurosci.* 18: 87–101.

Truman, J. W. (1996b) Insect nervous system metamorphosis. In L. I. Gilbert, B. G. Atkinson, and J. R. Tata (Eds.), *Metamorphosis: Postembryonic Reprogramming of Gene Expression in Amphibian and Insect Cells*. Orlando: Academic Press, pp. 283–320.

Truman, J. W., and Copenhaver, P. F. (1989) The larval eclosion hormone neurones in Manduca sexta: Identification of the brain-proctodeal neurosecretory system. *J. Exp. Biol.* 147: 457–470.

Truman, J. W., and Endo, P. T. (1974) Physiology of insect ecdysis. Neural and hormonal factors involved in wing spreading behavior of moths. *J. Exp. Biol.* 61: 47–55.

Truman, J. W., and Riddiford, L. M. (1970) Neuroendocrine control of ecdysis in silkmoths. *Science* 167: 1624–1626.

Truman, J. W., Rountree, D. B., Reiss, S. E., and Schwartz, L. M. (1983) Ecdysteroids regulate the release and action of eclosion hormone in the tobacco hornworm, *Manduca sexta* (L). *J. Insect Physiol.* 29: 895–900.

Truman, J. W., Taghert, P. H., and Reynolds, S. E. (1980) Physiology of pupal ecdysis in the tobacco hornworm, *Manduca sexta*. I. Evidence for control by eclosion hormone. *J. Exp. Biol.* 88: 327–337.

Truman, J. W., Ewer, J., and Ball, E. E. (1996) Dynamics of cyclic GMP changes in identified neurones during ecdysis behaviour in the locust, *Locusta migratoria. J. Exp. Biol.* 199: 749–758.

Truman, J. W., Talbot, W. S., Fahrbach, S. E., and Hogness, D. S. (1994) Ecdysone receptor expression in the CNS correlates with stage-specific responses to ecdysteroids during *Drosophila* and *Manduca* development. *Development* 120: 219–234.

Weeks, J. C., and Truman, J. W. (1984) Neural organization of peptide-activated ecdysis behaviors during metamorphosis in *Manduca sexta*. I. Conservation of the peristalsis motor pattern at the larval-pupal transformation. *J. Comp. Physiol.* 155: 407–422.

Weeks, J. C., and Truman, J. W. (1985) Independent steroid control of the fates of motoneurons and their muscles during insect metamorphosis. *J. Neurosci.* 5: 2290–2300.

Zitnan, D., Kingan, T. G., Hermesman, J. L., and Adams, M. E. (1996) Identification of ecdysis-triggering hormone from an epitracheal endocrine system. *Science* 271: 88–91.

Zitnan, D., Ross, L. S., Zitnanova, I., Hermesman, J. L., Gill, S. S., and Adams, M. E. (1999) Steroid induction of a peptide hormone gene leads to orchestration of a defined behavioral sequence. *Neuron* 23: 523–535.

Zottoli, S. J. (1978) Comparative morphology of the Mauthner cell in fish and amphibians. In D. Faber, and H. Korn (Eds.), *Neurobiology of Mauthner Cells*. New York: Raven Press, pp. 13–45.

18 Environmental Factors Influencing Hormone Secretion

Rae Silver and Lance J. Kriegsfeld

The sensory input that an animal receives can affect hormonal systems and, in so doing, affect reproductive function. Visual, tactile, olfactory, and auditory cues are all used in this regard, as is illustrated in this chapter. Most mammals are nocturnal, however, and rely heavily on the sense of smell to find food, to avoid danger, and even to find and select mates. Furthermore, odorants have powerful influences on reproductive physiology, including the maintenance of pregnancy and the acceleration of puberty. Many of the environmental cues that can affect hormonal secretion and, consequently, change the physiology or behavior of an individual will also be discussed.

How can environmental stimuli affect hormone secretion and reproductive status, and why might such responses be advantageous? What is the evidence that each of the senses can mediate such influences, and are these effects seen in humans?

Introduction

You should now be familiar with the idea that chemicals produced by our bodies (hormones and neurotransmitters, for example) influence how we feel, how we behave, and how we respond to our surroundings. In ancient times, personality traits were attributed to the body's chemical composition: people were thought to be sanguine, phlegmatic, bilious, or splenic according to the proportions of blood, mucus, bile, and spleen their bodies produced. Today we are much more knowledgeable about the ways in which hormones influence behavior, and there is no doubting the basic concept that body chemistry alters mood, behavior, and perception.

We are much less familiar, however, with the idea that our experiences can alter our body chemistry, though this topic is receiving serious scientific attention from the public, from researchers, and from the medical community (see National Center for Complementary and Alternative Medicine at http://nccam.nih.gov/). The aim of this chapter is to provide an overview of some of the remarkable ways in which the operations of our senses of sight, sound, smell, and touch can change endocrine functions. To illustrate this concept, we will focus on the chemical changes mediated by the reproductive system.

The plan of the chapter is first to describe the variety of environmental conditions under which hormone secretions can be altered in animal studies, with the goal of understanding the mechanisms mediating a range of phenomena. Experimental studies in animals allow us to isolate specific sensory systems and neural/endocrine pathways involved in particular hormonal effects. The second part of the chapter focuses on similar responses in human subjects and patients, where it is often difficult to isolate the specific contribution of individual factors.

We conclude with some reflections on how environmental stimuli are integrated to influence hormonal responses and physiology in natural populations in order to maximize survival. Here we emphasize the ways in which the various sensory and endocrine systems act in unison or in sequence in animals to insure the coordination between sex partners, and between parents and offspring, that is necessary if reproduction is to be successful in producing viable offspring.

Environmental Factors That Influence Hormones in Animals

Experimental research with laboratory animals permits the isolation and quantification of environmental stimuli that affect hormone production in carefully controlled studies. In the next section, four major sensory modalities (sight, smell, touch, and hearing) will be examined in turn. The effectiveness of stimuli from each modality on seasonal breeding, puberty, cycles of ovulation, pregnancy, and lactation in animals will be discussed in turn.

Visual

ONSET OF REPRODUCTION

Puberty

Numerous factors change with the progression of the seasons. One factor that reliably and predictably changes throughout the year is day length (number of hours of light per day). Animals use this information to time breeding seasonally (see below) as well as to guide reproductive development. When a female rat reaches puberty, the membrane covering the vagina ruptures. The age at which the vaginal membrane ruptures is therefore a convenient measure of the onset of puberty. Female laboratory rats exposed to normal seasonal fluctuations of light and dark demonstrate an influence of light upon attainment of puberty. The females born in April show vaginal membrane rupture at an average of 40 days, while those born in November do not show rupture until they are 47 days of age. Further evidence for an effect of light on puberty in rats comes from experiments in which females are raised under conditions of constant artificial light from the day of birth. Their vaginal membranes rupture 4 to 7 days earlier than those of females housed in conditions of alternating periods of artificial light and dark each day. It is interesting to note that the effects of light on puberty are in opposite directions in rats, which are nocturnal, from humans, who are diurnal. In diurnal birds such as white-crowned sparrows, light has a delaying effect on puberty (Yokoyama and Farner 1976).

The influence of light on the age of puberty, as measured by testicular descent, has also been studied in male rats. At the time of birth, the testes of rats lie in the abdominal cavity. Sometime before puberty, the testes descend from the abdominal cavity into the scrotum. The time of descent of the testes is advanced by several days in rats housed in constant light compared to control males housed in an environment of alternating periods of light and dark.

In reproductively photoperiodic mammalian species, puberty is attained more rapidly when animals are exposed to long day lengths than to short days (e.g., Edmonds and Stetson 1983; Forger and Zucker 1985; reviewed in Bronson 1989). Presumbly this modulation of puberty by photoperiod allows animals in nature to delay reproductive development if they are born late in the breeding season (i.e., late summer) and are unlikely to reach maturity and reproduce prior to the onset of inclement conditions. Although photoperiod manipulations lead to alterations in pubertal development in the laboratory, animals in nature probably use a variety of environmental cues to weigh the costs and benefits of delaying versus attaining reproductive maturity (see below).

Seasonal Regulation of Reproduction

Species inhabiting temperate latitudes typically breed during well-defined periods of time throughout the year and refrain from breeding at other times of the year. Prior to the cessation of reproduction, animals experience a dramatic regression of the internal reproductive glands concomitant with a decrease in reproductive hormones (see below). In advance of the breeding season, the reproductive system becomes fully functional. This seasonal reproductive function (and neural mechanisms regulating reproductive behavior) is equivalent to the onset of puberty, and light also regulates the seasonal regression and recrudescence of the reproductive system in seasonally breeding animals.

The first experimental demonstration that external stimuli affect the seasonal development of reproductive glands was reported by William Rowan in 1925. Rowan kept two groups of migratory birds called juncos in outdoor cages during the cold winter in Edmonton, Alberta. One group was exposed to extra periods of artificial light while the other group experienced only the normal periods of sunlight and darkness of a Canadian winter. At regular intervals after Christmas, Rowan autopsied the birds. He found that the ovaries or the testes of the birds exposed to additional periods of light were enlarged. This remarkable effect was caused by the extra light despite temperatures that dropped to $-45\,^{\circ}\mathrm{C}$. In later experiments, Rowan released birds and watched the direction they took as they flew away from the aviary. Juncos that had been exposed to the extra artificial light traveled north as though it were summer, while those kept in normal winter light headed south. These studies show that the additional light to which the caged birds were exposed produced gonadal growth and determined the direction in which the birds migrated.

Photoperiodic information is used to ensure that breeding coincides with optimal environmental conditions (e.g., favorable ambient temperature and readily available food). In recent years the analysis of the effects of light on the gonads has reached a very sophisticated level. Substantial evidence indicates that animals are able to measure time, using a "biological clock" in the brain (see chapter 12). These "clocks" allow animals to be awake and alert when they should be—during the daytime for such animals as seed-eating pigeons, at night for such nocturnal predators as rodents. In mammals, all known photoreceptors lie in the retina (Nelson and Zucker 1981; Yamazaki et al. 1999). The photoreceptor that communicates photic (light:dark) information to the brain's clock located in the SCN of mammals is different from the rods and cones used in vision. Mice lacking retinal rods and cones are behaviorally blind, yet continue to adjust the phase of their clock in response to light (Freedman et al. 1999; Lucas et al. 1999). This sensitivity to light is achieved by specialized ganglion cells that contain melanopsin, the protein found in amphibian melanophores that causes color changes (Hattar et al. 2002; Provencio et al. 2002). These ganglion cells send axons directly to the suprachiasmatic nucleus (Berson et al. 2002; Hannibal et al. 2002).

In birds and other nonmammalian vertebrates, interestingly enough, the reproductive system receives information via light-sensitive receptors in the brain itself, and not via the eyes or the pineal gland (reviewed in Foster and Soni 1998; Wilson 1991). If the eyes of a bird such as the white-crowned sparrow are covered by a lightproof shield, the growth of the gonads in response to the light proceeds normally, as if the shield were not present. On the other hand, shielding the brain from light (by injecting an opaque substance such as india ink under the skin overlying the skull) prevents normal gonadal growth even when the eyes are exposed to light (Menaker 1972). The brain's clock responds to light only during a certain phase of the animal's day, and not to the total amount of light (Follett and Sharp 1969). Animals kept in short day lengths (e.g., 6 hours of light and 18 hours of darkness) have regressed gonads. Exposure to an additional 15-minute period of light each day is sufficient to produce full growth of the testes if the light exposure is correctly timed. If the 15-minute period does not occur during the clock's sensitive period, no testicular growth occurs. Foster et al. (1985) showed that the spectral sensitivity of the brain photoreceptor is like rhodopsin, with a peak sensitivity around 492 nm. This protein was later identified as opsin; opsin-containing cells lie in hypothalamic regions (Silver et al. 1988) and send projections to the median eminence where they contact gonadotropin-releasing hormone (GnRH) terminals (Saldanha et al. 2001).

Mammals also exhibit pronounced alterations in reproductive function and behavior in response to light information (Bronson 1989; Bronson and Heideman 1994). Individuals of different photoperiodic mammalian species are often regarded as "long-day" breeders or "short-day" breeders. Long-day breeders are typically small mammals that are short-lived; these animals renew breeding activities when the amount of daylight increases (i.e., begin mating in spring). Short-day breeders are typically large mammals such as

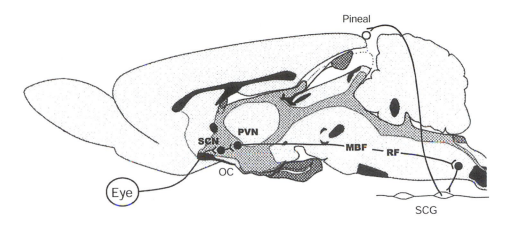

Figure 18.1 Input pathway from the retina to the pineal gland in mammals. Light information is transduced into a neural signal in the retina and transmitted via a direct retino-hypothalamic tract to the supra-chiasmatic nucleus (SCN). From the SCN, fibers synapse in the paraventricular nucleus of the hypothalamus (PVN). From the PVN, fibers travel through the medial forebrain bundle to the superior cervical ganglion (SCG). Postganglionic fibers from the SCG then project to the pineal gland to modulate melatonin production and secretion. OC, optic chiasm; MFB, medial forebrain bundle; SCG, superior cervical ganglion; RF, reticular formation.

ungulates; these animals begin reproductive activities when the amount of daylight begins to decrease (i.e, begin mating in autumn) (Bronson and Heideman 1994). Thus, in long-day breeders such as ferrets (*Mustela putorius*) and Syrian hamsters (*Mesocricetus auratus*), exposure to winter day lengths (i.e., short days) leads to a decrease in the secretion of the gonadotropins (i.e., LH and FSH). (Jallageas et al. 1994; Swann and Turek 1988). In short-day breeders such as minks (*Mustela vison*) and ewes (*Ovis aries*), the opposite pattern emerges; short-day exposure produces increased secretion of LH and FSH (Bittman et al. 1985; Jallegeas et al. 1994). These changes in the secretion of LH and FSH result in changes in gonadal maintenance, function, hormone secretion, and, in turn, behavior (Turek and Van Cauter 1994; Berndston and Desjardins 1974). The pathway by which light information affects reproductive function has been extensively studied (figure 18.1).

ADULT REPRODUCTIVE PHYSIOLOGY AND BEHAVIOR

Ovulatory Cycles
Visual stimuli more complex than light also affect hormone production in animals. A very good example is provided by the factors affecting ovarian development in certain adult female lizards, *Anolis carolinensis*. As discussed in chapter 7, the male lizard courts the female by bobbing his body up and down in a manner resembling push-up exercises and by extending his dewlap, a semicircular flap of tissue under his throat. In one experiment, the dewlaps of some males were painted with blue india ink, thereby masking the normal red color. In other males, the dewlap was surgically prevented from extending from the throat. This surgery did not interfere with his ability

to perform the bobbing movements. If a female were courted by a male that could not extend his dewlap, her ovaries did not grow. The color of the male's dewlap did not influence the female's ovarian response. Clearly, ovarian development in a female lizard of this particular species is not induced merely by seeing a male, but by seeing it court by bobbing and extending its dewlap. As Crews (1975) points out, while courtship by the male promotes ovarian development, aggressive displays are inhibitory.

In some species of birds, ovarian growth and ovulation are influenced by visual stimuli. For example, both the sound (see below) and the sight of a courting male are effective in producing ovarian growth. Female birds kept alone in soundproof cages show little ovarian growth, but if the sounds from a breeding colony are piped into the cage, then significant ovarian growth occurs. If, in addition, the female can see a courting male and if he responds to her behavior, then ovarian growth is even greater (Friedman 1977). In mammalian species, ovulation in induced ovulators appears to be more dependent upon olfactory stimuli (see below) during the social interaction than on visual stimuli.

Pregnancy

A final example of the effects of visual stimuli on reproductive hormones involves the effect of light on pregnancy (Mitchell and Yochim 1970). The total length of pregnancy and the timing of delivery were measured in rats kept on three schedules of artificial light: short (2 hours light/day), long (22 hours/day), or intermediate (14 hours/day). The results show that the duration of pregnancy was 12 hours longer in animals exposed to long periods of light each day than in animals exposed to short or intermediate light-length schedules. The time of delivery (parturition) was also influenced by light because all three groups of animals tended to give birth during the time of day in which the lights were turned on.

Lactation

Numerous studies of visual stimuli and lactation have been conducted to help increase milk production in dairy cattle. Bovine somatotropin (bST) leads to increased milk yield in dairy cattle. This potentiation of milk production is further enhanced if animals are also exposed to long day lengths (Miller et al. 1999; Reksen et al. 1999). The endocrine basis for the phenomenon is unknown, but recent evidence suggests that a hormone called insulin-like growth factor (IGF)-I may be modulated by day length. IGF-I is one of several molecules included in the IGF family (Jones and Clemmons 1995). IGF-I stimulates milk production in dairy cows, and cows exposed to a long photoperiods have greater circulating concentrations of IGF-I than cows exposed to natural day lengths shorter than the artificial light cycle (Dahl et al. 1997). These results hint at a potential endocrine mechanism responsible for photoperiodic modulation of milk yield in dairy cows and may provide a means of increasing milk yield without manipulating photoperiod.

From the above accounts of animal research, it is obvious that photic and visual stimuli are capable of affecting reproductive processes such as the onset of puberty, growth of the gonads, adulthood reproduction, duration of pregnancy, and lactation. We will see that the senses of smell, touch, and hearing also affect these processes.

Olfactory and Chemical Cues

Chemical substances released by one animal that affect the behavior and/or physiology of another animal are called pheromones (see Vandenbergh 1988 for review). Pheromones are detected by an olfactory system that is distinct from that which is typically considered the system responsible for detecting and decoding odors. The olfactory system of rodents has two components, the main and the accessory systems. The main olfactory system is responsible for the detection of volatile odors, and the accessory olfactory system is responsible for the detection of nonvolatile odors (including pheromones). In mammals, some pheromonal stimuli must be actively investigated so that the pheromone comes into contact with specialized receptors located on the roof of the mouth in the vomeronasal organ (VNO) (reviewed in Tirindelli et al. 1998). Receptors from the VNO synapse onto neurons in a subdivision of the olfactory bulbs termed the accessory olfactory bulbs (AOB). From here, neurons from the main olfactory bulbs and the AOB diverge onto different regions in the CNS (figure 18.2). Dogs use pheromones when they deposit chemical cues by urinating on tree trunks and fire hydrants, for example; other dogs are very interested in these deposits and spend substantial amounts of time sniffing them. Likewise, male moths of a certain species fly from considerable distances to approach the source of an odorous substance released by a conspecific female.

Pheromones are capable of acting at all stages of the reproductive life of an animal. They have been shown to affect the timing of puberty (Vandenbergh effect), the suppression of ovulation (known as the Lee-Boot effect), the induction of ovulation (Whitten effect), and the maintenance of pregnancy (Bruce effect) in a number of rodent species, particularly mice.

ONSET OF REPRODUCTION

Puberty

Female mice attain puberty earlier when they are exposed to a pheromone in adult male urine than when they are not (Vandenbergh effect). Immature mice dabbed between the nose and mouth with a small quantity of urine from adult males reach puberty sooner than females dabbed with a control substance such as water (Colby and Vandenbergh 1979). Additional research indicates that the pheromones are produced only by animals that have androgen in adequate quantities in their circulation. The pheromone that accelerates puberty is not volatile, and therefore is not carried by the air from the male to the female. Rather, the female must directly contact the urinary pheromone.

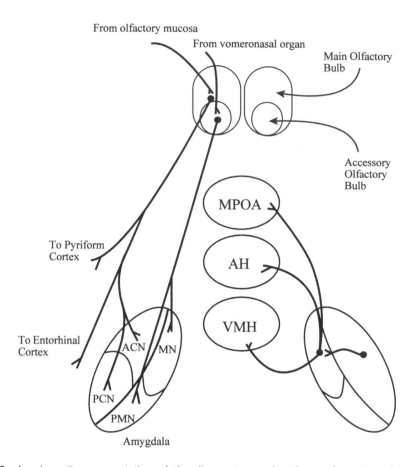

Figure 18.2 A schematic representation of the divergent neural pathways from the primary and accessory olfactory systems. Volatile odors are detected by the primary olfactory system and transduced into a neural signal that is transmitted to the main olfactory bulbs. From here, information is transmitted to cortical areas as well as to specific subdivisions of the amygdala. Nonvolatile odors are transmitted from the vomeronasal organ to the accessory olfactory bulbs. From here, information is transmitted to the specific subregions of the amygdala (areas that do not receive input from the primary olfactory system. Information from the cortical nuclei of the amygdala (receiving primary olfactory information) innervates the medial nuclei of the amygdala (receiving accessory olfactory information). Fibers from the medial nuclei then project to the medial preoptic area and hypothalamic nuclei. ACN, Anterior cortical nucleus; PCN, posterior cortical nucleus; MN, medial nucleus; PMN, posteromedial nucleus; MPOA, medial preoptic area; AH, anterior hypothalamus; VMH, ventromedial hypothalamus. (Modified from drawing by Ruth Wood.)

Social factors that presumably cause decreases in the production of androgen also cause decreases in the production of the pheromone. Among these social factors are subordination by other males and the presence of pregnant or lactating females. The pheromone itself is not an androgen: column chromatography of male urine suggests a factor with a molecular weight of 860 daltons (Vandenbergh et al. 1976). Recently, a urinary constituent (5,5 methyl-2-ethyltetrahydrofuran-2-ol) of male mice that accelerates puberty has been identified (Novatny et al. 1999). This substance may be partly (or wholly) responsible for the puberty acceleration seen in female mice housed with exposure to male conspecifics.

A pheromone produced by adult female mice may inhibit the onset of puberty in young females. The first indication that this might be so came from a study showing that isolated female mice reach puberty earlier than female mice kept in groups. By itself, this finding does not necessarily mean that a pheromone is involved; the effect could be due to crowding, to tactile contact among females, to auditory stimuli or to visual stimuli. Proof of the involvement of a pheromone was shown by brushing a small amount of urine taken from grouped female mice on the noses of isolated immature females. When this procedure was followed for 7 consecutive days, puberty occurred later than in control females that had water brushed on their noses (McIntosh and Drickamer 1977). Further studies showed that this puberty-retarding pheromone is produced by adult, as well as juvenile, female mice that are in physical contact with one another.

It has been suggested that the male pheromone (that favors onset of puberty) and female pheromone (that inhibits onset of puberty) help to regulate population density. Thus, the total amount of male pheromone released will be low when many males are present because production of male hormones is stifled in males that become subordinate during intense male-male aggressive interactions. The total amount of female pheromone present should theoretically increase with increasing population density, and this should have the effect of increasing the likelihood that immature individuals will reach puberty later when population density is high and earlier when population density is low.

Not only is more female pheromone present when population density is high because of increased numbers of females, but there is also some evidence that the potency of the pheromone (i.e., its ability to delay puberty) may actually be affected by population density (Coppola and Vandenbergh 1985; Massey and Vandenbergh 1980). Urine collected from wild female mice living in high-density populations, or laboratory mice that are group-housed, delays puberty in experimental female mice. However, urine collected from wild female mice living in sparsely populated areas, or singly-housed in the laboratory, fails to delay puberty in experimental females (Coppola and Vandenbergh 1985; Massey and Vandenbergh 1980). Thus, females may actively produce more (or more potent) puberty-delaying pheromone when population density becomes high.

Seasonal Regulation of Reproduction

In many rodent species, males and females often prefer urinary odors of long-day, reproductively competent conspecifics relative to short-day, reproductively quiescent conspecifics. One mechanism regulating the "attractiveness" of conspecific urine may be photoperiodic regulation of reproductive hormones. For example, in meadow voles (*Microtus pennsylvanicus*), females prefer the urine of long-day males to that of short-day males. If long-day males are castrated, this preference disappears, yet it can be reinstated if these castrated long-day males are given testosterone replacement (Ferkin et al. 1992). These findings suggest that preference for long-day versus short-day male urine may be a function of photoperiod-mediated alterations in gonadal steroids that, in turn, modulate pheromone production. The same preference for female odors is seen in male meadow voles; males prefer the odors of females held in long days compared to the urine of short-day females. As with males, this odor preference for female urine is abolished when long- and short-day females are ovariectomized, suggesting that day length affects odor cues emitted by females by altering ovarian hormone activity. (Ferkin et al. 1991).

In many mammals, chemosensory cues can override photoperiodic alterations in reproductive function. In one study of male lesser mouse lemurs (small primates), exposure to female urine was able to reverse the effects of short-day lengths on the reproductive system; it led to rapid increases in testosterone and eventual development of the reproductive system (Perret and Schilling 1995). Taken together, the findings presented here suggest that animals use numerous environmental cues to regulate reproduction and that one cue alone does not dictate the state of the reproductive system or the probability of engaging in sexual behavior.

ADULT REPRODUCTIVE PHYSIOLOGY AND BEHAVIOR

Male Reproductive Behavior

One of the best-known signaling pheromone systems involves the behavioral responses of male hamsters to odor cues (Johnston 1990). If the olfactory system is destroyed, the male hamster will neither court a female nor show sexual behavior (see Johnston 1990 for review). Male hamsters that are sexually experienced prefer the odor of estrous females to that of pregnant or lactating females. This is an adaptive response, as female hamsters are larger than males, and lactating and pregnant hamsters are very aggressive to males.

It has been established that the vaginal discharge from the female hamster contains chemosignals that attract and stimulate the sexual behavior of the male (Murphy 1980). If hamster vaginal discharge is applied to the hindquarters of a male hamster—either anesthetized or awake—it becomes sexually attractive to other males. In addition to eliciting male sexual behavior and related responses such as approaching and sniffing at the odor, hamster vaginal discharge produces a short-latency rise in testosterone and a lowering of aggressive tendencies. This may involve learning, as responses to hamster vaginal discharge can be conditioned (Johnston et al. 1978). Finally, early androgen exposure influences responses to hamster vaginal discharge. Females that receive testosterone neonatally have a significant preference for hamster vaginal discharge following gonadectomy (Gregory and Pritchard 1983).

Ovulatory Cycles

An early example of pheromonal or social environment influencing hormones was noted by van der Lee and Boot (1955). These researchers found that female mice that are group-housed exhibit longer estrous cycles than females that are singly-housed. This suppression of the estrous cycle was due to a lengthening of the diestrus stage of the cycle. As mentioned above, pheromones in the urine of male and female mice may act to modulate population density. Thus, when population density becomes high, the "stress" of being in a high-density area may contribute to the potency of the "estrus-suppressing-hormone." Evidence for this theory comes from a recent study in which urine from adrenalectomized singly-housed or group-housed females failed to suppress estrus in female mice (Ma et al. 1998). One hormone produced in response to stressful situations in mice and other rodents is called corticosterone (see chapter 10). Adrenalectomy removes this hormone and abates the effects of stress. When adrenalectomized females were given corticosterone, this treatment reinstated the ability of their urine to suppress estrus in experimental females (Ma et al. 1998). These findings suggest that increased corticosterone concentrations in response to the stress of living in high-density areas may be one of the mechanisms by which female mice regulate pheromone production and, in turn, population density.

As with puberty, estrus can be hastened in female mice by exposure to a male (Whitten 1957). This estrus-advancing substance is found in the urine of males; application of conspecific male urine to the nostrils of female mice accelerates the onset of estrus. Apparently the estrus-modulating effects of this substance is androgen-dependent; urine from castrated male mice fails to alter the estrus cycles of females.

As will be shown below for human menstrual cycles, the estrous cycles of female rodents become synchronized with exposure to other females (McClintock 1984). The pheromonal signals that act to synchronize estrus among female mice appear to be volatile; females sharing an air supply become synchronized to the cycle of the "donor" (McClintock 1984). Apparently, a pheromone released during the ovulatory stage lengthens estrous cycles, while preovulatory pheromones act to shorten estrous cycles. This finding led to the proposal of a coupled oscillator model of synchrony (Shank and McClintock 1984), whereby estrus synchrony is a function of exposure to both the estrus-lengthening and estrus-shortening pheromones of a number of female rodents.

Interestingly, some species do not exhibit spontaneous ovulatory cycles, and olfactory cues are necessary for estrous cycles and ovulation. For example, female prairie voles (*Microtus ochrogaster*) require stimuli from a male conspecific in order to become estrus (Richmond and Conaway 1969; Richmond and Stehn 1976). Female prairie voles do not exhibit a patent vagina or behavioral estrus until stimulated by male chemosensory factors found in male urine (Carter et al. 1980). Prior to estrus induction, female voles have extremely low concentrations of circulating luteinizing hormone (LH) and estrogen (Carter et al. 1980). After exposure to a conspecific male or male urine, females exhibit a rapid increase of LH concentrations followed by an increase in serum estrogen concentrations; progesterone is generally elevated within 72 h of mating (Carter et al. 1989; Cohens-Parsons and Carter 1987; Dluzen et al. 1981).

Females of some species require exposure to males in order to be induced into behavioral estrus and for ovulation to occur. For example, female musk shrews do not exhibit spontaneous estrus or ovulation. Typically, mating starts within an hour after a male is introduced to the female, and ovulation is stimulated after mating has occurred (Rissman et al. 1988). One recent study suggests that olfactory inputs are necessary to induce ovulation in musk shrews; ovulation was suppressed in mated female musk shrews that had their olfactory bulbs removed (Rissman and Li 2000). Interestingly, olfactory bulbectomized female musk shrews continued to exhibit receptive behavior and mate successfully. Because the entire olfactory bulbs were removed in this study, future studies are necessary to determine the relative contribution of the primary and accessory olfactory systems in mating-induced ovulation in musk shrews.

Pregnancy

The best-known experiments on the effects of pheromones on reproductive hormones were carried out by H. M. Bruce (1959). She noticed that pregnancy failed in mice that were exposed to a male other than the inseminator (the Bruce effect). If the new male belonged to the same strain ("strange male") as the inseminator, pregnancy failed in 30% of cases, but if the new male belonged to a different strain ("alien male"), pregnancy failed in 80% of the cases. The role of pheromones in this phenomenon is shown by several types of experiments. When the sense of smell was eliminated in females before mating, the presence of alien males did not result in pregnancy failure. Furthermore, pregnancy failure did occur in female mice with an intact sense of smell when they were exposed to bedding material that had been soiled by alien males. The pheromone was in the urine of animals that had adequate quantities of androgen.

The primary way in which the pheromone disrupts pregnancy appears to involve a decrease in prolactin (Marchlewska-Koj 1983). Pheromonal stimuli from an alien male decrease prolactin release, preventing formation of corpora lutea. The consequent decrease of progesterone prevents implantation. Administration of exogenous progesterone prevents the male-induced pregnancy block. Finally, column chromatography indicates that the active fraction of the pregnancy-blocking pheromone is approximately the same as the puberty-accelerating pheromone, suggesting that they may be the same agent (Vandenbergh et al. 1976).

It appears that the Bruce effect is a factor of the "memory" of the initial male with which the female mated. As mentioned above, pregnancy is terminated in females exposed to a novel male, yet female rodents maintain a memory of the male they mated with, and subsequent exposure to this male will not result in pregnancy block. This memory is short-lived, and female mice will terminate the pregnancy if they are exposed to the familiar male after 10 days of being singly housed. However, exposure to the familiar male will not result in pregnancy block if the animals are separated for 1 to 8 days.

The hippocampus is responsible for various forms of memory, including olfactory memory (e.g., Eichenbaum, Fagen, and Cohen 1986) (see chapter 14). However, lesions of the hippocampus fail to abolish the "memory for mate" in prairie voles (*Microtus ochrogaster*) and house mice (Demas et al. 1997; Selway and Keverne 1990). Importantly, cells from the VNO project to the AOB and then to a structure in the CNS called the amygdala (Brennan et al. 1990). In prairie voles, amygdala lesions abolish the memory for a mate, and the familiar male is as effective as an unfamiliar male at inducing pregnancy block, even if the male is reintroduced several days after mating (Demas, Williams, and Nelson 1997). Thus, the amygdala may represent an important structure for olfactory memory for mate.

Lactation and Parental Care

The onset of maternal behavior is mediated by hormones, yet the maintenance of maternal behavior during the first few postpartum weeks depends on experiences acquired while the dam interacts with pups (Rosenblatt 1990). As little as two hours of exposure to pups within 36 hours of parturition, facilitates maternal behavior tested ten days postpartum (Orpen and Fleming 1987). Maternal behavior seems to require exposure to olfactory stimuli rather than social interactions associated with exposure to pups. Female rats with vomeronasal or olfactory transections exhibit increased latencies to maternal behavior in maternal induction tests (Fleming et al. 1992). Taken together, these data suggest an interplay between hormones (necessary to initiate maternal behavior) and olfaction (necessary to facilitate and potentially maintain maternal behavior).

A Sense of Touch

The sense of touch or pressure has been shown to be involved in the alteration of hormone levels at all stages of reproductive life in nonprimate mammals. The effect of tactile stimulation on the hormones involved in ovulation in adult animals of certain species is very well documented (see chapter 4).

ONSET OF REPRODUCTION

Puberty

It is difficult to tease apart the effects of pheromonal cues and tactile stimuli on puberty acceleration in laboratory studies. However, one study suggests that cohabitation with a male mouse hastens the onset of puberty in female mice (Bronson and Maruniak 1976). Introduction of male urine to the bedding of the cage of a female leads to a rapid increase in the gonadotropins (i.e., LH and FSH) within 30 minutes (Bronson and Maruniak 1976). This increase in LH and FSH is potentiated if the male is physically placed into the cage of the female mouse. Although this study cannot definitively determine the tactile/social stimuli that lead to a further increase in the hormones responsible for puberty onset, the results suggest that some sort of interaction with the male is responsible. This tactile stimulation is unlikely to be mating because pre-pubertal female mice are not sexually receptive to a male conspecific.

ADULT REPRODUCTIVE PHYSIOLOGY AND BEHAVIOR

Ovulatory Cycles

Rabbits and ferrets generally do not ovulate unless they are mounted and the male achieves intromission. If the female's ovaries are adequately developed and in a state of readiness to ovulate, this tactile contact during copulation provides the neuroendocrine signal that causes a surge of LH from the pituitary. Ovulation then occurs within a few hours. How do we know that such "reflex ovulation" is caused by tactile cues from the male rather than visual, olfactory, or auditory cues? There are several ways to establish this. For example, the nerves leading from the genital area of the female can be severed or anesthetized so that the nerve impulses caused by tactile stimulation of the genitals do not reach the brain. When this is done, intromission by the male fails to cause reflex ovulation. Another approach is for the experimenter to stimulate the cervix of a cat, rabbit, or ferret with a glass rod. This tactile stimulation causes ovulation even though the male of the species cannot be seen, smelled, or heard by the female.

Of course, females of many species do not require contact by other members of their species in order to ovulate. These species, of which humans are one, are known as "spontaneous ovulators." In some instances we can change a spontaneous ovulator into a reflex ovulator by experimental manipulation. For example, female rats kept in continuous light fail to ovulate spontaneously, as rats normally do. When a male copulates with a continuous-light-exposed female rat, she ovulates reflexively. Stimulation of the female's cervix with a glass rod produces the same result.

Pregnancy

When a male mouse copulates with a female that is about to ovulate "spontaneously," the female usually becomes pregnant. If the male is vasectomized before he copulates, the tactile stimulation provided to the female's cervix by the male's penis causes changes in the female's hormonal conditions that are quite similar to the hormonal conditions that prevail early in pregnancy. This condition, induced by the vasectomized male, is called pseudopregnancy. These findings suggest that hormonal changes characteristic of the start of pregnancy or pseudopregnancy arise as the result of tactile stimulation of the female's cervix at about the same time as she is spontaneously ovulating. If this is so, an experimenter should be able to stimulate the cervix of a mouse with a glass rod or mechanical vibrator and induce a state of pseudopregnancy. However, many attempts to do this have failed.

Diamond (1970) sought to understand the basis of these pregnancy failures. He observed that when male mice copulate they intromit into the female about 5 to 13 times before they ejaculate, and there are intervals of 90 to 215 seconds between intromissions. Diamond reasoned that this pattern of repeated intromissions with characteristic intervals between them constitute a kind of "vaginal code" of tactile stimulation. He then imitated this code with mechanical stimulation of the female's cervix. When this code was imitated, pseudopregnancy was induced, but when the vaginal code was not imitated (i.e., too few insertions of the mechanical vibrator or inappropriate intervals between insertions), pseudopregnancy was not induced.

Apparently, not only the amount but also the pattern of tactile stimulation of the cervix is important for starting the changes in hormone secretion that accompany the early stages of pregnancy in mice. Similar findings have been made with rats and hamsters, with each species of rodent having a different "vaginal code." The importance of vaginal stimulation in human sexual behavior has become a topic of intense research interest by the drug industry (see below). Further descriptions of the function of pacing intromissions are provided in chapters 4 and 13.

The importance of tactile cues from the cervix in the initiation of the hormone changes of pregnancy has been shown in other ways. For example, the nerves leading from the cervix to the brain were severed in female rats. The females were then allowed to mate with male rats. Even though mating and spontaneous ovulation occurred, no pregnancy or pseudopregnancy ensued in the female rats. Further experimentation showed that a deficit in prolactin secretion caused by the severance of the nerves first became apparent about 8 hours after mating. If nerve-severed female rats were given an injection of prolactin 8 hours after mating, pregnancy occurred. Prolactin seems to potentiate the release of progesterone from the corpus luteum and thereby facilitate pregnancy. From these experiments one can conclude that tactile stimulation of the cervix of rats somehow signals the brain to release prolactin from the pituitary gland. Without this tactile signal, prolactin is not released in adequate quantities to ensure sufficient progesterone release, and pregnancy does not ensue in the rat.

Not only does tactile stimulation of the cervix serve an important role in starting the production of hormones in early pregnancy, but it also seems to influence the later stages of pregnancy in at least some rodents. In hamsters, artificial insemination fails to produce pregnancy (Diamond 1972). If a hamster is artificially inseminated and then given an injection of progesterone, pregnancy results, but only 25% of the offspring are born alive. If a hamster is artificially inseminated and her cervix is mechanically stimulated at the same time, pregnancy ensues, and all the offspring are born alive. In some unknown way, tactile stimulation of the cervix (perhaps by causing release of prolactin, which maintains the production of progesterone) ensures the well-being of the fetuses. It seems truly remarkable that the information provided by tactile stimulation of the vaginal cervix during copulation of the hamster should be translated and stored in such a way as to influence the viability of the offspring.

Lactation and Parental Care

We have now seen that tactile stimuli influence the onset of puberty, the occurrence of ovulation, and the start and maintenance of pregnancy. The sense of touch also has an influence on hormones at yet another stage of the reproductive process, the nursing phase. The sense of touch is important for the initiation of adequate mammary growth for lactation. This has been shown in experiments with rats. Pregnant rats that had a kind of Elizabethan ruffle collar placed around their necks had much smaller mammary than rats without such a collar. Apparently, this was because collared females could not lick their own bellies, and this failure to self-lick the teats resulted in a failure to produce hormones that encourage mammary gland growth. When collared, pregnant female rats had their teats mechanically stimulated, mammary growth was similar to that in normal rats. In fact, mechanical stimulation or massage of the teats induced mammary gland growth even in virgin rats.

In addition to providing stimulation for mammary growth during pregnancy, numerous hormones are released in response to suckling by pups, presumably to facilitate lactation and the adaptation to the lactation condition by the female (Li et al. 1999). Suckling by pups stimulates oxytocin, prolactin, and corticosterone secretion (Tucker et al. 1967; Walker et al. 1992). In addition, LH secretion is inhibited by suckling (Fox and Smith 1984). Thus, suckling helps to stimulate milk production and letdown (oxytocin and prolactin) in addition to mobilizing the energy resources necessary for the energy demands of milk production (corticosterone).

Not only is tactile stimulation necessary for lactation, but in some species, the vaginocervical stimulation (VCS) of childbirth may be necessary to initiate the maternal "bond" necessary for appropriate care of offspring. In ewes (*Ovis aries*), a strong maternal bond is usually formed after childbirth and allows the ewe to discriminate her offspring from other lambs (Kendrick et al. 1992); a recently parturient ewe will only allow her own offspring to approach her. Because parturition is associated with a prior increase in the ratio of estradiol to progesterone, early studies attempted to mimic this relationship in order to induce maternal behavior in virgin ewes. This treatment did not result in the initiation of maternal behavior. When ewes were treated with this same hormonal regimen and given vaginocervical stimulation, they rapidly became maternal (Keverne and Kendrick 1994). Apparently, VCS induces an increase in oxytocin production in the brain areas involved in maternal behavior, and the administration of oxytocin into the cerebrospinal fluid initiates maternal behavior in ewes (Keverne and Kendrick 1994).

The Sense of Hearing

Although auditory signals are important during courtship and in sexual behavior, their effects on reproduction have not been examined as intensively as the effects of other environmental factors such as light, odor, and touch. For this reason, we will have to depart from discussing, in order, the effects of sensation on hormones involved in puberty, seasonality, ovulation, start of pregnancy, maintenance of pregnancy, and lactation.

In some species, sounds produced by one member affect the production of hormones by a reproductive partner. Some interesting examples of the way these intraspecific (within species) sounds function as a normal component of reproductive cycles have been reported in birds. For example, Kroodsma (1976) tape-recorded the songs of male canaries. One group of female canaries heard a large repertoire of songs while the other group heard a smaller song repertoire. Females that heard the larger repertoire built nests sooner and laid more eggs than females that heard only a small variety of songs. Evidently, female reproductive hormone production and female reproductive behavior are stimulated by the content of the song of the male canary.

A similar conclusion can be drawn from Brockway's work with an Australian parrot, the budgerigar (1965). Female budgerigar vocalizations were recorded on tape and played daily to the females in 2-hour sequences for a total of 6 hours, or in one continuous 3-hour sequence. When the tape consisted of males singing a "soft warble," the females' ovaries grew and ovulation resulted. When the tape consisted of other male vocalizations such as "squacks," "chedelees," "whedelees," "tuks," and "loud warbles," the ovaries were not stimulated. Later work with budgerigars showed that females reach a higher degree of reproductive development when exposed to male song during the first half of a day than during the second half.

With the use of computers to parse and manipulate songs for playback studies of individual song elements, recent research has uncovered species-specific "sexy" phrases or syllables that lead to large reproductive responses (i.e., copulation-solicitation displays) and other phrases within the song that do not (Vallet and Kreutzer 1995). In one study in female canaries, "sexy" phrases (i.e., phrases that initiated copulation-solicitation displays in females) elicited more sexual response but were unrelated to nest building or egg laying (Lebaucher et al. 1998). This finding suggests that song may function to initiate courtship and semen transfer but may not be important for postcoital events and stimulation of female reproductive physiology or development. Thus, while copulation-solicitation displays may require highly selective song elements, ovarian development and nesting behaviors may not require such specific song patterns.

In fact, recent evidence suggests that heterospecific song (male song from a different species) may be as effective as conspecific song in stimulating ovarian follicular development, while heterospecific song is less effective than conspecific song at inducing oviposition (Bentley et al. 2000). Likewise, in white-crowned sparrows (*Zonotrichia leucophrys oriantha*), females show a clear preference for songs of their "natal" dialect over "foreign" dialect or heterospecific song for copulation-solicitation displays, while reproductive physiology (luteinizing hormone concentrations and ovarian growth) is equally stimulated by songs of natal and foreign dialects (MacDougall-Shackleton et al. 2000). Taken together, these findings suggest that certain aspects of mating in birds may require highly selective song elements to initiate, while other stages of reproduction do not. It is noteworthy that copulation-solicitation display are most selective because this would be the critical stage of courting for potential mating/insemination to occur.

Not only does the male budgerigar stimulate the ovaries of females by his song, but his song may also cause stimulation of his own testes. Brockway (1967) cut the nerves and muscles involved in song production by male budgerigars. The devocalized males had smaller testes and a lower sperm count than intact males. This difference was apparent even when the devocalized males were allowed to hear the songs of normal males. Thus, the male budgerigar seems to stimulate his own gonads by singing. The component of the song that seems to be involved is the long warble.

A few studies on the effects of intraspecific audible sounds on hormone production by mammals have also been performed. In one such study, a lactating female (female A) rat exposed to the stimuli emanating from another lactating rat (female B) with her litter ejected more milk in response to suckling than a control lactator (female C) not exposed to these stimuli. However, if female A was surgically deafened, no difference in ejection of milk occurred between female A and female C. From this, one would suppose that auditory stimuli from female B and her litter somehow increased release of the hormone that regulates the ejection of milk in female A.

Ultrasounds (i.e., sounds of too high a frequency to be heard by humans) have been shown to form part of the intraspecific communication mechanism in several mammals, but so far, no reports of the effects of ultrasonics emitted by one member of a species on the hormone production of another member of the same species have appeared.

Energy and Survival

In their natural environment, animals appear to use cues that predict changing seasons and further fine-tune the timing and extent of these adaptations based upon current conditions (Winfield 1983; Wingfield and Farner 1980). It has been suggested that that animals use two types of cues to phase reproductive efforts (Wingfield 1983; Wingfield and Kenagy 1991). One type provides long-term predictive signals (initial predictive information, e.g., photoperiod) and initiates gonadal alterations weeks in advance of changing seasons. The second type of cue provides information from the immediate environment (e.g., food and temperature) in order to provide short-term predictive signals (supplementary information). The latter cues would speed up or slow down gonadal changes regulated by the former.

The assumption based on this model is that animals will rely more heavily on supplementary information when the breeding season is less predictable from year to year (Cohen 1967). Some further modifications in adaptive behaviors and physiology must occur in response to unpredictable alternations in environmental conditions, and these events have been termed "modifying information" (Wingfield et al. 1998; reviewed in Wingfield et al. 2000). Finally, fine-tuning of adaptive behaviors and physiology occurs in response to behavioral interactions termed "integrating and synchronizing information" (reviewed in Wingfield et al. 2000).

Individuals of all species have evolved to maximize reproductive success. If environmental conditions were always favorable for reproduction, animals could maximize reproductive success by breeding more or less continuously. However, due to transient, unpredictable decrements in favorable environmental conditions, or more predictable seasonal fluctuations in environmental conditions in temperate regions, it is not advantageous for animals to breed continuously. Thus, animals have evolved to use environmental cues that signal whether or not conditions are currently favorable for reproduction (ultimate cues), or cues that predict, in advance, the onset of favorable/unfavorable conditions (proximate cues) (Baker 1938).

Perhaps the most significant alterations in the environment occur in temperate latitudes on a seasonal basis. Although the focus here is on well-studied mammalian and bird species, recent evidence indicates that modern *Homo* may maintain the "machinery" necessary for seasonal breeding, so humans may exhibit patterns of seasonal breeding as a result (reviewed in Bronson 1995; see below).

ENVIRONMENTAL CONTROL OF ENERGY ALLOCATION
Ecologists typically agree that the environmental factor most important for the regulation of seasonal breeding is food availability (Negus and Berger 1987). From an energetic perspective, animals (including humans) are faced with the task of allocating a limited energy "budget" (i.e., assimilated energy stored as fat or in the liver) to various behavioral and physiological demands. Certain demands, such as cellular maintenance, thermoregulation, and immune function, receive high priority, while nonessential demands such as reproduction and growth receive low priority (reviewed in Schneider and Wade 2000). Thus, when environmental conditions result in food shortages, animals shunt available energy into high-priority demands while nonessential functions are curtailed (reviewed in Bronson and Heideman 1994). As mentioned above, environmental cues act upon animals to regulate hormones. In turn, alterations in hormones lead to changes in physiology and behavior.

Ultimate environmental factors such as ambient temperature and food availability can act directly to influence the allocation of energy rapidly (within hours or days). Proximate factors (e.g., day length) allow animals to predict, well in advance, the onset of particular conditions in order to phase adaptations that require a significant amount of time to develop with the appropriate time of year. For example, in temperate latitudes, food is typically scarce during winter. Thus, animals must use proximate cues to initiate adaptations and alterations in energy allocation prior to conditions in which food is less available. As will be shown below, animals in the wild are capable of anticipating predictable changes in environmental conditions, as well as of assessing immediate conditions, to exquisitely time breeding and other energetically costly activities with the most favorable time of year.

Because animals in the wild must constantly appraise their available energy (or prospects to obtain food), many laboratory studies have evaluated how food availability may act to regulate the alterations in reproduction seen in the natural environment. The available data on the effects of food restriction on reproductive function have come primarily from laboratory strains of rats and mice (e.g., Brinkworth et al. 1992; Bronson 1987; Bronson and Marsteller 1985; Woodside 1991). In male rats and mice, sex steroid production (i.e., steroidogenesis) is considerably more sensitive to food restriction than is sperm production (i.e., gametogensis). Three factors determine the extent to which food restriction affects gametogenesis and steroidogenesis: (1) the degree of food restriction, (2) the length of time that food restriction is continued, and (3) the stage of the life cycle at which food restriction is imposed. Food restriction affects spermatogenesis only if the food restriction is prolonged and severe (e.g., Brinkworth et al. 1992; Nelson et al. 1985). These findings suggest that animals in the wild shunt energy temporarily away from reproduction when food becomes unavailable, yet maintain the ability to rapidly initiate reproduction when food again becomes more plentiful. However, prior to or during long-term food shortages (i.e., winter), animals may further conserve energy by an inhibition of spermatogenesis (in addition to steroidogenesis), and sacrifice the ability to rapidly reinitiate breeding when conditions improve. The interplay between ultimate factors and the proximate factors necessary to precisely time breeding and other energetically expensive activities will be discussed further below. Because food becomes less abundant as winter approaches, food can be used as either a proximate or an ultimate factor (reviewed in Bronson and Heideman 1994). However, current food availability may not provide an accurate assessment of future conditions.

Because ambient temperature also changes on a seasonal basis at temperate latitudes, animals can use changes in ambient temperature to phase seasonal adaptations. Ambient temperature can act directly to influence hormones and other physiological adaptations rapidly. Thus, temperature information (like food availability) can function as either a proximate or an ultimate factor. Low temperatures can inhibit testicular function alone (e.g., Desjardins and Lopez 1983), or in combination with other inhibitory extrinsic factors, including short day lengths (Dejardins and Lopez 1983; Nelson et al. 1989). Although temperature becomes lower as winter approaches, daily fluctuations in temperature make it an unreliable cue for animals to use to phase adaptations with the correct time of year.

Environmental Factors That Influence Hormones in Humans

The foregoing research, done in carefully controlled conditions, has clarified the contribution of each of the sensory systems to the modulation of the hormone secretions that regulate puberty, ovulation, sexual behavior, pregnancy, lactation, and care of young. In the next section, each of these systems will be examined in humans. We will see that many of the same mechanisms regulate human and animal reproduction, though in humans it is much more difficult to isolate the precise mediating mechanisms.

Onset of Reproduction

PUBERTY

The stage of puberty is the time at which an individual becomes capable of reproduction. Epidemiological data indicate that there is a secular trend toward greater height and earlier maturation in both men and women (Tanner 1992). These data were described as evidence of a substantial decline in the age at which girls reached puberty from about 1840 to 1950 (Tanner 1968). In the mid-1840s, the average Norwegian girl began menstruating at 17 years of age. Today the average age is 13 years (figure 18.3). A similar decrease in the age of puberty of girls has occurred in many other European countries and in the United States. The trend seems to have leveled off in the past 50 years, suggesting that girls may now be reaching sexual maturity at the earliest possible age, at least in these countries.

It is difficult to isolate the environmental factors involved in this interesting shift in the age of puberty, because the lives of people today differ in many ways from those of people one hundred years ago. One obvious difference is the increase in the percentage of people living in urban, rather than rural, settings. If urbanization plays a role in the advancement of human puberty, one might expect to see a difference in the average age of puberty between girls living in urban centers and those living in rural communities. This notion is supported by evidence that during the last century the average age of puberty for girls living in Warsaw has been earlier, by almost two years, than for girls living in rural parts of Poland. However, this demographic approach to the question of accelerated puberty is only marginally helpful in the search to isolate the particular environmental factors involved in the acceleration of puberty. After all, urban and rural people may differ in the amount and type of work they do, in the nutritional content of their food, and in the sights, sounds, smells, and temperatures to which they are exposed.

There is some evidence that the senses are involved in the onset of puberty in girls. Blind girls with some perception of light reach puberty earlier than normally sighted girls (Zacharias and Wurtman 1964). Totally blind girls

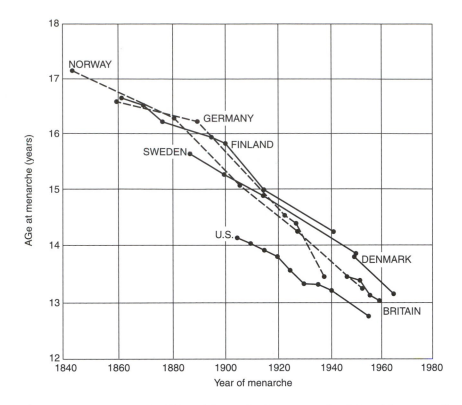

Figure 18.3 On the average, girls in the U.S. and Europe begin menstruation 2.3 to 3.3 years earlier than they did a century ago. (From Tanner 1976.)

with no light perception reach puberty even earlier than minimally sighted girls. Furthermore, in the springtime, when daylight is present for more than 12 hours of each 24-hour period (and the proportion of light is increasing), fewer girls start to menstruate than during seasons of reduced or decreasing amounts of daylight (Bojlen and Bentzon 1974). Increasing day lengths, or light, appears to inhibit gonadal development in human beings. In fact, light has complex effects on a multitude of endocrine secretions including melatonin, cortisol, growth hormone, and gonadal hormones, many of which can affect the onset of puberty in both sexes (Bellastella et al. 1998). While photic factors are likely to modulate puberty, they are not the only relevant cues.

While it has been suggested that changes of temperature characteristic of the seasons influence the onset of puberty, this seems unlikely. Eskimo and Nigerian girls reach puberty at the same age, indicating that the influence of climate on puberty is a small one. But a strong statement to this effect cannot be made based on available correlational data on humans. We do not know the effects (if any) on puberty caused by the increase in mean world temperature that occurred between 1850 and 1940. In fact, we have no puberty data on equally nourished groups of people living in environments that differ only in climate.

Perhaps improvements in living standards have influenced puberty. Over the last century and a half, there has been a dramatic improvement in nutrition and health in industrialized Western societies, dramatic changes in standards of living are continuing today (Houspie Vercauteren, and Susanne 1996). In order for females to reach puberty, sufficient energy must be available (Rosetta 1993). While most girls in the United States reach menarche between 11 to 13 years (see above), females in third-world subsistence societies, where malnutrition is prevalent, reach menarche much later, at 15 years for age (Groos and Smith 1992; Gopalan and Naidu 1972). These findings suggest that improvements in living standards (and improved nutrition) may be involved in the reduction in the age of menarche.

One interesting hypothesis devised to account for the decline in the age of menarche in industrialized societies ascribes this trend to alterations in the pheromonal environment that prepubertal females have been exposed to over the last century (Burger and Gochfeld 1985). As mentioned earlier, pheromones are airborne chemical substances released by one individual that affect the behavior and/or physiology of another animal (see Vandenbergh 1988 for review). It is well-established that pheromonal cues from female laboratory rodents delay the onset of puberty, while male pheromonal signals accelerate the onset of puberty (see above). Burger and Gochfeld (1985) suggest that similar mechanisms may account for the decline in puberty seen over the last century and a half. They suggest that mothers are home less because of an increasing trend for women to work, and fathers are home more, because of a decline in the number of working hours required, thereby changing the pheromonal conditions to which daughters are exposed. These correlational data provide a parallel between animal studies and trends seen in humans.

Finally, there is evidence that social factors can influence the timing of puberty, raising questions about the possible mediating mechanisms. Specifically, it has been shown that the quality of early family relationships affect the timing of puberty, with later pubertal timing associated with increased parental supportiveness indexed by such factors as the father's presence in the home and mother-daughter affection (Ellis et al. 1999) Conversely, earlier menarche (women) and spermarche (men) has been associated with greater stress in parental marital relations (Kim and Smith 1998).

SEASONAL REGULATION OF REPRODUCTION

In a review of annual cycles of human reproduction, Roenneberg and Aschoff (1990) have integrated data on climatic and photoperiodic information for 380 geographical locations. They show that on a global scale, photoperiod influences the physiology of human reproduction. Thus, conception rates are highest during the vernal equinox at high latitudes where changes in day length are pronounced. Temperature also appears to be a major influencing factor. Conception rates are above the annual mean when temperatures fall between 5 °C and 20 °C, and conception rates fall when temperatures lie beyond these extremes. Roenneberg and Aschoff note that the influence of environmental factors is decreasing in recent decades as people become increasingly shielded from photoperiodic cues (by indoor work) and from temperature (by heating and air conditioning).

More recently, Bronson (1995) has reviewed the potential environmental factors responsible for seasonal alterations in human reproduction. Again, high conception rates around the vernal equinox in human populations from middle to higher latitudes suggest that photoperiod may regulate seasonal changes in reproduction. As previously mentioned in the discussion of puberty, nutrition can dramatically affect the reproductive cycle of females (e.g., Groos and Smith 1992). Not only can puberty onset be influenced by the nutritional state, but the reproductive state can also be transiently influenced by the current availability of energy (see below). In some subsistence societies, annual variability in rainfall is associated with annual changes in food availability. There is some evidence that seasonal reductions in the rate of ovulation and prolonged lactational amenorhea are associated with times of low food availability in these societies.

There is also evidence that seasonal variation in human conception rates may be due to temperature effects. Sperm production in scrotal mammals is extremely sensitive to minor rises in temperature (reviewed in Bergh 1991). Thus, correlational evidence suggests that seasonally high temperatures may result in suppressed spermatogenesis, particularly if clothing is worn that does not allow scrotal cooling. Again, the epidemiological data is excellent in highlighting a phenomenon that must be examined, and less useful in elucidating the mediating mechanisms. There are reports of seasonality in triplet births, with peak numbers of triplets born in the early spring in the United States (Elster and Bleyl 1991). These findings suggest that humans may experience seasonal alterations in fecundity similar to those seen in the animal studies above. Likewise, human females may also exhibit differences in fertility associated with ambient temperature or some other factor that varies latitudinally.

We might imagine that if seasonal effects impact reproductive processes, we would find differences between individuals living at high latitudes and in equatorial regions. In keeping with this notion, the frequency of birth of fraternal (or dizygotic, from two separate eggs) twins has been reported to be higher in northern countries than in tropical countries. Also, the rate of twinning in the southern parts of France and Japan is lower than in the northern parts of these countries (Kamimura 1976). In much of the foregoing work in humans it has been difficult to determine whether the relevant climatic cue is day length or some correlated factor, like temperature.

Adult Reproductive Physiology and Behavior

OVULATORY CYCLES
Stimuli from the environment affect the reproductive functions of the adult as well as of the immature individual. The possible role of olfactory stimuli

in regulating the timing of the menstrual cycle of women received a prominent place in the imagination of scientists with the work of McClintock (1971) (see chapter 6). She studied the timing of menstruation in a group of women students living together in a college dormitory. She reasoned that if each woman's menstrual cycle was determined strictly by internal factors, then living together would not change the timing of menstruation. However, as the semester proceeded, the scatter in the timing of the menstruation decreased in roommates and close friends. That is, the menstrual cycles of women who had spent a lot of time together became synchronized. Of course, people who spend a lot of time together have many shared experiences. They probably keep similar hours, engage in the same activity cycles, eat similar foods, and experience the stresses of exams and other problems at about the same times. Nevertheless, it is reasonable to hypothesize that the synchronization of menstrual cycles in these college women might be due to olfactory stimuli.

In the years since McClintock's original observation was made, there have been numerous attempts to evaluate whether perspiration could synchronize menstrual cycles. In one study, perspiration from a donor was mixed with alcohol and applied to the upper lip of experimental subjects (Russell et al. 1980). Alcohol alone was applied to the upper lips of control subjects. At the beginning of the study the menstrual periods of the experimental subjects started about 9 days away from the donor's. Four months later, the difference had been reduced to about 3 days. The control group showed no such shift.

Subsequent experiments exploring the mechanism of menstrual synchrony have confirmed a role for pheromones. Odorless compounds from the armpits of women late in the follicular phase of the menstrual cycle accelerated the preovulatory surge of GnRH of recipient women and shortened their menstrual cycles. Odorless compounds collected later in the menstrual cycle delayed the GnRH surge of recipients and lengthened their menstrual cycles (Stern and McClintock 1998). These results demonstrate that odors can change the timing of the menstrual cycle. The fact that the odors are not consciously experienced is important because this is part of the classic definition of a pheromone.

Unconscious olfactory cues are thought to act on a specialized sensory system in the putative human vomeronasal organ, rather than through the classical olfactory system. It is remarkable to find that in the modern era, previously unknown sensory systems are still being discovered in the human body. The discovery of a vomeronasal system in humans has intensified the interest in the role(s) of human pheromones, since this may be the route for the communication of unconscious sensory information to the brain. Indeed, there is evidence that activation of the vomeronasal organ results in modulation of autonomic nervous system function and the release of gonadotropins from the pituitary gland (reviewed in Monti-Bloch et al. 1998).

The foregoing data showing a role for olfactory stimuli does not preclude environmental factors such as light, temperature, sound, nutrition, and stress

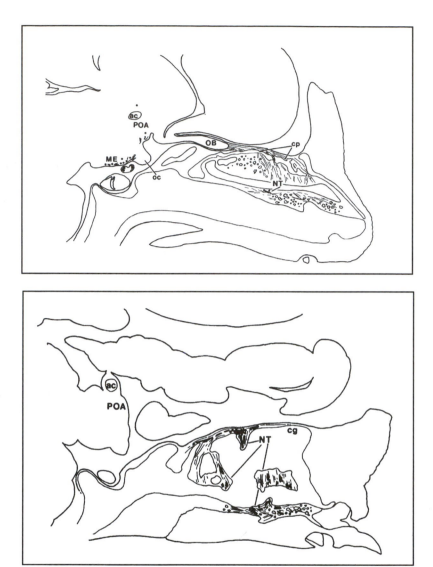

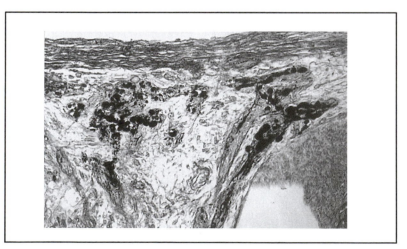

as additional influences on menstrual cycle. In fact, some of these other environmental factors may have altered the chemical quality of the sweat of the donors. It is likely that factors in addition to odors are indeed important. To mention one such example, the menstrual synchrony phenomenon is more likely to occur between close friends and in women with intensive social contact than in those who are roommates but not close friends (Weller 1995). A somewhat different slant on the role for olfactory stimuli in menstrual synchrony is seen in the data suggesting that menstrual synchrony does not occur among women basketball players, who are assumed to sweat in synchrony, nor among lesbian couples, despite their reported intimate interactions (Weller and Weller 1995; Trevathan et al. 1993).

While the foregoing studies emphasize responses to unconscious odors, the ability to detect odors has also been associated with reproductive function. In one study, olfactory acuity was measured in 96 women with menstrual irregularities and in 500 women with normal menstrual cycles (Marshall and Henkin 1971). A high percentage (83%) of the women with menstrual abnormalities had subnormal olfactory acuity. Many of the subjects were not aware of this lack of sensitivity to smells though a substantial percentage (20%) of those with irregular menses were virtually unresponsive to odors.

A parallel effect arises in Kallman's syndrome in men, where an inability to smell (anosomia) is accompanied by small testicular size. For a long while the "nasogentital" relationship was hard to understand (Rosedale 1945). While the data might indicate that a poor sense of smell results in hormone levels that are too low to insure normal testicular development and regular menses, they could just as well be taken to suggest that a low hormone level causes a poor sense of smell, or that there is no causative, but only a correlative, relationship between hormone levels and acuteness of the sense of smell.

An explanation for the association between olfactory and gonadal function has emerged, first in studies of mice and later in related work in humans (Schwanzel-Fukuda and Pfaff 1989; Wray et al. 1989; reviewed in Schwanzel-Fukuda 1999). In ontogeny, GnRH-expressing cells migrate from the epithelium of the olfactory placode to the hypothalamus (figure 18.4). The principal

Figure 18.4 Kallmann syndrome interferes with the normal migration of GnRH cells from the olfactory placode to the hypothalamus during development. (*Top*) Microprojection drawing, slightly lateral, of the midline in the sagittal plane of a normal 19-week-old fetus. This drawing shows the distribution of GnRH-expressing cells (large dots) and fibers (smaller dots). GnRH-expressing cells and fibers are seen among fibers of the nervus terminalis (NT) on the floor of the nasal septum, above the anterior commissure (AC), in the preoptic area (POA), and in the median eminence (ME). (*Middle*) Microprojection drawing of a sagittal midline section through the brain and nasal region of a 19-month-old fetus with Kallmann syndrome, showing abnormal migration of GnRH-expressing cells. The crista galli (cg) is shown in this section. A thick fascicle of GnRH fibers, which appears to be part of the NT, emerges from the nasal septum onto the cribiform plate, accompanied by a dense cluster of GnRH-expressing cells that failed to migrate to the POA and hypothalmus. (*Bottom*) Photomicrograph of a brain from a 19-week-old fetus with Kallman syndrome. Thick clumps and clusters of GnRH-immunoreactive neurons are visible on the dorsal surface of the cribiform plate. (Photomicrograph by Marlene Schwanzel-Fukada.)

endocrine deficit in Kallman's syndrome is a failure of secretion of GnRH. In Kallman's syndrome, the agenesis of the olfactory bulbs early in development results in a failure of GnRH neuronal migration from the olfactory region to the hypothalamus. That is, abnormal olfactory bulb development results in a failure of normal development and/or migration of GnRH-expressing neurons, resulting in small testes in men and irregular menses in women. That these gonadal and olfactory functions are indeed associated with anatomical anomalies has been shown with the use of modern brain imaging techniques. Magnetic resonance imaging revealed that all patients with Kallman's syndrome had abnormalities in the olfactory bulbs or tracts (Vogl et al. 1994) (see figure 18.4).

COITUS AND PREGNANCY

Hormonal changes associated with copulation occur in both men and women. In one study, the relationship between hormone levels and sexual activity was determined (Fox et al. 1972). Serum testosterone concentrations were higher in men during and immediately after intercourse than under resting conditions. In contrast to the changes that accompanied coitus, testosterone levels either increased slightly or not at all after masturbation, indicating that stimuli associated with sexual arousal by a partner is more reliably correlated with changes in testosterone than is ejaculation.

The idea that ejaculation need not precede an increase in male hormone production seems to be supported by an amusing and widely cited letter to the editor of *Nature* (Anonymous 1970). An anonymous author claimed that his beard growth was greater when he anticipated (and when he actually engaged in) sexual activity with his girlfriend than during periods when he was isolated on a remote island. The writer suggests that the enhanced beard growth can be explained by an increase in the production of testicular hormones, which are known to influence the rate of beard growth. Needless to say, this report elicited several critical letters to the editor noting that a number of factors, including water content of the skin, thickness of the skin (which changes 2 to 3 hours after awakening), and the degree of tension exerted by the muscles of the hair follicles, influence beard growth. It was suggested that the letter writer could do a better controlled study if he enticed his friend to drop in on him unexpectedly, or if she unexpectedly withheld her favors during randomly selected visits.

Despite the surreptitious giggling generally elicited by questions about how humans perform and think about sex and sexuality, it is a topic that is bound to receive increasing attention. Part of the increased visibility in the press of human sex behavior derives from the understanding of nitric oxide (NO) in the control of penile erection. Early pharmacological studies in which the enzymes for the formation of NO were inhibited suggested that NO is necessary for sexual behavior. These studies suggested that while sexual motivation was unaffected by blocking NO production, penile erection did not occur (Hull et al. 1994). Subsequent studies using electrophysiology to stimulate the nerves involved in erection, suggested that blocking NO abolished electrically stimulated erections in rats (Burnett et al. 1992).

These basic research findings rapidly turned into a bonanza for Pfizer, the drug company that makes Viagra, a drug that functions to maintain penile erection. Given that most of the sales of Viagra are to individuals who had no prior medical condition, we must conclude that the availability of a prolonged erection with the use of drugs is promoting sexual behavior in the population at large. The interest on the part of the public in purchasing such products as Viagra (see also chapter 5) has stimulated a broad-based search for other agents that allow sexual healing for dysfunction, and enhanced sexual performance for the unimpaired. Sales of Viagra topped $1 billion in its first year on the market (see website at http://www.nytimes.com; Article title: The Second Sexual Revolution; February 20, 2000). The success of Viagra has heightened awareness that innervation of and blood flow to the genital region is important in sexual arousal, which has resulted in a great surge of research in drugs, creams, and pills that might increase blood flow to the vaginal region.

All this attention to blood flow and sensory stimulation in the genital region of humans has also served to highlight the astounding fact that we know very little about the innervation of the genital region in women; and a new era of interest in the role of peripheral sensory factors in sustaining sexual behavior has been launched. An interesting overview of "love as sensory stimulation" is available in a paper by Komisaruk and Whipple (1998), investigators who have done a great deal of research into the role of peripheral factors in sexual behavior.

NURSING

One of the most important and easily demonstrable contexts in which external stimuli are known to affect the production of hormones involved in human reproduction is nursing. Milk production begins 2 to 3 days after childbirth. When the baby suckles at the nipple, tactile information from the nipple is transmitted from nerves in the breast to the brain, causing the release of oxytocin and prolactin, which circulate in the blood and ultimately reach the breast to promote milk production and release (see chapter 9). If the baby does not suckle, the mother becomes unable to produce milk. On the other hand, if suckling continues, the mother can continue to produce milk for her own child (or for other children) for many years.

Milk production and milk release, which together constitute lactation, can occur in women without a suckling infant. Visual or auditory stimuli acting alone can also cause milk release in lactating mothers when they see or hear their baby crying. This response can become conditioned to other cues such as the sounds of a nurse opening the door to bring the baby into the mother's room. Suckling influences not only the mother, but also the infant and the mother-infant dyad (reviewed in Uvnas-Moberg and Eriksson 1996). Non-nutritive suckling can enhance growth in infants, which is most likely due to the release of gastrointestinal hormones. Skin-to-skin contact between the mother and the infant and breast-feeding are thought to promote the mother-infant bond. There is some support for the idea that the hormone oxytocin plays a mediating role in this bonding response. Taken together, studies on mother-infant interactions indicate that visual, auditory, and tactile stimuli have a substantial effect on hormone synthesis and release. These hormones, in turn, act to modify the responses associated with maternal behavior and with mother-infant bonding.

Summary

This chapter has focused on the role of environmental factors in regulating specific stages of the reproductive cycle, including puberty, ovulation, sexual behavior, pregnancy, lactation, and parental behavior. Animals in the wild rely on these (and other) environmental cues to time reproduction with changing seasons in order to coordinate breeding with the times of the year that are most favorable for reproduction (i.e., most likely to result in offspring/parent survival). The reader should now have an appreciation for how animals in nature integrate numerous environmental factors to regulate reproductive activities.

1. All the information available to an animal in its environment is integrated to influence long-term and moment-to-moment changes in hormones and behavior.
2. As described in detail in chapter 12, animals respond to day-length changes with alterations in reproductive hormones and behavior.
3. Numerous factors, such as food availability and temperature, can act to further modify the timing and extent of reproductive alterations.
4. Finally, as shown above, social interactions can lead to alterations in hormones and behavior by acting through pheromones.
5. By integrating numerous environmental factors to time breeding to occur when conditions are maximally favorable, animals can increase the likelihood of survival of themselves and their offspring.

This chapter has demonstrated that cues from the internal and external environment act on the senses and have important influences on neuroendocrine systems. Each of the 5 senses has been shown to exert such effects, often after altering reproductive hormones. These phenomena help to coordinate reproductive function with the animal's environmental conditions, including seasonality, food availability, and social context. Although this chapter focused on reproductive hormones, environmental factors that impinge upon the senses can influence numerous endocrine factors and help to coordinate a host of adaptations with current or predictable changes in the environment.

Study Questions

1. Can you think of any examples where the environment affected your hormones, which in turn influenced your behavior? Describe what happened

and why you think this is an example of environmental influences on hormones and behavior.

2. Environmental stimuli can impact hormones through all sensory modalities. Give examples of each.

3. How does environmental control of energy and survival interact with the effects of specific sensory stimuli on hormones and behavior?

References

Anonymous. (1970) Effects of sexual activity on beard growth in man. *Nature* 226: 869–870.

Baker, J. R. (1938) The evolution of breeding seasons. In G. R. DeBeer (Ed.), *Evolution: Essays on Aspects of Evolutionary Biology*. Oxford: Clarendar Press, pp. 161–177.

Bellastella, A., Pisano, G., Iorio, S., Pasquali, D., Orio, F., Venditto, T., and Sinisi, A. A. (1998) Endocrine secretions under abnormal light-dark cycles and in the blind. *Horm. Res.* 49: 153–157.

Bentley, G. E., Wingfield, J. C., Morton, M. L., and Ball, G. F. (2000) Stimulatory effects on the reproductive axis in female songbirds by conspecific and heterospecific male song. *Horm. Behav.* 37: 179–189.

Bergh, A. R. (1991) Is testicular function in immature rats increased rather than decreased by a moderate increase in temperature? *Adv. Exp. Med. Biol.* 286: 179–182.

Berndston, W. E., and Desjardins, C. (1974) The cycle of the seminiferous epithelium and spermatogenesis in the bovine testis. *Am. J. Anat.* 140: 167–179.

Berson, D. M., Dunn, F. A., and Takao, M. (2002) Phototransduction by retinal ganglion cells that set the circadian clock. *Science* 295: 1070–1073.

Bittman, E. L., Kaynard, A. H., Olster, D. H., Robinson, J. E., Yellon, S. M., and Karsch, F. J. (1985) Pineal melatonin mediates photoperiodic control of pulsatile luteinizing hormone secretion in the ewe. *Neuroendocrinology* 40: 409.

Bojlen, K., and Bentzon, M. W. (1974) Seasonal variation in the occurrence of menarche. *Dan. Med. Bull.* 21: 161–168.

Brennan, P., Kaba, H., and Keverne, E. B. (1990) Olfactory recognition: A simple memory system. *Science* 250: 1223–1226.

Brinkworth, M. H., Anderson, D., and McLean, A. E. (1992) Effects of dietary imbalances on spermatogenesis in CD-1 mice and CD rats. *Food Chem. Toxicol.* 30: 29–35.

Brockway, B. F. (1965) Stimulation of ovarian development and egg laying by male courtship vocalization in budgerigars (*Melopsittacus undulatus*). *Anim. Behav.* 13: 575–578.

Brockway, B. F. (1967) The influence of vocal behavior on the performer's testicular activity in budgerigar (*Melopsittacus undulatus*). *Wilson Bull.* 79: 328–334.

Bronson, F. H. (1987) Puberty in female rats: Relative effect of exercise and food restriction. *Am. J. Physiol.* 252: R140–144.

Bronson, F. H. (1989) *Mammalian Reproductive Biology*. Chicago: University of Chicago Press.

Bronson, F. H. (1995) Seasonal variation in human reproduction: Environmental factors. *Q. Rev. Biol.* 70: 141–164.

Bronson, F. H., and Heideman, P. D. (1994) Seasonal regulation of reproduction in mammals. In E. Knobil and J. D. Neill (Eds.), *The Physiology of Reproduction*. New York: Raven Press, pp. 541–584.

Bronson, F. H., and Marsteller, F. A. (1985) Effect of short-term food deprivation on reproduction in female mice. *Biol. Reprod.* 33: 660-667.

Bronson, F. H., and Maruniak, J. A. (1976) Differential effects of male stimuli on follicle-stimulating hormone, luteinizing hormone, and prolactin secretion in prepubertal female mice. *Endocrinology* 98: 1101–1108.

Bronson, F. H., and Rissman, E. F. (1986) The biology of puberty. *Biol. Rev. Camb. Philos. Soc.* 61: 157–195.

Bruce, H. M. (1959) An exteroceptive block to pregnancy in the mouse. *Nature* 184: 105.

Burger, J., and Gochfeld, M. (1985) A hypothesis on the role of pheromones on age of menarche. *Med. Hypotheses.* 17: 39–46.

Burnett, A. L., Lowenstein, C. J., Bredt, D. S., Chang, T. S., and Snyder, S. H. (1992) Nitric oxide: A physiologic mediator of penile erection. *Science* 257: 401–403.

Carter, C. S., Getz, L. L., Gavish, L., McDermott, J. L., and Arnold, P. (1980) Male-related pheromones and the activation of female reproduction in prairie vole (*Microtus ochrogaster*). *Biol. Reprod.* 23: 1038–1045.

Carter, C. S., Witt, D. M., Manock, S. R., Adams, K. A., Bahr, J. M., and Carlstead, K. (1989) Hormonal correlates of sexual behavior and ovulation in male-induced and post-partum estrus in female prairie voles. *Physiol. Behav.* 46: 946–948.

Cohen, D. (1967) Optimizing reproduction in a varying environment. *J. Theor. Biol.* 16: 1–14.

Cohens-Parsons, M., and Carter, C. S. (1987) Males increase serum estrogen binding in brain of female voles. *Physiol. Behav.* 39: 309–314.

Colby, D. R. V., and Vandenbergh, J. G. (1979) Regulatory effects of urinary pheromones on puberty in the mouse. *Biol. Reprod.* 11: 268–279.

Coppola, D. M., and Vandenbergh, J. G. (1985) Effect of density, duration of grouping and age of urine stimulus on the puberty delay pheromone in female mice. *J. Reprod. Fertil.* 73: 517–22.

Crews, D. (1975) Effects of different components of male courtship behaviour on environmentally induced ovarian recrudescence and mating preferences in the lizard, *Anolis carolinensis*. *Anim. Behav.* 23: 349–356.

Dahl, G. E., Elsasser, T. H., Capuco, A. V., Erdman, R. A., and Peters, R. R. (1997) Effects of a long daily photoperiod on milk yield and circulating concentrations of insulin-like growth factor-1. *J. Dairy Sci.* 80: 2784–2789.

Demas, G. E., Williams, J. M, and Nelson, R. J. (1997) Amygdala but not hippocampal lesions impair olfactory memory for mate in prairie voles (*Microtus ochrogaster*). *Am. J. Physiol.* 273: R1683–1689.

Desjardins, C., and Lopez, M. J. (1983) Environmental cues evoke differential responses in pituitary-testicular function in deer mice. *Endocrinology* 112: 1398–1406.

Diamond, M. (1970) Intromission pattern and species vaginal code in relation to the induction of pseudopregnancy. *Science* 169: 995–997.

Diamond, M. (1972) Vaginal stimulation and progesterone in relation to pregnancy and parturition. *Biol. Reprod.* 6: 281–287.

Dluzen, D. E., Ramirez, V. D., Carter, C. S., and Getz, L. L. (1981) Male vole urine changes luteinizing hormone-releasing hormone and norepinephrine in female olfactory bulb. *Science* 212: 573–575.

Edmonds, K. E., and Stetson, M. H. (1993) Effect of photoperiod and gonadal maintenance and development in the marsh rat (*Oryzomys palustris*). *Gen. Comp. Endocrinol.* 92: 281–291.

Eichenbaum, H., Fagan, A., and Cohen, N. J. (1986) Normal olfactory discrimination learning set and facilitation of reversal learning after medial-temporal damage in rats: Implications for account of preserved learning abilities in amnesia. *J. Neurosci.* 6: 1876–84.

Ellis, B. J., McFadyen-Ketchum, S., Dodge, K. A., Pettit, G. S., and Bates, J. E. Quality of early family relationships and individual differences in the timing of pubertal maturation in girls: A longitudinal test of an evolutionary model. *J. Pers. Soc. Psychol.* 77: 387–401.

Elster, A. D., and Bleyl, J. (1991) Seasonality of triplet births in the United States. *Hum. Biol.* 63: 711–8.

Ferkin, M. H., Gorman, M. R., and Zucker, I. (1991) Ovarian hormones influence odor cues emitted by female meadow voles, *Microtus pennsylvanicus*. *Horm. Behav.* 25: 572–578.

Ferkin, M. H., Gorman, M. R., and Zucker, I. (1992) Influence of gonadal hormones on odours emitted by male meadow voles (*Microtus pennsylvanicus*). *J. Reprod. Fertil.* 95: 729–736.

Fleming, A. S., Gavarth, K., and Sarker, J. (1992) Effects of transections to the vomeronasal nerves or to the main olfactory bulbs on the initiation and long-term retention of maternal behavior in primiparous rats. *Behav. Neural. Biol.* 57: 177–188.

Follett, B. K. S., and Sharp, P. J. (1969) Circadian rhythmicity in photoperiodically induced gonadotrophin release and gonadal growth in the quail. *Nature* 223: 968–971.

Forger, N. G., and Zucker, I. (1985) Photoperiodic regulation of reproductive development in male white-footed mice (*Peromyscus leucopus*) born at different phases of the breeding season. *J. Reprod. Fertil.* 73: 271–278.

Foster, R. G., Follett, B. K., and Lythgoe, J. N. (1985) Opsin-like sensitivity of extra-retinal photoreceptors mediating the photoperiodic response in quail. *Nature* 313: 50–52.

Foster, R. G., and Soni, B. G. (1998) Extraretinal photoreceptors and their regulation of temporal physiology. *Rev. Reprod.* 3: 145–150.

Fox, C., Ismail, A., Love, D., Kirkham, K., and Loraine, J. (1972) Studies on the relation of plasma testosterone levels and human sexual activity. *J. Endocrinol.* 52: 51–58.

Fox, S. R., and Smith, M. S. (1984) The suppression of pulsatile luteinizing hormone secretion during lactation in the rat. *Endocrinology* 115: 2045–2051.

Freedman, M. S., Lucas, R. J., Soni, B., von Schantz, M., Munoz, M., David-Gray, Z., and Foster, R. (1999) Regulation of mammalian circadian behavior by non-rod, non-cone, ocular photoreceptors. *Science* 284: 502–504.

Friedman, M. B. (1977) Interactions between visual and vocal courtship stimuli in the neuroendocrine response of female ring doves. *J. Comp. Physiol. Psychol.* 91: 1408–1416.

Gopalan, C., and Naidu, A. N. (1972) Nutrition and fertility. *Lancet* 2: 1077–1079.

Gregory, E., and Pritchard, W. S. (1983) The effects of neonatal androgenization of female hamsters on adult preferences for female hamster vaginal discharge. *Physiol. Behav.* 31: 861–864.

Groos, A. D., and Smith, T. A. (1992) Age at menarche and associated nutritional status variables in Karimui and Daribi census divisions of Simbu Province. *P N G Med. J.* 35: 84–94.

Hannibal, J., Hindersson, P., Knudsen, S. M., Georg, B., and Fahrenkrug, J. (2002) The photopigment melanopsin is exclusively present in pituitary adenylate cyclase-activating polypeptide-containing retinal ganglion cells of the retinohypothalamic tract. *J. Neurosci.* 22: RC191.

Hauspie, R. C., Vercauteren, M., and Susanne, C. (1996) Secular changes in growth. *Horm Res.* 2: 8–17.

Hattar, S., Liao, H. W., Takao, M., Berson, D. M., and Yau, K. W. (2002) Melanopsin-containing retinal ganglion cells: Architecture, projections, and intrinsic photosensitivity. *Science* 295: 1065–1070.

Hull, E. M., Lumley, L. A., Matuszewich, L., Dominguez, J., Moses, J., and Lorrain, D. S. (1994) The roles of nitric oxide in sexual function of male rats. *Neuropharmacology* 33: 1499–504.

Jallageas, M., Boissin, J., and Mas, N. (1994a) Differential photoperiodic control of seasonal variations in pulsatile luteinizing hormone release in long-day (Ferret) and short-day (Mink) mammals. *J. Biol. Rhyth.* 9: 217–231.

Jallageas, M., Mas, N., Boissin, J., Maurel, D., and Ixart, G. Seasonal variations of pulsatile luteinizing hormone release in the mink (*Mustela vison*). *Comp. Biochem. Physiol. C Pharmacol. Toxicol. Endocrinol.* 109: 9–20.

Johnston, R. E., Zahorick, D. M., Immler, K., and Zakon, H. (1978) Attractions of male sexual behavior by learned aversions to hamster vaginal secretions. *J. Comp. Physiol. Psychol.* 92: 85–93.

Johnston, R. E. (1990) Chemical communication in golden hamsters: From behavior to molecules and neural meacahnisms. In D. A. Dewsbury (Ed.), *Contemporary Issues in Comparative Psychology*. Sunderland, Mass.: Sinauer, pp. 381–409.

Jones, J. I., and Clemmons, D. R. (1995) Insulin-like growth factors and their binding proteins: Biological actions. *Endocr. Rev.* 16: 3–34.

Kamimura, K. (1976) Epidemiology of twin births from a climatic point of view. *Br. J. Prev. Soc. Med.* 30: 175–179.

Kendrick, K. M., Levy, F., and Keverne, E. B. (1992) Changes in the sensory processing of olfactory signals induced by birth in sleep. *Science* 256: 833–6.

Keverne, E. B., and Kendrick, K. M. (1994) Maternal behaviour in sheep and its neuroendocrine regulation. *Acta Paediatr. Suppl.* 397: 47–56.

Kim, K., and Smith, P. K. (1998) Childhood stress, behavioural symptoms and mother-daughter pubertal development. *J. Adolesc.* 21: 231–240.

Komisaruk, B. R., and Whipple, B. (1998) Love as sensory stimulation: Physiological consequences of its deprivation and expression. *Psychoneuroendocrinology* 23: 927–944.

Kroodsma, D. E. (1976) Reproductive development in a female songbird: Differential stimulation by quality of male song. *Science* 192: 574–575.

Leboucher, G., Depraz, V., Kreutzer, M., and Nagle, L. (1998) Male song stimulation of female reproduction in canaries: Features relevant to sexual displays are not relevant to nest-building or egg-laying. *Ethology* 104: 613–624.

Lee and Boot (1955) Spontaneous pseudopregnancy in mice. *Acta Physiol. Pharmacol. Neerl.* 4: 442–443.

Li, C., Chen, P., and Smith, M. S. (1999) Neural populations in the rat forebrain and brainstem activated by the suckling stimulus as demonstrated by cFos expression. *Neuroscience* 94: 117–129.

Lucas, R. J., Freedman, M. S., Munoz, M., Garcia-Fernandez, J. M., and Foster, R. G. (1999) Regulation of the mammalian pineal by non-rod, non-cone, ocular photoreceptors. *Science* 284: 505-507.

Ma, W., Miao, Z., and Novotny, M. V. (1998) Role of the adrenal gland and adrenal-mediated chemosignals in suppression of estrus in the house mouse: The lee-boot effect revisited. *Biol Reprod.* 59: 1317–1320.

Macdougall-Shackleton, S. A., Macdougall-Shackleton, E. A., and Hahn, T. P. Physiological and behavioural responses of female mountain white-crowned sparrows to natal and foreign dialect songs. *Canad. J. Zool.* (In press).

Marchlewska-Koj, A. (1983) Pregnancy blocking by pheromones. In J. G. Vandenbergh (Ed.), *Pheromones and Reproduction in Mammals*. New York: Academic Press, pp. 151–173.

Marshall, J. R. H., and Henkin, R. I. (1971) Olfactory acuity, menstrual abnormalities, and oocyte status. *Ann. Intern. Med.* 75: 207–211.

Massey, A., and Vandenbergh, J. G. (1980) Puberty delay by a urinary cue from female house mice in feral populations. *Science* 209: 821–822.

McClintock, M. K. (1971) Menstrual synchrony and suppression. *Nature* 229: 244–245.

McClintock, M. K. (1984) Estrous synchrony: Modulation of ovarian cycle length by female pheromones. *Physiol. Behav.* 32: 7015.

McIntosh, T. K., and Drickamer, L. C. (1977) Excreted urine, bladder urine, and the delay of sexual maturation in female house mice. *Anim. Behav.* 25: 999–1004.

Menaker, M. Nonvisual light reception. (1972) *Sci. Am.* 226: 22–29.

Miller, A. R., Stanisiewski, E. P., Erdman, R. A., Douglass, L. W., and Dahl, G. E. (1999) Effects of long daily photoperiod and bovine somatotropin (Trobest) on milk yield in cows. *J. Dairy. Sci.* 82: 1716–22.

Mitchell, J. A. Y., and Yochim, J. M. (1970) Influence of environmental lighting on duration of pregnancy in the rat. *Endocrinology* 87: 472–480.

Monti-Bloch, L., Jennings-White, C., and Berliner, D. L. (1998) The human vomeronasal system. A review. *Ann. N.Y. Acad. Sci.* 855: 373–89.

Murphy, M. R. (1980) Sexual preferences of male hamsters: Importance of preweaning and adult experience, vaginal secretion and olfactory or vomeronasal sensation. *Behav. Neural. Biol.* 30: 323–340.

Negus, N. C., and Berger, P. J. (1987) Mammalian reproductive physiology: Adaptive responses to changing environments. *Curr. Mammol.* 1: 149–163.

Nelson, J. F., Gosden, R. G., and Felicio, L. S. Effect of dietary restriction on estrous cyclicity and follicular reserves in aging C57BL/6J mice. *Biol. Reprod.* 32: 515–22.

Nelson, R. J. (1987) Photoperiod-nonresponsive morphs: A possible variable in microtine population density fluctuations. *Am. Nat.* 130: 350–369, 1987.

Nelson, R. J., Frank, D., Smale, L., and Willoughby, S. B. (1989) Photoperiod and temperature affect reproductive and nonreproductive functions in male prairie voles (*Microtus ochrogaster*). *Biol. Reprod.* 40: 481–485.

Nelson, R. J., and Zucker, I. (1981) Absence of extraocular photoreception in diurnal and nocturnal rodents exposed to direct sunlight. *Comp. Biochem. Physiol.* 69A: 145–148.

Novotny, M. V., Jemiolo, B., Wiesler, D., Ma, W., Harvey, S., Xu, F., Xie, T. M., and Carmack, M. (1999) A unique urinary constituent, 6-hydroxy-6-methyl-3-heptanone, is a pheromone that accelerates puberty in female mice. *Chem. Biol.* 6: 377–383.

Orpen, B. G., and Fleming, A. S. (1987) Experience with pups sustains maternal responding in postpartum rats. *Physiol. Behav.* 40: 47–54.

Perret, M., and Schilling, A. (1995) Sexual responses to urinary chemosignals depend on photoperiod in a male primate. *Physiol. Behav.* 58: 633–9.

Provencio, I., Rollag, M. D., and Castrucci, A. M. (2002) Photoreceptive net in the mammalian retina. *Nature* 415: 493.

Reksen, O., Tverdal, A., Landsverk, K., Kommisrud, E., Boe, K. E., and Ropstad, E. (1999) Effects of photointensity and photoperiod on milk yield and reproductive performance of Norwegian red cattle. *J. Dairy Sci.* 82: 810–6.

Richmond, M., and Conway, C. H. (1969) Induced ovulation and oestrus in *Microtus ochrogaster*. *J. Reprod. Fertil.* Suppl. 6: 367–376.

Richmond, M., and Stehn, R. (1976) Olfaction and reproductive behavior in microtine rodents. In R. L. Doty (Ed.), *Mammalian Olfaction, Reproductive Processes, and Behavior*. New York: Academic Press, pp. 197–217.

Rissman, E. F., and Li, X. (2000) Olfactory bulbectomy blocks mating-induced ovulation musk shrew (*Suncus murinus*). *Biol. Reprod.* 62: 1052–1058.

Rissman, E. F., Silveira, J., and Bronson, F. H. (1988) Patterns of sexual receptivity in the female musk shrew (*Suncus murinus*). *Horm. Behav.* 22: 186–193.

Roenneberg, T. A., and Aschoff, J. (1990) Annual rhythm of human reproduction: II. Environmental correlations. *J. Biol. Rhythm.* 5: 217–239.

Rosedale, R. S. (1945) Nasogenital relationship. *Arch. Otolaryngology* 42: 235–238.

Rosenblatt, J. S. (1990) Landmarks in the physiological study of maternal behavior with special reference to the rat. In N. A. Krasnegor and R. S. Bridges (Eds.), *Mammalian Parenting*. Oxford: Oxford University Press, pp. 40–60.

Rosetta, L. (1993) Female reproductive dysfunction and intense physical training. *Oxf. Rev. Reprod. Biol.* 15: 113–141.

Rowan, W. (1925) Relation of light to bird migration and developmental changes. *Nature* 115: 494–495.

Russell, M. J. S., G. M., and Thompson, K. (1980) Olfactory influences on the human menstrual cycle. *Pharmacol. Biochem. Behav.* 13: 737–738.

Saldanha, C. J., Silverman, A. J., and Silver, R. (2001) Direct innervation of GnRH neurons by encephalic photoreceptors in birds. *J. Biol. Rhythms* 16: 39–49.

Schneider, J. E., and Wade, G. N. (2000) Inhibition of reproduction in service of energy balance. In J. E. Schneider and K. Wallen (Eds.), *Reproduction in Context.* Cambridge, Mass.: MIT Press, pp. 35–82.

Schwanzel-Fukuda, M. (1999) Origin and migration of luteinizing hormone-releasing hormone neurons in mammals. *Res. Tech.* 44: 2–10.

Schwanzel-Fukuda, M., Bick, D., and Pfaff, D. W. (1989) Luteinizing hormone-releasing hormone (LHRH)-expressing cells do not migrate normally in an inherited hypogonadal (Kallman) syndrome. *Mol. Br. Res.* 6: 311–326.

Schwanzel-Fukuda, M. P., and Pfaff, D. W. (1989) Origin of luteinizing hormone-releasing hormone neurons. *Nature* 138: 161–164.

Selway, R., and Keverne, E. B. (1990) Hippocampal lesions are without effect on olfactory memory formation in the context of pregnancy block. *Physiol Behav.* 47: 249–52.

Silver, R., Witkovsky, P., Horvath, P., Alones, V. Barnstable, C. J., and Lehman, M. N. (1988) Coexpression of opsin- and VIP-like-immunoreactivity in CSF-contacting neurons of the avian brain. *Cell Tissue Res.* 253: 189–198.

Swann, J. M., and Turek, F. W. (1988) Transfer from long to short days reduces the frequency of pulsatile luteinizing hormone release in intact but not in castrated male golden hamsters. *Neuroendocrinology* 47: 343–349.

Tanner, J. M. (1992) Growth as a measure of the nutritional and hygienic status of a population. *Horm. Res.* 38(Suppl. 1): 106–15.

Tanner, J. M. (1968) Earlier maturation in man. *Sci. Am.* 218: 21–27.

Tirindelli, R., Mucignat-Caretta, C., and Ryba, N. J. (1998) Molecular aspects of pheromonal communication via the vomeronasal organ of mammals. *Trends Neurosci.* 21: 482–486.

Trevathan, W. R., Burleson, M. H., and Gregory, W. L. (1993) No evidence for menstrual synchrony in lesbian couples. *Psychoneuroendocrinology* 18: 425–435.

Tucker, H. A., Paape, M. J., and Sinha, Y. N. (1967) Ovariectomy and suckling intensity effects on mammary nucleic acid, prolactin, and ACTH. *Am. J. Physiol.* 213: 262–266.

Turek, F. W., and Vancauter, E. (1994) Rhythms in reproduction. In E. Knobil and D. D. Neill (Eds.), *The Physiology of Reproduction.* New York: Raven Press, pp. 487–540.

Uvnas-Moberg, K., and Eriksson, M. (1996) Breastfeeding: Physiological, endocrine and behavioural adaptations caused by oxytocin and local neurogenic activity in the nipple and mammary gland. *Acta Paediatr.* 85: 525–530.

Vallet, E., and Kreutzer, M. (1995) Female canaries are sexually responsive to special song phrases. *Anim. Behav.* 49: 1603–1610.

Vandenbergh, J. G., Finlayson, J. S., Dobrogosz, W. J., Dills, S. S., and Kost, T. A. (1976) Chromatographic separation of puberty accelerating pheromone from male mouse urine. *Biol. Reprod.* 15: 260–265.

Vandenbergh, J. G. (1988) Pheromones and mammalian reproduction. In *The Physiology of Reproduction.* New York: Raven Press.

Vogl, T. J., Stemmler, J., Heye, B., Schopohl, J., Danek, A., Bergman, C., Balzer, J. O., and Felix, R. (1994) Kallman syndrome versus idiopathic hypogonadotropic hypogonadism at MR imaging. *Radiology* 191: 53–57.

Walker, C. D., Lightman, S. L., Steele, M. K., and Dallman, M. F. (1992) Suckling is a persistent stimulus to the adrenocortical system of the rat. *Endocrinology* 130: 115–125.

Weller, L., Weller, A., and Avinir, O. (1995) Menstrual synchrony: Only in roommates who are close friends? *Physiol Behav.* 58: 883–889.

Whitten, D. K. (1957) Effects of exteroreceptive factors on the oestrous cycle of mice. *Nature* 180: 1456–1457.

Wilson, F. E. (1991) Neither retinal nor pineal photoreceptors mediate photoperiodic control of seasonal reproduction in American Tree Sparrows (*Spizella arborea*). *J. Exp. Zool.* 259: 117–127.

Wingfield, J. C. (1983) Environmental and endocrine control of reproduction: An ecological approach. In S. I. Mikami and M. Wada (Eds.), *Avian Endocrinology: Environmental and Ecological Aspects.* Berlin: Springer Verlag, pp. 149–166.

Wingfield, J. C., Breuner, C., Jacobs, J., Lynn, S., Maney, D., Ramenofsky, M., and Richarnson, R. (1998) Ecological bases of hormone-behavior interactions: The "emergency life-history stage." *Am. Zool.* 38: 191–206.

Wingfield, J. C., and Farner, D. S. (1980) Environmental and endocrine control of seasonal reproduction in temperate zone birds. *Prog. Reprod. Biol.* 5: 62–101.

Wingfield, J. C., Jacobs, J. D., Tramontin, A. D., Perfito, N., Meddle, S., Maney, D. L., and Soma, K. (2000) Toward and ecological basis of hormone-behavior interactions in reproduction of birds. In J. E. Schneider and K. Wallen (Eds.), *Reproduction in Context.* Cambridge, Mass.: MIT Press, pp. 85–128.

Wingfield, J. C., and Kenagy, G. J. (1991) Natural regulation of reproductive cycles. In M. Schreibman and R. E. Jones (Eds.), *Vertebrate Endocrinology: Fundamentals and Biomedical Implications*, vol. 4, part B. New York: Academic Press, pp. 181–124.

Woodside, B. (1991) Effects of food restriction on the length of lactational diestrus in rats. *Horm Behav.* 25: 70–83.

Wray, S., Grant, P., and Gainer, H. (1989) Evidence that cells expressing luteinizing hormone-releasing hormone mRNA in the mouse are derived from progenitor cells in the olfactory placode. *Proc. Natl. Acad. Sci. USA* 86: 8132–8136.

Yamazaki, S., Goto, M., and Menaker, M. (1999) No evidence for extraocular photoreceptors in the circadian system of the Syrian hamster. *J. Biol. Rhythms.* 14: 197–201.

Yokoyama, K., and Farner, D. S. (1976) Photoperiodic responses in bilaterally enucleated white-crowned sparrows, *Zonotrichia leucophrys gambelii. Gen. Comp. Endocrinol.* 30: 528–533.

Zacharias, L., and Wurtman, R. J. (1964) Blindness: Its relation to age of menarche. *Science* 144: 1154–1155.

Glossary

Accessory sex structures Tissues and organs that are part of the reproductive tract and important in the transport of gametes. In males these consist of the epididymis, vas deferens, prostate, seminal vesicles, and, in reptiles, the renal sex segment. In females these consist of the uterus and fallopian tubes.

Action potential An all-or-none change in the membrane potential of an axon which results in synaptic transmission for communication between neurons.

Activational effects of hormones Transient actions of hormones, usually in adulthood. Activational effects may be defined by the occurrence of a given behavioral response only in the presence of a given hormone.

Active avoidance A type of learning in which an individual must perform a response in order to avoid a noxious stimulation.

Active play (rough and tumble play) Juvenile play that has a high level of active behaviors.

Active space The distance one electric fish can be from another and still have its electric organ discharges detected.

Adenohypophysis The anterior pituitary.

Adrenal gland A gland located just above the kidneys. It is composed of an inner medulla and an outer cortex. Among the hormones secreted from the medulla are dopamine, norepinephrine, and epinephrine (also called adrenaline). Aldosterone and glucocorticoids are among the over 50 steroid hormones secreted from the adrenal cortex.

Adrenalectomy The bilateral surgical removal of the adrenal glands.

Adrenaline A hormone secreted by the adrenal medulla (see also **epinephrine**).

Adrenergic receptors Receptors for the hormone epinephrine (also called adrenaline).

Adrenocorticotropic hormone (ACTH) A tropic hormone secreted by the anterior pituitary gland; it controls the production and release of hormones of the adrenal cortex and may also have central actions.

Age-limited song learning Song learning that is confined to the first year of life; a characteristic of certain songbirds such as zebra finches.

Aggression A form of behavior that can result in one animal injuring or killing another animal. In humans, the behavior must be accompanied by an intent to do harm.

Agonist A synthetic chemical mimic that binds to receptors and causes a biological response that is indistinguishable from the response normally elicited by a neurotransmitter or hormone.

Aldosterone A steroid hormone secreted by the adrenal cortex that regulates the salt and water balance in the body.

Allele A specific version of a gene.

Alpha-feto protein (AFP) A protein found in plasma that can bind to estrogens but not androgens in rodents.

Alternative life-history strategies   The presence in the same sex of a species, different phenotypes and different behavioral characteristics, which may be either inherited or environmentally induced.

Altricial   Describes young birds or mammals born in an immature condition, with poorly developed vision, learning ability, and locomotion, and dependent upon a parent for nutrition.

Alzheimer's disease   A type of dementia that occurs in middle age or older and is accompanied by a constellation of brain changes that are recognizable at autopsy (neurofibrulary plaques and tangles).

Amnesia   A partial or total loss of memory. See also **anterograde amnesia** and **retrograde amnesia**.

Amphetamine   A drug that acts by stimulating catecholamine release and blocking catecholamine reuptake into synaptic terminals.

Amphibian and basilar papillae   The auditory organs of frogs; the hair cells are located within these structures.

Amygdala   An almond-shaped brain structure located deep within the base of the temporal lobe of the brain. The amygdala is involved in the integration of emotional responses that are important for many behavioral systems (e.g., aggression, sexual behavior, and certain types of conditioned emotional responses). It receives input from the vomeronasal system and limbic system.

Anabolism   A term in physiology that refers to metabolic features that involve the building up of molecules, cells, and tissues. See **catabolism**.

Analgesia   The blunting of the perception of pain.

Androgen   A class of steroid hormones that are secreted primarily from the testes; it includes testosterone, dihydrotestosterone, and androstenedione.

Annual rhythms (type I)   Annual rhythms that are dependent to some degree upon the environment for their expression; type I rhythms do not persist in constant environmental conditions (i.e., constant light, temperature, food availability, etc.)

Annual rhythms (type II)   Annual rhythms that are generated independently of the environment by an endogenous clock, but rely upon the environment for entrainment to a period of 365 days; type II rhythms free run in constant environment conditions.

Anorexia   Loss of appetite.

Antagonist   A substance that binds to receptors and thereby blocks natural hormones and neurotransmitters from acting at the receptor.

Anterograde amnesia   The inability to form new memories that begins with the onset of the disorder.

Antibody   A protein substance produced in the blood or tissues in response to a specific antigen. Antibodies destroy or weaken foreign pathogens, thus forming the basis of immunity.

Antigen   A substance that stimulates the production of an antibody when it is introduced into the body. Antigens include toxins, bacteria, foreign blood cells, and the cells of transplanted organs.

Anti-Müllerian hormone (AMH)   A protein hormone secreted by the developing testes, which inhibits development of the Müllerian ducts into patent ducts; also called Müllerian regression factor (MRF).

Anurans   Frogs and toads.

Aphasia   An impairment in the production and comprehension of speech or written language following brain damage.

Apolipoprotein E (ApoE)   A gene that codes for a protein that plays a central role in lipid metabolism in the nervous system and other organs. The gene exists in 3 forms or alleles. The ApoE2 and ApoE3 forms are associated with a lower risk of Alzheimer's disease while the ApoE4 allele confers a greater risk.

Apomorphine   A dopamine receptor agonist.

Apoptosis   Programmed, orderly cell death that does not activate the immune system.

Appetively motivated   Describes tasks in which work is done in exchange for a positive reward, like food, water, or access to a mate.

Apraxia   An impairment in the production of manual or oral movements following brain damage, which may reflect an underlying motor programming disorder; it occurs in the absence of of paralysis or paresis.

Aromatase   An enzyme that catalyzes the conversion of testosterone into estradiol.

Assay   A method for determining the quantity of a substance present in a sample.

Associated reproductive pattern   A close temporal relationship between the maturation of the gametes, an increase in circulating concentrations of sex hormones, and the display of mating behaviors.

Ataxia   Lack of motor coordination.

Atrophy   The shinkage of a cell or the withdrawal of axons or dendrites.

Attractivity   The value of a given individual as a stimulus capable of eliciting sexual responses from an individual of the opposite sex.

Autoimmune disease   A disease characterized by abnormal immune system function that causes it to produce antibodies against antigens from its own body's cells.

Autonomic nervous system   The branch of the nervous system that controls functions that are not readily controlled consciously (e.g., heart rate, blushing, and gooseflesh). It includes sympathetic and parasympathetic components.

Autonomic responses   A pattern of bodily responses governed by the autonomic nervous system.

Autoradiogram   An image recorded on a photographic film or emulsion; it is produced by the radiation emitted from a section of brain tissue that has been treated or injected with a radioactively labeled isotope.

Axon   A single small extension of a neuron that (usually) branches many times and serves to transmit information from that neuron to target cells via the propagation of action potentials. Bundles of axons form nerves.

Bag cells   Two clusters of about 400 neurons each that are located on the anterior connectives of the abdominal ganglion in the sea slug *Aplysia*. The cells in a cluster are electrically coupled and secrete egg-laying hormone and associated peptides.

Basal forebrain   Refers collectively to cholinergic cells in the medial septum, the diagonal band of Broca, and the nucleus basalis magnocellularis.

Basal ganglia   A functional group of brain nuclei, consisting of the caudate nucleus, the putamen, and the globus pallidus. The basal ganglia are involved in voluntary limb movement, eye movement, and cognition.

B cells   A type of lymphocyte that arises from the bone marrow; it plays an important role in generating antibodies.

BDNF   Brain-derived neurotrophic factor.

Bed nucleus of the stria terminalis   A forebrain region that has interconnections to the amygdala and the hypothalamus.

Behavioral facilitation of reproduction   The stimulation of reproductive processes in one sex by the behavior of a member of the other sex.

Bioassay   An assay that uses a biological response to detect the presence and quantity of a substance in a sample.

Biogenic amines   Small aromatic amines that include epinephrine, norepinephrine, dopamine, octopamine, and serotonin. They may act locally as a neurotransmitter or neuromodulator, or systemically as a neurohormone.

Biphasic effects of progesterone   The ability of progesterone to facilitate and later inhibit sexual behavior in female vertebrates.

Blood-brain barrier   A cellular barrier consisting of brain blood vessels and surrounding glial cells that prevent free passage of components of the blood into the brain.

Bradykinesia   A neurological symptom characterized by a reduction of the speed of movements.

Brain nucleus   An aggregation of neuron cell bodies within the central nervous system.

Bruce effect   The blocking of pregnancy in a female rodent by the odor of a strange male.

Cannula   A small-diameter tube used to deliver a drug or hormone to a specific site, usually in the brain.

Castration   The removal of gonads; it usually refers to testes.

Catabolism   A term in physiology that refers to metabolic features that involve the breaking down of molecules, cells, and tissues. See **anabolism**.

Catecholamines   The neurotransmitters epinephrine (also called adrenaline), norepinephrine (also called noradrenaline), and dopamine.

Caudate nucleus   Brain structure (nucleus) that, together with the putamen and globus pallidus, forms the basal ganglia. See also **basal ganglia**.

cDNA (copyDNA)   DNA exists as a double strand of nucleic acids where one strand contains the genetic code for a protein and the other strand is the cDNA.

Cell-mediated immunity   The part of the immune response in which complement is mobilized to attack an invasive agent.

Central actions   Drugs or hormones that have effects within the central nervous system.

Central pattern generator   A functional group of central neurons that produces a sequence of temporally and spatially coordinated motor activity. The patterned activity can occur in the absence of sensory feedback and provides the basis for many rhythmic behaviors.

Cerebral lateralization   The specialization of one or the other cerebral hemisphere for a particular function.

Chaperone protein   A protein or group of proteins that facilitates the binding of a steroid hormone and its receptor to the DNA binding site.

Chemokine   Cytokines that are chemotactic for leucocytes.

Chemoreceptors   Receptor cells that detect changes in the chemical environment. This can be the external environment, such as when chemoreceptors in the vomeronasal organ detect pheromones, or the internal environment, such as when chemoreceptors in the hypothalamus respond to a decrease in glucose utilization.

Chirps   Electrical signals used in male courtship in the glass knife gymnotid fish *Eigenmania virescens*.

Cholinergic   Refers to cells that use acetylcholine as their synaptic transmitter.

Chorea   Refers to rapid, dancelike movements of the limbs or facial features that result from a neurological disorder.

Chorea graviderum   A rare complication of pregnancy in which a woman spontaneously exhibits rapid, dancelike contorted movements.

Chromosome   A long, filament-like structure found in cell nuclei, consisting of twisted coils of DNA.

Circadian clock   Mechanism(s) generating a master circadian rhythm; it is located in the suprachiasmatic nucleus in mammals.

Circadian rhythm   An endogenous, self-sustained oscillation with a freerunning period of approximately 24 hours.

Circadian time 12   Arbitrary designation of the time (phase) of locomotor activity onset of a freerunning, nocturnal animal. The time is relative to a circadian "day" that consists of 24 circadian hours, each of which may be longer or shorter than 60 minutes, depending upon whether the freerunning "day" is longer or shorter than 24 hours.

Circannual rhythm   A rhythm generated by a self-sustained, endogenous clock that has a period approximating 365 days.

CNS   Central Nervous System.

Complement   A complex cascade of immune messengers secreted in response to an infectious challenge and capable of killing such pathogenic invaders.

Complementarity   The combination of parts required for completion. Examples of complementarity are stimulus and response, signal and receiver, hormone and receptor, and mounting and receptivity.

Congenital   Present at birth as a result of either heredity or environmental influences.

Congenital adrenal hyperplasia (CAH)   An inherited adrenal enzyme deficiency that results in the overproduction of androgens, beginning in the prenatal period and continuing until controlled with appropriate medications. The condition, if not corrected, causes stunted growth and precocious puberty in males and females. In females, the additional androgens cause various degrees of masculinization of the external genitals and the brain.

Consolidation   A stage of memory formation in which information in short-term or intermediate-term memory is transferred to long-term memory.

Conspecific   A member of the same species.

Constraints   Factors that restrict or limit the development of new adaptations.

Copulation   An act in which individuals exchanging gametes.

Corpora allata   Endocrine glands situated behind the brains of insects that secrete juvenile hormone.

Corpus callosum   A fiber pathway in the brain that connects the two cerebral hemispheres.

Cortex   An external layer, e.g., in the brain or adrenal gland.

Corticosteroid binding globulin   A protein that binds and transports most glucocorticoids in the bloodstream. Because of the hydrophobic nature of steroid molecules, protein transporters keep the steroids in solution in the bloodstream, which is primarily aqueous.

Corticosterone   The major glucocorticoid secreted by rodent and bird adrenal glands.

Corticotropin-releasing factor (CRF)   A hormone released by the hypothalamus that stimulates the pituitary to secrete adrenocorticotropic hormone (ACTH).

Cortisol   The major glucocorticoid secreted by the primate adrenal gland.

Courtship   Actions of a member of one sex that induce a member of the opposite sex to mate with the individual performing the behavior.

Crystallized song   The final stage in song development in which birds produce songs with a well-defined structure and a stereotyped manner in successive renditions.

Cushing's syndrome   A condition in which levels of adrenal glucocorticoids are high, often arising from pituitary tumors, adrenal tumors, or deliberate therapy involving corticosteroids.

Cytokine   A chemical released by immune cells that serve as messengers between immune cells and also influence events within the brain and endocrine organs.

Cytoplasm   The interior of cell body; it surrounds and is separate from the nucleus.

Declarative memory   The memory of events, people, and things that can be recalled consciously.

Dehydroepiandrosterone (DHEA)   An androgenic steroid hormone secreted by the adrenal cortex.

Dendrite   Branchlike extensions of a neuron that receive information, usually from many cells.

Dentate gyrus   The part of the hippocampal formation that receives inputs from the entorhinal cortex and projects to the field CA3 of the hippocampus.

Deoxyribonucleic acid (DNA)   The chemical repository of genetic information. The sequence of nucleotides in DNA specifies a specific sequence of nucleotides in RNA for the production of a protein.

Dexamethasone   A synthetic mimic of the hormone corticosterone, the major glucocorticoid in rodents.

Diabetes insipidus   A disorder caused by the absence (or ineffectiveness) of vasopressin and the consequent loss of its antidiuretic actions in the kidneys. The disorder is characterized by an excessive excretion of water in urine and compensatory large increases in water intake.

Diabetes mellitus   A disorder caused by the absence (or relative ineffectiveness) of insulin and the consequent loss of the ability to store ingested calories as glycogen in the liver and triglycerides in adipose tissue. The disorder is characterized by elevated levels of blood glucose (hyperglycemia) and the appearance of glucose in urine (glycosuria).

Dichotic listening   A type of perceptual test in which different auditory stimuli are presented simultaneously to the two ears.

Diethylstilbestrol (DES)   A synthetic estrogen agonist. DES was administered clinically for the prevention of miscarriage, which may have had masculinizing or defeminizing effects on the brains of female children born to these mothers.

Dihydrotestosterone (DHT)   Metabolite of testosterone formed from testosterone by the action of the 5α-reductase enzyme. DHT has androgenic effects on the brain, accessory sex structures and peripheral secondary sex characteristics.

Dilantin   A drug that is a mimic or agonist of GABA; it binds to GABAergic receptors.

Dioecious   The characteristic of having two structurally distinct sexes (also called gonochorism).

Dissociated reproductive pattern   When the maturation of gametes and the display of mating behaviors occur at different times of the year.

DNA fingerprinting   A method for describing individual differences in patterns of DNA expression.

Dopamine   A neurotransmitter; a member of catecholamine family.

Dyadic   Involving two individuals.

Dynorphin   An opioid compound produced by the brain. See **opioids**.

Ecdysis   The event in arthropods of shedding the old exoskeleton at the end of each molt.

Ecdysteroids   A family of steroid hormones that triggers molting in insects.

Eclosion   The final ecdysis to the adult stage in insects that have a complete metamorphosis.

Eclosion hormone   A 62 amino acid neuropeptide found in insects. Its principle target is the CNS on which it acts to trigger the ecdysis behavior programs.

Egg-laying hormone   A 36 amino acid neuropeptide first found in the sea slug *Aplysia californica*. It triggers the stereotyped sequence of behaviors seen during egg laying.

Ejaculation   The pulsatile expulsion of semen during copulation.

Electric organ discharge (EOD)   A general name for the electrical signals made by mormyrid and gymnotid fish.

Electrocytes   Modified muscle cells in some fish that can produce electrical discharges.

Electroreceptors   Modified hair cells that can respond to electrical signals. In some fish species, electroreceptor organs are called "knollenorgen." See **knollenorgen**.

Encoding   A process of memory formation in which the information entering sensory channels is passed into short-term memory.

Endocrinology   The study of endocrine glands, their functions, and their products.

Endogenous   Originating from within. Describes hormones or neurotransmitters produced by an individual itself. See **exogenous**.

Endogenous clock   Any of a variety of possible mechanisms in an organism that may generate a self-sustained rhythm, regardless of period length.

Endorphin   A 31 amino acid protein that serves as an endogenous morphine or opioid by acting as a neurotransmitter in the brain and a hormone in the pituitary and gut. A class of neurotransmitter/hormones which are secreted in response to stress and can blunt pain perception, inhibit reproductive physiology, and alter immunity. (The pain-blocking abilities of beta-endorphin contribute to "runner's high.")

Enkephalin   A 5 amino acid peptide neurotransmitter with opioid properties.

Entorhinal cortex   A region of the cortex that provides neuronal inputs to the hippocampal formation.

Entrainment   The process by which a rhythm is synchronized to a periodic time-giving stimulus. See **Zeitgeber**.

EOD   Electric organ discharge form a weakly electric fish.

Eosinophil   A type of white blood cell.

Epigamic or intersexual selection   The evolutionary result of organisms choosing a mate nonrandomly from many different available individuals. In many species, epigamic selection has led to the evolution of male courtship signals, and females choose among many potential mates on the basis of these traits.

Epilepsy   A brain disorder in which neurons exhibit a dramatic increase in firing rate in the absence of increased stimulation; in other words, the threshold for excitation is reduced.

Epinephrine   A hormone released by the adrenal medulla that increases heart rate, releases glucose into the blood, and has direct effects on the brain; it is critical for adapting to stress. Its secretion is regulationed by the sympathetic nervous system (also called adrenaline). See **catecholamines**.

Estrogen   A class of steroid hormones secreted primarily from the ovaries; it includes estradiol, estrone, and estriol.

Estrous cycle   Cyclic events associated with the maturation of ovarian follicles and characterized by a distinct period of female sexual receptivity (estrus). Estrus is usually coordinated with ovulation, either through patterns of ovarian hormone secretion or by induced ovulation.

Estrus   The period of sexual receptivity in females.

Eukaryotic   Cells that have a distinct nucleus containing genetic information.

Excitatory amino acids   Amino acids that cause dramatic increases in neuronal activity. If they are administered in large amounts, neurons become overexcited and die.

Exocytosis   A process by which internal vesicles fuse with the external membrane of a cell, and then open to release chemicals outside the cell or into the intercellular space.

Exogenous   Originating from outside. Describes hormones introduced by an experimenter into an individual.

External fertilization   Eggs fertilized by sperm after being released into the environment.

Extrapyramidal motor system   The brain areas involved in the control of movement that are not part of the pyramidal system. They include the basal ganglia and the cerebellum.

Facultative   Describes a response that is flexible and contingent upon suitable environmental conditions; e.g., female ground squirrels terminate hibernation facultatively when food becomes available above ground. It does not imply causation.

Fallopian tube   A structure through which the ovum travels to reach the uterus, where in mammals the fertilization usually occurs.

Fat deposition   The storage of excess metabolic fuel as triglyceride in adipose tissue; the opposite of fat mobilization.

Fat mobilization   The release of stored metabolic energy from adipose tissue as glycerol and fatty acids; the opposite of fat deposition.

Fear conditioning   An unconditioned stimulus (e.g., a tone) is associated with a conditioned stimulus (e.g., a fear-producing event like an electric shock) so that typical behavioral and physiological reactions to fear come to be elicited by the unconditioned stimulus.

Feedback   Describes the way a physiological system is controlled. Negative feedback involves maintenance of a steady state or homeostasis (e.g., the regulation of body temperature). Positive feedback refers to the movement away from a set point (e.g., ovulation or spermiation).

Fimbria-fornix   A pathway of axons from the basal forebrain to the hippocampus.

Fistula   An opening that allows material to flow from one passage to another. An abnormal condition, usually the result of a congenital defect or surgery.

Follicle   An ovarian compartment housing an individual ovum. In the process of development and maturation, the follicle produces the hormonal changes necessary for ovulation and sexual behavior.

Follicle stimulating hormone (FSH)   A glycoprotein hormone released by the pituitary, FSH stimulates follicular development in the ovary and sperm formation in the testis and is, therefore, referred to as a gonadotropin.

Follicular development   The process by which a follicle evolves from a primordial state through growth, ovulation, and subsequent change into a corpus luteum.

Freerunning   A rhythm that is not entrained by (synchronized to) a timing-giving stimulus. See **Zeitgeber**.

Frequency   The number of rhythm cycles per unit of time (e.g., a circadian rhythm with a freerunning period of 24.5 hours has a frequency of 1.02 cycles/day).

GABAergic   Refers to gamma aminobutryic acid (GABA), the major inhibitory transmitter in the mammalian nervous system.

Gamete   Specialized cells for contributing genetic material from parents for sexual reproduction, i.e., sperm or eggs.

Gametogenesis   Egg or sperm production by the gonad.

Ganglion (invertebrate)   A discrete collection of neurons that may make up part of the CNS or may be found in the periphery.

Gender identity   The sex role people assume in their private thoughts.

Gender role   The sex role a person assume in social interactions.

Gene   A particular stretch of DNA that codes for a specific string of RNA nucleotides, which codes for a particular protein. Such a protein may be cleaved into several different active proteins.

General adaptation syndrome   Term invented by Hans Selye to describe the stress-response.

Genotype   The sum of all the genetic information possessed by an individual. See **phenotype**.

Gestation   The period from fertilization of the ovum to delivery of the young in viviparous animals.

Glia   Nonneural cells that provide the structural, nutritional, and other supports to the brain (also called neuroglia).

Globus pallidus   Together with the putamen and the caudate nucleus, the globus pallidus forms the basal ganglia in the brain.

Glucagon   A pancreatic hormone released during stress that contributes to the mobilization of energy from storage sites.

Glucocorticoids   A class of steroid hormones released by the adrenal cortex that affects carbohydrate metabolism and acts centrally to alter cognitive function. It is critical for adapting to stress. The primary glucocorticoid in primates and humans is cortisol, and in other animals it is corticosterone. Glucocorticoids aid adaptation, but chronic exposure to them can cause disease. A variety of synthetic glucocorticoids (such as prednisone or dexamethasone) are used clinically, taking advantage of the ability of glucocorticoids to suppress immunity and inflammation.

Gluconeogenesis   The ability of the liver to generate new glucose, typically by conversion of amino acids to sugars. The process is stimulated by glucocorticoids and catecholamines, and is part of the metabolic stress-response.

Glucoprivation   A decrease in the metabolic utilization of glucose in cells.

Glutamate   The major excitatory synaptic transmitter in the central nervous system.

GnRH pulse generator   A mechanism in the brain, presumably in the hypothalamus, that generates an ultradian clocklike output that controls the pulsatile release of GnRH (gonadotropin releasing hormone).

Gonad   An organ that produces gametes (i.e., the ovary and testis).

Gonadectomy   Removal of the gonads; i.e., ovariectomy or castration. See **orchidectomy**.

Gonadotropin releasing hormone (GnRH)   A peptide produced in the hypothalamus that modulates secretion of pituitary hormones (also called LH-RH).

Gonadotropins   Pituitary hormones that stimulate the gonad (i.e., the glycoprotein hormones luteinizing hormone (LH) and follicle stimulating hormone (FSH)). See **luteinizing hormone (LH)** and **follicle stimulating hormone (FSH)**.

Gonochorism   Having separate sexes in separate individuals (also called dioescious).

G-protein   The mediator of the response to ligand binding at a membrane receptor. G-proteins are responsible for activating a chain of events that alters the concentration of intracellular signaling molecules (i.e., intracellular messengers) such as cyclic amp.

Granule cell   A small, granular cell that is found in the dentate gyrus. It sends its axons to the field CA3 of the hippocampus.

Gravid   Pregnant; full of ripe ova or, in egg-laying animals, shelled eggs.

Growth factors   Target-derived chemicals that feed neurons to help them survive and grow (also called neurotrophic factors or trophic factors).

Growth hormone (GH)   A pituitary hormone whose actions promote normal growth in developing organisms, and tissue repair and energy metabolism in adults. Its release is stimulated by growth hormone releasing hormone and inhibited by somatostatin. Many growth hormone actions are mediated by its triggering the release, by the liver, of a class of hormones called somatomedins (also known as insulin-like growth factors). See **Somatomedin** and **Somatostatin**.

Growth hormone–releasing hormone (GHRH)   A hypothalamic hormone that stimulates the pituitary secretion of growth hormone.

Habituation   A simple type of learning that involves the loss of response after repeated presentations of a stimulus.

Hair cell   A sensory receptor found in the vestibular (balance) organ, the ear, and in modified form, the lateral line system and electroreceptor organs of aquatic organisms.

Haloperidol   A dopamine receptor antagonist; a neuroleptic drug used in the treatment of schizophrenia.

Handling   A procedure in which rats or mice are taken away from their mothers for a few minutes each day during early development. When the infants are returned to the nest, mothers lick and handle them more than infants that have not been momentarily removed.

Heritable   The relative amount of variance in a trait that is due to genetic factors and therefore can be passed on to offspring.

Hermaphrodite   Describes individuals that possess both male and female reproductive structures. It can occur either simultaneously or sequentially at different stages of the life cycle.

Heterogametic   Having different sex chromosomes; e.g., XY or ZW.

Hibernaculum   The underground burrow or den in which hibernating animals spend the winter.

Hierarchical control of rhythms   The concept that a master clock acts as a pacemaker generating a primary output rhythm. This primary rhythm then generates one or more secondary rhythms which can, in turn, generate tertiary rhythms, and so forth.

Hippocampal formation   A forebrain structure deep within the temporal lobe that includes the hippocampus proper (also called Ammon's horn), the dentate gyrus, and the subiculum.

Hippocampus   The area of the brain involved in learning and memory.

Homeostasis   The coordinated physiological and behavioral mechanisms by which animals maintain a relatively constant internal state despite living in an environment that fluctuates widely. Among the many variables that are homeostatically regulated are body temperature, blood glucose, blood pressure, and extracellular fluid osmolality.

Homogametic   Having similar sex chromosomes.

Hormone   A chemical released from cells that travels to and affects other cells.

Hormone replacement therapy   The administration of exogenous hormones to supplement deficient levels of endogenous hormones (e.g., estrogen therapy in postmenopausal women).

Hormone-sensitive genes   Genes whose expression is regulated by hormones, often by the binding of the activated hormone receptor complex to a particular DNA sequence in the gene's regulatory region.

HPA   Hypothalamic pituitary adrenal system.

HPG   Hypothalamic pituitary gonadal system.

Humoral-mediated immunity   The part of the immune response in which antibodies are formed as a defense against an invasive agent.

Huntington's disease   A hereditary disease of the basal ganglia characterized by progressive cell loss in the striatum and other brain regions; it is characterized by chorea and progressive dementia.

Hybrid   The offspring of parents of different species.

Hydrocortisone   A synthetic version of cortisol often administered in replacement studies.

6-Hydroxydopamine (6-OHDA)   A substance that is selectively toxic to catecholamine neurons.

Hyperprolactanemia   Increased or excessive release of prolactin.

Hypoglycemia   Low blood sugar.

Hypogonadism   Lack of gonads or gonadal secretions.

Hypophysectomy   Removal of the pituitary gland.

Hypophysis   The pituitary.

Hypothalamus   Brain structure (group of nuclei). A neural center at the base of the diencephalic region of the brain involved in the control of rhythmic and regulatory functions, including pituitary hormone release.

Hypotonia   Loss of muscle tone.

Hypovolemia   Low blood volume.

Hypoxia-ischemia   Lack of oxygen combined with lack of blood flow.

Hysterectomy   Surgical removal of the uterus in mammals.

Ibotenic acid   A neurotoxin used in the brain to produce lesions of cell bodies while sparing fibers of passage.

Implantation   The attachment of a fertilized egg to the wall of the uterus by the formation of a placenta in mammals.

Incubation   A period of development, usually referring to shelled eggs.

Indifferent gonad   An early stage in development when a gonad appears structurally intermediate between a testis and an ovary.

Induced estrus   Estrus that occurs only after exposure to stimuli from a male.

Induced ovulation   Ovulation in response to stimulation by a male.

Infradian rhythm   A self-sustained, endogenous oscillation with a freerunning period greater than the circadian but less than the circannual (e.g., 28-day menstrual cycle).

In situ hybridization   The use of a DNA or RNA probe to detect the complementary mRNA or DNA sequence.

Insulin   A pancreatic hormone released in response to increases in circulating glucose concentrations, or in response to stimulation of the parasympathetic nervous system. Insulin promotes uptake and storage of glucose and other energy substrates, and thus is a classically anabolic hormone.

Intact   A term used to indicate that no surgery has been done to remove tissues or organs.

Internal fertilization   Eggs fertilized by male sperm while still inside a female's body.

Interneurons   Neurons whose axons do not leave the brain nucleus where the cell body is found.

Intrasexual selection   Competition among members of the same sex for access to mates. Fights usually involve ritualized aggressive displays.

Intromission   Insertion of a penis into a vagina.

Involution   Reduction in size. Describes the functional inactivity and reduced size of the gonads during the nonreproductive portion of an annual cycle.

Ion channels   Pores formed by proteins that cross the cell membrane. These channels permit ions (typically sodium, potassium, and calcium) to travel into or out of the cell.

Juvenile hormones   A family of sesquiterpenoid hormones that act in the larval stages of insects to prevent metamorphosis.

Kallman's syndrome   A pathology in humans that is characterized by an inability to smell and a lack of gonadal development.

Klinefelter's syndrome   A syndrome in which externally masculine individuals possess two X chromosomes and a Y chromosome.

Knockout   An individual, often a mouse, that has a specific gene that has been inactivated or deleted.

Knollenorgen   Specialized sensory receptors for detecting EOD in weakly electric fish.

Lactation   Milk production and its release during the suckling of young.

Larynx   A sound-producing organ in vertebrates. In the clawed frog, contraction of the laryngial muscles cause sound-producing disks to pop apart, resulting in a click.

Lateral line organs   Organs located on the body surface of aquatic organisms that detect water movements; the sensory receptor is a hair cell.

Lateral ventricles   The most lateral portion of the ventricular system within each hemisphere of the brain that contains cerebral spinal fluid.

Lee-Boot effect   A suppression of estrous cycles in females due to overcrowding.

Leptin   A protein hormone that reduces food uptake and increases energy expenditure.

Leucocyte   A white blood cell.

Leydig cells   Specialized cells located in the testes between the seminferous tubules; the source of androgens.

Ligand   Any molecule that binds to another molecule; e.g., a hormone or neurotransmitter act as a ligand when binding to a receptor.

Ligand-gated ion channels   Receptors that change their conformation allowing ions to pass through when bound by their ligand.

Ligand-independent activation   Receptors that are activated in the absence of the presumptive ligand.

Light : dark cycle   The natural or experimental environmental photoperiod.

Limbic system   A constellation of interconnected brain areas that regulate social and sexual behaviors. It includes the hypothalamus, amygdala, septum, hippocampus, and bed nucleus of the stria terminalis (also called the emotional brain).

Lipolysis   The physiological process that breaks down stored triglycerides from adipose tissue into glycerol and fatty acids in adipose tissue.

Locomotor activity   Unit of measure of activity, usually in open-field tests or on running wheels.

Long-term potentiation (LTP)   A long-term increase in the excitability of a neuron to a particular synaptic input caused by repeated high frequency activity of that input.

Lordosis   A sexual posture characterized by immobility with a species-typical posture that facilitates vaginal penetration by the penis of the male. In rodents this usually consists of an arching of the back by extending the hindlegs and a lateral deflection of the tail.

Luteinizing hormone (LH)   A glycoprotein hormone released by the pituitary. LH stimulates estrogen and progesterone secretion by the ovary, and testosterone secretion by the testes; it is referred to as a gonadotropin.

Lymphocyte   A class of white blood cells that includes B- and T-cells.

Macrophages   Relatively long-lived phagocytic cells of mammalian tissues derived from blood monocytes. Macrophages play an important role in killing some bacteria, protozoa, and tumor cells; they release substances that stimulate other cells of the immune system and are involved in antigen presentation.

Mate call   A vocalization displayed during courtship.

Maternal aggression   The high level of aggression displayed by females soon after delivering young or laying eggs.

Melatonin   The primary hormone of the pineal gland; it is thought to be important in biological rhythms.

Menstrual cycle   Cyclic changes in the output of reproductive hormones in women that revolve around the maturation of egg follicles in the ovaries.

Menstrual phase   The portion of the menstrual cycle that is characterized overtly by menstruation (i.e., the shedding of the uterine lining).

Metabolic fuel   Any chemical substance derived from food that can be oxidized by cells to produce energy. Glucose and lipids are the main such fuels when animals are well nourished, but ketone bodies and free fatty acids derived from energy stores (fat) also become important fuels during fasting.

Metabotropic receptors   Receptors that when bound activate a second messenger or G-protein-mediated response.

Metamorphosis   The process by which a transition is made between life stages (e.g., a tadpole turning into a frog or a caterpillar into a moth).

Microdialysis Method by which small amounts of neurotransmitters in the extracellular fluid are collected for later analysis; it involves diffusion across a semipermeable membrane at the base of a cannula.

Midluteal phase A portion of the menstrual cycle characterized by high concentrations of estradiol and progesterone; it occurs about midway between ovulation and the onset of menstruation.

Modality The sensory domain of a particular stimulus (e.g., the visual modality or the auditory modality).

Molting The series of events in arthropodes that are involved in the production of a new exoskeleton and the shedding (ecdysis) of the old one.

Monocytes A class of white blood cells.

Monogamous species A species in which a male and female form a breeding pair that may last for one breeding season or for a lifetime.

Mormyrids and gymnotids Two orders of weakly electric fish.

Motoneuron A neuron whose cell body is located in the spinal cord and whose axonal terminal synapses on muscle fiber(s).

Motor pattern generator A nucleus or set of nuclei in the central nervous system that produces a patterned discharge that affects the activity of motoneurons.

Motor tape The representation of a stereotyped sequence of behaviors that is stored in the central nervous system.

Müllerian ducts A duct system connecting the gonad to the external body wall, present in both sexes early in development, but differentiating in females into the fallopian tubes, uterus, and inner vagina. See **wolffian ducts**.

Multiparous Having had multiple previous pregnancies.

Naloxone An opioid receptor antagonist.

Natural killer cells A certain type of white blood cell that attacks infected cells by binding to them and releasing lethal chemicals.

Natural selection An evolutionary process whereby traits which provide adaptational responses to the social, ecological, or physical environment are retained.

Neocortex The newest, most recently evolved portion of the cerebral cortex (this excludes cortical regions like the hippocampus).

Neonatal Occurring soon after birth.

Nephrectomy Surgical removal of the kidneys.

Neuroeffectors Motorneurons and the muscles they innervate.

Neurogenesis The mitotic division of non-neuronal cells to produce neurons.

Neurohormone Chemical released by a neuron into general circulation or into the hypothalamic-pituitary-portal system.

Neurohypophysis The posterior portion of the pituitary gland where axon terminals from neurons in the hypothalamus secrete oxytocin and vasopressin into the blood (also called posterior pituitary).

Neuroleptic Dopamine receptor antagonists with antipsychotic therapeutic value used for the treatment of schizophrenia.

Neuromodulation A rather loose classification of the action of many neuropeptides and biogenic amines. These actions are characterized by a slower time-course and actions over a broader area than those seen in classical neurotransmission.

Neuron A nerve cell capable of receiving and transmitting information.

Neuropeptides   Small chains of amino acids produced in the brain and used in neurotransmission or neuromodulation.

Neuropsychological test   Sensory, perceptual, cognitive, or motor tests which have been shown experimentally to depend on particular regions of the brain.

Neurosecretory cell   Specialized neuron that releases its neurotransmitter into the bloodstream rather than into a synapse.

Neurotransmitter   A chemical released by a neuron to relay information to other cells, usually other neurons.

Neutrophil   A white blood cell.

NMDA receptor   A specialized ionotropic glutamate receptor that controls a calcium channel that is normally blocked by MG^{2+} ions; it is involved in long-term potentiation.

N-methyl-D-aspartate (NMDA)   An excitatory amino acid that can be used as a neurotoxin to destroy the cell bodies of neurons.

Nonmnemonic factors   Factors that may influence performance on cognitive tasks but which are not directly related to learning and memory (e.g, sensory or motor factors, motivation, or attention).

Nonspatial maze learning   Learning to navigate in space using cues in the immediate or proximate environment (e.g., turn left at the corner with a stop sign; turn right after the large oak tree). See **spatial maze learning**.

Norepinephrine   A catecholaminergic neurotransmitter and hormone (also known as noradrenaline) that performs a variety of functions throughout the body. It is a major neurotransmitter of the sympathetic nervous system, and is a thought to be depleted in some parts of the brains of people with depression.

Nuclei   Collections of cell bodies in the central nervous system (i.e., the brain and spinal cord).

Nucleotide   One of several chemicals that make up DNA and RNA. The different nucleotides provide the specificity of information in such molecules. For DNA the nucleotides are thymine, guanine, cytosine, and adenine; RNA uses the same nucleotides except that uridine replaces thymine.

Nucleus   Either the spherical receptacle of genetic information in an eukaryotic cell, or a cluster of neuronal cell bodies found within the nervous system.

Nucleus of the solitary tract   A brain stem nucleus that receives information from the parasympathetic vagus nerve.

Nulliparous   A female that has never given birth.

Oophorectomy   Surgical removal of the ovaries. In rodents, this is also called an ovariectomy.

Open-ended song learning   The ability of certain bird species to learn new songs even as adults (i.e., beyond the first year of life).

Open-field activity   Standard measure for activity; refers to the locomotor behavior shown by an organism placed in a large, open arena.

Opioids   Compounds derived from opium, such as heroin and morphine; also compounds made in the body or synthesized exogenously that have opiate-like effects.

Orchidectomy   Surgical removal of the gonads. See **gonadectomy**.

Organizational effects of hormones   Actions during development, usually perinatally, which alter subsequent adult neural structures and functions. This term refers to the organizational/activational hypothesis, namely, that hormones, early in development, often have long-term, permanent effects on the nervous system that are activated later in life by the actions of circulating hormones. See **activational effects of hormones**.

Organizational hypothesis The proposal that androgens secreted by the developing testes permanently masculinize the developing nervous system, resulting in an adult which will more readily display male-typical behaviors.

Osmolality The concentration of osmotically active particles in solution.

Osmoreceptor Cerebral cells that detect changes in extracellular fluid osmolality (concentration of solute particles) that result from the induced movement of water by osmosis across the cell membrane.

Oviparity An egg-laying mode of reproduction with either internal or external fertilization.

Ovoviviparity The retention of a fertilized egg with reduced nutrient and waste exchange between the embryo and the mother and usually some kind of shell barrier.

Ovulation The physical release of a mature egg from the ovary. See **spontaneous ovulation**.

Oxytocin A peptide hormone secreted by the posterior pituitary gland that triggers milk let down in lactating females and may be involved in other reproduction and social behaviors.

Pacing behavior Behavior engaged in by a female rat to increase the interval between intromissions and enhance fertility.

Pain pathways Neural pathways carrying pain information, beginning with peripheral pain receptors, afferent projections to the spinal cord, ascending spinal pathways, and parts of the brain, including the raphe complex and the periaqueductal gray.

Parasympathetic nervous system Half of the autonomic nervous system. It subsumes the physiological functions associated with calm, vegetative states (such as slowing the heart while sleeping).

Parkinson's disease A neurological disease in which the dopamine neurons of the substantia nigra degenerate; it is characterized by motor and cognitive deficits.

Parthenogenesis A reproductive mode whereby fertilization is not required for a female to give birth; in parthenogenesis only daughters are produced and they contain only the mother's genes.

Passive avoidance A type of learning in which the individual must suppress some behavior that it would normally exhibit.

PCR Polymerase chain reaction.

Peptide A molecule consisting of about 50 or fewer amino acids.

Perceptual speed The ability to quickly and accurately perceive the details of a visual configuration or stimulus.

Periaqueductal gray See **pain pathways**.

Perinatal Occurring around the time of birth, including both the prenatal and neonatal periods. During this period many vertebrates, particularly rodents, are susceptible to the organizational effects of hormones.

Perineum The pelvic floor (i.e., the region including the genitalia and underlying structures adjacent to, but separate from, the abdomen).

Period The duration of a rhythm measured as the time between the appearance of an arbitrary phase point until the reappearance of that phase point; it is the inverse of *frequency*.

Peripheral   Describing the actions of a drug or hormone that take place outside of the central nervous system.

Phase   Any temporal location of a rhythm (e.g., each of the 360 degrees of a sine wave is a phase of that rhythm).

Phase advance   A shift of a rhythm caused by a Zeitgeber stimulus such that all subsequent phases of the rhythm occur relatively earlier than expected prior to the application of the stimulus. See **Zeitgeber**.

Phase delay   A shift of a rhythm caused by a Zeitgeber stimulus such that all subsequent phases of the rhythm occur relatively later than expected prior to the application of the stimulus. See **Zeitgeber**.

Phase response curve (PRC)   A curve showing the amount and direction of phase shift as a function of the circadian time of stimulus application. The PRC to light consists of a subjective day and a subjective night.

Phenotype   The sum of all physical characteristics of an individual that are expressed at a particular time. These traits are the result of the interplay of the genotype and the environment up to that point.

Pheromone   A chemical signal produced by one organism that is capable of altering the reproductive behavior or physiology of another member of the same species. Pheromones may act slowly (priming effects), may act quickly (releasing effects), or may communicate specific information (signaling effects).

Photoperiodic annual rhythms   Annual rhythms that are dependent to some degree upon seasonal changes in day length; photoperiodic annual rhythms, unlike circannual annual rhythms, do not persist or freerun when animals are kept in constant environmental conditions (also called photoperiodic time measurement or photoperiodism).

Pineal   A gland outside of, but attached to, the brain. The pineal secretes melatonin under the rhythmic control of the circadian clock to regulate environmentally sensitive reproductive activity.

Pitocin   A synthetic mimic of oxytocin that is sometimes given to women in order to increase uterine contractions and speed delivery at parturition.

Pituitary   An endocrine gland found beneath the brain and controlled by the hypothalamus.

Placebo control   An inert drug given to a patient that the patient does not know is ineffective. In clinical drug studies some patients receive the test drug and others receive a placebo drug to control for the psychological factors involved with knowing that you are receiving a drug treatment.

Plasmid vector   A small, independently replicating piece of extrachromosomal cytoplasmic DNA that can be transferred from one organism to another.

Plastic song   The intermediate stage of song development in which birds produce song syllables with a well-defined structure but which vary in order and number in successive renditions.

PNI   Psychoneuroimmunology.

POA   Preoptic Area of the hypothalamus.

Polygynous species   Species that have a mating system in which an individual mates with more than one other animal within a breeding season.

Postpartum estrus   The phenomenon where a female ovulates and becomes sexually receptive immediately or shortly after parturition, shown by a large number of mammals.

Preadaptation   Anatomical structure or behavior which appears in evolution or in development to serve one function but then serves another at a future time (also called exaptation).

Precocial   Refers to young birds or mammals born in a mature condition with well-developed vision, hearing, and locomotion, and has a relatively short period of dependence upon the parent for nutrition.

Preovulatory gonadotropin surge   A sudden large increase of luteinizing hormone (LH) that acts as the final hormonal stimulus for the next ovulation.

Preovulatory phase   The portion of the menstrual cycle just prior to ovulation in which estradiol levels reach peak concentrations.

Presynaptic terminal   The portion of the axon usually characterized by the concentration of synaptic vesicles containing neurotransmitter(s) which are released by exocytosis in response to the arrival of an action potential.

Primates   The order of mammals including monkeys, apes, and humans.

Procedural memory   Memory that is shown by performance rather than by conscious recall (also called nondeclarative memory).

Proceptive behaviors   Behaviors used to indicate the willingness of an organism to approach or solicit a member of the opposite sex.

Proceptivity   Extent to which an individual engages in behaviors likely to initiate mating from another individual. In female rats, ear-wiggling and hopping-and-darting appear to be proceptive behaviors.

Prolactin   A pituitary hormone secreted during nursing to promote lactation, during mating to promote progesterone release and successful implantation, and during stress to inhibit reproduction.

Propanolol   A drug that specifically blocks beta-adrenergic receptors.

Propylthiouracil   A potent blocker of thyroid hormone metabolism.

Prostaglandins   A class of fatty acid–derived compounds with a vast array of biological actions throughout the body.

Prostate gland   An accessory sex organ in male vertebrates that contributes fluid to semen, and is necessary for insemination to occur. The prostate has an absolute requirement for dihydrotestosterone for normal function.

Protein   A molecule consisting of a long string of amino acids. A short string of amino acids is referred to as a peptide.

Protein kinase   A diverse class of enzymes that transfer a phosphate group from ATP to proteins. Most second messengers alter cellular function through the activation of specific protein kinases.

Prothoracic glands   Insect endocrine glands that secrete the molting hormones, the ecdysteroids.

Proximate causation   Stimuli used by an organism to initiate, maintain, and terminate breeding.

Proximate mechanism   The genetic and physiological processes that contribute to behavioral expression.

Psychoneuroimmunology   A new scientific field concerned with the ways in which the brain and psychological states can alter immune function, and with how the immune system can, in turn, alter the brain and psychological states.

Puberty   Time at which an individual first becomes capable of reproduction.

Pulsatile release   Acute bursts of hormones released as pulses, usually 1 to 3 times per hour (e.g., the release of GnRH under the control of the GnRH pulse generator).

Pulse EOD   Type of electric organ discharge (EOD) in the weakly electric fish in which the interval between EOD pulses is long compared to the duration of the pulse itself.

Purkinje cells   Large cells in the cerebellum.

Putamen   Together with the caudate nucleus and the globus pallidus it forms the basal ganglia in the brain.

Pyramidal cell   A category of large pyramid-shaped cells that are found in the cerebral cortex and in fields CA1, CA2, and CA3 of the hippocampus.

Pyramidal system   Brain structure (fiber pathway). Output system connecting neurons in the motor cortex with spinal cord motoneurons for the activation of motor output (muscle movement).

Radial-arm maze   A complex maze composed of a central circular platform and arms radiating from it in a symmetrical fashion. The ends of the arms can be used as food sites to study how rodents learn and remember the location of food sites.

Radioimmunoassay (RIA)   A method of using antibodies and radiolabeled hormone to measure hormonal levels in a biological sample.

Radiolabeled   Describes a molecule in which one or more atoms are made up of radioactive isotopes, making it relatively easy to detect the molecule by detecting the radioactivity.

Receptive fields   The stimulus region and features that cause the maximal response of a cell in a sensory system.

Receptivity   Extent to which an animal will mate, often measured in female rodents by quantifying the frequency or duration of the lordosis reflex.

Reductase   5α-reductase catalyzes the conversion of testosterone into 5α-dihydro-testosterone (DHT).

Reflex ovulation   The ovulation of mature eggs in response to tactile (usually cervical) stimuli associated with copulation; it is a characteristic of cats, rabbits, and ferrets.

Releasing factor   One of many chemicals released by the hypothalamus into the hypo-thalamic-pituitary portal system that increase or decrease the release of specific hormones from the pituitary.

Reliability   The extent to which a biological phenomena is repeatedly observed.

Reproductive isolation   The prevention of interbreeding between species either by behaviors characteristic of the species (pre-mating mechanisms) or by infertility following mating (post-mating mechanisms).

Reproductive success   The extent to which a given individual's genes are present in succeeding generations. In practice, this quality is usually measured by determining the number of offspring that themselves survive to reproduce.

Reproductive synergism   Coordination and synchronization of hormonal, gonadal, and sexual events by behavioral interaction.

Resting potential   The electrical charge across a cell membrane. In neurons this refers to the charge seen in the absence of synaptic input.

Resting tremor   Regular, involuntary oscillating movement of a body part when it is at rest.

Retrograde amnesia   Loss of memory of events that occurred prior to some event such as a trauma.

Ribonucleic acid (RNA)   The chemical messenger, similar in structure to DNA, which is itself transcribed from DNA; it serves as the template for the translation of genetic directions into a specific string of amino acids to form a protein or peptide.

Rotational behavior   Persistent 360° circles or turns made in one predominant direction.

Running-wheel activity   Standard measure of activity in which the animal, usually a small rodent, turns a wheel while running.

Scoploamine   A drug that blocks muscarinic acetylcholine receptors.

Scrotum   The pouch of skin containing the testes.

SDN   Sexually dimorphic nucleus.

Seasonality (seasonal breeding)   The occurrence of various physiological and behavioral responses during a specific season (or seasons) of the year.

Secondary sex characteristics   Anatomical structures which may, or may not, contribute to reproduction and are usually sexually dimorphic. Examples include mammary glands and male pattern baldness.

Secretagogs   Term for a collection of hormones.

Seizures   Episodes in which a large group of neurons shows synchronized activation. These events have a wide array of causes including trauma and exposure to toxins or drugs.

Semialtricial   Refers to young birds or mammals born with vision and hearing but with poor locomotion and which are therefore dependent upon the parent for nutrition.

Seminal vesicles   An accessory sex organ in male vertebrates.

Seminiferous tubules   The site of sperm production in the testes.

Sensitive period   A limited time during development in which an organism can be permanently altered by a particular experience or treatment.

Sensory neurons   Neurons that respond directly to sensory stimuli or are excited by sensory receptors.

Sensory receptors   Cells that respond to external stimuli and alter the activity of adjacent sensory neurons.

Septal region   A region in the basal forebrain that provides inputs to the hippocampal formation.

Sex chromosome   A chromosome which contributes to sex determination (e.g., X and Y chromosomes for mammals, W and Z chromosomes for birds).

Sex determination   The point at which an individual begins developing as either a male or a female. In mammals this takes place at fertilization, depending on whether the sperm has contributed an X or a Y chromosome.

Sexual cycle   Cycle of ovarian follicular development, ovulation, and corpora lutea formation, including hormone secretion.

Sexual differentiation   The process by which a developing individual assumes the characteristics of either a male or a female. In vertebrates, gonadal hormones released following sex determination implement this decision by guiding developing somatic structures, including the brain.

Sexual dimorphism   The species characteristic of having males and females which are structurally different.

Sexual motivation   Interest in and attempts to engage in copulatory activity. A conceptual term referring to the inclination of an individual to seek out and approach another individual for the purpose of mating.

Sexual receptivity   The willingness to engage in copulatory behaviors. Receptivity in mammals is usually indexed by the probability that a female will show lordosis in response to flank stimulation or by the frequency or duration of female lordosis within a given time period.

Sexual selection   A counterpart to natural selection. Sexual selection arises when individuals of a species differ in their ability to compete with members of the same sex for access to mates (intersexual) or to attract members of the opposite sex (epigamic or intersexual selection).

Sexually dimorphic   Characters or behaviors that occur in different forms in the sexes.

Sexually dimorphic nucleus of the preoptic area (SDN-POA)   A region of the preoptic area of the hypothalamus which is larger in males than in females in both rodents and humans.

Silastic   A silicon rubber compound through which steroid hormones readily dissolve. Surgically implanted steroid-filled Silastic capsules slowly release the steroid into circulation.

SNB   Spinal nucleus of bulbocavernosus.

Social recognition memory   The ability of one member of a species to recognize another member of the same species via sensory cues.

Sodium appetite   A strong motivation to seek, obtain, and consume salty foods and fluids, typically as a consequence of sodium deficiency. It is a drive like hunger and thirst.

Somatic   Describes nonreproductive cells or tissues.

Somatomedins   A class of compounds released by the liver in response to growth hormone; somatomedins mediate some of the stimulatory effects caused by growth hormone.

Somatostatin   A hypothalamic hormone that inhibits the pituitary release of growth hormone.

Song repertoire   The number of different versions of species-specific song that an individual produces.

Spatial maze learning   The ability to navigate using 3-dimensional aspects of the distal environment rather than proximal cues. For example, learning to navigate by imagining or visualizing the location or orientation of objects, or features of objects, in three-dimensional space. See **nonspatial maze learning**.

Spinal nucleus of the bulbocavernosus (SNB)   A group of motoneurons in the spinal cord that innervate several muscles attached to the base of the penis.

Spines   Refers to small protrusions, about 1 to 3 μm in length, that densely cover the dendrites of the principal neurons in the hippocampus. In this structure, over 90% of the excitatory synapses occur on spines.

Spleen   An organ that produces lymphocytes, filters the blood, stores blood cells, and destroys cells that are aging. It is located on the left side of the abdomen near the stomach.

Splenium   The most posterior portion of the corpus callosum.

Spontaneous ovulation   Endogenous timing of ovulation occurring in the absence of stimulation from the male; it is often regulated by photoperiod.

Sprouting   The formation of new neuronal connections following neuronal injury.

Stereotyped behaviors   Any repetitive, seemingly aimless movements (e.g., repetitive movements of the head, mouth, facial features, or forelimbs).

Steroid hormone receptors   A family of proteins that act as transcription factors when bound to hormones. Members include receptors for sex steroids (androgens, estrogens, and progestins), thyroid hormones, and retinoic acid. These proteins have several domains, one of which binds the hormone and another which binds to DNA.

Steroidogenesis   The production and secretion of steroid hormones.

Steroids   Biologically active compounds that share a particular molecular structure resembling cholesterol; they consist of four linked rings of carbon atoms.

Stomatogastric ganglion   A small ganglion comprised of about 30 neurons and found in decapod crustaceans such as crabs and lobsters. It controls the movements of various regions of the stomach.

Stress dwarfism   A pediatric disorder in which children exposed to considerable amounts of stress cease growing. If a child is moved to a less stressful environment rapidly enough, growth may resume and catch up with normal levels (also called psychogenic dwarfism).

Stress-induced analgesia   The phenomenon that following exposure to certain types of stressors, organisms become less sensitive to pain.

Stressor   Any environmental challenge or perturbation that throws the organism out of homeostatic balance, or the psychological circumstances which lead an organism to believe that it is just about to be thrown out of homeostatic balance.

Stress-response   The endocrine and neural adaptations mobilized in response to a stressor which help to reestablish homeostasis.

Stretch receptor   Receptor cells located on the outside of an elastic vessel that detect changes in the tension of the vessel's walls (e.g., such receptors signal the brain when the stomach is empty or the bladder is full).

Striatum   One of a group of nuclei composing the basal ganglia with the globus pallidus. The putamen and caudate nucleus are referred to collectively as the striatum.

Subiculum   A rgion adjacent to the hippocampus that contributes to hippocampal formation (also called the hippocampal gyrus).

Subjective day   The portion of the circadian day in which a light stimulus produces neither phase advances nor delays. It corresponds to the time of low locomotor activity for nocturnal animals.

Subjective night   The portion of the circadian day in which a light stimulus produces a phase shift. During the early subjective night, these are phase delays which give way to phase advances during the late subjective night.

Subsong   The first stage of song development in which birds produce crude sounds that are highly variable in structure in successive renditions and bear little similarity to adult song.

Substantia nigra   The part of the brain nucleus that contains neurons that produce and deliver dopamine to the striatum.

Suprachiasmatic nucleus   The brain site of the mechanisms that generate "clock" activity; it controls circadian rhythmicity in mammals.

Sympathetic nervous system   One of two systems that compose the autonomic nervous system. (The other paired system is the parasympathetic nervous system.) The sympathetic nervous system subsumes physiological functions associated with arousal, such as increased heart rate and blood flow to the skeletal muscles.

Sympathoadrenal system   A division of the autonomic nervous system consisting of the sympathetic nerves and the adrenal medulla; it responds to conditions of stress by secreting catecholamine hormones (e.g., epinephrine or norepinephrine) that prepare the animal physiologically for attack, defense, or escape.

Synapse   Site between two neurons where presynaptic terminals connect with a postsynaptic cell.

Synaptic transmission   The passage of information between two cells across a synapse.

Synovial fluid   A viscous fluid that lubricates the joint (also called joint fluid).

Synthetic   Manufactured at the conscious direction of humans.

Systemic   Describes the hormones available throughout the body through the circulatory system. Also, describes the route of administration of drugs or hormone to the general circulation rather than directly into the central nervous system.

T cells   Lymphocytes that mature in the thymus glands.

Teats   Nipples of mammary glands.

Telencephalon   The frontal subdivision of the forebrain that includs the cerebral hemispheres, including the hippocampus and the striatum.

Temporal lobe   A region of the cerebral cortex located just behind the temple; it contains primary sensory regions for audition as well as modules for language.

Teratogen   An agent capable of causing malformations in embryos.

Testicular feminization mutation (TFM)   A genetic mutation that renders androgen receptors nonfunctional.

Testis determination factor (TDF)   The protein, a product of a gene on the Y chromosome, which instructs the indifferent gonad to develop as a testis.

Testosterone   A steroid hormone that is the principle secretion of the testes.

T-helper cell   Sets of T lymphocytes that are specifically involved in the differentiation of B lymphocytes into antibody-secreting cells.

Thermoregulation   The ability of animals to regulate their body temperature at an optimal temperature for physiological functioning.

Thiourea   A chemical inhibitor of thyroid hormone function.

Thymidine   A chemical precursor to thymine, the nucleotide found in DNA but not in RNA. In scientific experiments, when radioactively labeled thymidine is administered to animals with a developing brain it is incorporated into newly duplicated DNA of cells about to divide, marking the "birth date" of those cells.

Thymus   The lymphoid organ in which T lymphocytes are produced.

Ticking   A vocalization given by male and sexually unreceptive female clawed frogs; it results in release from the male's clasp.

Torpedo   The electric ray, a fish that can stun prey with shocks produced by the electric organ.

Torpor   A state of reduced metabolic functioning characterized by decreases in body temperature beyond the normal range of variability (e.g., mammals exhibiting shallow daily torpor, like Siberian hamsters or deermice reduce their body temperatures from $37\,°C$ to 15 to $20\,°C$ for up to several weeks.

Trace conditioning   A learning paradigm in which the conditioned stimulus (e.g., a tone) is separated in time from the unconditioned stimulus (e.g., the shock), but they are nevertheless paired by the animal when it learns the task so that the conditioned stimulus becomes predictive. This type of conditioning has been found to require hippocampal function.

Transcription   The creation of a specific string of RNA encoded by a gene.

Transgenic   Describes an animal, often a mouse, in which a gene has been inserted or altered.

Translation   The creation of a specific protein encoded by RNA.

Trophic relationships   A dependent relation between a neuron and the cell(s) it innervates. When one of these cells is removed, the remaining cell may die.

Turner's syndrome   A syndrome in which externally feminine individuals possess a single X chromosome but no Y chromosome.

Tyrosine hydroxylase   The rate-limiting enzyme in the biochemical pathway of catecholamine synthesis. It converts tyrosine to L-dopa, a precursor of dopamine, norepinephrine, and epinephrine.

Ultimate causation   Evolutionary factors that result in individuals within populations that behave or function in a particular way.

Ultradian rhythm   A class of rhythms with a range of periods shorter than the circadian range.

Urethra   A duct from the bladder that releases urine outside the body.

Uterus   A structure that connects the fallopian tubes to the vagina; it is usually the site of embryo implantation and fetal development.

Vaginal code   Refers to the number and patterning of intromissions characteristic of a species mating behavior. This code is essential for the induction of the progestational state (pregnancy). (It is possible to mimic the necessary tactile cues by mechanical means.)

Vagus nerve   The largest of the cranial nerves. The vagus nerve is made up of efferent fibers of the parasympathetic nervous system that carry information from the brain to various internal organs. The vagus also has sensory fibers that carry information to the brain from the internal organs.

Validity   The extent to which laboratory findings apply to situations outside of the laboratory.

Vandenbergh effect   The acceleration of puberty in a young female rodent due to odorant from an adult male.

Vasopressin   A hormone with a variety of effects throughout the body. A peptide hormone that is released from the posterior pituitary gland, it affects water balance. It can also be released from the hypothalamus where it acts as a secretagog at the pituitary, stimulating secretion of adrenocorticotropin (ACTH). Thus, hypothalamic vasopressin is typically released during stress. It also reduces blood pressure during serious blood loss, which stimulates the reabsorption of water, and it also has direct central actions that influence learning and memory systems.

Verbal fluency   Facility in generating words, phrases, or sentences that fulfill specific semantic or phonetic criteria.

Vesicle   A small, spherical-shaped structure for transporting protein(s).

Viral vector   Viral DNA that has been modified to serve as a vector for recombinant DNA.

Viviparity   A mode of reproduction whereby embryos are retained in the mother's body and nutrients and waste are exchanged.

Vole   A small, mouselike rodent that is often used for studies of the evolution of behaviors because there are many closely related species which have different breeding schemes and live in different environments.

Voltammetry The method by which the pattern of electrical current at the membrane is measured.

Vomeronasal organ A receptor organ for detecting chemical signals, particularly pheromones.

Ventral tegmental area (VTA) An area in the midbrain containing dopamine cell bodies whose axons project to the nucleus accumbens and other forebrain areas.

Wandering behavior Behavior shown by some caterpillars in preparation for metamorphosis. It involves the cessation of feeding and the display of sustained locomotion and other behaviors associated with the construction of a chamber for metamorphosis.

Water maze An apparatus ressembling a child's round swimming pool that can be used to assess learning and memory in rodents by having them locate a small platform hidden beneath the surface of water made murky by water-soluble paint.

Wave EOD A type of electric organ discharge (EOD) in which the interval between EOD pulses is short compared to the pulse duration itself.

Whitten effect The induction of estrus in a female rodent by the odor of a strange male.

Wolffian ducts A duct system connecting the gonad to the external body wall. It is present in both sexes early in development, but in males it differentiates into the epididymis, vas deferens, and seminal vesicles. See **Müllerian ducts**.

Working memory A short-term store of information that is useful for a few minutes, hours, or days but which is erased regularly (e.g., recalling where you parked your car at the mall today).

Xenopus African clawed frog.

Yerkes-Dodson law The finding in 1908 that the strength of a stimulus is related to the rate of learning via an inverted U-shaped function. This means that very high or very low stimulus intensities interfere with learning and that learning is best at moderate stimulus intensities.

Zeitgeber A stimulus used to impart information about time.

Zygote A fertilized egg; the single-celled beginning of an organisms.

Index